New Approaches to the Scientific Study of Religion

Volume 1

Introduction to the Series

This series presents new approaches to the scientific study of religion, moving from the first generation of studies that try to 'explain religion' towards a more critical effort to explore alternative paths in correspondence with this highly complex human and social feature. The series supports the development of new scientific models that advance our understanding of religious faith, emotions, symbols, rituals, meaning, and the anthropological and cultural dimensions of religions, integrating them into more complex models.

Recent decades have witnessed a growing interest in the study of religious mind and behavior from new disciplinary fields, such as cognitive psychology, neuroscience and bio-evolutionary science. The amount of published research is impressive and has reached a level that now calls for evaluation and revision of current models and developments. This new series supports this fast-moving development, encouraging the publication of new books that move on from current research towards larger horizons and innovative ideas.

This series:

- Increases academic communication and exchange in this multi-disciplinary research area.
- Provides a new impetus to the science and religion dialogue.
- Opens up new avenues of encounter and discussion between science and humanities traditions.

More information about this series at http://www.springer.com/series/15336

Hans-Ferdinand Angel • Lluis Oviedo
Raymond F. Paloutzian • Anne L.C. Runehov
Rüdiger J. Seitz
Editors

Processes of Believing: The Acquisition, Maintenance, and Change in Creditions

Springer

Editors
Hans-Ferdinand Angel
Institute of Catechetics and Religious Education
Karl-Franzens University of Graz
Graz, Austria

Raymond F. Paloutzian
Department of Psychology
Westmont College
Santa Barbara, CA, USA

Rüdiger J. Seitz
Department of Neurology, Centre for Neurology and Neuropsychiatry, LVR-Klinikum Düsseldorf
Heinrich-Heine-University Düsseldorf
Düsseldorf, Germany

Lluis Oviedo
Pontifical University Antonianum
Rome, Italy

Anne L.C. Runehov
Department of Theology
University of Uppsala
Uppsala, Sweden

ISSN 2367-3494 ISSN 2367-3508 (electronic)
New Approaches to the Scientific Study of Religion
ISBN 978-3-319-50922-8 ISBN 978-3-319-50924-2 (eBook)
DOI 10.1007/978-3-319-50924-2

Library of Congress Control Number: 2017934308

Printed on acid-free paper

This Springer imprint is published by Springer Nature
The registered company is Springer International Publishing AG
The registered company address is: Gewerbestrasse 11, 6330 Cham, Switzerland

Preface

This book addresses the notion of believing as a fundamental process determining the broad range of human behaviour. To intensify the scientific discourse on the "normal processes of believing", the *Credition Research Project* was inaugurated some years ago, culminating in the creation of this volume. The perspective is fully multidisciplinary.

The intention of the *Credition Research Project* (http://credition.uni-graz.at/) is to work out a "model of a normal process of believing" regardless of whether it may take place in religious or mundane contexts. In addition, possible applications of the model of credition in different fields of relevance (law, economic, religious science, communication theory, conflict resolution, education, and so on) are discussed.

There are three different but interdependent goals of research that cannot be considered in isolation, because they mutually influence each other. They are named and explained below.

- *Basic research*: to work out a model of credition in an interdisciplinary and transdisciplinary approach.
- *Applied research*: to review the scientific fields to which the model of credition may be applied and to test its validity.
- *Implementation research*: the focus of this type of research is to observe and to stimulate the integration of the model of credition in the context of conceptual work such as "concepts of sustainability" or "transitional justice", into communication processes (for instance, "development of education") or into organisations ("development of organisations" or "cross-culture exchange within organisations").

The structure of credition has been the title of a series of yearly conferences on basic research that have been held in Graz, Austria, since 2011. Additionally, a series of conferences was started in 2013, which opened the door to questions related to the application of the model of credition. The financial support of the Karl-Franzens University of Graz, the Government of Styria, and especially the continuous appreciation and financial contribution by the City of Graz are gratefully acknowledged.

The topics of the *Structure of Credition* conferences were:

2011 The Role of Cognition, Emotion, and Appraisal
2012 Memory, Space of Action, and Social Binding
2013 Formation, Causation, and Ideation
2014 Valuation, Association, and Decision Making
2015 Stabilisation, Awareness, and Attitude
2016 Epistemology, Networks, and Translation

The topics of the *Credition Applied Research* conferences which were held in different universities were:

2013 The Model of Credition and Its Possibilities of Application (Graz/Austria)
2014 The Application of the Credition Research Project in Economics and Social Sciences (Würzburg/Germany)
2015 How to Use the Model of Credition as Communication Tool in the Field of Politics and Education (Thessaloniki/Greece)
2016 Credition and Worldviews (Utrecht/The Netherlands)

The conference series of the Credition Implementation Research was inaugurated recently.

2016 The *Model of Credition* in Theology and Neuroscience (Rome/Italy)

This volume intends to give insights into our discussions of the recent years, and into the complexity of our interdisciplinary approach. All contributors to this book were speakers in the basic research conferences. Their contributions reflect their own scientific approach to and perspective on the topic. At the same time, they show that an interdisciplinary endeavour opens the door to a fundamental transformation of perspective without disregarding the foundational soil of traditional reflections. The book therefore highlights many perspectives which are connected to the question of what normal processes of believing – religious or not – might be. The intention is twofold:

- First, we intend to present approaches that integrate traditional discussions that are relevant for building a theory of normal believing processes.
- Second, we want to give the floor to a few contributions that explicitly integrate the process character of believing, shedding new light on the question of belief.

Of course, we know that much more research needs to be done. Therefore, this volume aims to encourage an interdisciplinary approach to research to develop a better understanding of what happens when people are believing.

The title of this book *Processes of Believing* intends to signify the conceptual switch from the noun "belief" to an expression suggesting the dynamic of the "process of believing". Similarly, the subtitle *Acquisition, Maintenance, and Change* outlines the broad perspective of this, highlighting such putative processes connected to believing.

It may sound grammatically strange to combine acquisition, maintenance, and change with the proposition "in" (i.e. "in Credition"). But many terms of our everyday language are not sufficient to express those processes that we want to highlight when using the term "credition". Importantly, we wish to indicate the need to integrate the question of credition into a theoretical frame, which will allow for a deeper understanding of the basic function of processes of believing in relation to human meaning-making system.

This book would not have been published without the dedicated cooperation of the editors at Springer. We especially want to thank Cristina Alves dos Santos and Anita van der Linden-Rachmat for their kind and empathetic support by which they followed the growing of the volume.

Finally, we want to express our special gratitude to two people who went the extra kilometre in helping this book come to completion. Katrin Staab, at the University of Graz, did a tremendous amount of work formatting all the chapters. Katelyn Mukai, at Westmont College in Santa Barbara, did a marvellous job of copy-editing all 31 chapters while accomplishing the dual goal of crafting correct English while keeping the author's native tone. The editors and authors appreciate their contributions very much. This book is the far better for it.

Graz, Austria — Hans-Ferdinand Angel
Rome, Italy — Lluis Oviedo
Santa Barbara, CA, USA — Raymond F. Paloutzian
Uppsala, Sweden — Anne L.C. Runehov
Düsseldorf, Germany — Rüdiger J. Seitz

Acknowledgments

The authors acknowledge the financial support by the University of Graz.

Contents

Part I Introduction

Introduction: What We Do Not Know About Believing – Approaching a New Scientific Hot Spot ... 3
Hans-Ferdinand Angel, Lluis Oviedo, Raymond F. Paloutzian, Anne L.C. Runehov, and Rüdiger J. Seitz

Credition: From the Question of Belief to the Question of Believing ... 17
Hans-Ferdinand Angel

Part II Psychology and Neuroscience

Believing, Remembering, and Imagining: The Roots and Fruits of Meanings Made and Remade ... 39
Raymond F. Paloutzian and Katelyn J. Mukai

Connection Between Scripts Embedding Motor Schemes and Decision Making ... 51
Gennaro Auletta

Beliefs and Believing as Possible Targets for Neuroscientific Research ... 69
Rüdiger J. Seitz

Neurobiological Factors Underlying Attachment and Trust in the Believing Process ... 83
Corina Aguilar-Raab and Beate Ditzen

New Concepts on the Motor System: Implications for Emotions and Credition ... 97
Giovanni Buccino and Ivan Colagè

Neural Underpinnings of the Human Belief System ... 111
Irene Cristofori and Jordan Grafman

Believing in the Effectiveness of Treatment: From Placebo to Credition and Back 125
Karin Meissner

The Power to Live with Disasters: Adaptive Believing Processes of the Self and World 139
Motoaki Sugiura

Belief and Belief Formation: Insights from Delusions 153
Michael H. Connors and Peter W. Halligan

Functional and Dysfunctional Religious/Spiritual Beliefs in Psychotic Disorders 167
Human-Friedrich Unterrainer

Part III Philosophy

The Theory of Credition and Philosophical Accounts of Belief: Looking for Common Ground 183
Aku Visala and Hans-Ferdinand Angel

Credition and Justification 195
Anne L.C. Runehov

Hume on the Origins of Religious Belief 209
Anders Kraal

The Structure of Credition in Whitehead's Metaphysics of Experience 217
Helmut Maaßen

Brain and Self – A Neurophilosophical Account 227
Georg Northoff

Creditions and Self-Identity: Embodiment Between Actions and (Life) Decisions 247
Ivan Colagè and Nicola Gobbi

A Process Pragmatist Heuristics of Believing 263
Michel Weber

Part IV Theology, Religious Studies, and Anthropology

Cognition, Emotion, and the Ethics of Authenticity 277
Oliver Davies

Recent Scientific Explanations of Religious Beliefs: A Systematic Account 289
Lluis Oviedo

Soul and Body According to "De Fide Orthodoxa" of St. John Damascene 319
Dorin Oancea

Music as a Medium of Personal Motion and Belief: Some Phenomenological Reflections ... 331
Peter Ebenbauer

Part V Social Sciences

Reconciliation After a Protracted Violent Conflict: Do Believing Processes Play a Role, and Which One? A Research Agenda ... 341
Joseph Marko

Understanding Young People's Worldview: A Practical Example of How to Work with the Model of Credition ... 363
Vasiliki Mitropoulou

Approaching Another Black Box: Credition in Economics ... 375
Richard Sturn

Credition in Business – Innovations with Crowdbusiness ... 387
Reinhard Willfort and Conny Weber

Part VI Natural and Computer Sciences

Creditions and Modern Computer Science ... 399
Horst Bischof

Public and Personal Causations of Creditions ... 405
Javier Leach

Wave-Particle Duality and Quantity-Quality Complementarity in Natural and Human Sciences: Implications for Credition Research ... 417
Sungchul Ji

Interoception and Gut Feelings: Unconscious Body Signals' Impact on Brain Function, Behavior and Belief Processes ... 435
Peter Holzer

Decision-Making and Credition Under a Microbial Perspective ... 443
Gabriele Berg and Maria Sensen

Part VII Conclusion

Structuring Credition ... 453
Hans-Ferdinand Angel, Lluis Oviedo, Raymond F. Paloutzian, Anne L.C. Runehov, and Rüdiger J. Seitz

Author Index ... 461

Subject Index ... 465

Contributors

Corina Aguilar-Raab Institute of Medical Psychology, Center for Psychosocial Medicine (ZPM), University Hospital Heidelberg, Heidelberg, Germany

Hans-Ferdinand Angel Institute of Catechetics and Religious Education, Karl-Franzens University of Graz, Graz, Austria

Gennaro Auletta Pontifical Gregorian University, Rome, Italy

University of Cassino, Cassino, Italy

Gabriele Berg Institute of Environmental Biotechnology, Graz University of Technology, Graz, Austria

Horst Bischof Institute for Computer Graphics and Vision, Graz University of Technology, Graz, Austria

Giovanni Buccino Dipartimento di Scienze Mediche e Chirurgiche, Università degli Studi Magna Graecia di Catanzaro, Catanzaro, Italy

Ivan Colagè Pontifical University Antonianum, Rome, Italy

Michael H. Connors ARC Centre of Excellence in Cognition and its Disorders, Department of Cognitive Science, Macquarie University, Sydney, NSW, Australia

Dementia Collaborative Research Centre, School of Psychiatry, University of New South Wales, Sydney, NSW, Australia

Sydney Medical School, University of Sydney, Sydney, NSW, Australia

Irene Cristofori Cognitive Neuroscience Laboratory, Brain Injury Research, Rehabilitation Institute of Chicago, Chicago, IL, USA

Department of Physical Medicine and Rehabilitation, Feinberg School of Medicine, Northwestern University, Chicago, IL, USA

Oliver Davies Department of Theology and Religious Studies, King's College London, London, UK

Beate Ditzen Institute of Medical Psychology, Center for Psychosocial Medicine (ZPM), University Hospital Heidelberg, Heidelberg, Germany

Peter Ebenbauer Institute of Liturgiology, Christian Arts and Hymnology, Karl-Franzens University, Graz, Austria

Nicola Gobbi Pontifical Gregorian University, Rome, Italy

Jordan Grafman Cognitive Neuroscience Laboratory, Brain Injury Research, Rehabilitation Institute of Chicago, Chicago, IL, USA

Department of Physical Medicine and Rehabilitation, Feinberg School of Medicine, Northwestern University, Chicago, IL, USA

Department of Neurology, Feinberg School of Medicine, Northwestern University, Chicago, IL, USA

Peter W. Halligan School of Psychology, Cardiff University, Cardiff, Wales, UK

Peter Holzer Institute of Experimental and Clinical Pharmacology, Medical University of Graz, Graz, Austria

Sungchul Ji Department of Pharmacology and Toxicology, Rutgers University, Piscataway, NJ, USA

Anders Kraal Department of Philosophy, University of British Columbia, Vancouver, BC, Canada

Javier Leach (Deceased) Facultad de Informática, Universidad Complutense, Madrid, Spain

Helmut Maaßen Heinrich-Heine-University Düsseldorf, Düsseldorf, Germany

Joseph Marko Institute of Public Law and Political Sciences, University of Graz, Graz, Austria

Karin Meissner Institute of Medical Psychology, Ludwig Maximilian University of Munich, Munich, Germany

Division Health Promotion, University of Applied Sciences Coburg, Coburg, Germany

Vasiliki Mitropoulou Aristotle University of Thessaloniki, Thessaloniki, Greece

Katelyn J. Mukai Department of Psychology, Westmont College, Santa Barbara, CA, USA

Georg Northoff Mind, Brain Imaging and Neuroethics Research Unit, Institute of Mental Health Research, Royal Ottawa Mental Health Centre, Ottawa, Canada

Dorin Oancea Facultatea de Teologie Andrei Saguna, Lucian Blaga University of Sibiu, Sibiu, Romania

Lluis Oviedo Pontifical University Antonianum, Rome, Italy

Raymond F. Paloutzian Department of Psychology, Westmont College, Santa Barbara, CA, USA

Anne L.C. Runehov Department of Theology, University of Uppsala, Uppsala, Sweden

Rüdiger J. Seitz Department of Neurology, Centre for Neurology and Neuropsychiatry, LVR-Klinikum Düsseldorf, Heinrich-Heine-University Düsseldorf, Düsseldorf, Germany

Maria Sensen Institute of Environmental Biotechnology, Graz University of Technology, Graz, Austria

Richard Sturn Institute of Public Economics, Karl-Franzens University of Graz, Graz, Austria

Motoaki Sugiura IDAC, Tohoku University, Sendai, Japan

IRIDeS, Tohoku University, Sendai, Japan

Human-Friedrich Unterrainer Institute of Psychology, Karl-Franzens University of Graz, Graz, Austria

University Clinic of Psychiatry, Medical University of Graz, Graz, Austria

Center for Integrative Addiction Research (Grüner Kreis Society), Vienna, Austria

Aku Visala Faculty of Theology, University of Helsinki, Helsinki, Finland

Conny Weber ISN – Innovation Service Network GmbH, Graz, Austria

Michel Weber Centre for Philosophical Practice, Brussels & Department of Educational Foundations, University of Saskatchewan, Saskatoon, Canada

Reinhard Willfort ISN – Innovation Service Network GmbH, Graz, Austria

Part I
Introduction

Introduction: What We Do Not Know About Believing – Approaching a New Scientific Hot Spot

Hans-Ferdinand Angel, Lluis Oviedo, Raymond F. Paloutzian, Anne L.C. Runehov, and Rüdiger J. Seitz

Abstract The human propensity to believe is one of the most fascinating phenomena of mankind. Since antiquity, philosophers have spent time and energy trying to understand how and why humans are touched and influenced by their beliefs. Nevertheless "belief" remains a strange phenomenon; it is both wanted and unwanted. Knowledge-based societies as well as either secular or strict religious worldviews can cast belief in a very negative light. Also, from a scientific point of view belief can be considered overly complex and heavily interwoven with religion. This chapter argues against the underestimation of the relevance of belief. It highlights the predominant use of the noun "belief" as one of the basic problems in both everyday speech and scientific research. But an understanding of belief that reduces it to only a noun is not sufficient. Beliefs are expressions and results of activities. This means that believing does not exist only as a noun, but also as a verb. We are active when we do what we call "to believe." The chapter explains that we are at the

H.-F. Angel (✉)
Institute of Catechetics and Religious Education, Karl-Franzens University of Graz, Graz, Austria
e-mail: ferdinand.angel@uni-graz.at

L. Oviedo
Pontifical University Antonianum, Rome, Italy
e-mail: loviedo@antonianum.eu

R.F. Paloutzian
Department of Psychology, Westmont College, Santa Barbara, CA, USA
e-mail: paloutz@westmont.edu

A.L.C. Runehov
Department of Theology, University of Uppsala, Uppsala, Sweden
e-mail: annerunehov@gmail.com

R.J. Seitz
Department of Neurology, Centre for Neurology and Neuropsychiatry, LVR-Klinikum Düsseldorf, Heinrich-Heine-University Düsseldorf, Düsseldorf, Germany
e-mail: seitz@neurologie.uni-duesseldorf.de

H.-F. Angel et al. (eds.), *Processes of Believing: The Acquisition, Maintenance, and Change in Creditions*, New Approaches to the Scientific Study of Religion 1,
DOI 10.1007/978-3-319-50924-2_1

crossroads of a change in perspective from examining "belief" to examining "believing". This change will foster our understanding of the more fundamental "process of believing" and enable us to analyze the process of how believing works in the human mind. Thus, the chapter provides an overview of the book, which starts with two introductory chapters and clusters the following chapters according to scientific disciplines ("neuroscience," "philosophy," "theology, religious studies, and anthropology," "social sciences," and "natural and computer sciences") though many of them reflect an interdisciplinary approach.

1 Belief: Between Crucial Importance and Neglect

1.1 The Crucial Importance of Belief

The human propensity to believe is one of the most fascinating phenomena of mankind. Since antiquity, philosophers have spent time and energy trying to understand how and why humans are touched and influenced by their beliefs. They pressed the "question of belief" – at least in the European tradition – which then became one of the central topics of philosophy and left its traces through all the history of the philosophical study of the mind. The nature of the mind remains an important issue in the twenty-first century, since myriad religious, metaphysical, and secular beliefs are widespread in developing countries, as well as in Eastern and Western societies. However, it is important to consider that when it comes to the question of what a belief is, it becomes obvious it has no common definition.

1.2 Belief: Over-Complex and Scientifically Isolated

It is difficult to understand what believing is due to its complexity. The topic of belief includes several partially-overlapping areas, such as "belief and knowledge" or "belief and delusion" – and can be especially divisive in cases of specific doctrinaire perspectives under the rubric of "belief and religion."

Thus, the question of what belief means (or should mean) is located in diverse fields of interest such as logic, the psychology of meaning-making, mental illness, religious experience, studies of the nature of truth, decision-making, law and jurisprudence, and in various religions and worldviews.

A consequence of this is that in every relevant field, one can find highly specified and elaborated discussions of belief. However, surprisingly, and rather unfortunately, these fields often seem to remain isolated from each other, with little genuine cross-field dialogue; this then limits the amount of collaboration that would allow them to affect each other in a serious way. This circumstance is a consequence of the highly specialized world of modern science, i.e., scientists are trained to examine a phenomenon (e.g., whether beliefs or believing as a process) from only their own fields of study. Many efforts to understand belief may be characterized as a "single-profile-approach." Specialists in the clinical relevance of belief may refer to an under-elaborated concept of doxastic logic; scholars of the relations between knowledge and belief may not consider the "formation of belief," since the latter topic is dealt with in the developmental and clinical fields. A consequence is that the concepts of belief and believing remain erratic and undefined. No discipline seems responsible for understanding them in all their complexity. Thus, research into the nature of belief and believing can be characterized as complex, as well as scientifically isolated.

1.3 Belief: Interwoven with Religion

A special problem with the concept of belief is that it is oftentimes automatically associated with religion. In some people's minds, it seems intrinsically intimate with religion – a unique relationship. No other concept relevant to understanding human behavior is as deeply tied to religion as belief. This connectedness becomes highly problematic, and fosters an unfortunate and inadequate understanding of belief. This is especially because (a) "religion" is often conceived of as a manifestation of Western tradition, whereas (b) in fact, people have beliefs about all manner of things in life, not only things called "religious."

Thus, restricting an understanding of belief and believing to only those phenomena that happen to be religious is short-sighted, as far as understanding the fundamental nature of believing is concerned. Making "belief" part of religion essentially allows "religion" to frame (and restrict) the various aspects of belief, when in fact, the range of aspects of believing can be far greater than that which is specified by a religion. As a consequence, under the overall umbrella "religious belief," concepts as different from each other as, e.g., delusion and knowledge, could be discussed in an unproductive manner because in any instance, either one may not connote anything religious; they would instead be arbitrarily forced to fit into a religion mold.

1.4 Belief: A Strange and Seemingly Unattractive Phenomenon

With regard to this complexity, it is understandable that in scientific reflections, belief – despite its long tradition – still appears ill-defined. Because of this, a general idea seems to be prevalent in many modern societies that what or how someone believes is not a public matter, so that its relevance might be either neglected or suppressed. There are several reasons why modern societies tend to underestimate the relevance of belief.

- Knowledge-Based Society
  In a modern knowledge-based society, the question of what people believe is less important than the question of what they know. For example, referring to personal beliefs in a job interview may be a deficit, not an advantage, especially from the perspective of a secular worldview where believing is seen as a relic of a past religious world, and employers may be leery of hiring someone they fear might be a religious fanatic.
- Secular Worldview
  In a secular society, questions about one's religion are typically of little public interest. That has an effect on the role that believing plays in life or in society because the presumed inherent connection between the concepts of belief and religion decreases any attention that people might give to the importance of beliefs – about anything – in their lives. A consequence is that there is little scientific interest in understanding the process of believing, which further contributes to the isolated scientific status of the topic. Because "religion" as a whole is a complex cultural concept with diverse and contested meanings, it is not, as such, something to be studied at the level of the natural sciences. A consequence is that the processes involved in believing have been largely left unexamined except for the role beliefs played in clinical contexts such as neurosis and delusions.
- Strict Religious Worldview
  Paradoxically, there are religiously-defined societies in the world that reflect an opposite extreme from the secular bases of modern societies, such that a specific religion defines all law, custom, and permissible behavior, and which is rooted in a specific doctrine in which all are required to declare belief. Such had been the nature of strict state-church societies in earlier times. Also in some current societies, religion is part of the state concept. The paradox is that although what a person declares belief in is important (sometimes it is a matter of life or death), the content of that belief in public and governmental affairs is assumed to be both accepted as well as true, and therefore is little impetus for scholarly debate about it or research into its psychological roots. It is essentially a "given" deemed truth, thus requiring assent by all and not subject to question. In such cases, examination of the process of believing seems of little importance.

  We have to realize the paradox of cultures in which belief matters to the point of defining the pivotal idea that the culture purports to stand for, while at the same time, the very rules of the game profoundly inhibit an inclination to question or test the roots of that idea. The consequence is that public declaration of a belief is important, but understanding its validity and the reasons why one would engage in believing it are not subject to question. The process of believing is discarded as something in need of understanding.
- Cognitive Science
  Progress in cognitive science suggests that many of our everyday ways of thinking reflect a built-in "folk-psychology." Folk-psychological ideas are

not expected to explain cognitive processes in a scientific sense, but do describe how the "ordinary mind" explains things. One term seen as especially avoidable is "belief," as illustrated by Stephen Stich in the subtitle of his book "From Folk Psychology to Cognitive Science: The Case against Belief." He explicitly claims "that this concept ought not to play any significant role in a science aimed at explaining human cognition and behavior" (Stich 1996: 5).

2 Belief as a New Hot Spot

2.1 Neglect of Belief: A Meander

Even though the social and natural sciences have neglected research and theory on the fundamental processes of believing, it is highly problematic to continue to do so. Closing our eyes to this phenomenon can even be seen as frivolous and short-sighted.

2.2 The Case Against the Underestimation of the Relevance of Belief

There is an increasing relevance of "belief" as a globalized word intended to handle seemingly insolvable problems. For example:

- The over-complexity of the modern world prevents anyone from having knowledge in all interconnected fields relevant to understanding the nature of believing. For example, in the social sciences, the so-called "expert dilemma" is well known, and is a consequence of this over-complexity.
- Another consequence is that political and social decision-making is undertaken under conditions of uncertainty.
- Planning for the future can refer only to previous knowledge. We simply do not have experience of future events to aid us in planning for the future. And there seems to be little chance of predicting the many incidental consequences of the decisions that are made.
- The current global situation highlights the relevance of religious belief in world affairs in an unusual and unexpected manner. Lacking understanding about not only what people believe, but also the fundamental processes involved in how and why they do so, is probably more dangerous to global peace and stability than lacking understanding about the phenomenon of "religion," because beliefs (whether religious or not) influence many domains of public life, including but not limited to politics and economics.

2.3 Crossroads: From Belief to Believing

One can dig deeper into the reasons for the oscillating, or perhaps neglected, attention given to the topic of belief. One of the basic problems is that in both everyday speech and scientific research, the noun "belief" is emphasized instead of the more fundamental phrase "process of believing." Thus, one can find discussions about "moral belief," "religious belief," "normative belief," "required belief," or "disbelief." Many book titles have included the world "belief" as noun (Hintikka 1962; Lipton 2008; Nilsson 2014). Scholars also talk about "belief systems" (Harkness and Super 1995) and "formation of belief" (Smith 2008). The question of how to maintain or change beliefs or belief systems seems to be attractive for the coaching of individuals and organizations (Green and Hayes 2003; Vieira 1994). And there is no doubt that to understand "belief" in the sense in which it is expressed as a noun is important for science. Moreover, traditional discussions in philosophy, psychology, and religious studies show important aspects of such an understanding of belief.

2.4 Believing as Process

Nevertheless, an understanding of "belief" that reduces it to only a noun is not sufficient. Beliefs are expressions and results of *activities*. This means that we have to realize that believing does not exist only as a noun, but also as a verb. We are active when we do what we call "to believe." Further, the *activity of believing* can be addressed as a question of what is going on inside a person's mind and emotions during the moments of believing (*while believing*). Also, any attempt to understand "believing" as a verb as an activity leads to important changes in perspective that open new horizons to understanding not merely what people's beliefs are, but why they engage in the processes that they do. In order to discuss such processes of believing in scholarly research, the term "creditions" was introduced as a neologism into the scientific debates some years ago [see Chapter 2: "Credition – From the Question of Belief to the Question of Believing" (Angel)]. By referring to the processes involved in believing instead of to the noun "belief," there is a profound change in the nature of the issues in need of research and answers that comes to the surface.

- Believing – knowledge
  Traditional philosophical issues such as the relationship between knowledge and belief are recast as the relationship between knowing and believing. The effect of this change is that novel and rarely discussed questions are raised. For example, what happens when we are engaged in "knowing"? And how can interdependence between knowing and believing be characterized and verified? [see Chapter 14: "Credition and Justification" (Runehov)].
- Believing – religion
  Even if questions about belief might be narrowly tied to religions, conceptualizing the mental process of believing as an aspect of a religion is normally not of

concern. But believing processes are as prevalent in religious contexts as they are in secular contexts. Religious beliefs are a special form of our general ability to engage in believing the meanings that we make. Thus, a deeper understanding of "religious beliefs" (see Chapter 21: "Recent Scientific Explanations of Religious Beliefs: A Systematic Account" (Oviedo)] can help us integrate relevant aspects of believing into the concept of credition.

- Believing – meaning-making
  Reflecting on a psychological approach, the process of believing can be understood as one of making and remaking meanings. What we call a "belief" has been constructed in the mind by fundamental meaning system processes. We act upon them mentally or behaviorally, appraise the outcomes in view of the expectations and predictions of our overall meaning system, and remake meanings based on those appraisals, whether similar or modified, and reappraise and remake them again and again through a continuous feedback cycle [see Chapter 3: "Believing, Remembering, and Imagining: The Roots and Fruits of Meanings Made and Remade" (Paloutzian & Mukai)]
- Believing as a subject of neuroscientific research
  This approach can be expected to open new dimensions of neuroscientific research. Evidence from neuroimaging and neurophysiology has shown that the intricately interwoven mental operations of perception, valuation, and generation of action affording believing are processed in extensive neural networks involving the dorsal medial and dorsolateral frontal cortex. Scientific approaches of this sort open strategies for an empirical exploration of the ethical guidance of human behavior [see Chapter 5: "Beliefs and Believing as Possible Targets for Neuroscientific Research" (Seitz)].

2.5 *Credition as a Normal Process of Believing*

The term "credition" was conceived in order to serve as a bridge between different processes such as cognition, affection, functions of believing, belief development, and even evolution. Under the general term "credition," we can reflect all verb-related aspects of beliefs and belief systems. Credition can be conceived from a cognitive neuroscience point of view as a normal "everyday" mental operation – at least in the sense of non-pathological believing. The concept of creditions as processes stresses the fluidity of the mental activity of believing, and is nevertheless open to being available to stabilize a belief for the sake of its ordinary continuity. Stable beliefs occur as a result of extensively repeated single processes of believing, which follow the rules of learning and are consequences of integrating individual experiences. From a psychological perspective, believing processes are embedded in a complex meaning-making procedure, and from a sociological perspective, they reflect in an accepting or withstanding way the impulses coming from a surrounding society. Creditions do not occur only within religions. On the contrary, they occur in all of life's contexts. In religious contexts, however, they may be manifest in particularly exquisite ways, as "religious experiences" may reflect processes of deep believing.

3 The Chapters of the Book

This book starts with two introductory chapters. Then, the chapters of the book are clustered according to scientific disciplines ("neuroscience," "philosophy," "theology, religious studies, and anthropology," "social sciences," and "natural and computer sciences") though many of them follow an interdisciplinary approach. Some of the chapters refer directly to aspects of the model of credition, while others intend to deepen the understanding of specialized but highly relevant aspects of the model. Most of the contributions demonstrate in a specific way the basic research program, but some are dedicated to the question of how to apply the model of credition in practical fields like pedagogics, economics, or political concerns. The following list of topical summaries provides a roadmap of the route this book will take, chapter by chapter.

I. *Introduction*

(2) *Hans-Ferdinand Angel* in his introductory chapter, "Credition: From the Question of Belief to the Question of Believing" traces the scientific developments that have led to the credition research project. He especially stresses the transformation of perspective, which is a consequence of a procedural approach (verb aspect) to the question of belief.

II. Psychology and Neuroscience

(3) *Raymond F. Paloutzian & Katelyn J. Mukai* in their chapter "Believing, Remembering, and Imagining: The Roots and Fruits of Meanings Made and Remade" explain how human and animal systems have developed so that they make meaning out of ambiguity. This occurs at the level of organs, organ systems, and overall mental processes. Psychologically speaking, a belief is what has been formed as a result of the meaning making process, and is constructed from incomplete bits and pieces of information.

(4) *Gennaro Auletta* describes in his contribution "Connection between Scripts Embedding Motor Schemes and Decision-making" that mental codes link the signals from the external physical world with the conceptualizing and execution of actions. He argues for a constructing role of the mind as it transforms operations into signals. It is of interest to learn what the relation of Auletta's code is to belief contents, or how the demonstrated flow of information is related to processes of believing.

(5) In his contribution "Beliefs and Believing as Possible Targets for Neuroscientific Research," *Rüdiger J. Seitz* will argue that the domains of perception, valuation, and generation of action are essential integrative human brain functions closely related to believing. Evidence from neuroimaging and neurophysiology has shown that these mental operations are processed in cortico-subcortical neural networks engaging the medial and lateral frontal cortex.

(6) Creditions occur in a social-interactional framework for which attachment and trust are important factors. This is highlighted by *Corinna Aguilar-Raab & Beate Ditzen* in their chapter "Neurobiological Factors Underlying Attachment and Trust in the Believing Process." Current research of the neuroendocrine system has primarily focused on the neuropeptides Oxytocin and Vasopressin as they have important regulatory

functions when people engage in social interactions and opens perspectives for future research on the relation between believing processes and the neuroendocrine system.

(7) *Giovanni Buccino & Ivan Colagè* focus in the chapter "New Concepts on the Motor System: Implications for Emotion and Credition" on the radical change of our conception of the brain motor system within the last two decades. As beliefs are assumed to play a major role at the root of action choice and selection of appropriate behaviors in social contexts they argue that a theory of credition may provide a conceptual framework helpful in integrating the "simulation theory" and the "theory-theory" approaches to mentalizing. Also, they suggest that explicit mentalizing processes may actually be grounded in more implicit mirror mechanisms.

(8) *Irene Cristofori & Jordan Grafman* present in their chapter "Neural Underpinnings of the Human Belief System" moral, legal, political and religious beliefs as important processes guiding human behavior. They summarize evidence showing that the prefrontal cortex in addition to the temporal cortex, reward networks and limbic regions are key players for social belief systems.

(9) In the chapter "Believing in the Effectiveness of Treatment: From Placebo to Credition and Back" *Karin Meißner* will present results of recent placebo research. She will show that the effectiveness of medical treatments depends not only on their specific pharmacological agents or physical properties, but also on contextual factors, including the patient's expectations, emotions, and beliefs. This chapter discusses possible interrelations with the framework of 'credition'.

(10) In his chapter "The Power to Live with Disasters: Adaptive Believing Processes of the Self and World" *Motoaki Sugiura* discusses the key personality factors related to the power to live after the Great East Japan Earthquake disaster, and connects them to the four fundamental functions of the credition process. Thereby, he highlights the role of beliefs in the power to live.

(11) *Michael H. Connors & Peter W. Halligan* explore in the contribution "Belief and Belief formation: Insights from Delusions" the nature of pathological beliefs as in delusions, and propose a five-stage non-recursive model which explains the formation of normal beliefs and pathological beliefs in neuropsychiatric diseases. In this model, beliefs are the basis for future acts.

(12) Creditions are understood as processes which can take place in mundane and in religious contexts. *Human-Friedrich Unterrainer* focuses in his contribution "Functional and Dysfunctional Religious/Spiritual Beliefs in Psychotic Disorders" on their religious dimension as religious/spiritual beliefs seem strongly related to parameters of mental health. Dysfunctional religious/spiritual beliefs have negative effects in different kind of disorders, but they also play a positive role in coping with mental diseases.

III. Philosophy

(13) *Aku Visala* and *Hans-Ferdinand Angel* introduce in their contribution some historical and contemporary philosophical discussions. They explore a number of ways in which the theory of credition could benefit from engaging with the philosophical literature on belief. They look at some historical and contemporary accounts of the relationship between belief and knowledge and address the perennial association of religion with belief. Finally, they make some preliminary suggestions as to how one could relate philosophical debates and discussions to the theory of creditions.

(14) *Anne Runehov* in her chapter "Credition and Justification" leans on the philosophical discussion of justified beliefs, and transforms the idea of justification from focusing on justified beliefs to justified processes of believing or justified credition. The authority relied upon is the philosopher Alvin Goldman.

(15) *Anders Kraal* highlights in his contribution "Hume on the Origins of Religious Belief" an influential idea of David Hume. In "*The Natural History of Religion*" (1757) he had argued that religious belief originates in and is sustained by a fear of misery coupled with mistaken beliefs as to the true causes of happiness. The interest of the chapter is to discuss how far recent neuroscientific findings, especially as they are provided by the model of credition, can contribute to understanding Hume's position.

(16) *Helmut Maaßen* bridges in his chapter "The Structure of Credition in Whitehead's Metaphysics of Experience" the credition research project with the work of Alfred North Whitehead, one of the most prominent philosophers of process thinking. As Whitehead refers to belief at one point of his analysis of feeling, it seems promising to focus on possible links between the concept of credition and the framework of Whitehead's metaphysics,

(17) *Georg Northoff* in his chapter "Brain and Self – A Neurophilosophical Account" suggests that the self is no longer characterized as a mental substance but as a cognitive function that can be studied empirically. He provides evidence from neuroimaging that the midline structures of the brain are critically engaged but not exclusive for the self. The discussion is open to speculate about the possible relation of the (empirical) self to belief formation and belief contents.

(18) In their paper "Creditions and Self-Identity: Embodiment between Actions and (Life) Decisions" *Ivan Colagè & Nicola Gobbi* describe connections between the theory of creditions and other recent neuroscientific and philosophical topics. In particular, the chapter will focus on those developments that give insights into the issue of self-identity and consciousness and showing that the theory of creditions is interestingly connected with other scientific and philosophical research. They point to new dimensions for future research perspectives that may profit from such connections.

(19) The concept of credition which rejuvenates the discussion of religion and faith inevitably refers to few long lasting debates in philosophy. *Michel Weber* in his contribution "A Process Pragmatist Heuristics of Believing" contextualizes the question of credition within a perspective that originated in Antiquity, as philosophy addressing the issue of believing has always relied to some extent on the antique bipolar juxtaposition of "gnôsis/pistis," His chapter aims at sketching a process pragmatist heuristics of believing.

IV. Theology, Religious Studies, and Anthropology

(20) For *Oliver Davies* the concept of creditions fosters an interesting new perspective on the extent to which emotion and reason combine to shape our beliefs. As religions characteristically emphasize the unity of reason and emotion he will argue in the chapter "Cognition, Emotion, and the Ethics of Authenticity" for a connection between the different religions. He will highlight as an overarching conceptualization of the human person in the light of the new self-knowledge that comes to us from contemporary neuroscience.

(21) *Lluis Oviedo* in his contribution "Recent Scientific Explanations of Religious Beliefs: A Systematic Account" describes a broad spectrum covering most studies published in the last 15 years that propose naturalist explanations of religion, in an attempt to outline their merits and limits.

(22) The Christian and particularly the Orthodox understanding of belief sometimes might be seen as a matter of the soul and not a matter of the body – an understanding that would not give any significance to the binomial "creditions – neuronal processes". But, such a view can be marked as reductionist when regarding positions of the Fathers. In his chapter "Soul and Body According to 'De Fide Orthodoxa' of St. John Damascene" *Dorin Oancea* will refer to one of the most influential theological thinkers who lived in the eighth century in Syria, and present some aspects of his comprehensive anthropological understanding of humans and their relations to God.

(23) Throughout history, chanting and music have been important resources concerning the anchorage of beliefs, or 'creditions,' as well as existential perspectives of life. In his chapter "Music as a Medium of Personal Motion and Belief: Some Phenomenological Reflections" *Peter Ebenbauer* discusses the interdependence of credition and music and describes how music constitutes an immediate expression of 'credition'.

V. Social Sciences

(24) *Joseph Marko* refers in his paper "Reconciliation after a Protracted Violent Conflict: Do Believing Processes Play a Role, and Which One? A Research Agenda" to the recent history of the Balkan countries which even 20 years after the conclusion of the Dayton Peace Agreement is little peaceful. The chapter tries to contribute to a better conceptualization for further research with regard to "ethnic" conflict and reconciliation by making use of the credition theory in order to explore which role "processes of believing" can play in the political mobilization of "ethnicity".

(25) In her chapter "Understanding Young People's Worldview: A Practical Example of How to Work with the Model of Credition" *Vasiliki Mitropoulou* shows in a very practical way in which the concrete educational work with young people can be influenced by introducing the model of credition. She will report that fter highlighting the emotional aspects of their processes of believing, research participants showed remarkable changes in self-understanding and understanding others.

(26) Credition processes are not a long–standing issue in economics, even though pertinent considerations never were completely absent from economic reasoning. *Richard Sturn* shows in his reflection "Approaching Another Black Box: Credition in Economics" some fruitful chances to implement creditions into a theoretical frame of economical thinking. Also, he characterizes the kinds of economic problems for which beliefs and creditions are not important but argues that credition theory may be relevant for a vast range of economic problems and approaches.

(27) *Reinhard Willfort* & *Conny Weber* in their chapter "Credition in Business – Innovations with Crowdbusiness" analyze which role beliefs play in innovation-management. Though most businesses believe that decisions are made rationally, the decision processes within an innovation management are often based on a

subjective assessment of different indicators including gut feelings and beliefs. By systematically taking into account the concept of credition this chapter takes a closer look at how to increase transparency and democratization of beliefs that influence decision-making processes within the field of innovation management.

VI. Natural and Computer Sciences

(28) *Horst Bischof* describes the relationship between computer science and creditions. Though computer science, like mathematics, is an exact science it is nevertheless more than just formalisms. It is also about the application of formal methods to real world data. The chapter shows that any subfield of computer science that deals with data needs to make assumptions which are based on creditions. Two simple examples from computer vision and machine learning demonstrate the effect of priors. Finally, Bayesian inference is introduced as a principle method to handle priors in a rigorous manner.

(29) *Javier Leach* classifies the causes of the processes of believing (creditions) into two types, public and personal processes. Each causal type of creditions corresponds to a kind of language. In his chapter he focusses on the use of language that tends to be formal and objective to express the causes of public creditions and symbolic to express the causes of the processes of personal creditions.

(30) In his chapter "Wave-Particle Duality and Quantity-Quality Complementarity in Natural and Human Sciences: Implications for Credition Research" *Sungchul Ji* shows that the Planckian distribution equation is suited to fit the observations of very different phenomena and events and, thus, is a powerful candidate to formulize basic brain functions underlying the credition processes.

(31) *Peter Holzer* in his paper "Interoception and Gut Feelings: Unconscious Body Signals' Impact on Brain Function, Behavior, and Belief Processes" makes the case for interoception, showing that signals from the gut affect cognition, emotion, and mood in healthy subjects as well as in neuropsychiatric diseases. He submits that by this "gut feeling," processes of believing are modulated.

(32) *Gabriele Berg & Maria Sensen* in their chapter "Decision-Making and Credition under a Microbial Perspective" highlight the microbiome as an important modulator for belief formation, owing to its vast presence in the intestine that, in turn, is heavily connected via the autonomous nervous system with the brain.

4 Conclusion

What do we know about believing – and what do we not know? First, there exists a long lasting discussion in the European History which makes the topic exhaustive. Second, nevertheless there was no major focus on the procedural aspect of the question of believing. This volumes will, that`s our hope, stimulate further research in a topic which is old and new at the same time. It opens a vast field for basic and applied research which might be interesting enough to fascinate especially younger fellows and encourage them for contributing to this scientific hotspot.

References

Green TB, Hayes M (2003) The belief system: the secret to motivation and improved performance. The Hayes Group International, Winston-Salem

Harkness S, Super CM (1995) Parents' cultural belief systems: their origins, expressions, and consequences. The Guilford Press, New York

Hintikka J (1962/2005) Knowledge and belief. An introduction to the logic of the two notions. London Christ College University Press, Ithaca

Lipton BH (2008) The biology of belief: unleashing the power of consciousness, matter & miracles. Hay House, Carlsbad

Nilsson NJ (2014) Understanding beliefs. The MIT Press, Cambridge, MA

Smith VM (2008) Environmental belief formation in children – a tool for environmental education improvement. VDM Verlag Dr. Mueller e.K

Stich S (1996) From folk psychology to cognitive science: the case against belief. MIT Press, Cambridge, MA

Vieira A (1994) Belief systems and your personal power. TPCS Publishers, New Port Beach

Credition: From the Question of Belief to the Question of Believing

Hans-Ferdinand Angel

Abstract This article will argue why belief can be seen as ill-defined phenomenon and highlight some especially problematic aspects of our understanding of belief. It will introduce into the discussion a fundamental change from a more static notion of belief to an understanding of believing as a fluent process. The term "credition" was conceived in order to serve as a bridge between different processes such as cognition, affection, functions of believing, belief development, and even evolution. Under the general term "credition," we can reflect all verbrelated aspects of beliefs and belief systems. Finally the chapter will give insights in the "model of credition" which seems to represent the believing process.

1 Belief as a Complex and Ill-defined Phenomenon

The nature of human belief is one of the main topics in the history of philosophy of the mind. In the European tradition it has been discussed since Antiquity. We can identify at least three partially overlapping topics that are covered by the term *belief*: belief and knowledge, belief and religion, and belief and faith (cf. Visala and Angel, this volume). Thus, it is not surprising that belief is an ill-defined phenomenon. This is easily seen when, for example, we examine the problematic issue of the relationship between the concepts *religion* and *belief*. Scientific discussions about religions may implicitly assume an understanding of what belief is, for example, by taking it to be part of religion and be a religious phenomenon (illustrated by the common phrase "religious belief"). This may explain the seemingly implicit and widespread idea that all beliefs are tightly associated with religions. Consistent with this, in recent decades some theologians emphasized a narrow link between faith and religion (Barth 1957; Rahner 2004), and the German theologian Max Seckler (1988) is well known for equating theology with "knowledge of the belief". Eventually, attempts were made to clarify the meaning of key concepts, for example, the distinctions between "belief" and "faith" (Kenny 1992; Mitchell 1994; Smith 1987) and

H.-F. Angel (✉)
Institute of Catechetics and Religious Education, Karl-Franzens University of Graz, Graz, Austria
e-mail: ferdinand.angel@uni-graz.at

H.-F. Angel et al. (eds.), *Processes of Believing: The Acquisition, Maintenance, and Change in Creditions*, New Approaches to the Scientific Study of Religion 1,
DOI 10.1007/978-3-319-50924-2_2

the relationship between "faith and reason" or "fides et ratio" (Helm 1999; Plantinga and Wolterstorff 1983). Importantly, the relationship between "belief" and "faith" is attracting the interest of modern scholars.[1]

2 Problematic Aspects of Belief

2.1 Conceptual Incompatibility of Overlapping Fields

Various problematic aspects of the concept of belief can be illustrated by listing bipolar word couplets of interdependence, such as:

> "belief – religion", "belief – spirituality", "belief – faith", "belief – knowledge", "belief – attitude", "belief – disbelief", "belief – illusion", "belief – delusion", "belief – neurosis", "belief – trust", "belief – placebo", "belief – aggression", "belief – forgiveness", "belief – decision", and so on.

Clearly, such approaches to understanding the phenomenon of "belief" are lacking depth and explanation, and seem more or less incompatible. A special problem is a strange pattern that combines knowledge and belief under the category of religion and includes a dichotomy between *religious belief* and *secular knowledge*. The religion + belief combination is underpinned by a traditional overinterpretation of religion (a systemic entity) in contrast to "religiosity" (a psychological and anthropological entity) – a problem that is partly a consequence of a lack of theoretical understanding of religiosity (Angel 2013b; Seitz and Angel 2014).

Considerations such as the above may nourish the notion expressed by highly influential authors within cognitive science that belief, at least as a folk psychology term, should be eliminated (Churchland 1979; Fodor 1975; Stich 1996). Stephen Stich argues, "that this concept ought not to play any significant role in a science aimed at explaining human cognition and behaviour" (Stich 1996, 5). Nevertheless, an increasing interest in understanding the academically neglected human ability to believe can be observed in the contemporary public as well as in scientific discourse.

2.2 Dominance of "Belief" as a Noun

One dominant problem is that in everyday speech as well as in scientific research the meaning or connotation of "belief" as a noun seems to be either assumed or at least emphasized. Common phrases that connote this include, for example, moral belief,

[1] This is occurring mainly within the English speaking tradition because such discussion is difficult in many other European languages (e.g., German) in which the linguistic preconditions of two different terms ("faith" and "belief") do not exist.

social belief, religious belief, formation of belief, political belief, brain-bases of belief, and so on. This kind of noun-oriented connotation of belief sounds as if it supports an assumption that belief is somehow static and can be a fixed element in a system of beliefs. Even the distinction generally known in philosophy and theology between "fides quae" (what we believe) and "fides qua" (the faith with which we believe) stresses a more static notion of belief. This distinction can be found in writings as early as those by St. Augustine, when he says: "Certainly we affirm with full truth that the faith which is etched in the heart of everyone who believes ... proceeds from a single doctrine, but it is one thing (ea quae creduntur), and another thing the faith with which we believe (fides qua credentur)" (De Trinitate, XIII, 2, 5).

There is a glaring problem, however. It is that using "faith" and "belief" as nouns does not emphasize the procedural aspect of *believing* as a general human ability. However, our language does include reference to belief in the sense of a verb (to believe), and as a potential mental act of any individual. Moreover, cognitive neuroscience aims specifically at understanding human behaviour with respect to interior mental processes. This corresponds to the recent argument that facts and knowledge are stored in the human brain (Krüger et al. 2009). Thus, there is an important conceptual distinction between doing research on beliefs versus doing research on the process of believing (cf. Visala and Angel, this volume). In order to create an intellectual bridge to connect the two sides of this distinction, scholars from both religious and secular fields recently began to work on understanding believing as a process rather than as only a mental construct connoting a faith/belief as a noun. This distinction may be fundamental, as suggested by research that shows that use of nouns versus verbs manifest in different ways, as evidenced by differing brain activities (Pulvermüller et al. 1999).

2.3 "Religious Belief" as a Prime Example of the "Belief-as-Noun" Problem

Because the phrase "religious belief" connotes a belief-as-noun idea, and because of the theoretical and practical lack of understanding of "religiosity" as a psychological and anthropological concept, the difference between religious belief and secular knowledge keeps the focus on the problematic narrow link between religion and belief instead of on the relation between believing and religiosity or religiousness. The conjunction of religion and belief even assumes that belief refers to a specific mental state rather than to believing as mental process. A strong emphasis on belief as a noun is evident in ecclesiastical contexts, whether termed "faith" or "belief", in reference to belief in God or the role of belief for Christians as faith in Christ. The same assumption is at the root of the idea that one can "pass on" a religious belief to one's children or other people.

3 Change to Credition: From Static Belief to the Process of Believing

In psychology and cognitive neuroscience, believing is understood as an act of generating and maintaining a mental construct as real or true based on previously stored information. There is increased interest in understanding this mental act in terms of adaptive significance, cognitive processes, and their neural implementation in the human brain (Krüger and Grafman 2013).

3.1 Signals of the Need for a Change in Perspective – The Path to Credition

Although the intellectual discussion about the nature of belief is old, new approaches are appearing. They can be heralded by the headline: "from static belief to the process of believing". They signal the need for a change in perspective.

- In clinico-pathological contexts, delusions have been defined as false beliefs that pertain to an assumed alternative reality. Similarly, religious experience has been described as a manifestation of epilepsy and stroke, affecting the right temporal lobe, thus supporting the notion that religious experience results from brain pathology. Now there is increasing interest in understanding mechanisms of deviance by implicitly or explicitly focusing on functional processes (Sugiura et al. 2015; Angel and Seitz 2016) and the "cognitive level analysis of belief per se" (Connors and Halligan 2015). For instance, Langdon and Coltheart (2000), who reviewed the reports of various types of bizarre delusions, proposed that two deficits must be present in such conditions – (1) damage to sensory and/or attention-orienting mechanisms, which causes aberrant perception and (2) a failure of belief evaluation (Langdon and Coltheart 2000). One result is that cognitive neuroscience and related disciplines show a new openness to understanding believing as human abilities and activities that can be approached empirically (Connors and Halligan 2015). But it seems that there is no acceptable definition what "belief" (as a noun) actually is and what, in comparison, a tentative taxonomy of a false belief or delusion is (Bell and Halligan 2013) (cf. Cristofori and Grafman, this volume; Connors and Halligan, this volume).
- Reviews of experimental studies of intuitive judgment propose two different systems of judgement (Morewedge and Kahnemann 2010), one in which automatic processes generate impressions and tentative judgments (System 1), another by which these first judgments might be accepted, blocked, or corrected by controlled processes (System 2).
- The nature of belief formation is, at least in neuropathology, discussed mainly in the context of adults (Langdon and Connaughton 2013). It has been shown that people form beliefs asymmetrically in that they "tend to discount bad news but embrace good news" (Sharot et al. 2012). But people of all ages form beliefs. Because of this, we have an opportunity to explore and build a bridge connecting

knowledge of the relationship between belief and ontogenetic development, belief in context of neuropathology, and belief in a neuropsychological and general anthropologic sense.
- Cognitive neuroscience implicitly discusses the notion that belief is a component of normal mental activity when attempting to explore the neural correlates of religious experience (Saver and Rabin 1999; Azari et al. 2001).
- Believing does not take place without valuation. The valuation process involves focusing attention on incoming information in a bottom-up fashion and forms our probabilistic accounts or beliefs about the event observed in the outside world. The comparison with knowledge acquired during infancy and childhood allows for the top-down attribution of personal affective loading to the new information using categories such as aversion, danger, pleasantness, utility, novelty, certainty, and mightiness (Seitz et al. 2009; Seitz and Angel 2014).
- Recent years have seen a rapidly growing interest within the cognitive science of religion in understanding the relationship between religion and psychological anthropology (cf. Oviedo, this volume).
- In the psychology of religion, there is increased interest in the processes that mediate both belief and unbelief, for religious and atheist orientations, respectively (Bullivant and Ruse 2013; Hills et al. 2004; Schnell 2012; Schnell and Keenan 2011), the relationship between religious belief and meaning (Paloutzian 2016; Park 2013), and definitional issues inherent in defining the concept of religion for psychological research and theory (Paloutzian and Park 2013a, b).

In order to highlight the process of believing as it might appear in a religious or secular manner and to stress this change in perspective, the neologism "credition" was coined (Angel 2006). The term "credition" stems from the Latin "*credere*" and is conceived as a psychological term analogous to emotion (lat. *Movere* = to move) and cognition (lat: *cogitare* = to think/to reflect) that denotes the mental activity related to what we mean when we say "he/she believes" (Angel 2013a; Seitz and Angel 2012).

3.2 *Illusion of an Easy Change*

To change the focus of theory and research on belief from a content-oriented to a process-oriented approach might seem like a small step that fosters the illusion of an easy change. But it is one task to conceptualize the role of belief as an attitude or as part of a "belief system"; it is quite another to try to understand what mental activity is actually going on and what it means when someone says he or she has a belief, came to believe, or is believing. Psycholinguistically, we want to understand the neurocognitive processes at the route of each step of the double change, from invoking the noun *belief* to the verb *to believe* to the progressive tense of the verb *to believe*.

Numerous challenges arise as a consequence of this change in perspective. Belief processes most likely differ with respect to the object, intensity, and subjective expression of believing. One of the major challenges is to filter the large number of noun-related reflections of "belief" through an innovative process perspective.

Because credition is conceived of as a process, questions emerge that may sound unusual in relation to concepts that reflect the notion of belief or faith as noun.

The reverse is also true. Re-articulating static concepts in terms of process concepts is a task that we must undertake. For example, starting from a procedural understanding of believing, every specific attitude or state of belief can be identified as the momentary end of a lifelong learning process that includes or summarizes many previous believing processes. The question of how beliefs form (i.e., "formation of belief") can be restated as a question of how repeated processes of believing lead to a more or less stable formation of belief. When we approach understanding belief with this perspective, the focus moves away from belief contents or dogma(s) – whether they belong to religions or other belief systems – and is directed towards inner mental activities and the modes by which individuals interact with their environment.

3.3 Focus on Process and Process Philosophy

Because the concept of creditions focuses explicitly on the elements of the process of believing, and because any process that happens can happen only through time, we must include time in however we come to understand believing. This may change how we approach doing research on belief. The act of believing guides behaviour in uncertain and ambiguous situations, and this usually has personal or social advantage over the risk of incorrect beliefs and inappropriate behaviour. Consistent with this active adaptive nature of the believing process, beliefs have been shown to influence reasoning as well as brain activity related to reasoning. This understanding implicitly refers to a theory of process and opens the door to philosophical questions of process. Since the model of credition is understood as a process in which the fluidity of beliefs is emphasized, it assumes that any description of normal believing is implicitly based on a process-theoretical foundation (Angel 2016). A theory of credition is, in effect, an applied theory of process.

The notion of process has been discussed in philosophy since antiquity. Two basic concepts (potentially contradictory) influenced the history of Western thinking. First, Heraclitus' (ca. 520–ca. 460 B.C.) idea that everything is in motion (Kahn 1981) was expressed by the neo-platonic philosopher Simplikios (ca. 490–560) in its most famous form "πάντα ῥεῖ" ("everything flows"). In contrast, Parmenides (ca. 520/515–ca. 460/455 B.C.) posited the idea of unchangeable being (Heitsch 1995; Graham 2013). The modern era has seen increased interest in the Philosophy of Process. On this topic the writings of Whitehead (1978), Bergson (1998), and Deleuze (1994) are especially relevant to a discussion of credition (cf. Maaßen, this volume).

To clarify, a process-oriented approach to believing will be able to include the notion "belief" (as a noun) – which can be metaphorically understood as a kind of stabilized snap-shot that might be either relevant for a short moment or be similar to a reliable old map underpinned by a stable attitude. Thus, this new focus on the process of believing is connected to but will modify traditional philosophical concepts, as illustrated in Gettier's famous paper about the relation between "true belief" and knowledge (cf. Runehov and Angel 2013). It will also open new questions such as whether notion of justification can be expressed within a concept of fluid believing (cf. Runehov, this volume) or how emotions may influence religious experience as illustrated by Hume's reflection on fear as an original basis of religions (cf. Kraal, this volume).

3.4 Focus on "Normal" Processes of Believing

Recent interdisciplinary research has begun to identify features of the psychophysiological processes that underlay believing. This means that a future task will be to shape a model of "normal" belief, or better stated, "normal processes of believing". This will further reflect a shift from a more pathologically oriented approach to a focus on a non-pathologic believing. Such a change in perspective will open new horizons and could be reminiscent of the period when the topic of "Emotions of Normal People" (Marston 1928) was introduced. This focus will open a field of research embedded in a framework that confronts the issue of what normality is. Both quantitative and qualitative research on the nature of normality could be developed with both synchronous and diachronic questions in mind. Thus, issues that span various time horizons could guide studies of normality across different cultures and different historical periods. Finally, our efforts to understand normality will of necessity require that we tackle allied challenges such as gaining a fuller understanding the notions of "norm" and "normativity".

3.5 Claims, Interdisciplinary Challenges, and Open Questions

With the lack of empirical effort to understand belief – sometimes called "neglect of belief" (Connors and Halligan 2015) – and the absence of theoretical attempts to understand "normal" belief, research on creditions could be seen as completely new. But actually, it makes explicit what has implicitly been going on for several years (cf. Sect. 3.1 above). The creditions model enables some old and implied questions to be put plainly on the table. What is a process? What is a process of believing? How can it be distinguished from other processes like the process of knowing, thinking, or having an intuition? What is the function of a process of believing for humans and how is it represented in the brain?

We still lack a definition of "normal believing process". Nevertheless, new questions emerge. For example, when does a believing process begin and end?" The notion that such a process begins and ends has never been raised in a theoretically sufficient way. More crucial is the question of what happens between the time when the process of believing begins and ends. These and related questions demonstrate the need for (a) theoretical efforts to conceptualize processes of believing, and (b) empirical research to test the ideas that emerge from those efforts. Such research activities mark a paradigm-shift.

We need to formulate a theoretical framework for "normal" believing that neither reflects pathological brain states nor applies only to religions. A credition model of processes of believing would do this by serving as an effective vehicle for discussing what happens at different scientific levels of analysis – that of transcendence, behavior and interaction with the environment, body, molecules, cells and neurons, genes, atoms, and subatomic entities or even the question of whether the Planckian Distribution Equitation may open new perspectives for credition research (Ji, this volume). To tackle this challenge, a theoretical framework has to be created that accounts for the fluidity of the believing process and that allows different scientific descriptions to be integrated, whether physical, biological, neural, or behavioral. For example, questions about the role of the motor system (cf. Buccino and Colagè, this volume) and the relation between body and self (embodiment) in prompting actions (cf. Colagè and Gobbi, this volume) can be articulated and researched.

The role of "computational" information processes (cf. Bischof, this volume), and how they relate to general information processing and energy consumption, modelled in the concept of "gnergy" (Ji 2012) are especially salient. Other issues also need to be addressed, for example, whether and in what sense emotions can be seen as information (Schwarz 2001, 2011), and how long it takes until emotional perception shows effects (Topolinski et al. 2015). A theory of creditions should be able to integrate such processes to formulate a procedural model that makes the interdependence of the fluidity and stability of beliefs clear and as well as integrate the above new findings on the dual cognitive model of intuitive and controlled judgment (Morewedge and Kahnemann 2010).

3.6 Credition: Model Building and Terminology

Despite the challenges noted above, an initial model can be presented that can be discussed and improved. When we change our focus from a static concept of belief to a concept of normal believing, the accent will be on the fluidity of those processes that merge internal and external reality and those that mediate their stable appearance. We cannot make this change within the boundaries of our past terminology and theoretical framework. Therefore, in order to develop the creditions model, it is necessary to introduce some new terms (e.g., "bab", "blob", "space of action", enclosure function, etc.). These terms make it possible to initially stress the process character of belief, and to eventually explain religious as well as non-religious believing.

4 Towards a Model of the Believing Process (Credition): Origin and Basic Assumptions

4.1 Psychological View on Religious Experiences

The concept of credition stems from a psychological view of religious experiences. It originated in a research project (Regensburg Symposia, 2002–2006) whose intent was to clarify our understanding of "religiosity/religiousness". Because the discussions took place in German, the main scope had been to understand the meaning of the German term *Religiosität* (Angel et al. 2006). This is an important historical detail because the German term Religiosität does not convey the same meaning as various concepts in the English language such as religiosity, religiousness or spirituality (Angel 2013b). Because the Regensburg Symposia situated the notion "religiosity" in the context of a general "interpretation of the word" (Hemel 1988) neuroscientific approaches to religious experiences were also examined (Angel 2006). The introduction of the term *credition* had a double intention:

- to strictly avoid the theoretical traps of a so-called "neurotheology" (Persinger 1987; d'Aquili and Newberg 1999; d'Aquili et al. 2001; Joseph 2002) because from a hermeneutic standpoint it is not possible to directly combine neurological findings with theological ideas. Or, to illustrate a related point, meditation is highly complex (Schmidt and Wallach 2014) and, for example, the effects of mindfulness meditation need not necessarily be rooted in religious experiences (La Cour and Peterson 2015).
- to bridge disparate neuroscientific results on the issue of where religious experiences are generated. Are they rooted exclusively in the limbic system (the limbic-marker theory) as suggested by Saver and Rabin (1999), or are they supported by cortical regions as found by Seitz and Azari (Azari et al. 2001)? This discrepancy in findings constituted a theoretical challenge. It was analyzed through the lens of a psychological anthropology based primarily on the concepts of emotion and cognition. But these two concepts alone were not sufficient to explain human religiosity (in the sense of the German term), a view later supported from an epistemological philosophy of science perspective (Runehov 2007). We concluded that as related to religiosity, creditions must be understood as interrelated with cognitions and emotions.

One outcome of the Regensburg Symposia proclaimed: No credition without cognition and emotion! We also suggested that creditions are part of an inner balance system. Given this conclusion, a model of credition would have to be linked to homeostatic concepts (Damasio 1998) and subliminal processes (Teske 2007; Smith 2011). Figure 1 illustrates the relationships among cognitive, emotive, and creditive processes.

The term *credition* was coined to denote believing processes that encompass both religious and secular beliefs. The "mental" or "cognitive" believing processes

Fig. 1 C-E-C triangle: No credition without cognition and emotion. "B" stands for "balance"

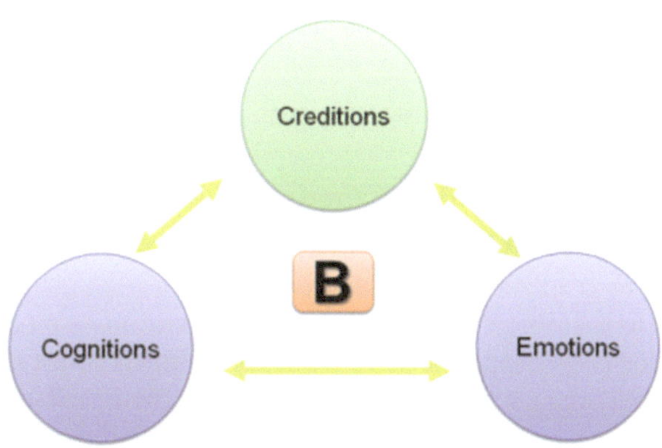

occur in the same way whether the content or context of experiences are religious or secular. Therefore, creditions are not restricted to beliefs about religious experiences; the concept of creditions is not unique to religions. However, understanding creditions is probably indispensable for understanding religiosity, religiousness, and religious experience.

4.2 Relations Between Credition, Emotion, and Cognition

Given this framework, the relation between cognition and emotion is of special interest (Angel 2015, 2017). The interdependence of emotional and cognitive processes has anthropological, psychological, and even theological implications (cf. Davies, this volume). The history of psychology includes a well-known discussion about whether cognition or emotion is primary; an aftermath was the formation of different scientific camps. The discussion started as a result of the so-called two-factor theory of emotion (Schachter 1964) and was pushed by its protagonists Richard Lazarus (1982) and Robert Zajonc (1984).

The debate came to serve a unifying function because of recent discoveries in neuroscience (Gray et al. 2002; Yarkoni et al. 2006; Schaefer and Gray 2007; cf. for the following see also Seitz and Angel 2014; Seitz et al. 2016). Although emotion and cognition are considered to be two different domains that serve separate and often opposite aspects of brain function, there is neuroimaging evidence that emotion and cognition are processed in overlapping areas of the lateral prefrontal cortex through which both can contribute to the control of thought and behaviour (Gray et al. 2002). Moreover, current data provide converging evidence that working memory and neural activity in the lateral prefrontal cortex can be influenced by affective variables. Although emotions have been shown to involve the amygdala and the orbitofrontal cortex (Rolls 2006), cognition comprises different aspects of mental activity such as speech production, memory, attention, and learning, which are processed across widespread circuits in the parietal, temporal, and frontal cortical areas as well as in the amygdala (Schaefer and Gray 2007). That is, the self-organization dynamics in the "perception-action-value triad" (Seitz et al. 2009) predicts the believing process as a personal cognitive-emotional function (Angel and Seitz 2016). From this perspective, it may be illuminating to envisage the role of music as a medium of personal motion and belief (cf. Ebenbauer, this volume).

4.3 Bab: Bridging the Gap Between What We Know and Lack of Terminology

The neuroscientific findings mentioned above on the processing of cognition and emotion in overlapping areas of the lateral prefrontal cortex support the idea of "hot cognition," which scholarship in psychology has considered for some time. But such findings have not yet been incorporated into a broader model because there has been no term to represent the cognitive-emotional interconnection until now. In order to express the meaning of "no credition without cognition and emotion", it seems both necessary and useful to introduce such a term, one that coveys the emotional tinge of propositions.

4.3.1 The Term "Bab"

As new umbrella-term to express the sense of a "proposition including its emotional tinge" at meta-theoretical linguistic level, let us use the term *bab*. The name "bab" is derived from the well-known Russian toy Babushka, which in some regions is known as Matryoshka, to indicate the similarity and comprehensiveness of their components, which we theorize to be one of four characteristics of babs. How is the character of babs best conceptualized?

4.3.2 Characteristics of "Babs"

Emotions can be of the same type but differ in intensity. Because of this, we need to be able to express the variability of the intensity of emotional loadings of a bab. Propositionally identical babs can differ by the "weight" or "mightiness" of their emotional loadings. To express this dynamic we introduce the terms *mega-bab* and *mini-bab* to signify the mightiness of an emotion. Thus we have a means to express the potential emotional fluidity of babs.

Within one person, the same propositional content might change from situation to situation and be "filled" or "coloured" with a different mightiness of emotional loadings. This fluid or dynamic character of the emotional mightiness of a bab might be called the babushka effect, an expression that may be found in different contexts but has lacked a clear scientific label until now. As mentioned, the term *bab* is derived from the Babushka metaphor. In analogy to the wooden toy babushka, which contains several figures of the same shape but different sizes, we can understand a bab as a fluid basic unit that transports content (i.e. an abstract proposition) in combination with the specific mightiness of emotional loadings. Owing to the mental function of attribution, we can postulate four different characteristics of babs (Sugiura et al. 2015; Angel and Seitz 2016). In the credition model, every bab includes all four aspects:

- The propositional content: a bab can be described as a proposition. For example: "I see something red" or "I feel something sharp". The proposition becomes explicit by statements such as: "I see this ball to be red" or "I feel this knife to be sharp".
- The emotional moment: For example, a red light may be perceived as beautiful, warm, or attractive, whilst a sharp item may be unpleasant, harmful, and, frightening. The term *bab* comprises the subliminal emotional moment in addition to the propositional content. When this information is expressed verbally, the bab will reach explicit awareness in both the speaker and listener.

- The sense of mightiness: The subjective perspective of a bab is not limited to the valence of an emotion. It also includes the intensity of emotions. This is reflected in the sense of mightiness or strength. And the notion that the mightiness of a bab can vary implies that we can scale emotions from strong to weak. The variability of bab mightiness yields the consequence that we can express the meaning of one person's bab differently than that of another person, even if they are propositionally identical. Degree of mightiness can be assessed by numerical or other scales.
- The sense of certainty: this characteristic reflects the conviction of an individual. A specific bab proposition can be believed with a high certainty by one person but with low certainty by another. For instance, "I see something red" or "I see something sharp" has a high degree of certainty in bright daylight but a low degree of certainty at dusk. The degree of certainty can be assessed by numerical or other scales.

4.3.3 Blob: The Subliminal Aspect of "Babs"

There is evidence that processes involved in believing are deeply influenced by factors that are subliminal and non-conscious (cf. Holzer, this volume, Meißner, this volume); there is an expanding list of phenomena so considered (cf. Berg, this volume). Because we usually are not conscious of most of the things we believe, a model of creditions must accommodate the subliminal aspects of believing (Teske 2007). The term *blob* is introduced to refer to a bab that remains subconsciously hidden. Blobs are non-conscious babs that mediate the influence of the content and degree of a belief on affects, motivations, and actions at a subliminal level.

In sum, the *bab* is a cover-term denoting aspects of belief including propositional content, emotion, mightiness, and certainty. In order to describe a single bab, it is necessary to name its propositional content, its emotional loading (for instance fear, joy, anger, and so on), its subjective importance (mega-bab vs. mini-bab) to the 'bab-owner', and its subjectively felt degree of certainty (e.g., doubt vs. certainty).

5 Credition: A Model of the Process of Normal Believing

5.1 Theoretical Challenges for a Model of Creditive Processes

There are many theoretical challenges that cannot be expanded upon in this one book. A few warrant comments here:

- Because understanding a process requires one to create an integrated picture of how its elements behave over time, a broad theoretical and philosophical discussion about the nature of time may be relevant. The model of credition allows for time-related discussions of the believing process.
- Introducing a time-based perspective into our picture of the process of believing leads to strange questions: When exactly does a creditive process begin? How is the end of a creditive process evident? We suggest that believing begins with an

initially novel perception and ends with preparing to take action (i.e. in the prefiguration of what we call "space of action") or to recover a self-determined control of oneself. Thus we conceptualize the term *credition* as located at the interface of attitude and action. Thus, thinking about doing something without any action is not understood to be credition.

- Processes of believing are interrelated with attitudes, influencing them as well as our actions. They are part of a complex meaning making process (cf. Paloutzian and Mukai, this volume). Thus, creditions are connected to perceptions, actions, attitudes, and convictions. These topics are subject to many theoretical and philosophical reflections, and many empirical findings on these topics are implicit contributions to an understanding of creditions. To screen the insights imbedded in this literature from the standpoint of the credition model is a major challenge for the future.
- Special attention should go to examining the role of the will. As a volitional procedure, will has to be discussed and integrated into the transformation process that occurs between perception and action.
- The model of credition identifies different functions as constituents of the process of believing. Thus the theoretical and philosophical questions related to function and functionality have to be discussed.
- The referential frame within which functions involved in believing take part (whether "body", "person", or perhaps a privileged candidate – "the self") are especially important to discussions of the process of believing. Concepts such as "body", "person", and "self" are relatively modern and have been discussed with controversy since the time of Enlightenment (Thiel 2014), and are prominent in the model of credition (cf. Northoff, this volume; Colagé and Gobbi, this volume). Many questions about the individual (Conway 2005) and the social self and its moral development (Han et al. 2008; Sugiura 2011, 2013; Potthoff and Seitz 2015) have emerged from these and related modern concepts.
- There are many additional topics that can be discussed within a theoretical framework of believing processes. These include action, truth, will, trust, and attachment (cf. Aguilar-Raab and Ditzen, this volume), codes and coding (cf. Auletta, this volume), and value, causality, and causation (cf. Leach, this volume).
- Evidence from neuroimaging and neurophysiology has shown that the intricately interwoven mental operations of perception, valuation, and generation of action affording believing are processed in extensive neural networks (cf. Seitz, this volume). This may provide new strategies for an empirical exploration of ethical guidance of human behavior (cf. Sugiura, this volume).

5.2 *Bab as Basic Unit of a Creditive Process*

In order to describe the aspects of the process of believing and build a model for it, we need to identify its basic units. A bab is such a unit. It refers to emotionally shaped propositions, or propositionally loaded and infected emotions that are indispensable to describing a process of believing.

5.3 *Bab-Blob-Configuration*

In all likelihood, a single bab does not by itself make a believing process. Doing so will require an ensemble of different babs. This ensemble might be called a bab-configuration. This configuration might be similar to what is better known as a mindset. The different babs in a bab-configuration can be thought of as interconnected. A bab-configuration is thus a structure that is modifiable but also somehow stabilized (Runehov and Angel 2013).

But let us not forget that most of the time, processes of believing occur below conscious awareness. Thus we need to include reference to the subliminal aspects of the process, and should better speak in terms of bab-blob-configurations instead of bab-configurations. We suggest that placebo (Meißner, this volume) and nocebo effects are clear examples of a subliminal, non-conscious believing process. Also, the non-conscious existence of an exaggerated hygienic "worriedness" might function as a blob in a bab-configuration. The babs and blobs in a bab-blob-configuration are interconnected. Those interconnections are relevant for different functions.

6 Credition: Poly-functionality of a Believing Process

The process of believing includes various mental operations that are heavily involved in the perception of events or objects in the external world and in the control of one's behavior (Sugiura et al. 2015). The bab-blob-configuration is relevant to the four different functions that constitute a believing process from its beginning to its endpoint. This configuration is not merely a "stable" or "ready" ensemble, but a mixture of relatively stable and more "fugitive" elements. Thus, a bab-blob-configuration can be thought of as a subset of a more general overarching mindset that is activated the moment a process of believing begins. The believing process, or credition, consists of a bundle of four conceptually successive and heavily interwoven mental functions.

6.1 *Enclosure Function*

In his influential Cognitive Dissonance Theory, Festinger (1957) included believing in the class of dissonance reduction processes. Accordingly, believing involves changing, adding, or eliminating a cognitive element in order to reduce dissonance with or between other cognitive elements. For example, the dissonance between two ideas (e.g., a belief that people are good in general, and knowledge that children may display aggressive behavior), is reduced by believing in the existence of malevolent ghosts who enter children and cause them to behave aggressively. The concept of dissonance reduction seems compatible with the explanation of human brain function in light of the free-energy principle as optimization-machinery for valuation and its counterpart, surprise (Friston 2010). Fundamental to this notion are probabilistic predictions of value or reward based on perceived information, of expected error, and of cost of future actions; these predictions can drive the system to the next state by the simple principle of reducing the free energy.

Believing is one expression of such a self-organizing process. This aspect of believing is intimate with its so-called *enclosure-function*. The enclosure-function is a cognitive process that constitutes or modifies propositions (bab-configurations) such as vague ideas, confirmed knowledge, values, or claims about what is moral. The bab-blob-configuration is involved when one questions whether a certain aspect can be believed; i.e., whether that aspect can be propositionally and emotionally integrated into an existing bab-blob-configuration. Thus the enclosure function is intricately interwoven with the process of perception. Any vague or doubtful (acoustical, optic, olfactory, sensual) percept of an external or internal event can be understood as a bab, which may be either included in or excluded from someone's bab-configuration. For example, if someone does not trust the quality of drinking water offered in a glass, the qualification "non-drinkable" might become a bab. The enclosure function determines whether this bab will be enclosed within the person's bab-configuration. If so, the person will be prompted to not drink the water; if not, the person is more likely to drink the water. If a non-conscious but exaggerated hygienic "worriedness" or concern exists, it might function as a blob in a bab-configuration. As a result, its influence on the enclosure process will lead to the exclusion of the bab "drinkable" in favor of the bab "non-drinkable" – and, as a result, the person will refuse to drink the water. This might happen according to Morewedge and Kahnemann's "System 1" which works as automatic operations of associative memory. Whether such a process can be understood as synonymous with self-organization while activating the enclosure function is a matter for future discussion.

6.2 Converter Function

The probabilistic assignment of attributes to an object or event constitutes a believing process. The converter function of credition is set in motion when bab-blob-configurations are activated, which is a complex transformation and which is preliminary to decision-making. A particular bab-blob-configuration does not force a certain decision or action, but rather, it prepares a space of action wherein the decision can take place. For example, when the bab "my cat is divine" is in someone's bab-configuration, if a fire breaks out the person will be prepared to rescue the cat from the fire. This preparation process is interdependent with several systems. One of them is the predictive system, which provides the individual with information about the feasibility of various responses and thereby modulates the preparation of actions (Delevoye-Turrell et al. 2010). The impulses coming from the bab-blob-configuration will not provoke single acts; rather, the converter function is preliminary to the concrete act of sketching out a space of action. The term "space of action" is introduced to mark a middle stage between motivation (I love my cat) and action (rescue the cat). Creditions support the preparation of actions via the converter function by reducing the number of choices and abbreviating the time it takes to make a decision. This transformation is complex; many issues discussed in Theory of Mind might be relevant to this concept.

6.3 Stabilizer Function

Whereas the enclosure process can produce bab-configurations, the stabilizer process has the ability to maintain them. The stabilizer function calms the bab-configurations, which are continuously modified by the subject's new experiences, and reduces the volatility of irritating impulses sent by the enclosure process to the converter function. The stabilizer function by repetition changes fluid bab-configurations into stable attitudes and mindsets. This stabilizing process follows the Hebbian principle, as associations are learned through repeated experiences of an action with its perceived consequences (Hebb 1949).

Therefore, the stabilization of bab-blob-configurations is a necessary precondition for consistent *"spaces of action"*. The stabilizer function brings creditions in touch with attitudes and mindsets. Many complex challenges of everyday life, such as decision making, planning, and building or rebuilding trust, are possible only on the basis of coherently shaped spaces of action. Most likely these functions are implemented on different stabilized neural circuits. In terms of the model of creditions, a "belief" (used as a noun) refers to a stabilized bab-configuration.

6.4 Modulator Function

This function of credition highlights how a creditive process can occur differently in specific ways, between individuals and between situations. Obviously, creditions are interrelated with an individual's bodily processes including his or her memory, gender, health, disability, and degree of psychic integrity, and are bound to the individual's level of cognitive and emotional development whether conscious or nonconscious. They may have a modulating effect at the cellular level, for example, in influencing of neural synchronizing processes. One the other hand, creditive processes might be modulated by bodily states such as stress, loss of trust, arches and pains, sadness, sexual arousal, or psychotic disorder (cf. Unterrainer, this volume). Examining the influence of emotions and appraisal on the modulation of creditions opens up a whole new set of intriguing questions. In addition, it may be profitable to explore whether or not the modulator function should be regarded more as a general principle that influences the other three functions (Fig. 2).

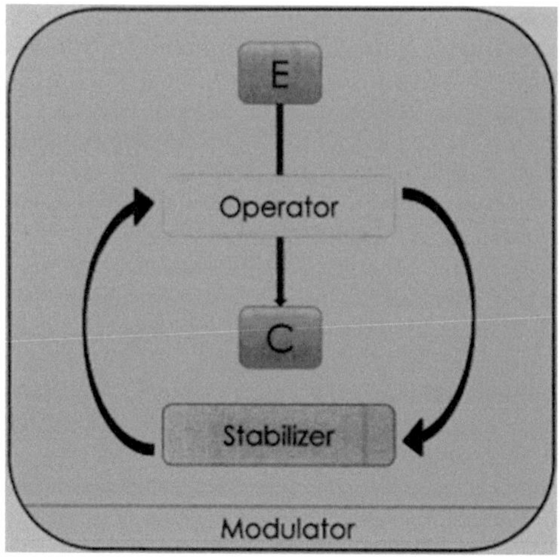

Fig. 2 The credition model describing the functions of the process of believing in relation to the "bab-blob configuration" (i.e. "semi-fluid mindset") which is stabilized by repeated operations (Stabilizer function): The Enclosure function (E) defines the representation of the stimulus and the Converter function (C) provides the appropriate action in response to the stimulus. Creditions are modulated (Modulator function) by the internal state of the individual (© HF Angel; conference presentation 2012, for the first time published in Angel and Seitz 2016)

6.5 Conclusion

The integrated model of credition introduces an interdisciplinary scientific field as a new perspective such that believing might be understood as an adaptive adjustment process that structures the interface of the inner representations and probabilistic estimates of the outside world according to a personal valuation matrix. The self-organization dynamics in the perception-action-value triad predicts the believing process as a personal cognitive-emotional function. Due to the equivalence of selecting belief and selecting action, what one believes ought to reflect a more congruent correspondence to personal valuation processes (Seitz et al. 2006, 2009).

Finally, the model of creditions can easily serve as a referential pattern or as a communication tool that may be useful when confronting questions about economics (cf. Sturn, this volume; Willfort and Weber, this volume), politics (cf. Marko, this volume), education (cf. Mitropoulou, this volume), and religious science and theology (cf. Oancea, this volume), or to reflect on religious fundamentalism (Hood et al. 2005).

References

Angel HF (2006) Religiosität als menschliches Potential. Ein anthropologisches Modell der Re-ligiosität im neurowissenschaftlichen Horizont. In: Angel HF et al (eds) Religiosität. Anthropologische, theologische und sozialwissenschaftliche Klärungen. Kohlhammer, Stuttgart, pp 62–89

Angel HF (2013a) Credition. In: Runehov ALC, Oviedo L (eds) Encyclopedia of sciences and religion, 1. Springer, Dordrecht, 536–539 (= Angel 2013a) http://www.springerreference.com/docs/html/chapterdbid/357430.html
Angel HF (2013b) Religiosity. In: Runehov ALC, Oviedo L (ed) Encyclopedia of sciences and religion, vol 4. Springer, Dordrecht, 2012–2014 (= Angel 2013b) http://www.springerreference.com/docs/html/chapterdbid/357427.html
Angel HF (2015) No believing without emotion. The overlapping of emotion and cognition in the model of credition. Studies in Science and Theology 15:215–222
Angel HF (2016) Process and creditions. How to understand the process of believing? In: Dziadkowiec J, Lamza L (eds) Recent Advances in the Creation of a Process-Based Worldview (European Studies in Process Thought 4). Cambridge Scholars Publishing, Newcastle upon Tyne, pp 194 – 205
Angel HF (2017) A process of merging interior and exterior reality: a short view on the structure of credition. In: Teixeira MT (ed) Mind in nature. European Studies in Process Thought. Cambridge Scholars Publishing. [in press]
Angel HF et al (eds) (2006) Religiosität. Anthropologische, theologische und sozialwissenschaftliche Klärungen. Kohlhammer, Stuttgart
Angel HF, Seitz RJ (2016) Processes of believing as fundamental brain function: the concept of credition. SFU Res Bull 1:1–20. doi:10.15135/16.4.1.1-20
Azari NP, Nickel J, Wunderlich G, Niedeggen M, Hefter H, Tellmann L, Herzog H, Stoerig P, Birnbacher D, Seitz RJ (2001) Neural correlates of religious experience. Eur J Neurosci 13:1649–1652
Barth K (1957) Kirchliche Dogmatik, ausgewählt und eingeleitet von Helmut Gollwitzer, Frank-furt/M
Bell V, Halligan PW (2013) The neural basis of abnormal personal belief. In: Kruger F, Grafman J (eds) The neural basis of human belief. Psychology Press, Hove, pp 191–223
Bergson H (1998) Creative evolution (orig. 1907/1911). Dover Pubns, Mineola
Bullivant S, Ruse M (eds) (2013) The Oxford Handbook of Atheism. Oxford University Press, Oxford
Churchland P (1979) Scientific realism and the plasticity of mind. Cambridge University Press, Cambridge
Connors MH, Halligan PW (2015) A cognitive account of belief: a tentative roadmap. Front Psychol 5:1588. doi:10.3389/fpsyg.2014.01588
Conway MA (2005) Memory and the self. J Mem Lang 53:594–628. doi:10.1016/j.jml.2005.08.005
D'Aquili E, Newberg A (1999) The mystical mind: probing the biology of religious experience. Fortress Press, Minneapolis
D'Aquili E et al (2001) Why God won't go away. Ballantine Books, New York
Damasio AR (1998) Emotion in the perspective of an integrated nervous system. Brain Res Rev 26:83–86
Deleuze G (1994) Difference and repetition (orig. 1968). Columbia University Press, New York
Delevoye-Turrell Y, Bartolo A, Coello Y (2010) Motor representation and the perception of space: perceptual judgements of the boundary of action space. In: Gangopadhyay N, Madary M, Spicer F (eds) Perception, action, and consciousness. Oxford University Press, Oxford, pp 217–242
Festinger LA (1957) Theory of cognitive dissonance. Stanford University Press, Stanford
Fodor JA (1975) The language of thought. MIT Press, Cambridge, MA
Friston K (2010) The free-energy principle: a unified brain theory? Nat Rev Neurosci 11(2):127–138. doi:10.1038/Nrn2787
Graham DW (2013) Science before Socrates: Parmenides, Anaxagoras, and the new astronomy. Oxford University Press, Oxford
Gray JR, Braver TS, Raichle ME (2002) Integration of emotion and cognition in the lateral prefrontal cortex. Proc Natl Acad Sci U S A 99(6):4115–4120. doi:10.1073/pnas.062381899
Han S, Mao L, Gu X, Zhu Y, Ge J, Ma Y (2008) Neural consequences of religious belief on self-referential processing. Soc Neurosci 3:1–15

Hebb DO (1949) The organization of behavior. Wiley, New York
Heitsch E (1995) Parmenides. Die Fragmente. Griechisch-deutsch. Artemis, Zürich
Helm P (1999) Faith and reason. Oxford University Press, Oxford
Hemel U (1988) Ziele religiöser Erziehung. Lang Verlag, Frankfurt/M
Hills P, Francis LJ, Argyle M, Jackson CJ (2004) Primary personality trait correlates of religious practice and orientation. Personal Individ Differ 36:61–73
Hood RW, Hill PC, Williamson WP (2005) The psychology of religious fundamentalism. Guilford, New York
Ji S (2012) Molecular theory of the living cell. Springer, New York
Joseph R (ed) (2002) NeuroTheology: brain, science, spirituality, religious experience. University Press California, San Jose
Kahn CH (ed) (1981) The art and thought of Heraclitus. An edition of the fragments with translation and commentary. Cambridge University Press, Cambridge
Kenny A (1992) What is faith? Essays in the philosophy of religion. Oxford University Press, Oxford
Krüger F, Barbey AK, Grafman J (2009) The medial prefrontal cortex mediates social event knowledge. Trends Cogn Sci 13:103–109
Krüger F, Grafman J (2013) I believe to my soul. In: Kruger F, Grafman J (eds) The neural basis of human belief. Psychology Press, New York, pp 225–236
La Cour P, Peterson M (2015) Effects of mindfulness meditation on chronic pain. Pain Med 16:641–652
Langdon R, Coltheart M (2000) The cognitive neuropsychology of delusions. Mind Lang 15(1):184–218. doi:10.1111/1468-0017.00129
Langdon R, Connaughton E (2013) The neuropsychology of belief formation. In: Krüger F, Grafman J (eds) The neural basis of human belief systems. Psychology Press, Hove, pp 19–42
Lazarus RS (1982) Thoughts on the relation between emotion and cognition. Am Psychol 37:1019–1024
Marston WM (1928) Emotions of normal people. Kegan Paul Trench Trubner and Co. Ltd., London
Mitchell B (1994) Faith and criticism. The Sarum lectures. Oxford University Press, Oxford
Morewedge CK, Kahneman D (2010) Associative processes in intuitive judgment. Trends Cogn Sci 14(10):435–440. doi:10.1016/j.tics.2010.07.004
Paloutzian RF (2016) Invitation to the psychology of religion, 3rd edn. Guilford Press, New York
Paloutzian RF, Park CL (2013a) Directions for the future of psychology of religion and spirituaity: research advances in methodology and meaning systems. In: Paloutzian RF, Park CL (eds) Handbook of the psychology religion and spirituality. Guilford Press, New York, pp 651–665
Paloutzian RF, Park CL (2013b) Recent progress and core issues in the science of the psychology of religion and spirituality. In: Paloutzian RF, Park CL (eds) Handbook of the psychology religion and spirituality. Guilford Press, New York, pp 3–22
Park CL (2013) Religion and meaning. In: Paloutzian RF, Park CL (eds) Handbook of the psychology religion and spirituality. Guildford Press, New York, pp 357–379
Persinger MA (1987) Neuropsychological bases of God beliefs. Praeger, New York
Plantinga A, Wolterstorff N (1983) Faith & rationality. Reason & belief in God. University of Notre Dame Press, Notre Dame
Potthoff D, Seitz RJ (2015) Role of the first and second person perspective for control of behavior: understanding other people's facial expressions. J Physiol Paris. doi:10.1016/j.jphysparis.2015.12.003. Epub ahead of print
Pulvermüller F, Lutzenberger W, Preissl H (1999) Nouns and verbs in the intact brain. Evidence from event-related potentials and high-frequency cortical responses. Cereb Cortex 9(5):497–506. doi:10.1093/cercor/9.5.497
Rahner K (2004) Grundkurs des Glaubens. Herder, Freiburg/Basel/Wien
Rolls ET (2006) Brain mechanisms underlying flavour and appetite. Philos Trans R Soc Lond Ser B Biol Sci 361(1471):1123–1136. doi:10.1098/rstb.2006.1852
Runehov ALC (2007) Sacred or neural? The potential of neuroscience to explain religious experience. Vandenhoeck & Ruprecht, Göttingen
Runehov ALC, Angel HF (2013) The process of believing: revisiting the problem of justifying beliefs. Studies in Science and Theology 14:205–218

Saver JL, Rabin J (1999) The neural substrates of religious experience. In: Salloway S et al (eds) The neuropsychiatry of limbic and subcortical disorders, Washington, DC/London, pp 195–207
Schachter S (1964) The interaction of cognitive and physiological determinants of emotional states. In: Berkowitz L (ed) Advances in experimental social psychology. Academic, New York
Schaefer A, Gray JR (2007) A role for the human amygdala in higher cognition. Rev Neurosci 18(5):355–363. doi:10.1515/REVNEURO.2007.18.5.355
Schmidt S, Walach H (eds) (2014) Meditation – neuroscientific approaches and philosophical implications. Springer, Cham
Schnell T (2012) Spirituality with and without religion. Arch Psychol Relig 34:33–62
Schnell T, Keenan WJF (2011) Meaning-making in an atheist world. Arch Psychol Relig 33(1):55–78. (download PDF: www.sinnforschung.org)
Schwarz N (2001) Feelings as information. Implication for affective influences on information processing. In: Martin LL, Clore GL (eds) Theories of mood and cognition. A user's guidebook. Psychology Press, London, pp 159–176
Schwarz N (2011) Feeling-as-information theory. In: Van Lange P, Kruglanski A, Higgins ET (eds) Handbook of theories of social psychology, Sage Publishing, Los Angeles
Seckler M (1988) Theologie als Glaubenswissenschaft. In: Kern W et al (eds) Handbuch der Fundamentaltheologie, vol 4. pp 180–241
Seitz RJ, Angel HF (2012) Processes of believing – a review and conceptual account. Rev Neurosci 23(3):303–309. doi:10.1515/revneuro-2012-0034
Seitz RJ, Angel HF (2014) Psychology of religion and spirituality: meaning-making and processes of believing. Relig Brain Behav 5:139–147
Seitz RJ, Nickel J, Azari NP (2006) Functional modularity of the medial prefrontal cortex: in-volvement in human empathy. Neuropsychology 20(6):743–751. doi:10.1037/0894-4105.20.6.743
Seitz RJ, Franz M, Azari NP (2009) Value judgments and self-control of action: the role of the medial frontal cortex. Brain Res Rev 60(2):368–378. doi:10.1016/j.brainresrev.2009.02.003
Seitz RJ, Paloutzian RF, Angel HF (2016) Processes of believing: where do they come from? What are they good for? F1000Research 2017, 5:2573 (doi: 10.12688/f1000research.9773.2) .
Sharot T, Kanai R, Marston D, Korn CW, Rees G, Dolan RJ (2012) Selectively altering belief formation in the human brain. PNAS 109(42):17058–17062. doi:10.1073/pnas.1205828109
Smith WC (1987) Faith and belief. Princeton University Press, New York
Smith ML (2011) Rapid processing of emotional expressions without consciousness awareness. Cereb Cortex 22:1748–1760
Stich S (1996) From folk psychology to cognitive science: the case against belief. MIT Press, Cambridge
Sugiura M (2011) The multi-layered model of self: a social neuroscience perspective. In: Kawashima R, Sugiura M, Tsukiura T (eds) New frontiers in social cognitive neuroscience. Tohoku University Press, Sendai, pp 111–135
Sugiura M (2013) Associative account of self-cognition: extended forward model and multi-layer structure. Front Hum Neurosci 7:535. doi:10.3389/Fnhum.2013.00535
Sugiura M, Seitz RJ, Angel HF (2015) Models and neural bases of the believing process. J Behav Brain Sci 5:12
Teske J (2007/2008) Bindings of the will. The neuropsychology of subdoxastic faith. Stud Sci Theol 11:27–43
Thiel U (2014) The early modern subject: Self-consciousness and personal identity from Descartes to Hume, 2nd edn. Oxford University Press, Oxford
Topolinski S, Erle TM, Reber R (2015) Necker's smile: immediate affective consequences of early perceptual processes. Cognition 140:1–13. doi:10.1016/j.cognition.2015.03.004
Whitehead AN (1978) Process and reality. Free Press, New York
Yarkoni T, Gray JR, Schaefer A (2006) Individual differences in amygdala activity predict response speed during working memory. J Neurosci 26(40):10120–10128
Zajonc RB (1984) On the primacy of affect. Am Psychol 39:117–124

Part II
Psychology and Neuroscience

Believing, Remembering, and Imagining: The Roots and Fruits of Meanings Made and Remade

Raymond F. Paloutzian and Katelyn J. Mukai

Abstract Without believing, there is no human life as we know it. Processes of believing are fundamental to how all people function. Although more often nonconscious than conscious, believing is the guide that leads humans and animals through the myriad options to settle upon or test the next action, reaction, possibility, or hunch. What we call a "belief" is a meaning that has been made. This chapter begins by explaining the substrates of meaning systems and relates them to all matters of believing whether religious or spiritual, unusual versus routine, or narrow versus broad in scope. Processes of believing enable us to navigate all life domains. In order to explain the development of the substrates of meaning systems, the chapter summarizes evolutionarily rooted aspects of human and animal functioning for which the emergence of some form of meaning making, assessment, and remaking is essential. The sequence goes from micro to macro in level of analysis. Each step reflects meaning system processes more developed than those prior to it. The propensity for meaning making, appraisal, and remaking is increased as one goes up the steps, from relatively rudimentary to complex global human meaning systems. The steps include perceiving, learning, intuiting, implementing, remembering, and imagining. The process of believing is multi-layered, consisting of making and remaking meanings, acting upon them mentally or behaviorally, and appraising the outcomes in view of the expectations and predictions. The process continues, as one remakes meanings, whether similar or modified, re-appraises them, and remakes them again through a continuous feedback cycle. The processes are integral to basic psychological functions including learning, perception, motivation, development, social cognition, human interaction, and human information processing, and show myriad effects across the spectrum from normal to abnormal mental states and behavior.

A friend who is deeply committed to less killing and more peace in the world asked me (RFP) an important and blunt question: "How do you change a person?" What followed was a long communication about social psychological research on attitude

R.F. Paloutzian (✉) • K.J. Mukai
Department of Psychology, Westmont College, Santa Barbara, CA, USA
e-mail: paloutz@westmont.edu; kmukai@westmont.edu

H.-F. Angel et al. (eds.), *Processes of Believing: The Acquisition, Maintenance, and Change in Creditions*, New Approaches to the Scientific Study of Religion 1,
DOI 10.1007/978-3-319-50924-2_3

change, persuasion, and behavior change.[1] Then came an elaborated discourse on a penultimate example of human change – psychological research on religious conversion and spiritual transformation (Paloutzian 2005; Paloutzian et al. 2013). Then he asked, "OK, but how do you change a person?" Academic psychological information was not providing the answer. It was necessary to dig deeper into what processes, at micro and macro levels, are most foundational to the regulation of human behavior. What emerged from this digging was that processes of believing were crucial, fundamental not only to human behavior but to all of life. In what ways are such processes integral to what has to happen to change a person from being a believer in one thing to re-believing, and doing, something else?

1 Strange Ways in Which Humans Work

Let us begin by observing some strange things about how humans and other animals work. Here are four simple examples:

1. The eye: We ordinarily think that when two people look at the same thing, they see the same thing. As an example with some precision, it makes common sense that if you stand at spot X and look at painting P, and one moment later your friend, who is exactly the same height as you so that his or her eyes are at exactly the same height and distance from the ground and the painting, and whose head is exactly oriented towards the painting in the same direction as yours was, so the same painting is literally what you see. This is false. We will explain later (see the section on perceptual capabilities, below). For now keep in mind that your eyes do not see the same thing as your friend's eyes (Goldstein 2010a, b), although you proceed as if your minds contain the same percept.
2. An atheist: Atheists were asked to dare God to do terrible things (Lindeman et al. 2014). After they did so, they felt anxious compared to controls. This sounds odd because by raw Aristotelian logic, if one does not believe that there is a god, then there is no rational reason to feel anything when making such a request because there is no belief that there exists a being capable of doing anything. The person "believes" the request does nothing. Why, then, does the person feel anxiety?
3. Placebos: Someone who takes a placebo while believing it is a drug may show effects similar to those produced by the real drug, especially when the effect is a changed mental state (Nash and Barnier 2008). A reliable example of this is the report of pain relief after taking a placebo while believing it was a pain relieving drug. This phenomenon may or may not seem strange nowadays, given that knowledge of it has become somewhat common. More strange, however, is that a placebo may produce a placebo effect when someone takes it knowing it is a placebo (Kaptchuk et al. 2010). That is, a person takes an inert pill with knowl-

[1] Space constraints preclude elaborating on this point, but ample documentation is evident upon examination of graduate or undergraduate texts in social psychology.

edge that it is not a drug – it is "nothing" – but feels pain relief anyway. How can believing and knowing that you are doing "nothing" cause effects?

4. A person experiences an unusual mental event during a so-called "near death experience" (NDE). NDEs often include white light, a sense of oneness with everything, feelings of connectedness with dead loved ones, and a vision of a long tunnel through which one is moving with bright light at the end, all culminating in feelings of peacefulness (Cardeña et al. 2014; Greyson 2014). Later, the person "believes" not only that there is life after death, but also that there are no such things as coincidences; the person "knows" it. For example, when seeing a cloud in the sky shaped like a straight line with a small round cloud at the end of it (so that the cloud configuration looks like an explanation point), the person "knows" this pattern is not a "mere" coincidence; it is her dead son communicating with her that he is alive and well in the afterlife – she is sure of it (Barlev et al. 2015; Kinsella and Barlev 2014).

2 We Are Left with Questions

What are the psychological roots of believing – anything? What happens at various levels of analysis to feed processes that constitute believing, which recently is called "creditions"[2]? Why is the capability of believing adaptive? The above four cases are examples of some of the fruits of believing. But what inputs made processes of believing develop at all? What functions do such processes involve, and serve? And to what range of phenomena do such processes apply?

The above four illustrations may sound unusual; they are all true. They are the smallest tip of a gigantic iceberg of the processes of believing – how humans, organs and organ systems, other animals, and groups make meaning out of ambiguity, appraise it, respond to those appraisals, and remake it again in a lifelong feedback cycle (Park and Folkman 1997; Park 2010). They are part of the evolutionarily selected processes that enable survival. Each of the above examples may not necessarily make logical sense, but they make psychological sense when we observe that each one involves someone being confronted with ambiguous information which, through one mechanism of another, had to be dealt with. Some meaning, some kind of psychological "whole" had to be made out of bits and pieces of data. In each case, the person, organ, or relevant system within the person responded not to the stimuli but to their meaning after being integrated and appraised in the person's cognitive system (Park 2010). Each of those meanings can be understood as "beliefs", and the whole set of processes by which meanings are made out of ambiguity can be understood as processes of believing (Paloutzian 2017; Seitz and Angel 2012, 2014).

In order to unpack the ideas summarized above, let us examine the roots of the processes of believing. These are found in making, appraising, responding to, and

[2]The term "creditions" is coined by Angel (see Chap. 2) as analogous to emotions: Creditions are to the processes of believing as emotions are to the processes of feeling.

remaking meanings. Such processes occur in systems that that range from micro to macro levels of analysis. Along the way, we will examine some ordinary and unusual fruits of the processes of believing. To what degree is human and animal behavior mediated by such processes?

3 Evolutionary Development of Meaning Making Is Foundational to Believing

In order to conceptualize how meaning systems operate and to understand the evolutionary process through which they came about, let us examine a sequence of steps in the development of the psychological substrates of meaning making, appraising, and remaking. At each step, an essential aspect is the capability of some information processing system, whether highly developed cognitively or not, to make a whole appropriate to its level of analysis out of ambiguous bits and pieces of information. The illustrations that follow start from a relatively micro level and in graded fashion move to a more macro level of analysis. The meaning system properties become more developed with each step. The more developed the step, the closer the psychological capabilities get to those that enable the abstract forms of believing manifest in human beings, as occurs in religions, spiritualities, and other complex creeds and codes (Park 2005, 2013).

3.1 Perceptual Capabilities

Consider visual perception. The meaning of a visual stimulus is not automatically deposited in an unchanged form onto the surface of the retina or in the occipital lobe of the brain. Instead, at least two processes operate, both constantly changing, that transmit information to the rest of the perceptual system to crate meaningful percepts. First, a narrow band of wavelengths of the electromagnetic spectrum (light) bounce off an object (e.g., a red apple) and enter the eye through the pupil. Then, these light rays hit the retinal rods and cones, whose network of cells partially processes this incoming stimulation and converts it to neural impulses compatible with the circuitry of the brain's visual pathway. Second, the eye saccades (Wolfe et al. 2009). This means that when the eye is looking at an object, the eye is not stationary, as if to "see" (or photograph) the entire object at once. Instead, the eye makes small movements approximately every one-half seconds. We can make saccades deliberately, but whether or not we do, they will happen automatically up to four times per second every minute of every hour that we are awake. At each movement, it detects the stimulation from one spot of the whole object – as illustrated in scenario 1 near the beginning of this chapter. Thus the eye never "sees" the whole, but is instead constantly picking up bits and pieces of data and sending them for further processing through the visual system (Goldstein 2010a b). This means that a percept is formed from a large amount of ambiguous information.

Thus, our perceptual system has made a meaningful percept from a bombardment of various wavelengths of light detected in small bits via the saccades of the eye. The result enables us to assume (hopefully correctly) that the object is a red apple that we can eat, throw, or balance on top of our head as a target for someone with a bow and arrow. At its most basic level, a percept of a whole is a meaning made out of smaller elements. These initial, rudimentary percepts are foundational to further interpretation of perceptual information. At the most encompassing levels, along with the increased complexity of global meaning systems comes abstract elements, such as goals, attitudes, identity, and one's worldview (Paloutzian and Park 2005, 2013, 2014; Park 2010). And the construction of symbols as meaningful abstract percepts is inherent to the realms of ideologies and worldviews of all kinds.

As summarized above, the meaning making properties of the visual system sound unidirectional, and therefore relatively simple. The causal direction is bottom-up; information comes in from the outside and is interpreted on the inside. But there is another layer of complexity that makes for top-down processing. The brain/mind not only interprets information sent to it; it also contains schemata, or pre-set or pre-learned patters or forms, which shape the percepts that are made (Goldstein 2010a, b). Thus, meaning systems both make sense out of information sent to them, and make the sensed information take one shape or another.

Percepts are actually the product of the interaction between the information entering the system from the outside and the inside schemata that the person's cognitive system brings to the interpretive task. If information entering the system is congruent with existing schemata, the system is stable and there is little need for it to change. However, if the information entering the system is in conflict with existing schemata, then the system may react – by rejecting the information, accommodating to it, or, in the most extreme case, converting to it. The latter case would be an instance of someone becoming a believer in something that he or she formerly rejected – an instance of a radical religious conversion, spiritual transformation, or becoming a follower of a previously forbidden political movement (Paloutzian et al. 2013).

The rudimentary processes summarized above seem minimally complex. However, as we go one step up the ladder of complexity, we will begin to see how a process that seems only slightly more nuanced actually requires more developed meaning-making and appraisal abilities. Learning is a small psychological step from perceiving; both of them involved meaning making as foundational to believing – in what is perceived, and in what has been learned (Paloutzian 2017).[3]

3.2 *Learning*

Meaning-making and appraisal, and therefore processes of believing, are integral to animal and human learning. To begin with a simple form of animal learning in a laboratory, consider a rat in a T-maze first being food deprived, and then being put

[3] Perceiving and learning both involve the enclosure function of creditions (see Chap. 2).

in the start box of the maze for the first trial of the experiment. The rat (presumably) does not know why it is being placed there, what a start box and the straight runway of a T-maze are, nor that food reinforcement has been placed in a goal box at the end of one arm of the T. The rat faces completely unknown stimuli. What capabilities are necessary for the rat to learn to make the correct turn at the choice point and receive food reinforcement?

The animal must have the capability to "connect the dots." In this example, this means that after multiple attempts and vis-à-vis the process of trial and error, the rat has perceived and followed the pattern in the stimulus complex that culminates in the food reward. Doing so requires the rat's cognitive system to engage in pattern construction over a sequence of trials (and therefore have a rudimentary mechanism for time perception), gradually retaining the elements of the correct pattern and eliminating those in incorrect patterns. Thus the rat gradually makes the "correct" meaning from the series of exposures to the twists, turns, and unknowns of the maze, and learns to make the "correct" turn at the choice point. We presume, but do not know, that a rat does this non-consciously; we make no speculation about whether rats have any cognitive function akin to human consciousness. However, in human terms we would say that making the correct turn assumes the rat's believing that doing so leads to food.

Operant conditioning, or learning by reinforcement, is another instance of meaning-making (Paloutzian and Park 2013). Because operant conditioning requires not only perceptual capability, but also sensory-motor, neuro-muscular, and appraisal-of-success skills above and beyond rudimentary sense perception, the meaning system processes in this illustration can be understood as more developed than those involved in vision alone. Of course, reward-based learning is not limited to animals only, because it is also a major form of learning in humans. All reward-based systems of behavior management or control assume that fundamental meaning making processes are operative, and that therefore those who are subject to those systems believe that if they perform certain behaviors, then certain rewards will follow. When we extrapolate the principles of learning to include more complex human cognitive learning, it becomes difficult to envision the transmission of value systems such as those at the root of religions and spiritualities from one generation to the next without the new generation constructing their own new meanings with, and therefore believing, the attitudes, teachings, and values at issue.[4]

3.3 *Intuiting*

Next, imagine a rabbit sitting in a forest clearing, in a situation in which evolutionary processes are salient. Suddenly, the leaves at the edge of the clearing rustle. The rabbit's head immediately looks up toward the direction of the noise and sees the

[4] In terms of creditions, we would say that the stabilizer function enabled the rat to settle into the state of having learned the correct response and enabled humans to hold the same attitudes and values in a consistent, continuous way over time.

leaves moving. What caused this disturbance? The wind? A hungry wolf? A human hunter? The rabbit does not have a clear answer to these questions; it is faced with an ambiguous pattern of stimuli that gives it no definitive signal about how to respond. Worse, an incorrect inference about what the stimulus pattern may mean could prompt the animal to perform the "wrong" behavior (i.e., stay in the clearing), a choice that could mean life or death, and thereby reproducing or not.

What "should" the rabbit do? Because of their environment, size, and place in the food chain, evolutionary processes have selected for rabbits the advantageous behaviors of running and hiding when faced with an uncertain, potentially lethal stimulus pattern. Of course, the response of running and hiding will be technically unnecessary in many instances because the rustling leaves may have been caused by wind. However, it is evolutionarily unfair to say that fleeing behavior on the part of the rabbit is erroneous; if the rustling leaves signal a wolf, the rabbit will certainly die. A rabbit gets to make the "error" of not running away only once (Kirkpatrick 205). In language used primarily for humans, we could say that evolution has selected for animals to believe in potential danger when confronted with certain configurations of ambiguous stimuli.

Due to the natural selection processes illustrated in the rabbit scenario, many organisms evolved to perform safety-enhancing responses to possible danger. In the case of the rabbit, what meaning system capabilities would have to have evolved in order for it to attribute dangerous meaning to particular stimulus patterns, and thereby perform the safest response? Again, using language normally applied to humans, the rabbit has developed the ability to be alert to potential alternative outcomes from a specific set of uncertain circumstances, and to intuit (i.e., engage in the process of believing) that one of those outcomes poses a threat. In addition, as evidenced by the typical "freeze" response displayed by many rodents upon encountering a startle stimulus, the rabbit may be experiencing what humans would call fear or anxiety, suggestive of the preparation of its system for a flight or fight response. In this particular example, the rabbit has developed a way to "imagine" that there could be a wolf or a lion with a lethal bite or a human with a deadly arrow, and that safety could be gained by "getting out of here." That is to say, the rabbit has to have developed what we label in humans as the ability to "intuit" or make the best guess about what might be lurking behind the bush, engage that intuition by believing it, and then choose the appropriate behavior in order to respond to what it believes.

The rabbit has evolved such that it will sometimes make meanings that are technically incorrect for that specific instance (e.g., the rabbit intuits danger when the leaves rustle, but on that occasion there is no danger because it is only the wind rustling the leaves). At such occasions the animal runs to safety even though it is not required, because by doing so in the long run it is more likely to live and reproduce.

Certain evolved meaning system intuitions produce responses that facilitate survival on the part of an individual, and hopefully to a larger extent, a species. There are many developmental steps on the ladder spanning the gap between rabbits and humans, but fundamental meaning-making processes are developing because evolutionary processes are selecting for them. And if, like the rabbit, humans have developed ways to intuit possible danger, unseen as well as seen, then it is not surprising that they can intuit other unseen presences such as gods, spirits, or other entities, which like danger are unseen and may or may not be there, but can nevertheless prompt profound human responses.[5]

3.4 Implementing

It is well established that nonhuman primates can create and use tools. A psychological substrate for such capabilities includes some sort of complex meaning system whose mechanisms engage the animal in believing that doing a particular thing now is good for something else in the future. Meaning system processes enable believing something yet to be, thus involve basic elements of intuiting over time.

An illustration can be seen in the way an animal implements a stick to draw ants out of a log, or uses a rock to crack open shells to reveal the meat inside. An animal so capable has to have some psychological mechanism that enables it to plan ahead, if only by a small amount of time, in order to successfully and intentionally make tools for future purposes. Thus, instead of waiting around in the hopes of finding the carcass of a dead animal for immediate consumption, the nonhuman primate might use objects found in its environment to prepare or conserve freshly found or freshly killed food for subsequent meals.

This type of behavior suggests a rudimentary ability to think outside of the box of time, to "see ahead" into the probable future, plan accordingly, and then remember which behaviors to exhibit at the right time and in the right context. Mental abilities such as these, which reflect a modulator function, contribute to the development of layers of meaning making capabilities, so that those that are phylogenetically older remain in place and function as they always have, while new meaning system processes evolve that meet the needs of more advanced and complex species. With this in mind, one starts to consider that these kinds of processes underlie the human ability to imagine and remember—abilities central to functioning of religions and spiritualities at the individual and group levels.

3.5 Remembering

The process of remembering is, of course, a matter of time. In meaning system terms, it is reconstructing a previously believed body of information (whether it be a picture in mental space, sounds, words, or other sensory-perceptual episodes) and re-believing it – or more specifically, believing the reconstructed version of it.

In the example noted above, a nonhuman primate's ability to use tools for preparation of future food assumes the existence of an appropriately complex memory system. Although greatly more developed, it is this kind of complex memory system

[5] Such responses, in creditions terms, are enabled by the converter function.

that is present in humans. Therefore, even the phenomena of human memory and all of our believing and behaving based upon this memory system depends on, and is actually rooted in, meaning-making processes. Research on memory retrieval tells us that a memory is not "pulled out" from its location in the mind in the same form in which it was stored, but rather is "reconstructed" (a meaning-making process), and its content can be changed by that process; the original meaning that was made and called a memory can be reconsolidated, or reconfigured, and stored in a new form (Cabeza and Nyberg 2000; Daniels 1986; Debiec et al. 2002). Therefore, as the capacity for memory expands, its involvement with aspects of the meaning system become more complicated, thereby fostering further development of the ability for believing, remembering, and re-believing.

3.6 Imagining

The ability to imagine was prerequisite for and concurrent with making the human mind capable of believing systems of thought, teaching, and speculation – the forerunners of complicated belief systems. Other human achievements can also be approximately linked to the same time period – the beginning of human language, communal living in complex (and somewhat hierarchical) social groups, and the establishment of what have been termed global meaning systems. At a minimum, the global meaning systems would have to be comprised of elements such as worldviews, personal and group values, specific goals and broader purposes, future planning, and the tendency to infer what is on other's minds by putting oneself "in the shoes" of others (what is referred to as *theory of mind* by psychologists; Park 2010, 2013). People thus developed the ability to not only remember (and by doing so, reconstruct) the past, but to imagine things that had not yet happened and to conceptualize the steps to take to pursue step-by-step goals in order to make what they imagine into a reality.

Believing in the existence of invisible deities with minds, otherworldly superhuman beings with feelings and preferences for what humans do and to what they give their allegiance, and the ability to make and interact in "make believe" worlds (as when children play a "let's pretend" game of "Doctor and Nurse"; Taves 2013) are all rooted in the fundamental processes of imagining and believing. This includes the temporary believing required for such behaviors and children's "pretend" games, and for adult analogues to them as exemplified in theatre and cinema. The reason an adult can have an intense emotional reaction to a movie or play, even though the person knows it is "only a movie or a play," is that the person is capable of believing the imagination. The same processes are at work when someone imagines a religious teaching (e.g., imagine Jesus doing X, or the Buddha doing Y) and responds in a genuinely believing way. The processes at work in the above examples are the same ones that are foundational to making meaning out of ambiguity and believing anything – whether lofty and ethically laden such as most religions or as specific and mundane as believing that if you sit down in a chair, it will hold you. Whatever else the lofty or the mundane do for humans, they feed the development and sustain the role of meaning systems and their intimate role in the processes of believing.

4 Conclusion

Humans do indeed behave in strange ways. In our daily routines, each of us feels as if we exist as one unit, but we don't. Our minds typically think it is a primarily rational organ, but it is far more constructive and assumptive. We talk as if there is a meaning inherent in a stimulus or a circumstance, when we more often attribute that meaning than detect it. We say something is sacred when it in fact the property of sacrality is something that, psychologically, we impute rather than it being given to us. The meanings upon which our lives hang and to which we commit our mundane and lifelong affairs are our constructions. Our ability to make and believe them are rooted in our evolutionary past, for given the stuff out of which we are made there would have been no survival without it.

These and other puzzling aspects of human behavior are as they are because we are creatures that are surrounded by unclear, ambiguous stuff. Our living depends upon continuing to receive and make meaning out of that information, appraise it in view of the global meaning system that we have developed, and respond to that appraisal. And this process is continuous at the levels of organs, organ systems, individuals, and groups. Believing means that a meaning has been constructed out of incoming information.

References

Barlev M, Kinsella M, Taves A, Paloutzian RF, German T (2015) Meaning making in a New Age spirituality group: pattern detection predicts anomalous experiences and paranormal interpretations. Paper presented at the meeting of the Society of Personality and Social Psychology, Psychology of Religion Preconverence, Long Beach, CA

Cabeza R, Nyberg L (2000) Imaging cognition II: an empirical review of 275 PET and fMRI studies. J Cogn Neurosci 12:1–47

Cardeña E, Lynn SJ, Krippner S (eds) (2014) Introduction: anomalous experiences in perspective. Varieties of anomalous experience: examining the scientific evidence, 2nd edn. American Psychological Association, Washington, DC, pp 3–20

Daniels PJ (1986) Cognitive models in information retrieval—an evaluative review. J Doc 42:272–304

Debiec J, LeDoux JE, Nader K (2002) Cellular and systems reconsolidation in the hippocampus. Neuron 36:527–538

Goldstein EB (2010a) Sensation and perception, 8th edn. Wadsworth/Cengage, Belmont

Goldstein EB (ed) (2010b) Sage encyclopedia of perception. Sage Publishers, Thousand Oaks

Greyson B (2014) Congruence between near-death and mystical experiences. Int J Psychol Relig 24(4):298–310

Kaptchuk TJ, Friedlander E, Kelley JM, Sanchez MN, Kokkotou E et al (2010) Placebos without deception: a randomized controlled trial in irritable bowel syndrome. PLoS One 5(12):e15591. doi:10.1371/journal.pone.0015591

Kinsella M, Barlev M (2014) Meaning making in the afterlife movement. Paper presented at the Society for the Scientific Study of Religion Annual Meeting, Indianapolis, 3 October–1 November 2014
Kirkpatrick LA (2005) Attachment, evolution, and the psychology of religion. Guilford Press, New York
Lindeman M, Heywood B, Riekki T, Makkonen T (2014) Atheists become emotionally aroused when daring God to do terrible things. Int J Psychol Relig 24(2):124–132
Nash MR, Barnier AJ (2008) Oxford handbook of hypnosis. Oxford, Oxford
Paloutzian RF (2017) Invitation to the psychology of religion, 3rd edn. Guilford Press, New York
Paloutzian RF (2005) Religious conversion and spiritual transformation: a meaning-system analysis. In: Paloutzian RF, Park CL (eds) Handbook of the psychology of religion and spirituality. Guilford, New York, pp 331–347
Paloutzian RF, Park CL (2005) Integrative themes in the current science of the psychology of religion. In: Paloutzian RF, Park CL (eds) Handbook of the psychology of religion and spirituality. Guilford Press, New York, pp 3–20
Paloutzian RF, Park CL (2013) Recent progress and core issues in the science of the psychology of religion and spirituality. In: Paloutzian RF, Park CL (eds) Handbook of the psychology of religion and spirituality. Guilford Press, New York, pp 3–22
Paloutzian RF, Park CL (2014) Religiousness and spirituality: the psychology of multilevel meaning making behavior. Relig Brain Behav 4:49–61
Paloutzian RF, Murken S, Streib H, Rößler-Namini S (2013) Conversion, deconversion, and spiritual transformation: a multilevel interdisciplinary view. In: Paloutzian RF, Park CL (eds) Handbook of the psychology of religion and spirituality, 2nd edn. Guilford Press, New York, pp 399–421
Park CL (2005) Religion and meaning. In: Paloutzian RF, Park CL (eds) Handbook of the psychology of religion and spirituality. Guilford Press, New York, pp 295–314
Park CL (2010) Making sense of the meaning literature: an integrative review of meaning making and its effects on adjustment to stressful life events. Psychol Bull 136:257–301
Park CL (2013) Religion and meaning. In: Paloutzian RF, Park CL (eds) Handbook of the psychology of religion and spirituality, 2nd edn. Guilford Press, New York, pp 357–379
Park CL, Folkman S (1997) Meaning in the context of stress and coping. Rev Gen Psychol 1:115–144
Seitz RJ, Angel HF (2012) Processes of believing – a review and conceptual account. Rev Neurosci 23:303–309
Seitz RJ, Angel HF (2014) Psychology of religion and spirituality: meaning-making and processes of believing. Relig Brain Behav 5(2):118–178
Taves A (2013) Building blocks of sacralities: a new basis for comparison across cultures and religions. In: Paloutzian RF, Park CL (eds) Handbook of the psychology of religion and spirituality, 2nd edn. Guilford Press, New York, pp 138–161
Wolfe JM, Kluender KR, Levi DM (2009) Sensation and perception, 2nd edn. Sinauer, Sunderland

Connection Between Scripts Embedding Motor Schemes and Decision Making

Gennaro Auletta

Abstract Codes are crucial for biological systems because they allow control. The biological codes are interfaces between signals (whether external or internal) and functions. They codify a signal in order to give rise to appropriate functions or functional actions. Humans impose codes on external signals, thus influence biological (neural) functions in themselves and others. They do this through the mental codification of operations on physical items with the purpose of making these a codified system. The mind is a function of biological-neural processes and for this reason is able to put signals and functions in a feedback loop. Focusing on actions, we can distinguish three levels: Scripts (rational plans), schematic scenes (programming), and motor categories (execution of behavior). We can further distinguished a level of more basic motor acts, like prehension, pulling, pushing, etc. All motor categories expand in scenes while all scenes are organized in scripts. Through this code the mind maps possible operations on signals in an informational space such that the result is itself a combination of external physical units according to a code. In this way the mind can influence both its own and conspecifics' neural excitation patterns and functions.

1 Basic Elements of Codification

The present contribution has a cybernetic character and explores the connection between motor-decisional, emotional, and cognitive aspects. My final goal will be to show that the result constitutes a conceptual framework that is relevant to the foundations of a model of credition. So, the goal of the paper is to show which are the essential constituents (with their interconnections) of credition.

The first issue to consider is that the human brain is a biological system that reproduces basic functions that are present in all organisms at a higher level of complexity (Auletta 2011a). For this reason, it is important to briefly focus on what is fundamental of all organisms in order to understand what makes the human brain so peculiar.

G. Auletta (✉)
Pontifical Gregorian University, Rome, Italy

University of Cassino, Cassino, Italy
e-mail: gennaro.auletta@gmail.com

H.-F. Angel et al. (eds.), *Processes of Believing: The Acquisition, Maintenance, and Change in Creditions*, New Approaches to the Scientific Study of Religion 1,
DOI 10.1007/978-3-319-50924-2_4

Life could not exist without *control*. In fact, living organisms are characterized by a significant amount of chemical reactions. When considered from the point of view of the complexity of the chemicals involved, however, they represent a tiny amount of all the reactions that could spontaneously occur. For example, the number of proteins that can theoretically exist are likely to be about 10^{390}, yet the number of those that are produced by living organisms are a tiny part of that: about 10^6–10^8 in the case of humans (Uhlen and Ponten 2005). This means that chemical reactions are driven through sophisticated check and repair mechanisms (Alberts et al. 2008, Chap. 2). A splendid example is given by the production of selenocysteine, a crucial component for the selenoprotein, which is necessary for life. Since such an amino acid is not codified by the genetic code, in order to produce this protein without introducing any change in the code, the cell has developed a very complex molecular machinery that allows the "reading" of one of the stop codons (UGA) as a triplet codifying for the selenocysteine (see Fig. 1). The reason is that codes are upstream of all regulations in the organism and so it is extremely dangerous to change them but it is safer to intervene downstream.

For understanding the role of codes, let us consider the sensory activity: all organisms are able to catch specific classes of signals (according to their environment and needs) in order to monitor environmental variations and act accordingly. A cybernetic theorem tells us that there is no controlling instance without a *model* of the system to be controlled (Conant and Ashby 1970). From the start, this sets cognition in strict connection with action. Now, no model and controlling instance is possible without *codes*, in particular without imposing endogenous codes on the

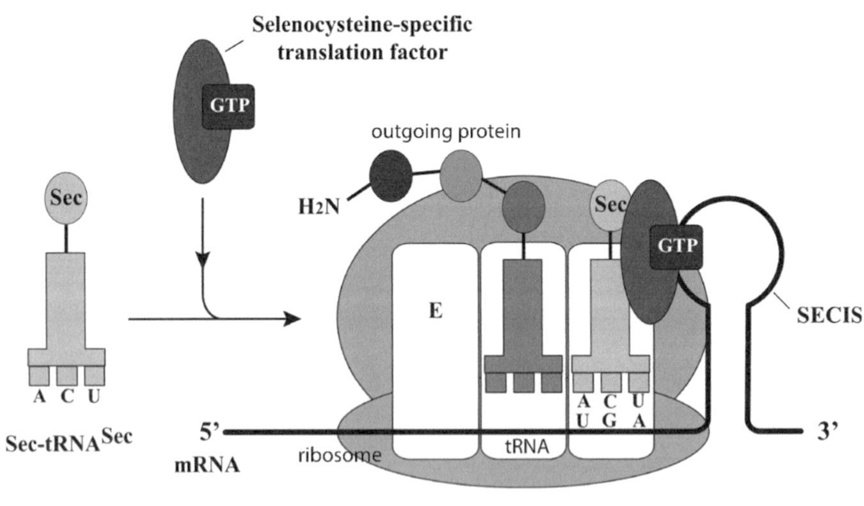

Fig. 1 The complex machinery for recoding the stop codon UGA into a code for selenocysteine. Here, recoding is performed by a modified tRNA (having the triplet ACU but with a selenocysteine (Sec) attached) thanks to the influence of (i) a stem loop structure (SECIS element, including a GTPase enzyme) downstream the UGA codon and a (ii) specific translation factor. Adapted from (Ramon Fuentes NP 2012)

system (e.g. the environment) to be controlled. A code is defined through three different aspects (Ling and Xing 2004):

- There exist (at least) two different elements (like 0 and 1 for the binary code) that are mutually exclusive. These two (or more) elements can be taken to be the code *alphabet*.
- These elements can be combined according to some rules, and these combinations can be understood as *codewords* constituting the code used.
- Codes can exist only if there is a *plurality* of them (not necessarily in the same system) allowing "translations" from one code to another.

The necessity for organisms to use codes is simple: if the reactions or actions of the controlling instance depended on the physical-chemical nature of the signal (whether external or internal) received, the former would depend on the latter and become in fact controlled, as happens for most devices of our technology which are controlled, directly or indirectly, by ourselves (Auletta and Jeannerod 2013). At the opposite, imposing a code on the controlled instance allows the biological controller to attribute functional and vital meaning to the different signals according to its intrinsic needs. (This is one of the main differences between the British associationist view of the brain and the continental school.) Such a process is necessarily *top-down*, where with such a term in such a context I understand the capability of the controller to canalize biochemical reactions occurring spontaneously (Auletta et al. 2008; Auletta 2012).

Thus, we speak of control when an organism is able to treat several environmental factors as functionally *equivalent*, that is, satisfying some functional need plus or minus in the same way. This is necessary, since those classes represent the grid (the code) that the organism "imposes" on the world in order to be able to exert control at all. For instance, the bacterium *E. coli* divides its whole universe of signals in attractants and repellents on a background of neutral signals, as displayed in Fig. 2 (Auletta 2011b and 2013 and literature quoted there). It is attracted by various sugars and amino acids and repelled by fatty acids, alcohols, and other potentially noxious

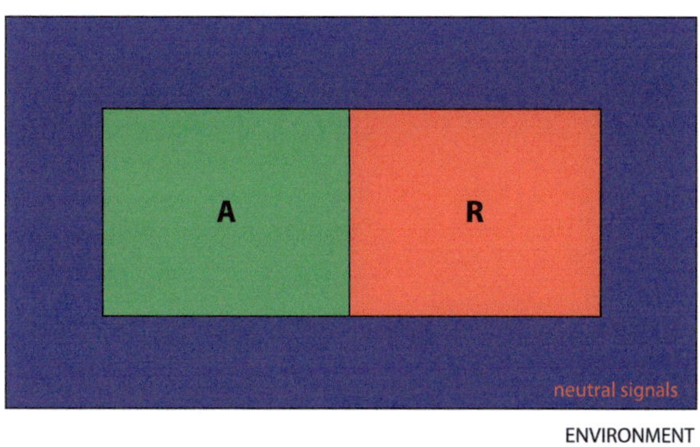

Fig. 2 The world of the *Escherichia coli* (Note that in such a way the organism establishes equivalence classes between different kinds of signals)

compounds. Note that, the two classes of signals regroup chemicals of different sorts, whose common denominator is represented only by the needs of the organism. Obviously, during its evolutionary history, some, possibly random, associations that for one reason or the other turned out to work well where selected.

The second crucial aspect is that the emerging and the manipulation of codes is in fact impossible without mechanisms that allow the organism to be partly shielded relative to the external (but similar arguments are true also for the internal) environment. Only partly, because, the organism needs also to be sensitive to changes occurring in the exterior in order to act appropriately. This means that in general these two aspects (i) respond to different mechanisms but (ii) need to be integrated for finding a quasi-optimal trade-off (optimality is in fact rarely attainable and even dangerous for survival). This is accomplished through the fact that any organism (and any significant part or subsystem of an organism) can be represented as a Markov blanket, as displayed in Fig. 3. The structure of the Markov blanket allows a *filtered sensitivity* to the exterior, i.e. a limited-range sensitivity such that the information is received, coded, re-elaborated (often in connection with endogenous signals), and canalized through the sensory-metabolic network of the organism giving finally some output (often some kind of action). Recent free-energy models show that fundamental physical and chemical processes may have spontaneously generated this kind of structures whose prototype is the external bacterial membrane (Friston et al. 2014).

In this way, even the humble bacterium can display a complex regulatory system as shown in Fig. 4. Here, the input environmental signal ψ (that has been influenced by some previous action of the organism) is codified by the sensory system S, which is now in the state s_t and delivered to the regulatory system R that simultaneously receives inputs from the memory slot M represented by a previous sensory input s_{t-1}, and the decisional system D in the state d_t. Both the decisional system and the regulatory system contribute to the final action a_{t+2} of the action system A.

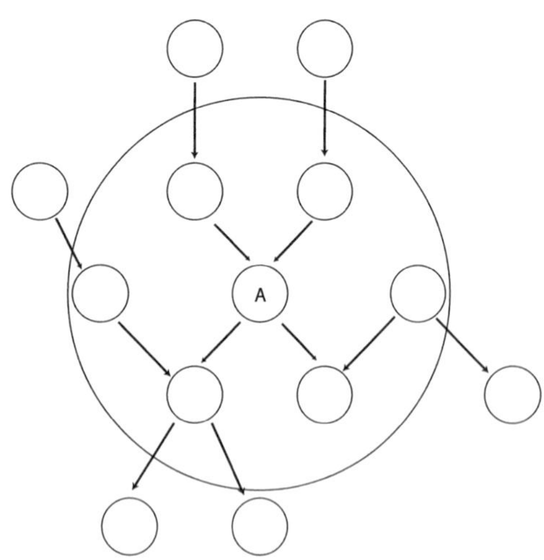

Fig. 3 The Markov blanket of node A is displayed by the *large circle*. It encompasses the node A itself, its parents (the nodes above that influence it), its children (the nodes below that it influences) and other parents of those children (nodes that have influences on the latter and are on the sides of A). All other nodes are excluded. In other words, the function of a Markov blanket is to introduce a protective belt around its central node

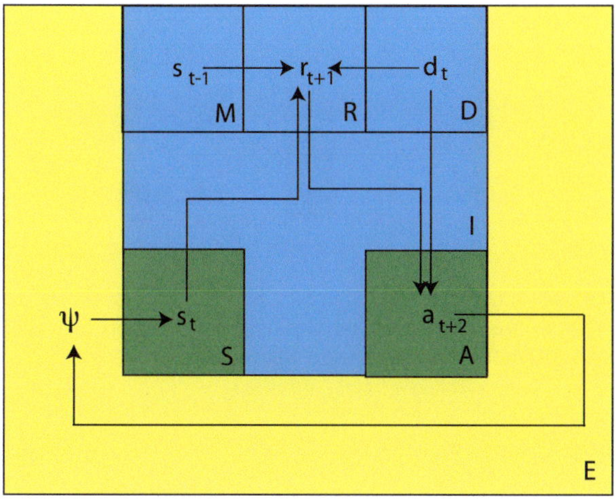

Fig. 4 The organism as a Markov blanket. In *blue* the internal system I (the cell in the easiest case), in *yellow* the external part (the environment E giving rise to a signal ψ). The internal blanket I has two sub-blankets that are shown in *green*: S stands for sensory subsystem, A for action subsystem. M stands for the memory slot, R for representational (model-building) and D for some "decisional" subsystem. The memorized state is the result of a previous input. The symbols *s, a, r, d* denote the state of the relative subsystem at time *t*, while s_{t-1} denotes the sensory input at the previous time $t_{-}1$ that has been memorized

This complex mechanism through which a physical-chemical signal is classified according to the needs of the organism and evaluated for possible responses is in fact a semiotic mechanism, as shown in Fig. 5 (Auletta 2011a): a signal is taken as a sign for something else (like something that either is good if food source or bad in other cases) and therefore as an index of appropriate action (either swimming in that direction or tumbling for moving away: see Fig. 6). Note that to tumble determines a pure random "choice" of a new direction. Nevertheless, a combination of subsequent tumblings interspaced by comparisons of sensory inputs (the current one with the previous one occurred about 3–4 s before) allows in most cases to get the food. Note also that the first scholar to have pointed out this kind of semiotic processes is the mathematician and philosopher C. S. Peirce (CP, 2.228, 2.247–48, 2.304, 1.540; 1903, 1907).

2 The Human Brain and Symbolic Systems

When we pass to the human brain, we obviously attain a huge increase in complexity. It is not my intension to present here a structural or functional sketch of the brain, an issue that is far beyond the scope of this contribution. I shall rather focus on the basic cybernetic aspects that characterize it. Note that the human brain is essentially structured like all other mammalian brains, with three fundamental

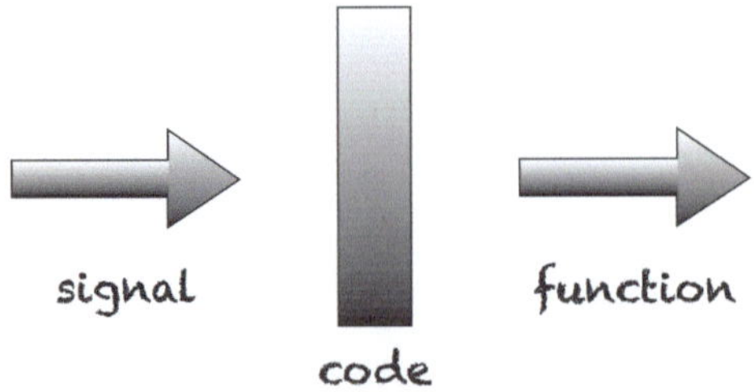

Fig. 5 The code as codifying a signal as a sign for a function (or a functional action) (Note that a signal can be understood as a variation in a physical-chemical medium, like a wave produced by a chemical oscillatory system like in the Belousov–Zhabotinsky reaction)

Fig. 6 *E. coli*'s motion. *Above*: Straight swim. In this case, the flagella turn counter–clockwise. *Below*: Tumbling. In this case, the flagella turn clockwise. When tumbling, the bacterium takes a random direction that in general is different from the previous one (Adapted from Auletta 2011a)

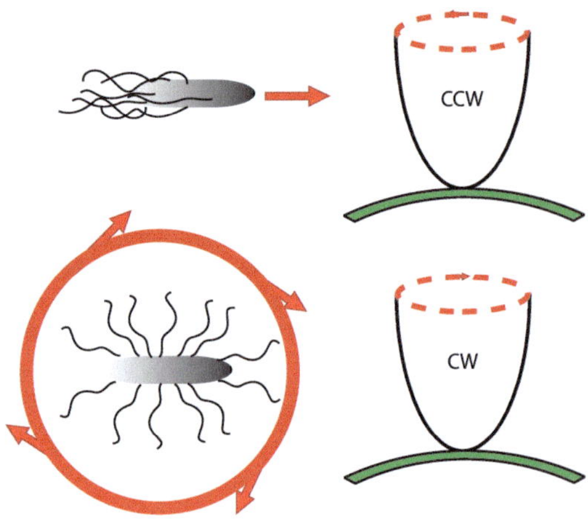

systems: a sensory-cognitive, a motor-decisional and an emotional network. These huge systems (which are very complex and stratified in themselves) collaborate for many basic functions, of which the main ones are (Auletta 2011a, Sec. 17.6):

- *Memory*, understood as the fixation of past experiences, especially when emotionally charged. This means that sensory and emotional aspects are necessarily involved here.
- *Learning*, i.e. the ability to acquire competencies that will turn out useful in the future. It requires therefore contributions from the sensory-cognitive and motor-decisional systems.
- *Behavior*, the sum of different dispositions that help the organism in the natural and social context and are reinforced according to the received feedback. Here, both emotional and motor aspects are involved. Often, learning and behavior or also learning and memory are confused. The reason is that behavior was initially studied through conditioning techniques, while the studies on memory were in fact initially performed on more elementary organisms like mollusks (see Kandel 2006), in which these different functions cannot be so clearly distinguished.

Note that this triad expresses an elementary functionality of life that already exists at a bacterial level (in fact, they have a sensory, a motor and a regulatory system and are in fact able to memorize, to learn, and to acquire some habituation). In general, as we have seen, life is characterized by the ability to acquire information about the environment, to correct responses, and to consolidate those patterns that (to a certain extent) fit with external conditions. Although the above functions, ad high-level cognitive abilities, are common to all mammals, humans are a very special case. In fact, while all organisms (included humans) display a semiotic activity, only humans (at least on the Earth) have built symbolic systems (Auletta 2011a, 3rd part). The issue of the symbolic systems is not to exert control on other systems (like for semiotic activity) but rather to verify and improve the matching between the (Bayesian) hypotheses generated by the brain and external (both natural and social) reality (Friston and Kiebel 2009). We say that an inference is Bayesian when it fulfills the so called Bayes rule for probabilities. The so called a posteriori probability that we choose the hypothesis or select the event denoted by j on the basis of the data k, is given by $p(j|k) = p(k|j)p(j)/p(k)$, where $p(k)$ is the probability distribution of the parameter k, $p(j)$ represents the a priori probability that the chosen hypothesis j is true, and $p(k|j)$ expresses the probability that the values k of the parameter have indeed occurred supposing that the hypothesis j is true, and is related to the previous one by $p(k|j) = p(k)p(j|k)/p(j)$. In other words, Bayesan probabilities (and inferences) allow to infer not only an output j from an input k but also, inversely, the input k from the output j, what is really crucial for human cognitive functions since it allows us to continuously compare what we know a priori or previously with what we learn on experiential basis.

Over a century ago, von Helmholtz (1896: 586–89) correctly pointed out that every sensory activity (of humans and other organisms) is a kind of hypothesis generating or testing. Nevertheless, in all organisms but humans this matching has only been a consequence of natural selection and is in general biologically hardwired. In other words, while models generated by other organisms have uniquely a biologically adaptive significance, the models generated by humans need to be *faithful* to the external reality, and here the comparison allowed by Bayesian inferences is crucial. Although higher animals like mammals display, for example, motor schemes that are plastic, a closer look shows that only the *assembly* of motor subsegments is plastic (typically during a battle) while the subsegments themselves (like showing teeth or inarching the back for a cat) are hardwired. Only the other primates show behavioral schemes that can be considered as provided of some plasticity as a whole (Marshall-Pescini and Whiten 2008), as displayed by their ability to reproduce (emulate) the action of other agents, as it is evident through the results of the research program on mirror neurons (Fogassi et al. 2005; Rizzolatti et al. 1990). Note that monkeys can "reflect" in their neural circuitry the action of another agent only when this action has a purpose (like ingesting food rather than bringing it near the mouth). Nevertheless, characteristic of the human brain and mind is what evolutionists have called *improvisional intelligence* (Cosmides and Tooby 2002; Cosmides et al. 2010): any environmental resource or signal is evaluated on the grounds of the contingent and variable necessities of the human culture. In other words, the same stuff could be a poison to certain purposes but a drug for others. This is why our hypotheses need to be faithful: the enormous variability of the possible models of the *same* object would generate disastrously contradictory behaviors if the models were not "theoretically" organized. This implies, as it is notorious, that the functional needs of the human being are in part detached from the biological substrate and this is what makes of the functions of the human brain *second-level* functions, i.e., abstract functions of biological functions.

To deepen the latter point, let us consider some main characters of symbolic systems:

1. Symbols are not bound to experience: concepts like infinity in mathematics or force in physics (force is in fact never directly perceived but inferred given some effects that we take as induced by its presence) or even beauty or truth have no immediate empirical substrate. This is crucial, since improvisional intelligence requires the capability to extract information from the environment that is most of the time *hidden* to direct experience, since otherwise humans would still depend on hardwired perceptions (on the sensory manifestations of the objects). In other words, by looking at the external aspect of a mushroom often we cannot say if it is comestible or poisonous. Obviously, also many animals can make this distinction but again thanks to mechanisms that re hardwired.
2. This capability to expand the universe in which we live far beyond the immediate perceptual limits makes of all symbolic systems means that are potentially *infinite* (Chomsky 2000; Hauser 2009): with our ordinary language or mathematics we can in principle express any possible concept. This is crucial, since there are no a priori limits on the possible understanding and manipulation of an object.
3. Conventional systems of such a complexity cannot exist without the capability to *share* these codes with our conspecifics. This is crucial: since there is no longer a biological "guarantee" of the correctness of our models, only their sharing in a common culture or social practice ensures the survival of our species. Thus, all symbolic systems have necessarily a social-pragmatic dimension (they are conventional).

Let us briefly consider the latter point. One of the distinctive traits of humans relative to, for example, chimpanzees is our capability to share intentions: a child learning a language tries to follow the gaze of the mother and find eye-contact (Tomasello 2008, 2009, 2014). Humans show a basic capability to be empathic with conspecifics (and even other animals). This is crucially connected with our ability to read the mind of others (Frith 2007). In fact, human communication confers an important role to facial expressions as representing emotions (Seitz et al. 2008; Prochnow et al. 2013). Also, early *homo sapiens*'s societies were characterized by a significant amount of cooperation and even altruism (Fehr and Gächter 2002; Fehr and Fischbacher 2003; Gintis 2003). This would be impossible without a strong connection of the cognitive dimension with emotions, in particular without the human empathy that makes this sophisticated system of communication and collaboration possible. Empathy in short is the human capability to understand (and participate to) the cognitive-emotional state of the other.

Let us briefly focus on the connection between the cognitive and the decisional-motor dimensions. To catch hidden information and to make social use of it demands in fact a crucial capability to *manipulate* the external world according to our codes (Auletta 2011a, Chap. 24). Simple small stones can become element of a computing "machine", representing in this way numbers to add or subtract; emission of phonemes and even gestures combined in appropriate ways become a symbolic communication system like the human natural language, and so on. This makes symbols very different relative to signs. In fact, we impose symbolic codes to signals by manipulating them directly in order to mold actions and biological functions (included neural excitation patterns) of ourselves or our conspecifics. For instance, we are the only species whose members can voluntarily submit themselves to some kind of physical or mental training in order to modify their cognitive abilities or even their behavior. This is precisely how the mind is a function of functions and displays motor cognition. In other words, we impose a code in advance in order to determine the further steps (as displayed in Fig. 7) instead of the code being a mediator between signal and function, as it happens in semiotics. Summarizing, we accomplish this through the manipulation of elements of the physical world according to our code with the purpose of producing a codified signal capable to have influence on our own functions or on functions of others, in our social exchanges.

The involvement of symbols in the human dimension needs to be understood on the basis of a triple dissociation concerning the three basic systems of the brain – motor, emotional, and sensory:

- The first dissociation is between goals and means. Coming back to other primates and the issue of mirror neurons, several studies show that e.g. chimpanzees can emulate an action but not imitate it (Fig. 8): see Auletta (2011a, Secs. 18.6 and 20.2 and literature quoted there). In fact, what this animal does, when seeing an action having a good result, is that it tries to do the same with its own means: the chimp has understood the behavior (and its consequences, so its general "meaning") but cannot understand the abstract *goal* that is behind that action, which would require a theory of mind. At the opposite, any human child understands very quickly that a certain action can be performed with other (and perhaps better) means, what requires that dissociation. Without this capability,

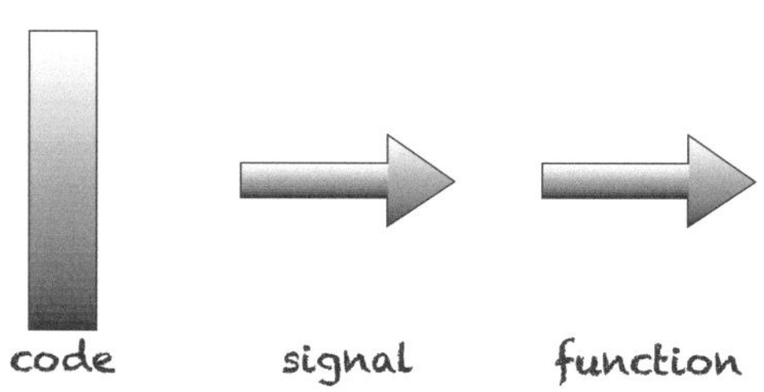

Fig. 7 The way in which symbolic codes work. Compare this mechanism with that displayed in Fig. 5. The basic elements are the same (more complex biological systems rarely change basic systems). They have only been remolded conferring to the codes the leading role

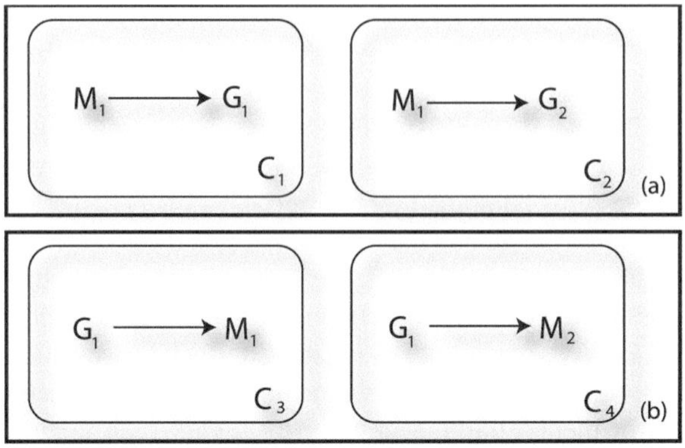

Fig. 8 The difference between doing the same or emulation and a true imitation. (**a**) By observing the same action (the means M1) in a certain context (either C1 or C2) it is possible to infer a certain context-specific goal (G1 or G2). In this way, it is possible to try to do a similar action (choose the same means) in order to fulfill the same goal (G1 or G2) in a particular context. This is emulation. (**b**) In order to truly imitate (to choose a means appropriate to an arbitrary context for pursuing the same goal), it is necessary first to understand what the goal is (here G1) of the other agent in a given context (C3 or C4) and that the choice of the means, which could be different (either M1 or M2), must be appropriate to the context and is only instrumental to the abstract-goal realization. This presupposes true empathic mind reading and symbolic sharing of intentions

we cannot understand the ratchet effect of the human culture (Tomasello 1999): the overall accumulation of the most effective products, procedures, and so on, while all other primates show a fundamental incapability to improve the means that they have.

- The second dissociation is between reward and fruition. We can see this typical behavior also among other primates who often conceal food and decide to postpone their fruition because of the dangerous presence of a conspecific. Obviously, in the case of the other primates, this dissociation is only for short time and is in fact a simple delay of immediate enjoyment. In the case of humans, this dissociation can last very long and be sometimes even permanent. Again, we could barely understand human society without such dissociation. Obviously, also e.g. some insects cumulate food for the winter, but in such a case it is again hardwired behavior, while in the case of humans, due to our improvisional intelligence, there is no connection of this kind.
- The third dissociation concerns that between sensory manifestations and possible use or function or even meaning of the percept. In other words, our models of the world no longer depend on their sensory manifestations only. This is what in fact improvisional intelligence consists in.

3 Three Levels of Action

How can a symbolic machine work? It is here that Jeannerod's work becomes particularly interesting. Following the contribution of Bernstein (1967), already from his early work (Jeannerod 1988) he stressed the fact that the motor system is hierarchically organized (in fact in the brain we distinguish three main levels working in top-down way). The most basic level is that of specific motor performances and is connected with very elementary motor segments, like pushing or pulling an object. This part is still present in our brain and is more directly connected with the cerebellum and the spinal cord. It is likely to be very ancient and in fact we can assume that also elementary brained animals have it. In fact, this is the level of *biological goals* (in a neural context) aiming at the survival of the organism.

An intermediate layer that has certainly been acquired by mammals, due to the strong contribution of the emotional system (see Fig. 9), allows programming of several actions. We can call such a level that of *intentions in actions*. However, since intentions in action are those goals that tend to give rise to a coordinated sequence of actions and single movements with a practical and immediate result, we may assume that, for example, reptiles are able to work at this level. It is when those intentions express or are related to purposeful and socially interactive behavior that they likely require mammalian complexity.

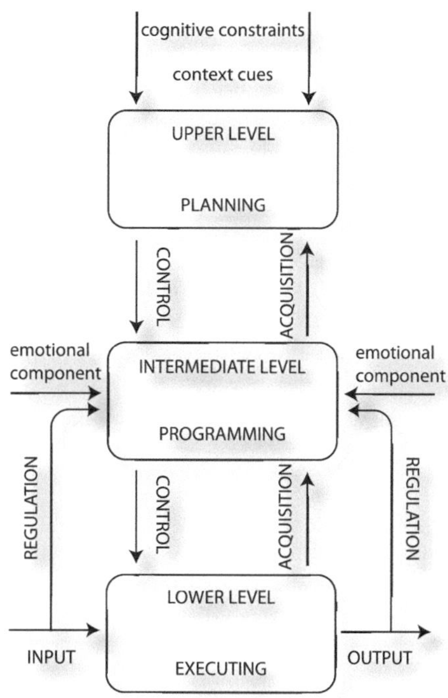

Fig. 9 Jeannerod's distributed model for the generation of actions. It is likely that inputs mediated by the affective system also go to the intermediate level (Adapted from Jeannerod 1999)

Jeannerod (2006) had learnt the distinction between intentions in action and prior intentions (on which I shall say more below) from the philosopher J. Searle (1983) who had in turn elaborated on an original idea of the philosopher E. Anscombe (1957). *Intentions in actions* are still instantiated in motor segments, but with a higher complexity than those of the first level, since here there is a coordination and a purpose. The highest point of these intentions in action is represented by the capability of primates to understand the complex and meaningful behavior of their conspecifics and to neurally react as the action would be performed by themselves, where I recall that only *meaningful* actions are targeted in this way.

Finally, the highest level is that of rational planning, which Jeannerod considered as dealing with *prior intentions*. While the intentions in action, although purposeful, are elaborated and implemented in the course of the action (and therefore do not require a conscious agency), rational plans are consciously elaborated before the action starts and demand in general abstract aspects and items that are not (neither spatially, nor temporally) immediately present. In general, they do not deal with the details of the execution and are therefore fully independent of the action as such, what can give the false impression that they play no role at all. In fact, many (e.g. Libet 1985) have pointed out that consciousness is a too slow agency to be able to influence the course of action. Nevertheless, due to the hierarchical nature of the motor system, rational plans are able to frame single programmed subsegments (which in turn embed single execution subsegments) in such a way to establish a long-lasting and intentionally directed course of action. This also means that rational plans are "located" not only before the start of the action, but also after (as suggested by Libet), or at least at check points where corrections and amendments are needed. Suppose that I desire to go from Rome to Berlin. Many programming subsegments are necessary, like to buy a ticket or go to the airport if I have decided to fly (which obviously collect themselves many different kinds of lower level motor performances). All these subsegments would not lead to expected final result (me being in Berlin) if they were not coherently organized. This is the function of planning. Note that for planning many of these subsegments are interchangeable. For instance, to travel with a company or another is to a certain extent equivalent, to travel one hour before or later could be considered equivalent, and so on. It is only the rational plan (or the intentions of the agent) and its corrections to determine these equivalence classes.

Jeannerod's model can be combined with studies coming from another approach which allow us to come back to the issue of symbols. A hierarchical structures of (i) motor tools, (ii) sensory tools, and (iii) brain tools has been established (Iriki and Taoka 2012), which resemble the hierarchy of representations from indexical (motor) to iconic (sensory) to symbolic (brain) structures of development. Non–human animals use mostly motor tools and rarely use the class of 'sensory tools'. In monkeys, previous studies have demonstrated that they can be trained to use a sort of endoscope only after having acquired an ability to use a motor tool (a rake). This training must imply the ability to reorganize the image of the body to one in which the rake is incorporated as an extension of the forearm.

It is evident, then, that sensory tools cannot be dissociated from context understanding. If we looked at ourselves through our own externalized eyes (the second layer of the tools), we would observe ourselves as external objects by shifting from the first-person to the third-person perspective, i.e., a 'self-objectification'. This leads to the perception of our own intrinsically intransitive movement as transitive, i.e. to the acquisition of a sense of the self (as the subject), and leading to the movement of ourselves or our body parts perceived as objects. We may hypothesize that once the 'self' has been bifurcated into a subjective self and an objective self, the mind and/or intentionality emerges as a function that bridges those fragmented 'selves' and reunites them, producing the recognition of a self that continues across time from the past through the present towards the future. We have thus reached the level of planning, that is, of a coherent temporally history that frames different actions and decisions of the subject (Jeannerod 2009). Once the future self is recognized as having a core that is identical to that of the present self, one might wish to save the present information for future use. This can be accomplished by, e.g., taking notes or drawing pictures, which requires an external device for memorizing facts; thus, an 'externalization of the brain' is produced as the tool class of the third layer, and this is crucial for both (i) the characteristic symbolic manipulation of the external world that is typical for humans in general and (ii) the way in which we formulate and realize our plans in particular. In this case, the environment, which is adapted to our needs, becomes also the receptacle of human information for later use, a kind of extended mind Bruner and Iriki 2015), what shows again the relevance of the social aspect for human culture.

4 The Mental Organization and Codification

Jeannerod's tripartition finds also an interesting counterpart in the studies on memory (Schank 1999), where, as mentioned, emotional aspects play an important role. Starting from the basic level that we can call with Jeannerod that of *motor goals*, we can further distinguish *scenes* that we can associate with intentions in action and in particular as organizers of motor programs, and *scripts*, that we can associate with prior intentions. A script is:

- A temporal collection of specific memories (schemata of situations)
- Organized around common points (purposeful programs);
- Being therefore an active (symbolic) memory organizer.

In Fig. 10 an example is shown. A script goes very well together with the notion of plan or prior intention as far as is both hierarchically and temporally organized: it supposes a relative long sequence of related motor subsegments that can happen themselves in different locations and moments of time. Such a script organizes the motor programs, including our social-emotional interactions. Note that each of the three levels here can be in turn hierarchically organized. Actually, scenes are in most cases not single motor programs but are instead clusters of motor programs representing pur-

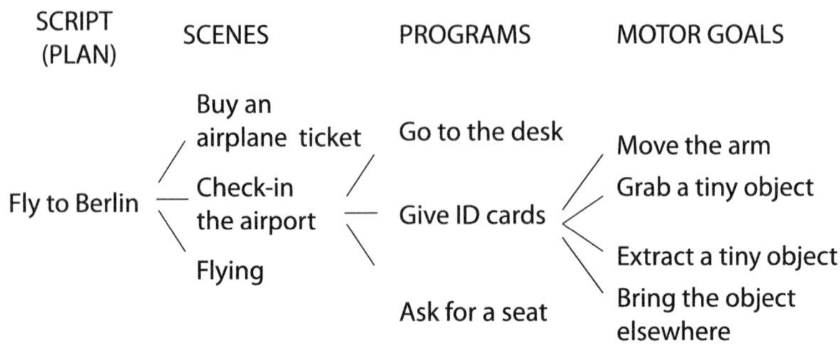

Fig. 10 The script fly to Berlin is schematically shown

poseful actions. What is crucial here and makes the association scenes-programming is the notion of contextuality. I have already stressed that monkeys can emulate the behavior of other agents but the necessary condition is represented by their understanding the "meaning" of the action. This means to understand the context of the action (for instance, eating, driving, and so on). The level of the motor programs is represented by the sequence of actions going to the desk, give the ID card, ask for a (specific) seat, and so on. These purposeful actions consist of coordinated sequences of motor executions representing motor goals, like moving an arm, extracting a tiny object, and so on. Obviously, also here there can be a whole hierarchy: for instance extracting a tiny object can itself be a relative complex action. The crucial point is that such motor segments and subsegments represent very general categories of action that do not constitute by themselves a complete meaningful act, which pertains to programming. It may disputed whether extracting a tiny object satisfies such a criterion. Considering the significant number of possible *different* contexts in which this can occur, it seems that we cannot attribute a functional-contextual relevance to this level of action.

From an evolutionary point of view, a relatively ancient biological layer (motor goals) is not removed by successive developments but integrated into a new symbolic system through meaningful motor programs. Scenes are the schematic but semantically consistent combinations of the general structures that are themselves devoid of specific purposes, and a script is a specific way of temporally organizing scenes and actions.

Through this code the mind maps possible operations on signals in an informational space such that the result is itself a combination of external physical units according to a code. In this way the mind can influence both its own and conspecifics' neural excitation patterns (the first-level functions here).

5 Credition

What I have proposed is to integrate Jeannerod's motor cognition research program with the involvement of mnemonic and emotional aspects. To understand this, let us come back to the triple dissociation characterizing humans. The first dissociation discussed above, that between means and goals, means that our behavior is socially characterized in new ways: it is intentional behavior, i.e. pursuit of *ends* that can be socially shared.

The second dissociation, that between reward and fruition, opens the world of *values* (see Seitz et al. 2009). Acts and happenings are no longer judged only in accordance with the individual advantage but are again permeated by social instances (I recall here what said on altruism). Note that although values and rewards are not completely dissociated, being both rooted ultimately in the emotional part of the brain, the system of values tends, as all other symbolic systems, to be hierarchically organized, while in general such a hierarchy is not observed in the case of basic emotions.

The third dissociation, that between sensory manifestations and model-significance of the object or event, makes *believing* necessary. Beliefs are normally understood either as an issue of religion only or as a manifestation of a human incapability to be objective in the sense required by modern science. This is a deep misunderstanding. Among the most important outcomes of the epistemology of the twentieth century is the principle that our scientific theories be held to be true only subject to the test of evidence; they must in principle be falsifiable. This is also a manner of believing (see Auletta 2011c and literature quoted there). In general, it is impossible to conceive scientific activity without a significant amount of believing, both in the scientist's personal capability to be a good researcher as well as in the correctness of theories and models that dominate one's field and that are taken for granted (while subject to change based on contrary evidence). Examples from everyday life are uncountable: we do not normally have children with a partner without believing that our relationship with our partner will endure and that we are capable of taking care of the children; a student does not typically study a certain discipline at a university without believing that he/she can live with that in the future; and so on. The ultimate goal of science (and of symbolic activity in general) is to rationally justify beliefs -- in agreement with the idea that rational plans introduce amendments to previous strategies that in the best case make them more rationally grounded.

I think the issue at the heart of the credition model is in its capability to connect the three dimensions of beliefs, values, and ends. The crucial question for credition is: what are the beliefs, models, and values that make a certain behavior to be X instead of Y? I think the integrated symbolic proposal presented here could help future research on these issues.

6 Conclusion

If we want to understand the "code" of the mind, I suggest that we not search for a kind of "mentalese" or language of thought (Fodor 1975). I would rather focus on the operations that the brain makes on information from the external world and on the way that the human individual socially interacts with its conspecifics. The ultimate biological root of codes shows that they serve practical purposes and, although cognitive aspects are crucial, they always serve the sake of appropriate action of the organism in an ever-changing environment. Also, when the social environment is taken into account, they involve important emotional (empathic) components. For this reason, I support the development of a research program making the connection between Jeannerod's motor cognition and the social-emotional aspects considered in this chapter in a symbolic understanding of the human's brain activity.

References

Alberts B, Bray D, Lewis J, Raff M, Roberts K, Watson JD (2008) The molecular biology of the cell, 5th edn. Garland P, New York
Anscombe GEM (1957) Intentions. Blackwell, Oxford
Auletta G (2011a) Cognitive biology: dealing with information from bacteria to minds. Oxford University Press, Oxford
Auletta G (2011b) Teleonomy: the feedback circuit involving information and thermodynamic processes. J Mod Phys 2(3):136–145
Auletta, G, in collaboration with Colag'e I, D'ambrosio P, Torcal L (2011c) Integrated cognitive strategies in a changing world, G and B Press, Rome
Auletta G (2012) Causation upside down? Rev Port Filos 68(1–2):9–32
Auletta G (2013) Information and metabolism in bacterial chemotaxis. Entropy 15:311–326
Auletta G, Jeannerod M (2013) Introduction: consciousness as a top-down causal agency. In: Auletta G, Colagè I, Jeannerod M (eds) Brains top-down: is top-down causation challenging neuroscience? World Scientific, Singapore, pp 1–49
Auletta G, Ellis G, Jaeger L (2008) Top-down causation by information control: from a philosophical problem to a scientific research program. J R Soc Interface 5:1159–1172
Bernstein NA (1967) The coordination and regulation of movements. Pergamon, Oxford
Bruner E, Iriki, A (2015) Extending mind, visuospatial integration, and the evolution of the parietal lobes in the human genus. Quat Int:1–13
Chomsky N (2000) New horizons in the study of language and mind. Cambridge University Press, Cambridge
Conant RC, Ashby RW (1970) Every good regulator of a system must be a model of that system. Int J Syst Sci 1:89–97
Cosmides L, Tooby J (2002) Unraveling the Enigma of human intelligence: evolutionary psychology and the multimodular mind. In: Sternberg RJ, Kaufman JC (eds) The evolution of intelligence. Erlbaum, London, pp 145–198
Cosmides L, Barrett HC, Tooby J (2010) Adaptive specialization, social exchange, and the evolution of human intelligence. Proc Natl Acad Sci USA 107:9007–9014
Fehr E, Fischbacher U (2003) The nature of human altruism. Nature 425:785–791
Fehr E, Gächter S (2002) Altruistic punishment in humans. Nature 415:137–140
Fodor JA (1975) The language of thought. Harvester Press, Hassocks
Fogassi L, Ferrari PF, Gesierich B, Rozzi S, Chersi F, Rizzolatti G (2005) Parietal lobe: from action organization to intention understanding. Science 308:662–667
Friston K, Kiebel S (2009) Predictive coding under the free – energy principle. Philos Trans R Soc B364:1211–1221
Friston KJ, Sengupta B, Auletta G (2014) Cognitive dynamics: from attractors to active inference. Proc IEEE 102:427–445
Frith CD (2007) Making up the mind: how the brain creates our mental world. Blackwell, Oxford
Gintis H (2003) The Hitchhiker's guide to Altruism: gene-culture co-evolution, and the internalization of norms. J Theor Biol 220:407–418
Hauser MD (2009) The possibility of impossible cultures. Nature 460:190–196

Iriki A, Taoka M (2012) Triadic (Ecological, neural, cognitive) Niche construction: a scenario of human brain evolution extrapolating tool use and language from the control of reaching actions. Philos Trans R Soc B367:11–24
Jeannerod M (1988) The neuronal and behavioural organization of goal–directed movements. Oxford University Press, Oxford
Jeannerod M (1999) The cognitive way to action. In: Russell RJ, Murphy N, Meyering TC, Arbib MA (eds) Neuroscience and the Person: Scientific Perspectives on Divine Action. Vatican Observatory, Berkeley, pp 57–66
Jeannerod M (2006) Motor cognition: what actions tell the self. Oxford University Press, Oxford
Jeannerod M (2009) Le cerveau volontaire. O. Jacob, Paris
Kandel ER (2006) In search of memory: the emergence of a new science of mind. W. W Norton, New York
Libet B (1985) Unconscious cerebral initiative and the role of conscious will in voluntary action. Behav Brain Sci 8:529–539
Ling S, Xing C (2004) Coding theory: a first course. Cambridge University Press, Cambridge
Marshall–Pescini S, Whiten A (2008) Chimpanzees (*Pan troglodytes*) and the question of cumulative culture: an experimental approach. Anim Cogn 11:449–456
Peirce CS (1903) The Nature of Meaning. In Peirce (EP), II, 208–225
Peirce CS (1907) Pragmatism. In Peirce (EP), II, 398–433
Prochnow D, Kossack H, Brunheim S, Müller K, Wittsack AJ, Markowitsch AJ, Seitz RJ (2013) Processing of subliminal facial expressions of emotion: a behavioral and fMRI study. Soc Neurosci. doi:10.1080/17470919.2013.812536
Ramon Fuentes M (NP) (2012) The concept of function in molecular biology: a theoretical framework and a case study. Dissertation, Pontifical Gregorian University. Discussed May 2012
Rizzolatti G, Gentilucci M, Camarda RM, Callese V, Luppino G, Matelli M, Fogassi L (1990) Neurons related to reaching–grasping arm movements in the rostral part of area 6 (Area 6aβ). Exp Brain Res 82:337–350
Schank RC (1999) Dynamic memory revisited. Cambridge University Press, Cambridge
Searle JR (1983) Intentionality: an essay in the philosophy of mind. Cambridge University Press, Cambridge
Seitz RJ, Schäfer R, Scherfeld D, Friederichs S, Popp K, Wittsack KJ, Azarif NP, Franz M (2008) Valuating other people's emotional face expression: a combined functional magnetic resonance imaging and electroencephalography study. Neuroscience 152:713–722
Seitz RJ, Franz M, Azari NP (2009) Value judgments and self–control of action: the role of the medial frontal cortex. Brain Res Rev 60:368–378
Tomasello M (1999) The human adaptation for culture. Annu Rev Anthropol 28:509–529
Tomasello M (2008) Origins of human communication. The MIT Press, Cambridge, MA
Tomasello M (2009) Why we cooperate. The MIT Press, Cambridge, MA
Tomasello M (2014) A natural history of human thinking. Harvard University Press, Harvard
Uhlen M, Ponten F (2005) Antibody–based proteomics for human tissue profiling. Mol Cell Proteomics 4(4):384–393
von Helmholtz HLF (1896) Handbuch der physiologischen Optik, 2nd edn. L. Voss, Hamburg/Leipzig

Beliefs and Believing as Possible Targets for Neuroscientific Research

Rüdiger J. Seitz

Abstract There is a lack of a scientifically acceptable definition of "belief", although personal beliefs can be found with high prevalence in societies. Recently, cognitive neuroscience research has developed an interest in the neurophysiological processes underlying "believing". Central to the processes of believing is the notion of probabilistic representations of objects and events. As information from the complex outside world is explored interactively by the senses and evaluated in terms of personal meaning, the corresponding mental representations are inherently subjective but typically do not reach awareness. When they are reinforced and become conscious, they constitute personal beliefs. Belief contents may gain transcendent connotations and, thereby, anticipatory implications for the future. The neurophysiological processes underlying believing have been described tentatively by models of fundamental brain functions applying to the physical, interpersonal and societal dimensions. Evidence from neuroimaging and neurophysiology has shown that the intricately interwoven mental operations of perception, valuation, and generation of action affording believing are processed in extensive neural networks involving the dorsal medial and dorsolateral frontal cortex. Scientific approaches of this sort open strategies for an empirical exploration of ethical guidance of human behavior.

1 Introduction

In colloquial language the statement "I believe that ..." often is not used accurately when people are asked about an experience or a reason for an observation. Typically, they may say: "I believe this is so and so" or more carefully "I think this is so and so". Such propositions express the subjective perspective of a person. However, the individual becomes aware of the observed fact or event only with a limited degree of subjective certainty. In principle, these propositions can be verified by a second person. In contrast, the statement "I know that ..." pertains to the recall of world knowledge that has been acquired by the speaker. In fact, humans learn that their

R.J. Seitz (✉)
Department of Neurology, Centre for Neurology and Neuropsychiatry, LVR-Klinikum Düsseldorf, Heinrich-Heine-University Düsseldorf, Düsseldorf, Germany
e-mail: seitz@neurologie.uni-duesseldorf.de

H.-F. Angel et al. (eds.), *Processes of Believing: The Acquisition, Maintenance, and Change in Creditions*, New Approaches to the Scientific Study of Religion 1,
DOI 10.1007/978-3-319-50924-2_5

perceptions are structured, verified and reinforced by the report of other people, be that by conversation, education or the media. Examples are "I know that 3 times 4 equals 12" or "I know that the earth circulates on an orbital rotation around the sun". By contrast, the statement "I believe that God is the creator of the world" is a proposition resulting from many different perceptions. Importantly, this statement reflects a belief; it cannot be verified. Moreover, the statement "The earth circulates around the sun" cannot be verified by ordinary people. Rather, this is world knowledge which was brought about by the advancement of the sciences. These examples reveal that the sciences have heavily influenced our beliefs about the world.

When scientific discourse comes to the noun "belief", there is no acceptable definition of what this actually is and what, in comparison, a false belief or delusion is (Bell and Halligan 2012). Historically, "belief" has been related closely to "religion" as is described in detail by Angel in this volume. In the recent neuroscientific discussion this corresponds to the argument that facts and knowledge are stored in the human brain (Krueger et al. 2009). In contrast, the notion of creditions (Angel 2013) emphasizes the procedural aspect of "believing" similarly to other psychological processes. Specifically, "credition" has been conceived as a psychological term denoting the mental activity related to what we call "he/she believes". Thus, the relation of the term "believing" to human behaviour and to human brain function is of considerable neuroscientific interest. As only one illustration, believing and religious beliefs have been hypothesized to be by-products of normal human cognition (Boyer 2003; Kapogiannis et al. 2009). Accordingly, "believing" may be conceptualized as an expression of a number of psychological processes that are brought about by the human brain. Consequently, psychology of religion has recently earned much scientific interest (Paloutzian and Park 2013).

In the attempt to elucidate what believing denotes, it is assumed as a point of departure that each individual constantly interacts with the complex outside world. Humans are equipped with highly developed senses by which they can explore the physical environment and the people around them. Importantly, most of the incoming sensory information is processed below awareness, since the information is obscured by ambient distracters impairing the signal to noise ratio, or is accessible only for brief periods of time. Thus, the mental representations of sensory information are never a perfect match but rather reach only a certain degree of probability. There is a large body of literature on the characteristics, limitations, and neural coding of sensory perception (see reference books by Chaudhuri 2010; Barth et al. 2012). It is important to note that there is a tight link between perception and action, since people have to base their actions on the probabilistic, fuzzy mental representations of their perceptions. This chapter addresses the questions of how believing is related to perception and actions, and how results from neuroscience research of human brain function can advance our understanding of what believing and beliefs might be.

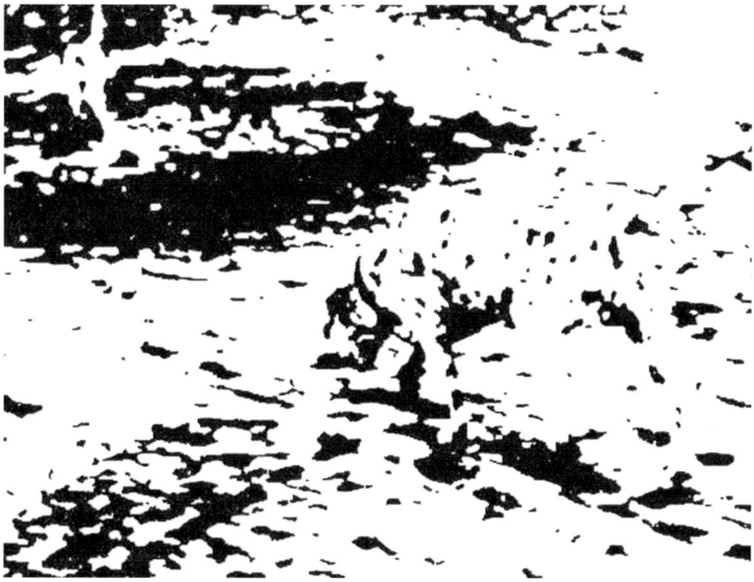

Fig. 1 Instable picture of a Dalmatian dog. The dog is obscured by image noise but its Gestalt becomes apparent upon prolonged inspection (Thurston and Carraher 1966)

2 Belief Formation Grounded in Perception

From one moment to the next, subjects are confronted with sensory information from the external world and internal information about their mood and momentary feelings. Different processing streams mediate the analysis of the physical properties of objects, their use, the spatial configurations between them, their relation to adjacent objects as well as the nature and temporal order of events (Tsuchiya et al. 2008; Schweisfurth et al. 2014). The quality and intensity of the sensed information determine the probability of the subject's mental representation of the perceived information.

Owing to the magnitude of the signal-to-noise ratio and the exposure time, these representations have a probabilistic character (Fig. 1). This has been formulated mathematically by Bischof in this volume. At the edge of awareness, humans are able to decode emotional face expressions which are typically transient, extending over some 30 to 40 milliseconds (Harry et al. 2012; Smith 2011; van Gaal et al. 2011). Typically, complex scenes or events are condensed into simplified perspectives. Nevertheless, subjects rely on these personal representations as valid, regarding them as components of the world around them. This corresponds to the notion of the neural code as presented by Auletta in this volume. The different features of objects are explored by dedicated exploration routines such that there is an intimate interaction of perception and action (Roland and Mortensen 1987; Jeannerod 1995; Binkofski et al. 2001). This formal analysis is mediated by the

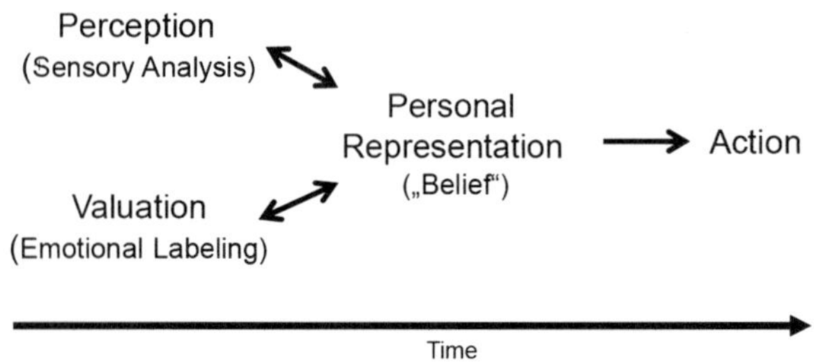

Fig. 2 Schematic model of the evolution of a person's probabilistic mental representations. The mental representations are generated by perpetuating interactions with the outside world (perception) and the inside world (valuation). These interactions involve cognitive functions such as exploration and comprehension in perception and attention and attribution in valuation. Actions are generated on the basis of these previously generated personal probabilistic representations which also build the basis for anticipating the cost and reward to achieve a goal

modality specific sensory cortical areas ultimately leading to comprehension of an object or event (Fig. 2).

In addition to the sensory information about the physical properties of objects and events, humans estimate in an interactive fashion to what extent these objects and events might have a personal value for them (Seitz et al. 2009). This probabilistic judgment is the default first-person perspective of "what does it mean to me?". Consequently, the relevance of external information is coded implicitly, with the emotional categories of happiness, anger, fear, surprise, and disgust constituting the so-called gut feeling, which is described in detail by Holzer in this book. In an explicit manner, subjects attribute the qualities of good, beautiful or adverse and dangerous to what they attend to (Fig. 2). Recently, it was described that these attributed values are coded according to the all-or-none theory in a contrasting bimodal fashion (Johnson et al. 2015). Moreover, the new information is attributed to categories such as credibility, novelty, proximity, utility and pleasantness. Notably, there is empirical evidence that repetitively occurring stimuli induce an illusion of truth (Chang et al. 2010; Henkel and Mattson 2011). Consequently, the formal sensory representations gain an explicit dimension of which the perceiving person becomes aware. This cognitive-emotional integration of information has a probabilistic nature owing to the continuing interaction of the subject with the external and internal world corresponding to the notion of a stabilized bab-configuration in the credition process as proposed by Angel (2013). In terms of neurophysiology, these different external and internal perceptions are combined into coherent representations in the brain that have been related to distributed gamma oscillations (Engel and Singer 2001; Roux et al. 2012). Also, evidence has accumulated that the valuation process occurs rapidly and involves different parts of the human brain, including the medial frontal gyrus (Seitz et al. 2006; Grabenhorst and Rolls 2011; Bzdod et al. 2012). Note that these mental processes cannot be reduced just to the brain but are integral to and brought about by the action of the brain which is embedded within the human body (Fuchs 2009).

Particularly in social interactions that typically span over seconds to minutes, the perceived events are set into a formal cognitive as well as subjective emotional perspective (Bird and Viding 2014). Humans may not only perceive an emotional facial expression but may engage in reasoning about the explanation for the emotion they are observing in their counterpart (Potthoff and Seitz 2015). These reflexive considerations critically involve the empirical self which is related to the engagement of the medial frontal cortex as presented by Northoff in this book. Importantly, humans may attribute abstract categories of social value such as moral, justice, and ethics to what they perceive. It should be noted that the subject's conclusion about the physical properties of objects and events is generally assumed to be virtually identical among different subjects, while in contrast it is well known that the personal relevance of the same object or event may be considered profoundly different among subjects. That is, the interactive processes of perception and valuation are weighted differently among different people. This individual valuation process may become abnormal as can be seen in neuropsychiatric patients (Veit et al. 2013) and in, for example, patients who were traumatized by what they perceived (Sartory et al. 2013). Notably, the midline structures of the human brain have been shown to be activated by symptom provocation in acute stress disorder (Cwik et al. 2014). Also closely related are the concepts of placebo, which will be highlighted by the chapter of Meissner in this book.

According to Morewedge and Kahneman (2010), the formation of mental representations involves a type 1 process which is intuitive and implicit, and overrules the abstract and rational type 2 process. It was hypothesized that type 1 processes represent a faulty intuition system that gives major biases to intuitive judgment controlling a person's rational operations. Such a dual pathway was shown to engage different brain areas (Kuo et al. 2009). It is important to emphasize, however, that the perceived information belongs to the past, since sensory perception takes time, and awareness about a perceived item or signal occurs subsequently to exploration of the item or the event. Accordingly, new information is compared with previously sampled information, i.e. the memory of the personal representations generated in the past. In fact, the subjective relevance of new information is judged in comparison to pre-existing knowledge. Thus, prior experience may be updated and modified. But likewise, new information may be rejected as incompatible with the prior representations. Interestingly, personal representations or beliefs have been reported to become so predominant that they overrule the perception of ongoing signals (Wiese et al. 2014).

The formation of probabilistic personal representations outlined here corresponds to the enclosure and stabilization processes as described for creditions in detail by Angel in this volume. In an integrated model, the self-organizing nature of the believing process was regarded as the basic principle of the system dynamics (Sugiura et al. 2015). This model was based on the perception-action-value triad applying to basic and increasingly more complex levels, namely the physical, interpersonal and social level. Connors and Halligan provide a five-stage model in this book which proposes that beliefs are formed by iterative circles involving search of meaning, evaluation of belief, and belief acceptance.

3 Role of Beliefs for Decision Making

In the preceding section it was described that sensory perception leads to corresponding representations in the human brain that are essentially probabilistic in nature and become personally meaningful by a simultaneously ongoing valuation process. It was suggested that the resulting probabilistic personal representations can be considered to be personal beliefs. Importantly, these probabilistic personal representations are used for the initiation of actions and control of behaviour (Fig. 2). The probabilistic mental representations or beliefs can be used by the individual in a prospective fashion to make predictions about the possible reward and costs when performing actions and, above that, how to optimize behaviour (Friston 2010; Vlaev et al. 2011). Accordingly, subjects have to make decisions to select an appropriate action. Driving forces are desires or appetite (Rolls 2006). When people set out to initiate and maintain certain behaviour, they have to identify the given situation, adapt to restrictions in their environment, and determine how to reach their goal without running into physical harm or evoking objections by competitors. These behavioural decisions have to take into account the physical environment and the actual personal situation. Nevertheless, such decisions are made spontaneously and with ease but can become painstaking when information is complex and only partially available, or suppressed by noise or competing computations. In fact, personal decisions concerning the control of actions and adaptive behaviour are subconscious or intuitive (Kahnt et al. 2010). The interesting question, therefore, is in which way the processing of subliminal information in the human brain differs from supraliminal information in decision making. Subliminal information is very briefly presented, for only 40 ms or less; information presented for 100 ms or more is supraliminal. It may nevertheless remain unconscious if attention is drawn away from it and focused on other targets (Potthoff and Seitz 2015). Nevertheless, the subjects have a sense of agency when making the decisions and undertaking the actions (Farrer and Frith 2002). Moreover, subjects typically take a positive stance to their decisions, since they believe to have made the right decisions.

It ought to be emphasized that decisions are based on implicit or explicit assumptions that are stored in the brain as personal probabilistic representations but influence acts in the near or far future. These assumptions rely on the person's past experience, moral and ethical standards, and current emotional situation or mood. Such decisions pertain to daily affairs of low impact, for example, the issue what to wear to the wedding of a good friend. The person in question may reason: "For the sake of my friendship with the bride I would like to avoid being underdressed when I go to her wedding". But the decisions can be more difficult, for example, when it comes to giving money to a charity foundation. The question then is: "What is the expected personal reward versus the cost of no longer having the money to spend for myself?" Possible rewards may include high social reputation, personal joy resulting from seeing the success of the charity organization as a result of my sponsorship, or the personal trust gained by having done something good, since the good deed may turn into something good for the sponsor him-or-herself some time in the future. Accordingly, behavioural decisions involve the discrimination of right from wrong, good from bad, and pleasant from unpleasant based on memories of prior experience, personal socialization, and ethical standards. They lead to predispositions such as attitudes, desires, and hopes that are instrumental for the selection of an appropriate and the suppression of inappropriate actions.

In numerous neuroimaging studies it was found that the prefrontal cortex plays a prominent role in executive functions such as manipulation of information, planning, and decision making (Duncan and Owen 2000; Niendam et al. 2012). There is evidence that a broad spectrum of executive functions involve an extensive circuit in the human brain including bilaterally the dorsolateral frontal cortex, the inferior frontal gyrus, the medial dorsal cortex and the ventrally adjacent anterior cingulate gyrus, the parietal cortex lining the intraparietal sulcus, the inferior temporal gyrus as well as subcortical structures such as the caudate nucleus, the thalamus and the neocerebellum. The dorsolateral prefrontal cortex is specifically involved in the discrimination of objects and emotional face expressions (e.g. Stoeckel et al. 2003; Prochnow et al. 2013). While symbolic discriminations as in speech processing and in arithmetic involve the left dorsolateral prefrontal cortex, spatial, sensory, emotional and abstract discriminations involve the right dorsolateral prefrontal cortex (Duncan and Owen 2000). Flexibility, inhibition and working memory show areas of overlap in the dorsolateral prefrontal cortex, the inferior frontal gyrus, the dorsal medial frontal cortex, and the cortex lining the intraparietal sulcus (Niedam et al. 2012). As evident from functional connectivity studies, the dorsolateral frontal cortex area relevant for the pre-decision phase is functionally connected bilaterally with the inferior frontal cortex implicated in lower-level empathy, and the medial dorsal frontal cortex, the so-called pre-SMA (Prochnow et al. 2014). This corresponds to the binding of visual social cues as present in facial expressions and gestures (Conty et al. 2012). In contrast, the slightly more anterior part of the dorsolateral prefrontal cortex that is specifically engaged with the discrimination process serves as part of a wide bilateral cortex involving a spatially distinct circuit including the inferior parietal lobule and the inferior temporal cortex (Prochnow et al. 2014). This is similar to the network that engages in false beliefs as compared with true beliefs (Döhnel et al. 2012). There is a clear correlation between the intelligence score and the degree of activation in the dorsolateral prefrontal cortex such that more demanding tasks result in higher activation (Duncan et al. 2000; Cole and Schneider 2007). Furthermore, the more items are maintained in working memory, the greater the gamma-band activity in Brodmann area 9 of the dorsolateral prefontal cortex (Roux et al. 2012). Notably, motor preparatory activity in the posterior parietal cortex was found to be modulated by subjective absolute value (Iver et al. 2010) reflecting the close association of motor programming and representations of success of the actions.

4 Role of Beliefs to Cope with the Future

An existential question for humans is: "How can I survive in the future?" As the future is not known, we do not know whether we will be exposed to physical harm, starvation or painful illness. Nor do we know when and how our family members or friends or even we ourselves will die. While the strategies to cope with questions of this kind probably vary among humans, most people are frightened by the unpredictability of their future. Nevertheless, humans need to make decisions regarding what to do in order to satisfy their immediate longings and long-term desires (Rolls 2006). To make such decisions, people have to weigh the potential future reward against the limitations and costs inherent in the possible choices. Cristofori and Grafman describe in this book that moral, legal, political and social beliefs are of critical importance for the person's decision making and guidance of behaviour. A particular motivation for behaviour is the belief that one ought to do something good for others, for example, when one helps or supports poor or disabled people. This belief is highly prevalent in Western societies (Pechey and Halligan 2012), and is probably related to the promises of present and/or future fulfillment or benefit provided by the Christian tradition. Similarly to other religions, the Bible provides grand promises that suggest an even and protected path in life, and ultimate justice and salvation after death. An example of this can be seen in a passage from Psalm 23.

The LORD is my shepherd; I shall not want.
He makes me lie down in green pastures.
He leads me beside still waters.
He restores my soul.
He leads me in paths of righteousness
for his name's sake.
Even though I walk through the valley.
of the shadow of death,
I will fear no evil,
for you are with me;
your rod and your staff,
they comfort me.
You prepare a table before me
in the presence of my enemies;
you anoint my head with oil;
my cup overflows.
Surely goodness and mercy shall follow me
all the days of my life,
and I shall dwell in the house of the LORD
forever.[1]

[1] Psalm 23 (https://www.biblegateway.com)

Each paragraph of the psalm constructs pictures of environmental encounters that suggest comfort, shelter, and eternal peace. Notice that the psalm also states that even if the present involves deprivation, hostility, and fright, there is the prospect of future salvation. Thus, the psalm utilizes the positive emotional loading of personal memories to provide a personal meaning to the individual life experience (Seitz and Angel 2014). In a functional neuroimaging study it was found that the recital of Psalm 23 led to activation in a number of higher-order brain areas. In fact, the activation pattern involved the precuneus, an area related to visual recall, and most heavily the dorsal medial frontal cortex including the pre-SMA, which is a supramodal brain area integrating cognitive, emotional and preparatory functions (Azari et al. 2001).

The individual's answer to the question of how to cope with the future is critically related to an existential meaning making, be it secular, spiritual, or religious (La Cour and Hvidt 2010). It is suggested that the mental processes described in this chapter represent fundamental human brain functions transforming cognitive and emotional perspective-taking into personal considerations of secular and likewise non-secular transcendence as elaborated by Mesulam (2008). It is hypothesized that these mental processes include dual implicit/intuitive and abstract/rational cognitive processing (Watts 2007) and afford the processing of the key elements of secular and religious belief systems which are myths, ritual actions and the feeling of transcendence (Schnell 2003). They correspond to the three dimensions of knowing, practice, and importance in existential meaning making as found in secular societies (La Cour and Hvidt 2010). These belief systems originate from the fundamental dualistic experience of the surrounding immanent physical world and the seemingly immaterial, non-accessible sky. As outlined above, promises for the future are provided by belief systems as, for example, by religions. For religious beliefs, these key elements are supplemented by the notion of creativity, almightiness and truth that have been attributed to deities or God (Fischbeck 2005).

Figure 3 depicts that secular and non-secular beliefs expand in time, linking the past to the future. Rituals play a key role in stabilizing beliefs, owing to their standardized practice on regular repetitions in the time being. These rituals are grounded

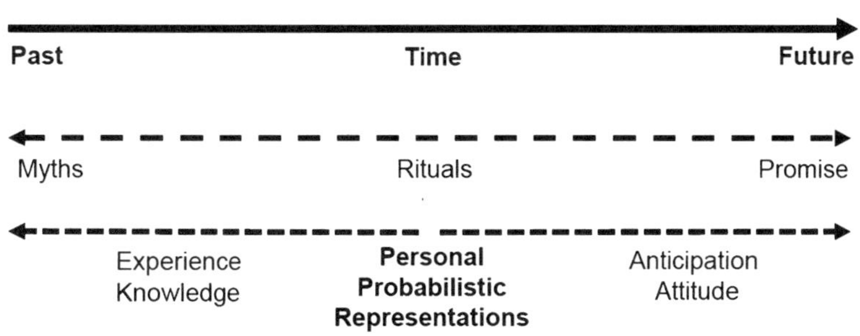

Fig. 3 Hypothetical model of formation and consequences of personal belief systems. Beliefs are generated by ritual practices that are perceived and valuated by the participating subjects. The thereby generated personal probabilistic representations build up the personal experience. Narratives (including myths) reinforce these representations by referral to tails beyond personal experience. For communities they provide the knowledge framework for entertaining rituals and guiding education and socialization. These beliefs that link the world's past with the individual's past also provide a promise for the future. This link makes the individual believe that the ultimate goal of the world can be anticipated by the learned narratives forming his/her attitude

by myths that refer to the past beyond the limits of personal experience. In fact, they constitute the experience and knowledge and, thereby, the belief systems of the individuals from childhood onwards (Seligman and Brown 2010). On this background the individual's experience gets linked with narrative knowledge. This combination of information generates trust into the promise provided by the narratives strengthening the subjects against perceived threats of their physical integrity (Boyer and Liénard 2006). Moreover, it leads to the acceptance of moral and ethical standards that are derived from such narratives and limit the possible actions to be selected. Furthermore, according to promises of the given belief system, the individuals are put into the position to anticipate their future accordingly, which is suited to the individual's attitude. With respect to the notion of expectation there are close connections to the concept of placebo outlined in the chapter by Meissner in this volume.

It is of note that religion has been conceived as a meaning making system as outlined by Paloutzian and Mukai in this book. This system comprises mental core processes that enable a person to evaluate incoming information, to regulate beliefs, affects, and actions, and to live with a sense of personal continuity throughout life (Emmons and Paloutzian 2003). Even further, Paloutzian and Park (2013) hypothesize that the processes of sacralisation belong to the meaning making system. Similarly, the recipients of rituals and myths are prompted to believe that the probabilistic representations of pleasant perceptions in the past are similarly valid for the time being and the future. Above that, the persons are persuaded to believe that the future will be peaceful and bright akin the sky at sunset on a clear summer evening. This belief content is both simplistic and transcendent, providing a large promise for the individual's future. The processes underlying this belief rely on the action-perception-value triad which loads the individual's past perceptions with positively-flavoured memories. In fact, many different mental representations are likely to be combined into belief systems that link the "golden" past with bright expectations for the future of the individual and, in a broader sense, of communities or even societies. In consequence, when people state to believe in God, this most often means that they attribute high subjective certainty to their mental representations of the frequently heard religious narratives. Mental processes related to believing have been shown to be related to enhanced neural activity in the medial frontal cortex (Seitz and Angel 2012).

This chapter has outlined a framework of the processes of believing that pertain to secular and non-secular belief systems. This framework provides a springboard for interdisciplinary exploration and hypothesis testing in terms of human brain physiology, but also in pathological states in patients with neuropsychiatric diseases. Furthermore, it opens new paths of interdisciplinary discussions on a wide range of traditional philosophical topics such as the relation of belief and faith, or the acquisition and behavioural consequences of secular and religious beliefs.

References

Angel HF (2013) Credition. In: Runehov ALC, Oviedo L, Azari NP (eds) Encyclopedia of sciences and religion. Springer Reference, Dordrecht. http://www.springerreference.com/docs/html/chapterdbid/357430.html

Azari NP, Nickel J, Wunderlich G, Niedeggen M, Hefter H, Tellmann L, Herzog H, Stoerig P, Birnbacher D, Seitz RJ (2001) Neural correlates of religious experience. Eur J Neurosci 13:1649–1652

Barth FG, Giampieri-Deutsch P, Klein HD (2012) Sensory perception – mind and matter. Springer Biomedical Sciences Neurosciences, Wien

Bell V, Halligan PW (2012) The neural basis of abnormal personal belief. In: Kruger F, Grafman J (eds) The neural basis of human belief, vol 10. Psychology Press, New York, pp 300–329

Binkofski F, Kunesch E, Dohle C, Seitz RJ, Freund HJ (2001) Tactile Apraxia: unimodal apractic disorder of tactile object exploration associated with parietal lobe lesions. Brain 124:132–144

Bird G, Viding E (2014) The self to other model of empathy: Providing a new framework for understanding empathy impairments in psychopathy, autism, and alexithymia. Neurosci Biobehav Rev 47(4):520–532

Boyer P (2003) Religious thought and behaviour as by-products of brain function. Trends Cogn Sci 7:119–124

Boyer P, Liénard P (2006) Why ritualized behaviour? Precaution systems and action parsing in development, pathological and cultural rituals. Behav Brain Sci 29:595–613

Bzdod D, Schilbach L, Vogeley K, Schneider K, Laird AR, Langner R, Eickhoff SB (2012) Parsing the neural correlates of moral cognition: ALE meta-analysis on morality, theory of mind, and empathy. Brain Struct Funct 217:783–796

Chang LJ, Doll BB, van 't Wout M, Frank MJ, Sanfey AG (2010) Seeing is believing: trustworthiness as a dynamic belief. Cogn Psychol 61:87–105

Chaudhuri A (2010) Fundamentals of sensory perception. Oxford university press, Don Mills

Cole MW, Schneider W (2007) The cognitive control network: Integrated cortical regions with dissociable functions. NeuroImage 37:343–360

Conty L, Dezecache G, Hugueville L, Grèze J (2012) Early binding of gaze, gesture, and emotion: neural time course and correlates. J Neurosci 32:4531–4539

Cwik JC, Sartory G, Schürholt B, Knuppertz H, Seitz RJ (2014) Posterior midline activation during symptom provocation in acute stress disorder: an fMRI study. Front Psychol 5:49. doi:10.3389/fpsyt.2014.00049

Döhnel K, Schuwerk T, Meinhardt J, Hajak G, Sommer M (2012) Functional activity of the right temporo-parietal junction and of the medial prefrontal cortex associated with true and false belief reasoning. NeuroImage 60:1652–1661

Duncan J, Seitz RJ, Kolodny J, Bor D, Herzog H, Ahmed A, Newell F, Emslie H (2000) A neural basis for general intelligence. Science 289:457–460

Duncan J, Owen AM (2000) Common regions of the human frontal lobe recruited by diverse cognitive demands. Trends Neurosci 23:475–483

Emmons RA, Paloutzian RF (2003) The psychology of religion. Annu Rev Psychol 54:377–402

Engel AK, Singer W (2001) Temporal binding and the neural correlates of sensory awareness. Trends Cogn Sci 5:16–25

Farrer C, Frith CD (2002) Experiencing oneself vs another person as being the cause of an action: the neural correlates of the experience of agency. NeuroImage 15:596–603

Fischbeck HJ (2005) Die Wahrheit und das Leben Wissenschaft und Glaube im 21. Jahrhundert, Herbertz Utz Verlag/München

Friston K (2010) The free-energy principle: a unified brain theory? Nat Rev Neurosci 11(2):127–138

Fuchs T (2009) Embodied cognitive neuroscience and its consequences for psychiatry. Poiesis Prax. doi:10.1007/s10202-008-0068-9

Grabenhorst F, Rolls ET (2011) Value, pleasure and choice in the ventral prefrontal cortex. Trends Cong Sci 15:56–67
Harry B, Davis C, Kim J (2012) Subliminal access to abstract face representations does not rely on attention. Conscious Cogn 21:573–583
Henkel LA, Mattson ME (2011) Reading is believing: the truth effect and source credibility. Conscious Cogn 20:1705–1721
Iver A, Lindner A, Kagan I, Andersen RA (2010) Motor preparatory activity in posterior parietal cortex is modulated by subjective absolute value. PLoS Biol 8:e1000444. doi:10.137/journal.pbio.1000444
Jeannerod M (1995) Mental imagery in the motor context. Neuropsychologia 33:1419–1432
Johnson SGB, Merchant T, Keil FC (2015) Predictions from uncertain beliefs. Proceeding of the 37th Annual Conference of the Cognitive Science Society, Austin, Texas, USA
Kahnt T, Heinzle J, Park SQ, Haynes JD (2010) The neural code of reward anticipation in human orbitofrontal cortex. PNAS USA 107:6010–6015
Kapogiannis D, Barbey AK, Su M, Zamboni G, Krueger F, Grafman J (2009) Cognitive and neural foundations of religious belief. Proc Natl Acad Sci U S A 106:4876–4881
Krueger F, Barbey AK, Grafman J (2009) The medial prefrontal cortex mediates social event knowledge. Trends Cogn Sci 13:103–109
Kuo WJ, Sjöström T, Chen YP, Wang YH, Huang CY (2009) Intuition and deliberation: two systems for strategizing in the brain. Science 324:519–522
La Cour P, Hvidt NC (2010) Research on meaning-making and health in secular society: secular, spiritual and religious existential orientations. Soc Sci Med 71:1292–1299
Mesulam M (2008) Representation, inference, and transcendent encoding in neurocognitive networks of the human brain. Ann Neurol 64:367–378
Morewedge CK, Kahneman D (2010) Associative processes in intuitive judgment. Trends Cogn Sci 14:435–440
Niendam TA, Laird AR, Ray KL, Dean VM, Glahn DC, Carter CS (2012) Meta-analytic evidence for a superordinate cognitive control network subserving diverse executive functions. Cogn Affect Behav Neurosci 12:241–268
Paloutzian RF, Park CL (2013) Recent progress and core isssues in the science of the psychology of religion and spirituality. In: Paloutzian RF, Park CL (eds) Handbook psychology spirituality, vol 1, 2nd edn. Guilford Press, New York, pp 3–22
Pechey R, Halligan P (2012) The prevalence of delusion-like beliefs relative to sociocultural beliefs in the general population. Psychopathology 44:106–115
Prochnow D, Kossack H, Brunheim S, Müller K, Wittsack H-J, Markowitsch H-J, Seitz RJ (2013) Processing of subliminal facial expressions of emotion: A behavioral and fMRI study. Soc Neurosci 8(5):448–486. doi:10.1080/17470919.2013.812536
Prochnow D, Brunheim S, Kossack H, Eickhoff S, Markowitsch HJ, Seitz RJ (2014) Anterior and posterior subareas of the dorsal lateral prefrontal cortex in socially relevant decisions based on masked affect expressions. doi:F1000research 3:212. doi:10.12668/f1000research/4734.1
Potthoff D, Seitz RJ (2015) Role of the first and second person perspective for control of behaviour: understanding other people's facial expressions. J Physiol (Paris) 109: 191–200
Roland PE, Mortensen E (1987) Somatosensory detection of microgeometry, macrogeometry and kinesthesia in man. Brain Res 434:1–42
Rolls ET (2006) Brain mechanisms underlying flavour and appetite. Philos Trans R Soc Lond Ser B Biol Sci 361:1123–1136
Roux F, Wibral M, Mohr HM, Singer W, Uhlhaas PJ (2012) Gamma-band activity in human prefrontal cortex codes for the number of relevant items maintained in working memory. J Neurosci 32:12411–12420
Sartory G, Cwik J, Knuppertz H, Schürholt B, Lebens M, Seitz RJ, Schulze R (2013) In search of the trauma memory: A meta-analysis of functional neuroimaging studies of symptom provocation in Posttraumatic Stress Disorder (PTSD). PLoS One 8:e58150

Schnell T (2003) A framework for the study of implicit religion: the psychological theory of implicit religiosity. Implicit Relig 6:86–104
Schweisfurth MA, Schweizer R, Treue S (2014) Feature-based attentional modulation of orientation perception in somatosensation. Front Hum Neurosci 14:519. doi:10.3389/fnhum.2014.00519
Seitz RJ, Nickel J, Azari NP (2006) Functional modularity of the medial prefrontal cortex: involvement in human empathy. Neuropsychology 20:743–751
Seitz RJ, Franz M, Azari NP (2009) Value judgments and self-control of action: The role of the medial frontal cortex. Brain Res Rev 60:368–378
Seitz RJ, Angel H-F (2012) Processes of believing - a review and conceptual account. Rev Neurosci 23:303–309
Seitz RJ, Angel H-F (2014) Psychology of Religion and Spirituality: Meaning Making and processes of believing. Relig Brain Behav. doi:10.1080/2153599X.2014.891249
Seligman R, Brown RA (2010) Theory and method at the intersection of anthropology and cultural neuroscience. SCAN 5:130–137. doi:10.1093/scan/nsp032
Smith MI (2011) Rapid processing of emotional expressions without conscious awareness. Cereb Cortex 22:1748–1760
Stoeckel MC, Weder B, Binkofski F, Buccino G, Shah NJ, Seitz RJ (2003) A fronto-parietal circuit for tactile object discrimination: an event-related fMRI study. NeuroImage 19:1103–1114
Sugiura M, Seitz RJ, Angel H-F (2015) Models and neural bases of the believing process. JBBS 5:12–23
Tsuchiya N, Kawasaki H, Oya H, Howard MA, Adolphs R (2008) Decoding face information in time, frequency and space from direct intracranial recordings of the human brain. PLoS One 3:e3892. doi:10.1371/journal.pone.0003892
Thurston JB, Carraher RG (1966) Optical illusions and the visual arts. Van Norstrand Reinhold, New York, p 18 (cited in Resnikoff HL. The illusion of reality. Springer Science, Heidelberg, New York, p 245)
van Gaal S, Scholte HS, Lamme VA, Fahrenfort JJ, Ridderinkhof KR (2011) Pre-SMA gray matter density predicts individual differences in action selection in the face of conscious and unconscious response conflict. J Cogn Neurosci 23:382–390
Vlaev I, Chater N, Steward N, Brown GDA (2011) Does the brain calculate value ? Trends Cogn Sci 15:546–554
Veit R, Konica L, Klinzing JG, Barth B, Yilmaz Ö, Birbaumer N (2013) Deficient fear conditioning in psychopathy as a function of interpersonal and affective disturbances. Front Hum Neurosci 7:706. doi:10.3389/fnhum.2013.00706
Watts F (2007) Emotion regulation and religion. In: Gross J (ed) Handb emotion regulation. Guildford Press, New York, pp 504–520
Wiese E, Wykowsky A, Müller HJ (2014) What we observe is biased by what other people tell us: beliefs about the reliability of gaze behavior modulate attentional orienting to gaze cues. Plos One 9(e):94529

Neurobiological Factors Underlying Attachment and Trust in the Believing Process

Corina Aguilar-Raab and Beate Ditzen

Abstract Credition – the cognitive process of believing – is embedded in a social-interactional framework. As soon as an individual becomes involved in a process of believing, he or she engages in motivational, cognitive, and affective processes based on the contact with and perception of an object of belief and the "community of believers" or "in-group members". Social cognition and social behaviour are the major constituents of these interactional processes. Apparently, attachment and trust – which are crucial for healthy outcomes throughout the lifespan – are strongly associated with one another. Psychobiological processes are important underlying factors that are entangled with the social-interactional dimension of credition. In social neuroscience, current research of the neuroendocrine system has primarily focused on the neuropeptides Oxytocin (OT) and Vasopressin (VP) as they have important regulatory functions when people engage in social interactions. For example, OT stimulates the motivation to develop an attachment to someone and increases qualities like trust. The effects are dependent on the influences of stress, as chronic and traumatic stress inhibits the motivation to attach while low levels of stress foster bonding behavior. In contrast, VP seems to be involved with increased vigilance, arousal, activation, and anxiety, which are required aspects of the flight-fight mechanism. Interestingly, whether OT and VP are associated with positive or negative social cognition and behavior depends on the (social) context and other contributing factors. We conclude that attachment and trust are important factors in the believing process. Combined with cognitive, emotional, and motivational processes, these factors influence behavior towards ourselves and others, which is in turn strongly influences neuroendocrine functions. Attachment and trust and their associated neurobiological foundations are reciprocally associated. Hence, a continuation of scientific progress needs to take place in order to produce more complex, high-quality, multi-dimensional and multi-disciplinary approaches. Only then will we be able to gain a more comprehensive understanding of these mechanisms and how we can effectively foster positive changes of social interactions related to health and well-being.

C. Aguilar-Raab (✉) • B. Ditzen
Institute of Medical Psychology, Center for Psychosocial Medicine (ZPM), University Hospital Heidelberg, Heidelberg, Germany
e-mail: corina.aguilar-raab@med.uni-heidelberg.de; beate.ditzen@med.uni-heidelberg.de

H.-F. Angel et al. (eds.), *Processes of Believing: The Acquisition, Maintenance, and Change in Creditions*, New Approaches to the Scientific Study of Religion 1,
DOI 10.1007/978-3-319-50924-2_6

> There is a strong current in contemporary culture advocating 'holistic' views as some sort of cure-all... Reductionism implies attention to a lower level while holistic implies attention to higher level. These are intertwined in any satisfactory description: and each entails some loss relative to our cognitive preferences, as well as some gain... there is no whole system without an interconnection of its parts and there is no whole system without an environment. (Varela 1977:77–85).

1 Introduction

Attachment and trust are important qualities that are certainly interrelated with social interactions. They are psychologically important throughout the lifespan as they are highly correlated with psychosocial wellbeing and health. The process of believing entails motivational, cognitive and affective aspects and it is embedded in a social framework. These components are related to neurobiological functioning that underlie social cognition and social behavior. Furthermore, attachment and trust as central social concepts are associated with a reduced responsiveness to stress and enhanced sense of control, with the latter referring to expectations about personal accomplishments and coincidental eventualities that effect performances and outcomes.

1.1 Social Neuroscience

Human social cognition, emotions and motivation, as well as social behavior are key elements of basic and applied research interests in the field of health, medical psychology and psychotherapy. In this context, the main aim is to shed more light on what are causal and contributable factors for the development and maintenance of mental and physical health, along with a focus on diseases and disorders and their most effective treatments. Recent research shows an increasing interest in the complexity of human functioning by taking into account the social context and framework. Influenced by a continuous increase in sophisticated methodology and technologies, research objectives have expanded towards more complex models. Not only does one witness linear and single-method but also non-linear and multi-method approaches that are partially based on interdisciplinary pathways operationalized in terms of social interactional paradigms; these reveal a deeper understanding of the depended arising nature of psychological phenomena (Ditzen and Heinrichs 2014; Ditzen et al. 2007, 2008; Insel 2013). This is also reflected in the relatively young field of "social" neuroscience, with an emerging body of substantial publications (Editorial 2012).

As social beings, we are interconnected with and interdependent on each other. We fundamentally rely on others. Along our lifespans, we experience social support and help towards survival and the fulfillment of the integrity of bio-psycho-social and even religious/spiritual aspects of life (Berkman and Kawachi 2000; Schwarz

2009; Uchino 2006). In this process, we are in need of affiliation with a caregiver (the mother, father, significant other), whereby this affiliation is rooted in a continuously reciprocal process that produces attachment (styles) and trust – first towards the primary caregiver (as an outer object), after which one can internalize towards oneself.

In this sense, research on human experience and behavior pays closer attention to (social) context and various contextual factors.

1.2 Believing – In What?

From a psychological point of view, beliefs or the act of believing contain various definitions that do not necessarily share a common understanding. Beliefs are part of our personality and importantly influence our perceptions and behavior. In order to understand how behaviors arise (Ajzen, 1985; Bandura 1982, 1997), the idea of how people perceive their capacity to control and influence results, reactions and the like is crucial to understand. In this sense, believing refers to the fact that individuals have diverse perspectives about if and how they might affect several outcomes.

As far as the cognitive process of believing is concerned – termed as "credition" by Seitz and Angel (2012) – attachment, bonding and trust emerge to be some of the crucial aspects. Nevertheless, one can begin the journey of reflection by questioning, "In what to believe, with regard to which object?" In theistic religions the object of belief is very often endowed with human characteristics (intellect, emotions; form/shape). This might be due to the boundaries of our cognitive processes. However, in non-theistic religions such as Buddhism, spiritual teachers and/or deities, who comprise and represent the refinement of inner mental qualities, are also equipped with it. The point is, it is easier to relate to something with which we are familiar and with which we share common grounds. At the same time, from an educational point of view, it is a skillful means to build up a "belief system" in such a way (in terms of being based on human mechanisms of perception, cognition etc.) so that we are able grasp, on the one hand, something that might be inconceivable and which is difficult to rationally explain or which is difficult to imagine at a stage of beginners; and, on the other hand, to benefit from the spiritual practices that are meant to be applied (in terms of commitment, continuity etc.).

With regard to the "Big Four" model of religious dimensions (4 Bs: believing, bonding, behaving, and belonging, Saroglou 2011) as a cross-cultural and universal model, believing can manifest in many different ways, but it is a "basic universal component of religion, (…) and connected with people's meaning-making process" (p. 1323). From a functional aspect, believing ensures the upholding of certain beliefs, convictions and views in more or less dogmatic and tolerant ways. Bonding is outlined by emotional aspects that essentially come about through an association with transcendence (nature, cosmos, god, deities etc.). As the triggered emotional experiences can be positive (e.g. love) or negative (e.g. guilt), emotional stability can vary across belief systems. The dimension of behaving is about ethics and norms that shape interactions such as altruism and pro-social behavior; but it can also refer to religious/spiritual practices (rituals etc.). Belonging is the source of social identity, which might lead to the feeling of interconnectedness, self-esteem and the like (Saroglou 2011). Furthermore, belonging to a religious sub-group is important for building social trust, and the stage of trust is dependent on contact with the group members and reliance on the belief system (Welch et al. 2004). It can be shown that informal social ties can enhance generalized trust. Additionally, health improvement is related to intensification of trust (Glanville et al. 2013).

1.3 Neurobiological Grounds

Based on animal and human research, it is well established that our neuroendocrine system regulates social cognition, emotion and motivation, and this in turn regulates behavior (McCall and Singer 2012). Various hormones have important regulatory functions in these mechanisms (Insel and Young 2001). In recent research, the neuropeptides Oxytocin (OT) and Vasopressin (VP) – of which the latter is also referred to as arginine vasopressin (AVP) or antidiuretic hormone (ADH; for its functioning in terms of water retention) – have been of foremost interest in social neurosciences (Ebstein et al. 2012; Ferri and Flanagan-Cato 2012; Young and Wang 2004). They share evolutionary origins and comprise similar biochemical structure of peptides (both have nine amino acids rings, though there are differences in two of nine amino acids) (Carter 2007). The term OT is rooted in Greek and means "quick birth" – as OT is an important promoter in delivery, milk letdown reflex, etc. It is found in all kinds of mammals, females and males alike, although gender differences have been shown (e.g. it seems as if VP is predominantly important in male behavior) (Carter 2007).

OT is produced in the hypothalamus; in particular, it is synthesized in the paraventricular and supraoptic nuclei of the hypothalamus. As a hormone, it is released into the blood stream and transported to pituitary gland (and further on in the course of systemic circulation), while as a neurotransmitter it is involved in the processes of emotional and behavioral responses in different parts of the brain (Smith et al. 2006; Sofroniew 1983; Stoop 2014). OT plays a significant role in the limbic system, which includes the amygdala among other structures. VP is secreted into the amygdala, olfactory bulb, bed nucleus of stria terminalis and the locus coeruleus (Stoop 2014). As OT and VP are released into the CNS, they affect receptors in various brain regions. OT and VP receptors are found in brainstem regions that are involved in reproductive and social behaviors, and are connected to the hypothalamic pituitary adrenal hypothalamic-pituitary-adrenocortical (HPA) axis, and furthermore to the ANS (Carter 2007; Landgraf and Neumann 2004).

The HPA and the sympatho-adrenal medullary axes maintain or reinstate homeostasis during stress. Both react interactively but there are differences in timing: The HPA axis reacts slower to the perception of stressors than the SNS and is mediated by corticotropin-releasing hormones (CRF), adrenocorticotropic hormone (ACTH) and cortisol. This reaction enables an assimilation to stress that possibly takes up to several days (Ulrich-Lai and Herman 2009). Studies on mice have shown that CRF in low to medium dose stimulates the release of dopamine in the nucleus accumbens (NAcc) and therefore increases approach behaviors – an effect that does not persist when exposed to chronic stress (Lemos et al. 2012). For humans, this indicates that low levels of stress influence bonding, which is mediated by CRF and dopamine positively while chronic or traumatic stress inhibits the motivation to attach. Dopamine-regulated reward mechanisms interact with the neuropeptide OT to mediate the motivation to attach to someone (Domes et al. 2014; Kanat et al. 2014). Strathearn assumes that the nigrostriatal dopamine system plays a mediating role as well: Parts of the striatum serve as a switchpoint for dopamine and project the influence of social stimuli to prefrontal areas that are involved in processing of affects and cognition. Learning experiences with positive social interactions stimulate the release of OT which then – mediated by dopamine mechanisms – enable the feelings of joy and emotional security (Strathearn 2011).

The systemic effects of OT are associated with the contraction of muscles and different kinds of outputs and fluids released from the body (of sperms/sperm interjection, fetus, placenta, milk; Buckley 2010). On an emotional and behavioral level, it supports the processes of love, pleasure, sexual activity, social behavior and bonding (maternal, infant etc.), relaxation, breast-feeding, nesting, aggressive protective behaviors etc. Emotions both activate and are activated by hormone production, which leads to physiological reactions of the parasympathetic and sympathetic nervous systems (Schmid and Downe 2010). As OT can be understood as a modulator, it fosters connecting and calming responses involved in the parasympathetic nervous system. In line with that, OT stimuli include touch, warmth, social interaction, security etc. Human brain regions, which are endowed with OT and VP receptors, show activation by maternal and romantic love (Bartels and Zeki 2004; Jenkins et al. 1984; Loup et al. 1991). For example, in social interactions, intranasal administration of OT reduces the neuroendocrine response to stress (Ditzen et al. 2009; Heinrichs et al. 2003) as well as the cortisol responses to a couple conflict discussion in women (Ditzen et al. 2009) and reduces anxiety (Kirsch et al. 2005). The administration of intranasal OT revealed also mediation effects in the framework of social cognition and perception (RME-Test: Domes et al. 2007). Qualities like generosity, cooperation and trust increased due to OT (Kosfeld et al. 2005; Theodoridou et al. 2009). Alternatively, VP might function in an anxiogenic way connected to the sympathetic nervous system, increasing behavioral and neuroendocrine levels of anxiety. VP seems to go along with increased vigilance, arousal, activation and anxiety, which are required aspects in the flight-fight mechanism (Carter 2007; Peichl 2009).

Current studies have shown that oxytocin cannot be regarded as a "love-hormone" per se (Guzman et al. 2013). Much depends on the context indicating strong social in- and out-group effects ("in-group trust" vs. defensive financial behavior towards out-groups; "in-group favoritism" vs. "out-group derogation") (De Dreu et al. 2010, 2011), as well as that intranasal oxytocin increases envy ("Schadenfreude": Shamay-Tsoory et al. 2009). Furthermore, the valence of its effects depends on personal experience (Bertsch et al. 2013; Heim et al. 2008).

2 Bridging Neurobiological Grounds to Processes of Believing

Attachment/bonding and trust are two of the main important qualities that build close and important relationships between (sentient) beings in the social world – as we have described before. These processes are notably connected with neurobiological factors. Here, the process of believing is pervaded by trust – trust in the object and in the practices of belief. The followers of religious or spiritual systems need to place their own trust in the guidance (and the grace) of the object, whether it is external or internal. In line with that, we can define this as an interactional process where the increase of trust – which as mentioned above can be induced by administration of OT – leads to higher benefits of this somehow "social" interactions. As described in Fig. 1, the process of believing is embedded in a triangle of cognition, emotion, and motivation, which are influenced by neuroendocrine mechanisms and vice versa. This is reciprocally connected to behaviors, as on the one hand behavior might have a more conscious impact on cognition, emotion and motivation, and on the other hand, experience might have an effect on endocrine responses. Indeed, the whole process is integrated in social and environmental cues and its interactive processes.

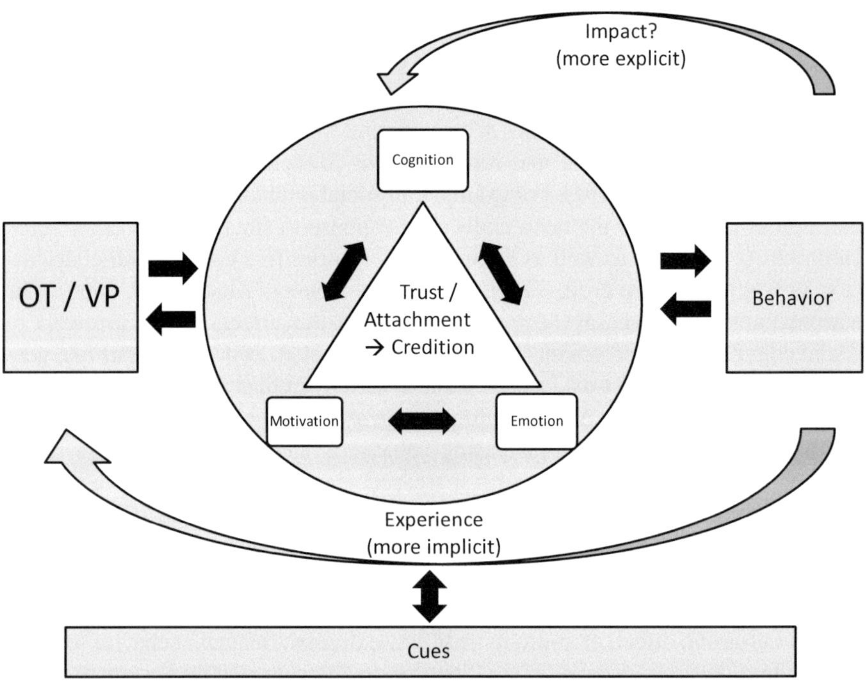

Fig. 1 Reciprocal connections between attachment/trust and the process of believing in the interplay of cognitive, emotional and motivational qualities influenced by OT/VP and social/environmental cues leading to behavior (inspired and based on (McCall and Singer 2012)

As far as the neurobiological foundation is concerned, OT is important for connecting and calming down responses, crucial, for example, in the process of pregnancy, giving birth and early mother-child interactions as it might influence the fetus/child in the genetic formation and epigenetic functioning (Pariante 2014; Puglia et al. 2015; Rodrigues et al. 2009). A lack of appropriate contextual factors and social responses in prenatal phase, delivery and early childhood might lead to "social suffering" in the sense of a lack of social interactional abilities (e.g. previous attachment insecurity might be the case in borderline personality disorder) (Barone 2003; Fonagy et al. 2000). Hypothetically, this in turn might lead to a higher need for emotional stability, trust, or security, which might foster compensation by turning towards religion and contemplative/spiritual practices (given that many religious/spiritual engagements are motivated by personal suffering and the drive for change). Based on the reciprocal nature of adaptation and influencing capacities (see also assimilation vs. accommodation: Piaget 1976) as well as the neuroplasticity of the brain, religion/spirituality – if trust is placed in its objects of worship and practice – might activate the synthesis of OT and reinforce pro-religious/spiritual behaviors.

In order to understand phenomena – whether in terms of internal states or external events – humans develop the skills and means to create models which are similar to human form and functioning. This leads to a societal interactional process – not only with the primordially involved object of belief and practice, but also – at least as a side-effect but sometimes as an essential matter – with the religious/spiritual community (e.g. the Sangha in Buddhist terms). From a social scientific perspective on religious communities and other social groups, believing includes shared motivations and actions because they are essential for a group to function. From the outside, third-person perspective, believing functions on a psychological level in terms of bonding and belonging (affiliation and identification), which is associated with in- and out-group effects (in this context e.g. referring to religious/spiritual dogmatism). This is similar to the early child-mother interactions and its underlying neurobiological factors. Therefore, we might conclude that the underlying neurobiological factors are also relevant for the interactional process with the object of belief as well as with members of the religious communities. On an individual level, the relationship between the believer and the object of belief manifests in similar ways as between humans in a social interactional framework. It can be assumed that similar neurobiological factors are correlated with processes in which attachment, a certain kind of bonding and trust play a causal role of the functional process of believing. On a social level, within centers of practice and worship, in- and out-group effects might be generally regulated by OT/VT. Religious/spiritual communities tend to strengthen the cohesion of the group of followers by exaggerating positive and beneficial aspects of their own concepts/practices and neglecting the value of diversity or otherness of non-members (Abrams and Hogg 2006; Hunsberger and Jackson 2005; Johnson et al. 2012).

With regard to the process of believing, one can think of the cognitive process in which certain functions evolve gradually and are correlated to various activities in certain brain regions (Seitz and Angel 2012). But one can also think of religious or spiritual practices (prayer, reading sacred texts, contemplation, meditation etc.) that are embedded in this process (see above "behaving").

When applying techniques of mind training, enhancing positive, prosocial emotions and cognitions which for example is the case for engaging in the four brahmaviharas or so called four immeasurables or virtues (loving kindness, compassion, joyous effort, equanimity; (Hinton et al. 2013; Hofmann et al. 2011), it might be concluded that OT mediates the effects of these practices or that they lead to an increased regulation of OT-receptors in the brain (Mascaro et al. 2015) – even under pathological conditions of impaired sociability as seen in Autism spectrum disorder (Lukas and Neumann 2011). Empathy, which is somehow related to the mentioned mental qualities, seems to be associated with genetic variation of OT receptors (Carter 2014; Rodrigues et al. 2009). This in turn, can be strongly related to reinforcing processes of believing being rooted in attachment and trust (Carter 2014).

Contemplative practices might lead to an alteration in the release of hormones like OT that might foster experiences of calming down and feelings of connectedness, which are the frequently self-reported effects of such techniques (Hutcherson et al. 2008; Torner et al. 2002).

3 Discussion

The paragraphs above illustrate the interconnections between social neurosciences emphasizing neuroendocrinological mechanisms in the social context and how motivation, cognition, and emotions, which are significantly involved in the process of believing, are rooted in these basic functions. Clearly, our intention was not to reduce the complexity of human experience and behavior and its causal rationalizations to bio-psychological agencies. Instead, we sought to offer a glimpse of neurobiological underpinnings and that this in itself, is far more complex, as the growing recent research in this specific field demonstrates.

Most importantly, research on OT/VP and the generalizability of its insights have to be handled with caution. There are highly interdepended and reflexive processes on every level beginning at micro up to macro cosmos; it is important to consider the dependency of outcomes and findings on distal and proximal circumstances (time, space, dynamic etc.). Therefore, more studies focusing on high external validity and ecologically valid methods are necessary in order to gain more insides in important real-life matters in/of humans, their social world and (ecological) environments.

With regard to endocrinology in particular, there is a need to investigate gender differences because significant gender interactions could be found in both OT and VP (Bartz et al. 2011). Furthermore, early positive and adverse life experiences and the formation of attachment styles might influence the OT synthesis and receptor expressions (Olff et al. 2013; Walum et al. 2012). In this sense, theories of psychoanalysis or psychodynamics in the field of psychotherapy appear in a different light and gain more evidence by neurophysiological findings, demonstrating some complementarity among sciences (Fonagy et al. 2007).

Accounting for these factors and in line with McCall and Singer (2012), the influence of neuropeptides and steroid hormones on motivation, cognition, emotion, and behavior is modulated by neurochemical interactions but also by intra-species variations in terms of receptor density in the brain, individual differences like sex, and environmental factors as well as context-specific aspects (like tasks etc.). The movement towards more complex, high-quality and multi-dimensional approaches, which are enriched by inter-disciplinarity, has already started (Insel 2013).

As the plasticity of the brain and neuropeptide functioning seems to be very promising in promoting beneficial changes for mental and physical health, we would like to risk a confident glance towards the future. Mental and physical well-being and health can be gained by a self-effective effort of applying different interventions and techniques which – whether there is a spiritual/religious or just a common health behavior dimension (or secular "spiritual"/"contemplative" practice such as stress reduction programs – like MBSR: Kabat-Zinn 1990) – credition (process of believing) is an important element being entangled with cognitive, emotional, and motivational aspects influencing behavior towards ourselves and others.

The potential for change, which is at the root of psychotherapy and other interventions and which may also be a part of belief systems, comes forth by the possibility of changing one's own attitude, viewing, and convicting/believing (based on insight and learning), and in turn positively influencing cognitive and emotional states. A positive, and possibly qualitative, shift in religious/spiritual view/perspective and belief can be essential in alleviating suffering – although we may narrowly focus on ourselves and take our perspective for granted, not realizing that suffering may enable us to grow with a deep feeling of interconnectedness.

The first person perspective, subjective experience, and understanding will always be the natural reference point in the process of believing, whether in the context of religion and spirituality or in the context of research. The problem might not be defined by the dualistic oscillation between subjectivity and objectivity, but how we gain a beneficial insight by taking into account first, second, and third person perspectives and their mutual interaction (Shear and Varela 1999). In this sense, science might improve to the extent that it is able to include first person perspectives, experience, and insights and their interrelationships by taking multiple perspective, multi-method, and interdisciplinary approaches, which have already become the promising horizon.

According to a salutogenetic approach (Antonovsky 1997), health is promoted by sense of coherence that includes meaningfulness, comprehensibility, and manageability. The process of believing also covers a phenomenon in which meaning making takes place. Taking this into account, meaning-centered coping or religious/spiritual-coping strategies play an important role; for example, in dealing with the existential breakdowns when facing insecurity, impermanence, and mortality (Pargament et al. 2000). To transform the perspective and attitude towards such a threat and finding ways of integrating it cognitively and emotionally helps to rebuild healthy minds and lives (Mehnert et al.2007; Vehling et al. 2011). In everyday terms, living a meaningful life rests upon investigating the nature of one's own realities. Healthy and compassionate relationships towards others and ourselves are crucial in this regard (Dalai Lama 2012).

To conclude, there is a positive link between process of believing and mental and physical health. Meaningfulness, positive emotions, attachment security and other states are significantly positively correlated (Saroglou 2011). They are not independent processes; mind and body are interdependent.

References

Abrams D, Hogg MA (2006) Social identifications: a social psychology of intergroup relations and group processes. Routledge, New York

Ajzen I (1985) From intentions to actions: a theory of planned behavior. In: Kuhl J, Beckmann J (eds) Action control. Springer, Berlin/Heidelberg, pp 11–39

Antonovsky A (1997) Salutogenese . Zur Entmystifizierung der Gesundheit. dgvt-Verlag, Tübingen

Bandura A (1982) Self-efficacy mechanism in human agency. Am Psychol 37(2):122–147. doi:10.1037/0003-066X.37.2.122

Bandura A (1997) Self-efficacy: the exercise of control. Macmillan, New York

Barone L (2003) Developmental protective and risk factors in borderline personality disorder: a study usingtheadultattachmentinterview.AttachHumDev5(1):64–77.doi:10.1080/1461673031000078634

Bartels A, Zeki S (2004) The neural correlates of maternal and romantic love. NeuroImage 21(3):1155–1166

Bartz JA, Zaki J, Bolger N, Ochsner KN (2011) Social effects of oxytocin in humans: context and person matter. Trends Cogn Sci 15(7):301–309. doi http://dx.doi.org/10.1016/j.tics.2011.05.002

Berkman LF, Kawachi I (2000) Social epidemiology. Oxford University Press, New York

Bertsch K, Schmidinger I, Neumann ID, Herpertz SC (2013) Reduced plasma oxytocin levels in female patients with borderline personality disorder. Horm Behav 63(3):424–429. doi:http://dx.doi.org/10.1016/j.yhbeh.2012.11.013

Buckley S (2010) Sexuality in labour and birth: an intimate perspective. In: Walsh D, Downe S (eds) Essential midwifery practice: intrapartum care. West Sussex UK, Wiley-Blackwell, pp 213–234

Carter CS (2007) Sex differences in oxytocin and vasopressin: implications for autism spectrum disorders? Behav Brain Res 176(1):170–186. doi:http://dx.doi.org/10.1016/j.bbr.2006.08.025

Carter CS (2014) Oxytocin pathways and the evolution of human behavior. Annu Rev Psychol 65(1):17–39. doi:10.1146/annurev-psych-010213-115110

Dalai Lama (2012) Beyond religion: ethics and happiness in a global world. Rider, London

De Dreu CKW, Greer LL, Handgraaf MJJ, Shalvi S, Van Kleef GA, Baas M, Feith SWW (2010) The neuropeptide oxytocin regulates parochial altruism in intergroup conflict among humans. Science 328(5984):1408–1411. doi:10.1126/science.1189047

De Dreu CKW, Greer LL, Van Kleef GA, Shalvi S, Handgraaf MJ (2011) Oxytocin promotes human ethnocentrism. Proc Natl Acad Sci 108(4):1262–1266

Ditzen B, Heinrichs M (2014) Psychobiology of social support: the social dimension of stress buffering. Restor Neurol Neurosci 32(1):149–162

Ditzen B, Neumann ID, Bodenmann G, von Dawans B, Turner RA, Ehlert U, Heinrichs M (2007) Effects of different kinds of couple interaction on cortisol and heart rate responses to stress in women. Psychoneuroendocrinology 32(5):565–574

Ditzen B, Schaer M, Gabriel B, Bodenmann G, Ehlert U, Heinrichs M (2009) Intranasal oxytocin increases positive communication and reduces cortisol levels during couple conflict. Biol Psychiatry 65(9):728–731. doi:http://dx.doi.org/10.1016/j.biopsych.2008.10.011

Ditzen B, Schmidt S, Strauss B, Nater UM, Ehlert U, Heinrichs M (2008) Adult attachment and social support interact to reduce psychological but not cortisol responses to stress. J Psychosom Res 64(5):479–486
Domes G, Heinrichs M, Michel A, Berger C, Herpertz SC (2007) Oxytocin improves "mind-reading" in humans. Biol Psychiatry 61(6):731–733. doi:http://dx.doi.org/10.1016/j.biopsych.2006.07.015
Domes G, Kumbier E, Heinrichs M, Herpertz SC (2014) Oxytocin promotes facial emotion recognition and amygdala reactivity in adults with Asperger Syndrome. Neuropsychopharmacology 39(3):698–706. doi:10.1038/npp.2013.254
Ebstein RP, Knafo A, Mankuta D, Chew SH, Lai PS (2012) The contributions of oxytocin and vasopressin pathway genes to human behavior. Horm Behav 61(3):359–379. doi:http://dx.doi.org/10.1016/j.yhbeh.2011.12.014
Editoral (2012) Focus on social neuroscience. Nat Neurosci 15(5):645–645
Ferri SL, Flanagan-Cato LM (2012) Oxytocin and dendrite remodeling in the hypothalamus. Horm Behav 61(3):251–258. doi:http://dx.doi.org/10.1016/j.yhbeh.2012.01.012
Fonagy P, Target M, Gergely G (2000) Attachment and borderline personality disorder: a theory and some evidence. Psychiatr Clin N Am 23(1):103–122
Fonagy P, Mayes L, Target M (2007) Developmental science and psychoanalysis: integration and innovation. Karnac Books, London
Glanville JL, Andersson MA, Paxton P (2013) Do social connections create trust? An examination using new longitudinal data social forces doi:10.1093/sf/sot079
Guzman YF, Tronson NC, Jovasevic V, Sato K, Guedea AL, Mizukami H, Radulovic J (2013) Fear-enhancing effects of septal oxytocin receptors. Nat Neurosci 16(9):1185–1187. doi:10.1038/nn.3465
Heim C, Young LJ, Newport DJ, Mletzko T, Miller AH, Nemeroff CB (2008) Lower CSF oxytocin concentrations in women with a history of childhood abuse. Mol Psychiatry 14(10):954–958
Heinrichs M, Baumgartner T, Kirschbaum C, Ehlert U (2003) Social support and oxytocin interact to suppress cortisol and subjective responses to psychosocial stress. Biol Psychiatry 54(12):1389–1398. doi:http://dx.doi.org/10.1016/S0006-3223(03)00465-7
Hinton DE, Ojserkis RA, Jalal B, Peou S, Hofmann SG (2013) Loving-kindness in the treatment of traumatized refugees and minority groups: A typology of mindfulness and the nodal network model of affect and affect regulation. J Clin Psychol 69(8):817–828
Hofmann SG, Grossman P, Hinton DE (2011) Loving-kindness and compassion meditation: potential for psychological interventions. Clin Psychol Rev 31(7):1126–1132. doi:http://dx.doi.org/10.1016/j.cpr.2011.07.003
Hunsberger B, Jackson LM (2005) Religion, meaning, and prejudice. J Soc Issues 61(4):807–826. doi:10.1111/j.1540-4560.2005.00433.x
Hutcherson CA, Seppala EM, Gross JJ (2008) Loving-kindness meditation increases social connectedness. Emotion 8(5):720–724. doi:10.1037/a0013237
Insel TR (2013) Transforming Diagnosis. http://www.nimh.nih.gov/about/director/2013/transforming-diagnosis.shtml
Insel TR, Young LJ (2001) The neurobiology of attachment. Nat Rev Neurosci 2(2):129–136
Jenkins JS, Ang VT, Hawthorn J, Rossor MN, Iversen LL (1984) Vasopressin, oxytocin and neurophysins in the human brain and spinal cord. Brain Res 291(1):111–117
Johnson MK, Rowatt WC, LaBouff JP (2012) Religiosity and prejudice revisited: in-group favoritism, out-group derogation, or both? Psychol Relig Spiritual 4(2):154–168. doi:10.1037/a0025107
Kabat-Zinn J (1990) Full catastrophe living: using the wisdom of your mind and body to face stress, pain, and illness. Delacorte, New York
Kanat M, Heinrichs M, Domes G (2014) Oxytocin and the social brain: Neural mechanisms and perspectives in human research. Brain Res 1580:160–171. doi:http://dx.doi.org/10.1016/j.brainres.2013.11.003
Kirsch P, Esslinger C, Chen Q, Mier D, Lis S, Siddhanti S, Meyer-Lindenberg A (2005) Oxytocin modulates neural circuitry for social cognition and fear in humans. J Neurosci 25(49):11489–11493. doi:10.1523/jneurosci.3984-05.2005

Kosfeld M, Heinrichs M, Zak PJ, Fischbacher U, Fehr E (2005) Oxytocin increases trust in humans. Nature 435(7042):673–676
Landgraf R, Neumann ID (2004) Vasopressin and oxytocin release within the brain: a dynamic concept of multiple and variable modes of neuropeptide communication. Front Neuroendocrinol 25(3):150–176
Lemos JC, Wanat MJ, Smith JS, Reyes BA, Hollon NG, Van Bockstaele EJ, Phillips PE (2012) Severe stress switches CRF action in the nucleus accumbens from appetitive to aversive. Nature 490(7420):402–406. doi:10.1038/nature11436
Loup F, Tribollet E, Dubois-Dauphin M, Dreifuss JJ (1991) Localization of highaffinity binding sites for oxytocin and vasopressin in the human brain. An autoradiographic study. Brain Res 555(2):220–232
Lukas M, Neumann ID (2011) Brain oxytocin is a main regulator of prosocial behaviour - link to psychopathology. In: Eapen V (ed) Autism – a neurodevelopmental journey from genes to behaviour. InTech, Rijeka. doi:10.5772/18841
Mascaro JS, Darcher A, Negi LT, Raison CL (2015) The neural mediators of kindness-based meditation: a theoretical model. Front Psychol 6:109. doi:10.3389/fpsyg.2015.00109
McCall C, Singer T (2012) The animal and human neuroendocrinology of social cognition, motivation and behavior. Nat Neurosci 15(5):681–688
Mehnert A, Müller D, Koch U (2007) Die Erfassung von sinnbasierten Bewältigungsstrategien und Lebenseinstellungen. Z Klin Psychol Psychother 36(3):176–188. doi:10.1026/1616-3443.36.3.176
Olff M, Frijling JL, Kubzansky LD, Bradley B, Ellenbogen MA, Cardoso C, van Zuiden M (2013) The role of oxytocin in social bonding, stress regulation and mental health: an update on the moderating effects of context and interindividual differences. Psychoneuroendocrinology 38(9):1883–1894. doi:http://dx.doi.org/10.1016/j.psyneuen.2013.06.019
Pargament KI, Koenig HG, Perez LM (2000) The many methods of religious coping: development and initial validation of the RCOPE. J Clin Psychol 56(4):519–543
Pariante CM (2014) Depression during pregnancy: molecular regulations of mothers' and children's behaviour. Biochem Soc Trans 42(2):582–586. doi:10.1042/bst20130246
Piaget J (1976) Piaget's Theory. In: Inhelder B, Chipman H, Zwingmann C (eds) Piaget and his school. Springer, Berlin/Heidelberg, pp 11–23
Peichl J (2009) Neurogene Reaktion auf Bedrohung, Liebensbindung und traumatische Opfer-Täter-Bindung. Trauma and Gewalt 1:18–33
Puglia MH, Lillard TS, Morris JP, Connelly JJ (2015) Epigenetic modification of the oxytocin receptor gene influences the perception of anger and fear in the human brain. Proc Natl Acad Sci U S A 112(11):3308–3313. doi:10.1073/pnas.1422096112
Rodrigues SM, Saslow LR, Garcia N, John OP, Keltner D (2009) Oxytocin receptor genetic variation relates to empathy and stress reactivity in humans. Proc Natl Acad Sci 106(50):21437–21441. doi:10.1073/pnas.0909579106
Saroglou V (2011) Believing, bonding, behaving, and belonging: the big four religious dimensions and cultural variation. J Cross-Cult Psychol 42(8):1320–1340. doi:10.1177/0022022111412267
Schmid V, Downe S (2010) Midwifery skills for normalising unusual labours. In: Walsh D, Downe S (eds) Essential midwifery practice: intrapartum care. Wiley-Blackwell, West Sussex, pp 159–190
Schwarz M (2009) Is psychology based on a methodological error? Integr Psychol Behav Sci 43(3):185–213. doi:10.1007/s12124-009-9089-8
Seitz RJ, Angel HF (2012) Processes of believing – a review and conceptual account. Rev Neurosci 23(3):303–309
Shamay-Tsoory SG, Fischer M, Dvash J, Harari H, Perach-Bloom N, Levkovitz Y (2009) Intranasal administration of oxytocin increases envy and Schadenfreude (Gloating). Biol Psychiatry 66(9):864–870. doi:http://dx.doi.org/10.1016/j.biopsych.2009.06.009
Shear J, Varela FJ (1999) The view from within: first-person approaches to the study of consciousness. Academic, Imprint
Smith MP, Ayad VJ, Mundell SJ, McArdle CA, Kelly E, Lopez Bernal A (2006) Internalization and desensitization of the oxytocin receptor is inhibited by Dynamin and clathrin mutants in human embryonic kidney 293 cells. Mol Endocrinol 20(2):379–388. doi:10.1210/me.2005-0031

Sofroniew MV (1983) Morphology of vasopressin and oxytocin neurones and their central and vascular projections. Prog Brain Res 60:101–114. doi:10.1016/s0079-6123(08)64378-2
Stoop R (2014) Neuromodulation by oxytocin and vasopressin in the central nervous system as a basis for their rapid behavioral effects. Curr Opin Neurobiol 29:187–193. doi:http://dx.doi.org/10.1016/j.conb.2014.09.012
Strathearn L (2011) Maternal neglect: oxytocin, dopamine and the neurobiology of attachment. J Neuroendocrinol 23(11):1054–1065. doi:10.1111/j.1365-2826.2011.02228.x
Theodoridou A, Rowe AC, Penton-Voak IS, Rogers PJ (2009) Oxytocin and social perception: oxytocin increases perceived facial trustworthiness and attractiveness. Horm Behav 56(1):128–132. doi:http://dx.doi.org/10.1016/j.yhbeh.2009.03.019
Torner L, Toschi N, Nava G, Clapp C, Neumann ID (2002) Increased hypothalamic expression of prolactin in lactation: involvement in behavioural and neuroendocrine stress responses. Eur J Neurosci 15(8):1381–1389
Uchino BN (2006) Social support and health: a review of physiological processes potentially underlying links to disease outcomes. J Behav Med 29(4):377–387. doi:10.1007/s10865-006-9056-5
Ulrich-Lai YM, Herman JP (2009) Neural regulation of endocrine and autonomic stress responses. Nat Rev Neurosci 10(6):397–409. doi:10.1038/nrn2647
Vehling S, Lehmann C, Oechsle K, Bokemeyer C, Krüll A, Koch U, Mehnert A (2011) Global meaning and meaning-related life attitudes: exploring their role in predicting depression, anxiety, and demoralization in cancer patients. Support Care Cancer 19(4):513–520
Walum H, Lichtenstein P, Neiderhiser JM, Reiss D, Ganiban JM, Spotts EL, Westberg L (2012) Variation in the oxytocin receptor gene is associated with pair-bonding and social behavior. Biol Psychiatry 71(5):419–426. doi:http://dx.doi.org/10.1016/j.biopsych.2011.09.002
Welch MR, Sikkink D, Sartain E, Bond C (2004) Trust in god and trust in man: the ambivalent role of religion in shaping dimensions of social trust. J Sci Study Relig 43(3):317–343. doi:10.1111/j.1468-5906.2004.00238.x
Young LJ, Wang Z (2004) The neurobiology of pair bonding. Nat Neurosci 7(10):1048–1054

New Concepts on the Motor System: Implications for Emotions and Credition

Giovanni Buccino and Ivan Colagè

Abstract Experimental studies carried out over the last two decades have radically changed our conception of the brain motor system. The discovery of mirror neurons in the monkey brain and the evidence in the human brain of a mirror mechanism, whose neural substrate most likely relies on mirror neurons, support the notion that the role of the motor system is not limited to the execution of actions, but also includes the ability to understand action and to code the intentions behind others' actions. This experimental evidence extends the role of the motor system to cover functions traditionally considered as cognitive. The mirror mechanism first described for mirror neurons seems to be a more general functional mechanism in the brain, extending also to emotions and sensations; the neural substrates active when we feel certain emotions and sensations are also active when we observe other people feeling those same emotions or sensations. Thus, these mechanisms may turn out to constitute a biologically grounded link between ourselves and other individuals. After reviewing the main data and theories about the mirror mechanisms for actions and emotions, this paper outlines how these mechanisms may be relevant for self-related processes, especially insofar as these processes are engaged in social interactions. From this, links with the relevance of credition theory are proposed. In particular, assuming that beliefs are at the root of action choice and selection of appropriate behaviours in social contexts, the theory of credition may provide a conceptual framework helpful in integrating the "simulation theory" and the "theory-theory" approaches to mentalizing, also suggesting how explicit mentalizing processes may actually be grounded in more implicit mirror mechanisms.

G. Buccino (✉)
Dipartimento di Scienze Mediche e Chirurgiche, Università degli Studi Magna Graecia di Catanzaro, Viale Salvatore Venuta - Loc. Germaneto, 88100 Catanzaro, Italy
e-mail: buccino@unicz.it

I. Colagè
Pontifical University Antonianum, Rome, Italy
e-mail: i.colage@antonianum.eu

H.-F. Angel et al. (eds.), *Processes of Believing: The Acquisition, Maintenance, and Change in Creditions*, New Approaches to the Scientific Study of Religion 1,
DOI 10.1007/978-3-319-50924-2_7

1 Introduction

As of 20 years ago, the motor system was thought to consist of three areas located in the frontal lobe: the primary motor area, largely corresponding to Brodmann area (BA) 4; the premotor area, corresponding to BA 6; and the supplementary motor area (SMA), situated in the mesial part of the frontal cortex. The main role attributed to the primary motor area was to execute movements, while the premotor and supplementary motor areas were considered to be mainly involved in action planning and motor imagery, respectively. This notion has been radically changed by experimental evidence derived from studies on neuroanatomy and neurophysiology (Rizzolatti et al. 1998). Anatomical studies have shown that motor areas may be subdivided into sub-areas that are now indicated by the letter F (which stands for "frontal"), followed by a number from 1 to 7 (F1–F7). Each of these areas is connected to a distinct area either in the parietal lobe or in the prefrontal cortex. Sub-areas F1–F5 are strictly connected to distinct sectors of the parietal lobe, while areas F6 and F7 are connected to distinct areas within the prefrontal cortex. Moreover, sub-areas related to the parietal lobe project into the spinal cord, while those related to the prefrontal cortex do not. Neurophysiological studies have shown that in each of these sub-areas, a part of the body (the mouth or the hand, for example) is motorically represented, such that the same biological effector may be represented several times for different motor purposes (Rizzolatti et al. 1998). Multiple motor representations of the upper limbs and mouth have been described in detail in areas F4 and F5. Several neurophysiological studies have focused on the motor properties of F5 neurons. Neurons found in this area are active during the execution of object-directed actions carried out by the hand and/or the mouth. Some neurons are active during grasping, object manipulation, or the act of bringing food to the mouth. These neurons are therefore considered able to build up a repertoire of actions, which, like a vocabulary of words, can be used in a number of contexts (Rizzolatti et al. 1988).

Experimental evidence supports the notion that areas within the motor system not only play a fundamental role in action planning and execution, but are also endowed with sensorial properties; some neurons in F5, in fact, are active during the presentation of visual stimuli. According to their visual properties, F5 neurons have been subdivided into two classes:

- Mirror neurons, which become active when an individual observes another who performs an action that is similar or logically related to that motorically coded by the same neuron (Gallese et al. 1996; Rizzolatti et al. 1996);
- Canonical neurons, which fire during the visual presentation of an object, provided that the object's form and/or dimension fit with the action motorically coded by that same neuron (Murata et al. 1997, 2000).

Mirror neurons may play a specific role in understanding as well as in processing and interpreting the intentions of others' actions (Rizzolatti and Craighero 2004; Buccino et al. 2004a). Canonical neurons may code the features of objects that are relevant for manipulation and/or for interacting with them. For the aim of this chapter, we will focus on mirror neurons and the mirror neuron system and leave aside the description of canonical neurons and their functions.

2 The Mirror Neuron System in the Monkey

Mirror neurons are active not only when a monkey performs a given goal-directed action (e.g. grasping a piece of food with the hand), but also when it observes a conspecific or an experimenter performing the same or a similar action (Gallese et al. 1996; Rizzolatti et al. 1996). Mirror neurons were first identified in the premotor area F5. Subsequently, they have also been described in other brain areas, such as the inferior parietal lobe. The set of areas where mirror neurons have been found are often described as the mirror neuron system (MNS). It is generally assumed that these neurons allow one to understand the actions performed by other individuals by means of a neural mechanism that maps the observed action onto the same neural population which controls the execution of that same action.

It has been proposed that the MNS is involved in coding the goal of an action. Since the observed action is mapped onto the neural network controlling the execution of the same action by the observer, and since the observer knows the meaning and the consequences of that action, this knowledge can be eventually transferred to the observed action. This notion is supported by the results of an experiment where the activity of F5 mirror neurons has been investigated in two different experimental conditions (Umiltà et al. 2001). In one condition, the subject, a monkey, could observe the entire sequence of an action – such as, for instance, hand-grasping an object. In the other condition, the monkey was prevented from observing the last part of the sequence by means of a panel: the animal knew that an object was hidden behind the panel but it could not observe the experimenter's hand-grasping it. More than half of the recorded mirror neurons kept on firing even when the animal could not see the last part of the action. This has been taken to indicate that mirror neurons are able to infer missing information, namely to simulate the last part of the action and then, through this simulation, infer the completion of the action.

Many actions performed upon objects are accompanied by a characteristic noise. Manipulating a set of keys produces a typical noise from which it may be possible to infer the action eliciting that noise, even if the action is not visible. An experimental study (Koehler et al. 2002) investigated the neural mechanism that underpins the capacity of recognizing actions from the noise they produce. Mirror neurons in area F5 of the monkey were recorded under different conditions, namely: when monkeys performed actions with a typical noise (e.g. cracking a peanut), when the animal both observed and listened to the same action, and finally when the animal could either observe or listen to that action. Results showed that during the condition of listening to the typical sound of an action, without observing that action, a significant number of recorded neurons presented a response similar to that recorded when the animal could both observe and listen to the action. These neurons were labelled "audio-visual mirror neurons". This finding indicates that mirror neurons are able to code the same action regardless of the sensory modality involved in its perception, as if they embodied an "abstract" representation of actions.

Subsequently, mirror neurons have been identified that activate during the execution and observation of actions performed with the mouth (Ferrari et al. 2003). They are abundant in the lateral part of area F5. As far as their motor properties are concerned, they respond when the monkey performs several mouth-related actions. According to their visual properties, they can instead be subdivided into two classes. The more representative class responds during the observation of ingestion actions, such as mouth-grasping of food, chewing, sucking, and so on (ingestion mirror neurons). The majority of ingestion mirror neurons are selective for a specific ingestion action and about one third of them show a strict congruence between the executed and the observed action that elicits the neuronal response. The other class responds during the observation of mouth actions with communicative functions, such as lip smacking (communicative mirror neurons). The latter class shows only a broad congruence between the observed and executed action, since the observed action is communicative while the executed action is related to food ingestion. However, it should be noted that also in this case, the executed ingestion action and the observed communicative action share a similar motor pattern. For instance, a neuron responding to the observation of lip smacking responds also when the monkey performs a similar action, such as sucking fruit juice.

Do mirror neurons contribute to encoding the visual perspective from which actions performed by others are seen? To answer this question, the visual responses of monkey mirror neurons of area F5 were recorded using a novel experimental paradigm based on the presentation of videos showing grasping actions from different visual perspectives (Caggiano et al. 2011). The authors found that the majority of the tested mirror neurons (75%) exhibited view-dependent activity with responses tuned to specific points of view. A minority of the tested mirror neurons (25%) exhibited view-independent responses. The authors proposed that the view-independent mirror neurons encode action goals, irrespective of the details of the observed actions, whereas the view-dependent mirror neurons might either form an intermediate step in the formation of view-independent mirror neurons or contribute to a modulation of view-dependent representations in higher-level visual areas, potentially linking the goals of the observed actions with their pictorial aspects.

3 The Mirror Neuron System in Humans

Several studies using neurophysiological – e.g. transcranial magnetic stimulation (TMS) – or brain imaging – e.g. functional magnetic resonance imaging (fMRI) – techniques have also demonstrated that the human brain is provided with a MNS able to map the observed actions onto the same neural structures involved in the actual execution of the observed actions. A pivotal study carried out by means of TMS (Fadiga et al. 1995) has shown that during the observation of hand actions, motor evoked potentials (MEPs) recorded from hand muscles actually involved in the execution of the observed actions show an increased amplitude. In keeping with this, by means of quantified electroencephalography (qEEG; Cochin et al. 1999) and magnetoencephalography (MEG; Hari et al. 1998), it has been shown that during the observation of hand actions, there is a decrease of mu-rhythm, similar, although less evident, to what is observed during the execution of the same actions. These experimental findings suggest that both action execution and action observation share common neural substrates. An fMRI study (Buccino et al. 2001) has shown that, in humans, the motor system is recruited not only during the observation of hand actions, but also during the observation of actions performed with the mouth or the foot. Moreover, the study has demonstrated that during action observation, different sectors of the premotor cortex become active depending on the biological effector (hand, foot, or mouth) involved in the execution of the observed action. This somatotopic organization is reminiscent of that which is classically described in the primary motor cortex when actions are executed (homunculus motorius). It is generally maintained that the MNS may allow individuals to understand actions through a mechanism that maps the observed action on the neural structures devoted to the execution of the observed action in the observer's brain (an observation-execution matching system for actions). Hence, a subject can understand an action performed by another individual (e.g. having a coffee) because the very same neurons normally recruited in the subject's brain during the actual execution of that action activate also during the observation of such an action. It is worth stressing that this kind of understanding does not depend on logical-deductive reasoning, but directly relies on the observer's experience and motor competence.

Another fMRI study has confirmed and extended the data reviewed so far (Buccino et al. 2004b). During the experiment, participants were asked to observe videos depicting mouth actions performed by three individuals belonging to distinct species: man, monkey, and dog. The observed actions were either ingestive (e.g. biting and chewing performed by all the individuals) or communicative mouth actions (namely silent speech performed by a man, lip smacking performed by a monkey, and barking performed by a dog). The findings have shown that during the observation of ingestive actions, there was an activation of the areas belonging to the MNS, independently of the individual performing the action. On the other hand, a different pattern of activation was found during the observation of communicative actions. In this case, only when the actor was a man performing silent speech, there was an activation of areas also recruited during the actual execution of speech. These data suggest that the MNS may contribute to understanding actions performed by other individuals (even when they belong to other species) through a mirror mechanism only if the observed actions are already part of the motor repertoire of the observer. When the observed actions do not belong to the motor repertoire of the observer, as in the case of barking, then the motor system is not active (there is no motor resonance) and the observed action is most likely described and understood in visual terms. In keeping with this notion, observation of barking activated an area within the superior temporal sulcus where neurons have been identified that discharge during the observation of biological motions, but not during their execution by the observer.

Further confirmation of these findings came by another fMRI study (Calvo-Merino et al. 2005) showing that the recruitment of the MNS during action observation is affected by the motor competence of the observer. For example, in capoeira dancers the recruitment of the motor system is greater if they observe capoeira dancers than classical ballet dancers; conversely, classical ballet dancers recruit their motor system more when they observe other ballet dancers than when observing capoeira dancers.

4 The Mirror Neuron System and the Understanding of Intentions

An action may be carried out in different contexts and for different aims. During breakfast, one may grasp a cup to drink coffee; after breakfast, one may grasp a cup to put it into the sink. An external observer can understand the different purposes of the same actions when carried out in different contexts.

Classically, it is maintained that understanding the intentions underlying the actions of others is a cognitive task based on a series of logical deductions about the individual performing the observed action and the context in which the action is carried out. As a whole, these cognitive operations are defined as "theory of mind" and, according to many authors, require the activation of specific areas in the brain distinct from those involved in action execution. The discovery of mirror neurons provides an alternative, although does not provide a mutually exclusive explanation for coding the intentions of actions performed by others. According to this alternative, we can understand intentions because when we attempt to understand them, the same neural structures become active in our brain as if we ourselves were to pursue the same intentions. We can therefore understand the aims of actions of others by internally rehearsing their pattern of motor expression, i.e. "*their* motor representations".

Two recent studies support the notion that the MNS may contribute not only in understanding an observed action but also in grasping the intention of the actor. To assess the role of the MNS in coding the intentions underlying the actions of others, Iacoboni and colleagues performed an fMRI study using different video-clips depicting an action (i.e. grasping a cup) in two different contexts, namely during and after breakfast (Iacoboni et al. 2005). Participants were divided into two groups. Subjects in the first group were simply requested to observe the presented actions carefully (implicit task); in the second group, subjects were asked to indicate the reason why the actor performed the observed action (explicit task). The results of the study showed that there was no differential activation between the two groups, which suggests that there are no specific areas in the brain devoted to solving the explicit task. These findings imply that coding the intentions of the actions of others does not require specific neural structures, but rather is an automatic process that intervenes in parallel with the recruitment of the neural structures devoted to the execution of those actions. In keeping with this, indeed, the study has shown the activation of areas within the MNS.

These findings have been recently extended in a study in which participants were requested to observe different actions that could fulfil an intention (intended actions) or not (non-intended actions, such as when an actor grasps a cup to drink, but the cup falls down) (Buccino et al. 2007). In this study, participants were divided into two groups as well: an implicit group, including participants who had simply to observe the presented actions carefully, and the explicit group, including participants who were required to report whether the action was intended or not. The results showed that in both groups there was a recruitment of areas within the MNS during action understanding and intention coding, thus confirming the role of this system in the processing of the intentions underlying the actions of others. Moreover, when directly comparing non-intended and intended actions, there was a differential activation in three distinct areas: the right temporo-parietal junction, a sector of the supramarginal gyrus in the left hemisphere, and a part of the mesial prefrontal cortex. These areas are classically included in the "theory of mind" circuit. However, they have also been reported to be involved in attentional tasks, when participants have to detect the sudden appearance of stimuli in a temporal or spatial sequence. Although the results of this study might support the "theory of mind" (because non-intended actions could more strongly recruit areas normally devoted to interpret the intentions underlying the actions of others), it cannot be excluded that the activation of these areas was just due to attentional reasons. Participants paid more attention to non-intended actions, compared to intended actions, because these actions depicted unattended events both in the temporal and in the spatial domains (such as, for example, a cup falling down).

In a monkey study, Fogassi and colleagues assessed the neurophysiological mechanisms through which mirror neurons may contribute to coding other's intentions (Fogassi et al. 2005). The study demonstrated that parietal mirror neurons in the monkey become active during the observation of an action depending on the type of action that follows. For example, mirror neurons have been identified that fire during both the execution and the observation of grasping an object, but only when the following action was to bring the grasped object to the mouth; a different set of mirror neurons was shown to be active only when the grasped object was put into a beaker. The authors propose the notion that mirror neurons may contribute to understanding the intentions underlying the actions of others because they would be included within motor chains aimed at specific motor goals and intentions. The recruitment of these motor chains in action observation would also automatically code the intentions behind the actions that they code motorically.

5 Mirror Mechanisms for Emotions

So far, we have described the neurophysiological mechanisms that allow us to understand actions (and underlying intentions) without a specific emotional content; so-called "cold" actions. In everyday life, however, we are often requested to understand the feelings of other individuals and to infer their emotional state on the basis of their behaviour. This is a crucial component of real social interactions, and has special relevance for processes of so-called social cognition. Is it possible to assume that a "mirror mechanism" (with properties similar to the mirror neuron system for action and intention understanding) exists also for emotions? Several studies have addressed this question.

For example, A. Damasio proposed the hypothesis that understanding the emotions of other individuals relies on the activation of the same neural structures active when we feel the same emotions (Damasio 2003). In this report, it was proposed that the recognition of emotions of others depends on the recruitment of a neural circuit coding the emotions of other people as if they were our own emotions (an "as if loop"). This "as if loop" includes the insula and somatosensory areas, thus suggesting that the recognition of emotions also requires the recruitment of those areas where body parts are represented.

In the same year, an fMRI study reported that the observation and imitation of facial expressions related to specific emotions (e.g. fear, anger, joy, disgust, etc.) involves the same neural structures underlying the manifestation of those emotions: insula, amygdala, and ventral premotor cortex (Carr et al. 2003). Analogous fMRI results have shown that the left anterior insula is active both when a subject actually feels disgust and when he/she observes other persons feeling disgust (Wicker et al. 2003). Even in the case of pain (which, although strictly speaking is not an emotion, is often accompanied by emotional feelings), it has been reported that neurons in the anterior cingulate are active both when pain is felt by a subject and when the subject sees painful stimuli applied to another person (Hutchison et al. 1999). A more recent fMRI study not only confirmed those findings – showing the activation of anterior insula and cingulate both when the subjects underwent painful stimuli and when they observed the same stimuli applied to other individuals – but also indicated that the activation of those brain regions was stronger when the observed individuals were affectively close to the subjects (Singer et al. 2004; see also Singer 2006 for review).

These findings and hypotheses prompted the idea that a mirror mechanism is also present in the cortical areas involved in coding emotions (Gallese et al. 2004) and that mirror mechanisms may be a crucial component of social cognition tout court. In other words, feeling emotions and recognizing the same emotions in other individuals are processes that share common neural structures. It is worth underlining that, from a cytoarchitectonic point of view, the anterior insula has a structure similar to motor areas. Moreover, electrophysiological studies show that in the monkey, the stimulation of this area causes the appearance of movements in different parts of the body. One may therefore consider the insula as another "mirror area" devoted to emotions and their bodily correlates.

These and other findings have prompted the proposal of a theoretical generalization stating that the brain is endowed with "shared circuits" (Gallese et al. 2004; Keysers and Gazzola 2006). Such shared circuits would be circuits active both when a subject performs actions or feels sensations and emotions, and when the subject perceives the actions, sensations and emotions of other individuals. The shared circuits, therefore, would match the actions, sensations and emotions of others with the subject's own, thus allowing the latter to understand – or, in some sense, to have access to – the state of the individuals she/he is observing. Therefore, this generalized perspective suggests that mirror mechanisms – or "shared circuits" – may also resort to self-related processing, and that social cognition mechanisms based on the mirror system(s) and self-related processing based on cortical midline structures (including medial prefrontal cortex, anterior cingulate and precuneus) may be substantially integrated (see Uddin et al. 2007 for review).

This suggestion is supported by recent findings that show that reading others' emotional facial expressions jointly involves mirror areas as well as cortical midline structures (Seitz et al. 2008; Prochnow et al. 2013a). In particular, as far as midline structures are concerned, these studies show a key involvement of medial frontal cortex in processing emotional face expression. The medial frontal cortex is considered as a fundamental hub in mentalizing and affective theory of mind (Frith and Frith 1999, 2003; Frith 2012).

It is well known that two distinct approaches may be identified in the literature on social cognition: the one emphasizing the role of automatic and implicit mirror-matching mechanisms (so-called "simulation theory" approach), and the other stressing the role of explicit, mentalizing mechanisms (so-called "theory of mind" approach). There have been recent, rather speculative, attempts at integrating the two approaches (Keysers and Gazzola 2007; Uddin et al. 2007; see also Frith and Frith 2012). These models propose that simulation theory and theory of mind are not separate and independent processes. Rather, they may be regarded as two stages of the same social-cognitive mechanisms. Under this view, the mentalizing processes would be triggered by the mirror processes in specific situations and tasks requiring explicit and reflective treatment of social cues, especially when this treatment also requires, or simply induces, conscious consideration of self-related aspects (see also Buccino et al. 2007; Gusnard et al. 2001; Gusnard and Raichle 2001 for review).

We think that processing of emotional and affective information may substantiate such an integrative approach, further suggesting that the higher-level, explicit and reflecting processes of mentalizing are anyway rooted and triggered by more automatic, mirror mechanisms. Although preliminary, key findings in this direction have been recently reported in a combined behavioural and fMRI study inquiring into the processing of emotional face expression (Prochnow et al. 2013b). The study indeed focused on subliminal face expressions (i.e. face expressions presented for 40 ms, thus very unlikely to be consciously accessed). The results show that both mirror areas (especially in the inferior frontal gyrus and anterior insula) and mentalizing areas (in particular the dorsomedial frontal cortex) are active in processing subliminal facial expression. These activations substantially overlap those found in studies involving the presentation of supraliminal face expression. These findings are in line with the idea that mirroring and mentalizing are two sides of the same coin, and that conscious and explicit processing of other's emotions (affective theory of mind) is rooted in automatic and implicit processing mediated by mirror mechanisms (or "shared circuits").

6 Conclusion: Implications for (and from) the Theory of Credition

In this concluding section we would like to outline some implications of what we have seen so far for the theory of credition. Before doing this, we shall briefly recap some aspects of this theory that are relevant for our task.

The theory of credition addresses the issue of the process of believing, i.e. the dynamic process of belief formation, evaluation and modification (Angel 2006, 2013). A credition is defined as a configuration of "babs" or "blobs". A "bab" is any internal or external perception, even a "vague or doubtful" one. Blobs would be "non-conscious babs", and are subliminal in kind though effective in bab/blob-configurations. Therefore, a credition may be considered as a network (configuration) of both subliminal and supraliminal neural representations (babs and blobs). Moreover, the theory of credition defines four functions acting on such configurations: enclosure function, converter function, stabilizer function, and modulator function (See also Angel's contribution in this volume). In what follows, we will focus only on the enclosure function, which is the function that actually forms or re-arranges creditions by assembling (new or existing) babs and blobs in a network. Recent research in credition theory has also proposed a possible neural instantiation of the enclosure function that, according to this proposal, may be supported by medial frontal cortex (Sugiura et al. 2015). Indeed, the medial frontal cortex is know to have a key role in integrating perception-related information mainly represented in posterior cortices, action-related information mainly coming from frontal regions, and emotion/value-related information in the (para-)limbic system (see also Seitz and Angel 2012).

Clearly, at least at the conceptual level, beliefs may be considered as the basis for selection of appropriate actions and behaviours, in the sense that we select actions on the basis of what we believe about the current situation, our capabilities and preferences, the expected consequences of our actions, etc. The theory of credition even suggests that selection of beliefs is virtually equivalent to selection of actions (Sugiura et al. 2015:20). In social contexts, this process is highly important and also concerns our beliefs about the (emotional) state of others (an essential element in choosing what to do in specific social situations). The theory of credition indeed acknowledges a key role to the mirror system in this process, as it may "explain why belief related to other's action allows efficient conversion to the believer's action plan" (Sugiura et al. 2015:16).

Now, we have seen that understanding the state of other people with which we are interacting – i.e. understanding their intentions (Sect. 4 above) and emotions (Sect. 5) – also involves the medial frontal cortex (which we have just seen to be a key brain region in the theory of credition) and happens in similar ways both in subliminal and supraliminal contexts (and we have seen that creditions – intended as bab/blob-configurations – involves both conscious and unconscious elements). This might suggest that the involvement of medial prefrontal cortex in mentalizing and theory of mind may not be due to the existence of a "specialized module" for these (higher-level) functions in social contexts, but may rather reflect the need for the subject to retrieve his/her beliefs in social interactions. The fact that the medial frontal cortex is active also during subliminal processing of facial emotional expressions may thus be explained, in keeping with the theory of credition, on the basis of its involvement in belief formation and re-arrangement (the enclosure function). From this perspective, the formation of beliefs may be conceived as a process that starts with implicit automatic processing in other brain regions (among which the mirror areas for intention and emotion), whose outputs are integrated in medial frontal regions.

This is a speculative suggestion that would require further empirical and theoretical work to be satisfactorily assessed. However, it may help in pursuing the task of integrating the two main approaches in current social cognition: the simulation theory and the theory of mind. Moreover, such an approach may even contribute to show how higher-level, explicit and reflective mechanisms of social cognition (such as mentalizing) are essentially rooted in more implicit and automatic, mirror mechanisms, thus also promoting a fundamentally embodied view of (social) cognition.

References

Angel HF (2006) Religiosität als menschliches Potential. Ein anthropologisches Modell im neurowissenschaftlichen Horizont. In: Angel HF, Broking-Bortfeldt M, Hemel U, Kunstmann J, Jakobs M, Pirner ML, Rothgangel M (eds) Religiosität. Kohlhammer, Stuttgart, pp 62–89

Angel HF (2013) Credition, the process of belief. In: Runehov ALC, Oviedo L (eds) Encyclopedia of sciences and religions. Springer, Dordrecht, pp 536–539

Buccino G, Binkofski F, Fink GR, Fadiga L, Fogassi L, Gallese V, Seitz RJ, Zilles K, Rizzolatti G, Freund HJ (2001) Action observation activates premotor and parietal areas in a somatotopic manner: an fMRI study. Eur J Neurosci 13:400–404

Buccino G, Binkofski F, Riggio L (2004a) The mirror neuron system and action recognition. Brain Lang 89:370–376

Buccino G, Lui F, Canessa N et al (2004b) Neural circuits involved in the recognition of actions performed by non-conspecifics: an fMRI study. J Cogn Neurosci 16:114–124

Buccino G, Baumgaertner A, Colle L, Buechel C, Rizzolatti G, Binkofski F (2007) The neural basis for understanding non-intended actions. NeuroImage 36(2):T119–T127

Caggiano V, Fogassi L, Rizzolatti G et al (2011) View-based encoding of actions in mirror neurons of area f5 in macaque premotor cortex. Curr Biol 21(2):144–148

Calvo-Merino B, Glaser DE, Grezes J, Passingham RE, Haggard P (2005) Action observation and acquired motor skills: an fMRI study with expert dancers. Cereb Cortex 15:1243–1249

Carr L, Iacoboni M, Dubeau MC, Mazziotta JC, Lenzi G (2003) Neural mechanisms of empathy in humans: a relay from neural systems for imitation to limbic areas. Proc Natl Acad Sci U S A 100:5497–5592

Cochin S, Barthelemy C, Roux S, Martineau J (1999) Observation and execution of movement: similarities demonstrated by quantified electroencephalography. Eur J Neurosci 11:1839–1842

Damasio A (2003) Feelings of emotion and the self. Ann N Y Acad Sci 1001:253–261

Fadiga L, Fogassi L, Pavesi G, Rizzolatti G (1995) Motor facilitation during action observation: a magnetic stimulation study. J Neurophysiol 73:2608–2661

Ferrari PF, Gallese V, Rizzolatti G, Fogassi L (2003) Mirror neurons responding to the observation of ingestive and communicative mouth actions in the monkey ventral premotor cortex. Eur J Neurosci 17:1703–1714
Fogassi L, Ferrari PF, Gesierich B, Rozzi S, Chersi F, Rizzolatti G (2005) Parietal lobe: from action organization to intention understanding. Science 308(5722):662–667
Frith CD (2012) The role of metacognition in human social interactions. Philos Trans R Soc Lond B Biol Sci 367:2213–2223
Frith CD, Frith U (1999) Interacting minds – a biological basis. Science 286:1692–1695
Frith U, Frith CD (2003) Development and neurophysiology of mentalizing. Philoso Trans R Soc Lond B Biol Sci 358:459–473
Frith CD, Frith U (2012) Mechanisms of social cognition. Annu Rev Psychol 63:287–313
Gallese V, Fadiga L, Fogassi L, Rizzolatti G (1996) Action recognition in the premotor cortex. Brain 119:593–609
Gallese V, Keysers C, Rizzolatti G (2004) A unifying view of the basis of social cognition. Trends Cogn Sci 8:396–403
Gusnard DA, Raichle ME (2001) Searching for a baseline: functional imaging and the resting human state. Nat Rev Neurosci 2:685–694
Gusnard DA, Akbudak E, Shulman GL, Raichle ME (2001) Medial prefrontal cortex and self-referential mental activity: relation to a default mode of brain function. Proc Natl Acad Sci U S A 98:4259–4264
Hari R, Forss N, Avikainen S, Kirveskari E, Salenius S, Rizzolatti G (1998) Activation of human primary motor cortex during action observation: a neuromagnetic study. Proc Natl Acad Sci U S A 95:15061–15065
Hutchison WD, Davis KD, Lozano AM, Tasker RR, Dostrovsky JO (1999) Pain related neurons in the human cingulated cortex. Nat Neurosci 2:403–405
Iacoboni M, Molnar-Szakacs I, Gallese V, Buccino G, Mazziotta JC, Rizzolatti G (2005) Grasping the intentions of others with one's own mirror neuron system. PLoS Biol 3:529–535
Keysers C, Gazzola V (2006) Towards a unifying neural theory of social cognition. Prog Brain Res 156:379–401
Keysers C, Gazzola V (2007) Integrating simulation and theory of mind: from self to social cognition. Trends Cogn Sci 11:194–196
Koehler E, Keysers C, Umiltà MA, Fogassi L, Gallese V, Rizzolatti G (2002) Hearing sounds, understanding actions: action representation in mirror neurons. Science 297:846–848
Murata A, Fadiga L, Fogassi L, Gallese V, Raos V, Rizzolatti G (1997) Object representation in the ventral premotor cortex (area F5) of the monkey. J Neurophysiol 78(4):2226–2230
Murata A, Gallese V, Luppino G, Kaseda M, Sakata H (2000) Selectivity for the shape, size, and orientation of objects for grasping in neurons of monkey parietal area AIP. J Neurophysiol 83(5):2580–2601
Prochnow D, Hoeing B, Kleiser R, Lindenberg R, Wittsack HJ, Schäfer R, Seitz RJ (2013a) The neural correlates of affect reading: an fMRI study on faces and gestures. Behav Brain Res 237:270–277
Prochnow D, Kossack H, Brunheim S, Muller K, Wittsack HJ, Markowitsch HJ, Seitz RJ (2013b) Processing of subliminal facial expressions of emotion: a behavioral and fMRI study. Soc Neurosci http://dx.doi.org/10.1080/17470919.2013.812536
Rizzolatti G, Craighero L (2004) The mirror-neuron system. Annu Rev Neurosci 27:169–192
Rizzolatti G, Camarda R, Fogassi L, Gentilucci M, Luppino G, Matelli M (1988) Functional organization of inferior area 6 in the macaque monkey. II. Area F5 and the control of distal movements. Exp Brain Res 71(3):491–507
Rizzolatti G, Fadiga L, Fogassi L, Gallese V (1996) Premotor cortex and the recognition of motor action. Brain Res 3:131–141
Rizzolatti G, Luppino G, Matelli G (1998) The organization of the cortical motor system: new concepts. Electroencephalogr Clin Neurophysiol 106:283–296

Seitz RJ, Angel HF (2012) Processes of believing – a review and conceptual account. Rev Neurosci 23(3):303–309

Seitz RJ, Schaffer R, Scherfeld D, Friederichs S, Popp K, Wittsack H-J, Azari NP, Franza M (2008) Valuating other people's emotion face expressions: a combined functional magnetic resonance imaging and electroencephalography study. Neuroscience 152:712–722

Singer T (2006) The neuronal basis and ontogeny of empathy and mind reading: review of literature and implications for future research. Neurosci Biobehav Rev 30:855–863

Singer T, Seymore B, O'Doherty J, Kaube H, Dolan RJ, Frith CD (2004) Empathy for pain involves the affective but not sensory components of pain. Science 5661:1157–1162

Sugiura M, Seitz RJ, Angel HF (2015) Models and neural bases of the believing process. J Behav Brain Sci 5:12–23

Uddin LQ, Iacoboni M, Lange C, Keenan JP (2007) The self and social cognition: the role of cortical midline structures and mirror neurone. Trends Cogn Sci 11:153–157

Umiltà MA, Kohler E, Gallese V, Fogassi L, Fadiga L, Keysers C, Rizzolatti G (2001) I know what you are doing: a neurophysiological study. Neuron 31:155–165

Wicker B, Keysers C, Plailly J, Royet JP, Gallese V, Rizzolatti G (2003) Both of us disgusted in my insula: the common neural basis of seeing and feeling disgust. Neuron 40:655–664

Neural Underpinnings of the Human Belief System

Irene Cristofori and Jordan Grafman

Abstract Human beings are wired to believe. These beliefs – including moral, legal, political, and religious beliefs – are extremely important because they can define a person's character and influence decision-making processes. Recent neuroimaging and lesion studies have shown that these beliefs have neural underpinnings in the human brain. This chapter reviews the current research on the human social belief system and its neural correlates. There is no evidence of dedicated brain systems uniquely devoted to a specific kind of human social belief. The studies reviewed in this chapter highlight a core set of regions within the prefrontal cortex, in association with the anterior temporal lobe, reward circuit, and limbic regions, that appear to critically mediate a variety of social belief systems.

1 Introduction

Philosophers defined beliefs as states of mind about the world. Some beliefs are based on our perception and *easy* to verify such as *I believe that the sky is blue today* and others are based on our abstract thoughts/ideology and *difficult* to prove such as *I believe in God*. Social beliefs refer to a particular set of beliefs including moral, legal, political, and religious beliefs by which individuals identify themselves. The

I. Cristofori
Cognitive Neuroscience Laboratory, Brain Injury Research, Rehabilitation Institute of Chicago, Chicago, IL, USA

Department of Physical Medicine and Rehabilitation, Feinberg School of Medicine, Northwestern University, Chicago, IL, USA

J. Grafman (✉)
Cognitive Neuroscience Laboratory, Brain Injury Research, Rehabilitation Institute of Chicago, Chicago, IL, USA

Department of Physical Medicine and Rehabilitation, Feinberg School of Medicine, Northwestern University, Chicago, IL, USA

Department of Neurology, Feinberg School of Medicine, Northwestern University, Chicago, IL, USA
e-mail: jgrafman@northwestern.edu

H.-F. Angel et al. (eds.), *Processes of Believing: The Acquisition, Maintenance, and Change in Creditions*, New Approaches to the Scientific Study of Religion 1,
DOI 10.1007/978-3-319-50924-2_8

same social beliefs are commonly shared between members belonging to the same group. Social beliefs root us in the world, shape our reality, allow us to navigate the world with a certain amount of confidence, and they influence our decisions. Why did neuroscientists start to study human social beliefs? First, they are uniquely human cognitive and social processes, and understanding their neural and cognitive foundations may illuminate aspects of human brain evolution. Second, there may be both common and distinct components or dimensions intrinsic to the moral, legal, political, and religious belief systems we adhere to whose identification may aid in advancing our theoretical ideas about the mediation of beliefs in individual brains around the globe. Third, it may lead to beneficial ways to evaluate the effects of brain injury on identity and social behavior, and suggest potential intervention methods to remediate social impairments. The aim of this chapter is to review where different beliefs systems are coded in the human brain. This chapter also focuses on four lines of research, examining moral, legal, political, and religious beliefs, including both neuroimaging and lesions studies. Finally, the chapter outline possible directions for future research of the human beliefs system.

2 Moral Beliefs

Human moral beliefs may underlie other forms of social belief systems including those concerned with politics, law and religion. Moral beliefs not only enable individuals to be concerned about their own behavior, but also allow these individuals to care about others. Moral beliefs are often quick and implicit (Moll et al. 2005). Key moral beliefs may have evolved out of rules that established stable individual, family, and tribal relationships *preceding* the developing of large-scale belief systems such as those concerned with markets, politics, and religion that helped larger societies become more stable. Moral beliefs – like other forms of belief – are complex cognitive processes likely composed of many sub-components that can be revealed by neuroimaging studies of healthy volunteers or studying patients with focal brain damage.

Recently, Moll and collaborators (Moll et al. 2011) suggested that distinct prefrontal cortical (PFC) and related subcortical structures underlie distinct moral sentiments. In addition to PFC structures, specific posterior cortical regions such as the temporo-parietal junction (TPJ) and intraparietal sulcus (IPS) have been shown to play a crucial role in moral sentiments (Robertson et al. 2007a, b). Moral sentiments play a key role in regulating social behavior and may be impaired following PFC and limbic system lesions in humans, as lesions in these areas have been shown to lead to impairments in the decision-making processes. In some circumstances, patients with a focal lesion to the PFC cortex accept dangerous actions to maximize *good* consequences [i.e. utilitarian moral judgments (Koenigs et al. 2007; Moretto et al. 2010)]. To determine whether specific brain lesions can affect selective aspects of moral sentiments, Moll and collaborators (2011) investigated the performance of patients with a behavioral variant of Frontotemporal Dementia (bvFTD) and normal matched controls on a Moral Sentiment Task. This task evaluates the understanding of *prosocial* (guilt, compassion, and embarrassment) and *other-critical* (anger, disgust) sentiments. The task requires reading 98 social scenarios (e.g., *Your mother called telling you she wasn't feeling well. You didn't take her seriously and the next day she died*) and selecting the appropriate sentiment from among three additional distracters. Prosocial and other-critical scores were computed and z-normalized. In addition, resting-state 18-Fluoro-Deoxy-Glucose Positron Emission Tomography (FDG-PET) was used to determine the relationship between neurometabolic abnormalities and bvFTD patient impairment on prosocial and other-critical judgments (controlling for dementia severity and other clinical scores). Neuropsychological and neuroimaging data were obtained from 21 bvFTD patients and 30 healthy volunteers. Patients with bvFTD suffer from progressive frontotemporal neurodegeneration, characterized by early social impairments (Neary et al. 1998). Several studies have linked the inappropriate social behavior and feelings in these patients to atrophy in the ventral and dorsomedial PFC and anterior temporal cortex (Liu et al. 2004; Rosen et al. 2005; Snowden et al. 2001; Takahashi et al. 2004). For these reasons, patients with bvFTD offer a unique opportunity to understand the specific role of different brain regions in enabling prosocial sentiments. In this study, Moll and collaborators (2011) found a decrease in resting scan glucose metabolism in the PFC, anterior temporal cortex, amygdala, inferior parietal lobe, midbrain and basal forebrain (including septum), hypothalamus, and medial thalamus in bvFTD patients compared to healthy volunteers. Moreover, evidence indicated that damage/dysfunction in specific PFC and limbic structures underlie impaired attributions of prosocial and other-critical sentiments in bvFTD patients, as measured by resting PET metabolism. Although bvFTD patients were equally impaired on both types of moral sentiment (prosocial and critical), using a functional neuroimaging measure, the data suggested that different components of moral sentiments are potentially anatomically dissociable.

Traditional studies on moral beliefs have used extreme or unfamiliar situations, such as moral dilemmas, to induce unusual thought processes rather than those used for more common moral judgments (Moll et al. 2005). To address this, Knutson and collaborators (2010) have recently standardized a set of common vignettes based on real-life events that can be used to study moral beliefs and judgments (Knutson et al. 2010). These researchers obtained the ratings of these moral vignettes on several dimensions including emotional intensity, degree of social norm violation, and level of harm or benefit caused. In addition, using factor analysis, researchers were able to define the underlying components of the moral vignettes. Three components accounted for most of the variance: norm violation, social affect, and intention. These moral vignettes can be used in future studies on moral judgment in behavioral, neuropsychological, and functional imaging experiments. Moral vignettes such as those standardized in the Knutson et al. study have the advantage of ecological validity that is extremely important when studying morality (Casebeer 2003). Vignettes bases on real-life scenarios are more relevant to individuals and are more likely to belong to individuals' personal experiences. Ecological validity is particularly relevant for moral beliefs studies, because moral beliefs are deeply dependent on situational and cultural context.

The evidence discussed above strongly implies that the neural mechanisms of moral beliefs system are not restricted to the PFC, limbic areas or any other brain region. The event-feature-emotion complex (EFEC) framework has been postulated to explain the functioning of moral beliefs (Moll et al. 2005). According to this model, moral and behavioral experiences arise from the synchronization of three main neural networks: the PFC (which stores structured event knowledge), the posterior and anterior regions of the temporal cortex (which regulate social perceptual and functional features) and the limbic regions (which process basic emotional states). The EFEC theoretical framework explains that the moral beliefs system and the three main components of the EFEC framework interact to produce moral emotions such as compassion. The PFC provides contextual event representations (e.g., the girl is an orphan and the odds of adoption are low), the superior temporal sulcus and anterior temporal cortex contribute social perceptual (e.g., sad facial expression of a child) and functional (e.g., the concept of helplessness) features, and limbic/paralimbic regions underpin basic emotional states (e.g., sadness).

The neuroscience of moral beliefs has the huge potential to improve the assessment, treatment, and progress of behavioral disorders. Understanding the neural basis of moral beliefs will help to shape environmental, psychological, and medical treatments aimed at fostering prosocial behaviors.

3 Legal Beliefs and Punishments

Legal third-party punishment in response to the violation of social norms is an evolved behavior that presumably was selected because it enabled individuals to live more securely and cooperatively in an intensely social human culture. Society expects that criminal behavior will be punished, usually by an unaffected third-party, to reinforce social norms. On the other hand, free will – the free choice to comply or violate social norms – is often associated with antisocial and criminal behavior including cheating, stealing, aggression and defection (Vohs and Schooler 2008; Baumeister et al. 2009).

Krueger first investigated the effects of belief in free will on third-party punishment (Krueger et al. 2014). The authors combined a third party punishment task with functional magnetic resonance imaging to study how belief in free will might affect their punishment of hypothetical offenses varying in emotional content, ranging from property destruction and theft to rape and murder. While in the fMRI scanner, 26 healthy subjects (13 females, 13 males) were asked to estimate how much punishment John deserved for each of the legal vignettes on a Likert-scale (ranging from No Punishment = 0, to Extreme Punishment = 100). As a control task, participants were asked to estimate the number of syllables for each of the vignettes on a Likert-scale (ranging from Approximately 30, to Approximately 95). For example, one hypothetical vignette was *"John knows the address of a woman who has highly offended him. As he had planned the day before, he waits there for the woman to return from work and, when she appears, John shoots her to death"* (Robinson and Kurzban 2007). In post-experiment questionnaires, participants were asked to rate their subjective affective experience elicited by the scenarios to control for brain activation changes due to emotional processing of the legal vignettes. Moreover, participants were divided into two groups based on their belief in free will: *libertarians* (believing more in free will) and *determinists* (believing less in free will and more in scientific determinism). The grouping was based on a median split approach of the difference score between belief in free will and determinism [measured by the FAD-Plus Questionnaire (Paulhus and Carey 2011)].

The findings showed that *libertarians* punished more severely than *determinists*, but only in the condition of low affective cases. This result was also associated with a stronger activation in the right temporo-parietal junction (TPJ). The TPJ is a region involved in attentional selection to salient stimuli and attribution of others' intentions and beliefs. However, in the condition of high affective cases, the belief in free will-based behavioral and neural differences disappeared. Both groups similarly punished high affective cases and showed higher activation in the right insula. The right insula is a key structure implicated in aversive interoceptive-emotional processing. Together, these results demonstrate that the impact of belief in free will on third party punishment is context-dependent. These results may have important and practical legal applications. For example, in low affective crimes, belief in free will might influence jurors' decisions in a way for which lawyers and judges as whole might have to account. On the other hand, for high affective crimes, judges and lawyers should be less concerned about jurors' belief in free will and more concerned about the emotional valence of the crime.

In a more recent study, Glass investigated third-party punishment in a large sample of patients with focal damage (Glass et al. 2015). They evaluated male combat veterans (N = 114) from the Vietnam Head Injury Study, which is a prospective, long-term follow-up study of veterans with focal penetrating traumatic brain injuries and veterans without focal penetrating traumatic brain injuries (healthy matched controls, N = 32). Participants were given a set of legal vignettes on separate cards, which were each composed of a header and a scenario consisting of two or three sentences. Each vignette described an event during which a named perpetrator (John) engages in criminal offenses including theft by taking, theft by fraud, property destruction, assault, burglary, robbery, kidnapping, rape, negligent, homicide, manslaughter, murder, and torture in a variety of situations (Robinson and Kurzban 2007). The offenses contained in the scenarios represent about 94.9% of the offenses committed in the United States (sexual assault, 0.8% of all offenses; robbery, 2.5%; assault, 19.0%; household burglary, 14.0%; and theft 58.6%). Participants were given complete discretion to punish John for his actions as an unaffected third-party, and asked to rank-order the cards to reflect the degree of legal punishment that the perpetrator deserved.

The study aimed to explore the psychological components of third-party punishment and its underpinning neural network. A whole-brain voxel-based lesion-symptom mapping approach was used in conjunction with a rank-order third-party punishment task to uncover brain regions necessary for third-party punishment. Patients who showed *atypical* third-party punishment behavior had lesions associated with brain region members of the mentalizing [dorsolateral PFC (dlPFC), ventromedial PFC (vmPFC)] and central executive (bilateral dlPFC and right intraparietal sulcus) networks. Moreover, altruism and executive functioning predicted third-party punishment: altruism was associated with third-party punishment in patients with lesions in the right dlPFC, whereas executive functioning was associated with third-party punishment in patients with lesion in the right dlPFC.

These results specify the neural network of the psychological components underlying third-party punishment and show that each of those components is modulated by a distinct cortical midline structure: intention behind norm violation (dlPFC), harm to the victim (parietal cortex), and outcome for the perpetrator (vmPFC). Moreover, these results confirm criminal law's two central tenets: with only rare exceptions, the law punishes only intentional acts that cause harm (tangible or intangible). These two requirements are not the only necessary conditions of punishment, as they are driven by an underlying vmPFC value system. Finally, these results are consistent with the arguments of evolutionary theory (especially given the PFC involvement), which has theorized that third-party punishment is an evolved behavior that was selected because it enabled us to live more securely and cooperatively in our intensely social human culture.

Legal beliefs can be influenced by external factors. For example, the hormone and neurotransmitter oxytocin facilitates complex social cognition and behaviors, such as empathy. Empathy, in terms of the interests and welfare of others, is a crucial factor in third-party decision-making (Zeelenberg and Breugelmans 2008). Krueger et al. investigated the effect of exogenous oxytocin in modulating the empathy of an unaffected third-party toward offenders and victims of crimes (Krueger et al. 2013). The authors investigated whether intranasal oxytocin modulates empathy of an unaffected third-party toward offenders and victims of criminal offenses. Fifty-four healthy male participants were randomly assigned to either the oxytocin or placebo group. The study was a double-blind and a between-subjects design. Participants were given a set of legal vignettes to read which described events during which an offender engaged in criminal behaviors against victims. The participants, in the role of an unaffected third-party, were asked to rate the criminal behaviors based on the degree to which the offender deserved punishment and on the degree of the harm received by the victim. Intranasal oxytocin increased third-party decision-makers' perceptions of harm for victims but not the desire to punish offenders of criminal offenses. The researchers argued that oxytocin promoted empathic concern for the victim, which corresponded in an increased tendency for prosocial behavior regarding the interpersonal relationship between an unaffected third-party and a victim. More research is needed in this topic, and future studies should investigate how the context- and person-dependent nature of intranasal oxytocin in individuals with antisocial personality disorder and psychopathy.

4 Political Beliefs

Most human societies are governed by political beliefs and organizations that emerged in conjunction with the establishment of moral and legal guidelines. As was the case with the identification of subcomponents of moral sentiment and legal punishment, are there underlying cognitive subcomponents that drive how people think about political beliefs?

Knutson and collaborators (2006) first conducted a neuroimaging study to investigate the neural correlates of political attitudes. In this study, participants belonging to different political orientations were asked to perform a modified version of the Implicit Association Task IAT (Greenwald et al. 1998) during fMRI. In this modified IAT, faces and names of Democratic and Republican American politicians were associated with positive and negative words. Participants were asked to categorize the faces of the politicians as either Democratic or Republican, and the sequence of words as either pleasant or unpleasant. Response keys were associated in a congruent and incongruent manner according to participants' political orientation. For instance, Democratic participants were involved in a congruent condition when Democratic candidates' faces and pleasant words required the same response key, and an incongruent condition when Democratic candidates' faces and unpleasant words required the same response key. The results showed that participants were faster to categorize the faces of the political candidates in the congruent condition. In addition, brain activity during the task was linked to the context in which the politician was presented. During the congruent condition the PFC network was involved, including the vmPFC and the anterior PFC, which is implicated in storing stereotypical knowledge and integrating emotion during decision-making. During the incongruent condition, additional brain regions were involved, including the dlPFC and the ACC, which are involved in conflict resolution and cognitive control. Moreover, this study showed that brain activity during the congruent condition correlated with participants' explicit ratings of the candidates. A positive correlation occurred between the activity in the PFC and the rating of candidate's face (i.e., the more positively the participant evaluated the candidate's face, the more the PFC was activated). Additionally, a negative correlation was found between the activity in the lateral PFC and the rating of the political party affiliation (i.e., the more the participant was affiliated with a party, the lower the activity in the lateral PFC). This first study showed that political beliefs are the results of two main systems: one involved in political preference, and the other involved in knowledge about politics (defined here by political candidates).

Other studies further investigated how beliefs can modulate political information. Amodio and collaborators (Zeelenberg and Breugelmans 2008) found that political predispositions underpin distinct neural structures. The authors recorded the event-related potentials (ERPs) of liberals and conservatives while they performed a go/no go task. The go/no go task requires that participants respond as quickly as possible to stimuli until the response becomes automatic. Some of the trials require detecting a situation of cognitive conflict, and thus withholding the learned response,. This task has been largely used to study conflict monitoring, i.e, a mechanism able to detect when a habitual response is suppressed (Zeelenberg and Breugelmans 2008). The study of Amodio and collaborators showed that ERP amplitudes correlated with political orientation. Liberals had greater conflict related brain activity, that is, larger ERP amplitudes and better performances at the go/no go task. These results suggest that a liberal orientation is linked to better conflict monitoring, while a conservative orientation is linked to better performance in tasks that require fixed responses.

The studies presented above divided participants and stimuli according to political orientation or affiliation; however, the liberal-conservative distinction might not be the only political dimension to determine responses to political stimuli. A multidimensional approach to understanding how people think about political beliefs may be useful instead of relying upon a single dimension concerned only with the conservatism/liberalism dimension. To this aim, Zamboni and collaborators identified a set of underlying dimensions that dominate how we think about political beliefs (Zamboni et al. 2009). These dimension are individualism, conservatism, and radicalism. In the first part of the study, the authors performed an exploratory multivariate analysis to discover the underlying criteria used to assess statements about political beliefs. They found that individuals – to explain political beliefs – use individualism, conservatism, and radicalism dimensions. In a second part of the study, a parametric fMRI design showed that when participants were asked to assess political statements, these dimensions were associated with different brain activity. The liberal-to-conservatism dimension was associated with activation in the dlPFC, a structure involved in social decisions and deliberative thinking; the moderate-to-radical dimension was associated with the ventral striatum, a structure involved in reward and cooperation; in this context, moderation can be perceived as a form of social reward. Finally, the individual-to-society dimension showed patterns related to two key structures: the dmPFC was more activated by more society-related statements while the vmPFC was more activated by individual-related statements. Other studies have supported the concepts that different regions of the PFC regulate different aspects of political beliefs, that the vmPFC is linked to the judgment of social beliefs similar to the people we trust, and that the dmPFC is linked to the judgment of social beliefs similar to people we distrust (Mitchell et al. 2006).

More recently, Gozzi and collaborators found that having a greater interest in politics is associated with greater activation in the amygdala and ventral striatum compared to individuals with little interest in politics when simply reading political opinions *in accordance* with their own views (Gozzi et al. 2010). This result suggests that political beliefs may share the same neural system involved with more *traditional* rewards (i.e, food, money).

The vmPFC plays a crucial role in evaluation processing, and patients with lesions involving the vmPFC have displayed abnormal social behavior and thinking (Mah et al. 2004, 2005). In a further study, Cristofori et al. (2015) examined whether the vmPFC also modulates how individuals rate political beliefs. Patients with penetrating traumatic brain injury ($N = 102$) and healthy controls ($N = 31$) were tested on the Political Belief Task. This task involved the rating of 75 statements expressing political beliefs concerned with welfare, economy, political involvement, civil rights, war and security. Participants rated each statement according to their level of agreement. The statements related to the three dimensions underlying political beliefs: radicalism, individualism, and conservatism. Voxel-based lesion symptom mapping (VLSM) analysis found that diminished scores for the radicalism dimension (i.e. statements that were rated as less radical than the norms) were associated with lesions in bilateral vmPFC. In a second part of the study, the authors divided the patients into three groups according to lesion location (i.e. vmPFC, dlPFC and parietal cortex, this latter area chosen as the location for control lesions). They found that the vmPFC, but not the dlPFC, group had reduced radicalism scores compared with parietal and healthy control groups. These findings emphasize the pivotal role of the vmPFC in appropriately valuing political beliefs and may explain more general inappropriate social judgments observed in patients with vmPFC lesions.

In conclusion, the studies presented above uncovered that a complex network of cerebral structures process the political belief system.

5 Religious Beliefs

Religious belief emerges in conjunction with moral beliefs, motivates political and legal beliefs, and has been thought to have a special status in the human brain.

Religious belief, like moral, legal and political belief, is embedded in different ways in different people and societies. Religious beliefs are often concerned with the existence of supernatural phenomena that are difficult to assess in the laboratory. What can be reliably measured is how humans process, act upon, and store/represent religious beliefs. Can religious belief be divided into dimensions or components like moral, legal or political beliefs? If so, can we determine whether there is something special about the emotional, social, cognitive, or neural architectures utilized when humans process religious beliefs compared to other social and cognitive processes?

In a pioneering study, Kapogiannis and collaborators (2009) started to answer these questions and identified brain areas underpinning religious beliefs: the bilateral frontal gyrus, right superior mediofrontal gryus, association areas within the temporal lobes, and right medial occipital and parietal regions (Kapogioannis et al. 2009). In the first part of the study, the authors presented statements about God's emotion and involvement (such as *"God is punishing", "Religion is moral guiding"*). A multidimensional scaling analysis revealed three psychological dimensions of religious belief: God's perceived level of involvement, God's perceived emotion, and doctrinal/experiential religious knowledge. Statements related to God's lack of involvement activated brain networks concerned with understanding an agent's actions, emotion processing, and self-relevance – all components required to understand the intentions of another agent (i.e., Theory of Mind, ToM). Statements reflecting God's perceived emotion involved brain regions of the ToM and higher order emotional regulation. Statements involving a low-imagery content of doctrinal knowledge activated more temporal-lobe regions than statements involving a high-imagery content of experiential knowledge.

For the first time, Kapoglannis et al. defined a psychological and neuroanatomical framework of religious belief. In this framework, religious beliefs involve brain regions underpinning abstract semantic processing, imagery, and intent related and emotional ToM. These neural processes can occur at implicit and explicit levels (Siegal and Varley 2002; Just et al. 2004; Cunningham et al. 2004). In addition, the results show that religious beliefs are based on cognitive-emotional interaction in the anterior insula, specifically in religious individuals. The results support the idea that religious beliefs are integrated in brain areas involved in cognition and social cognition (Boyer 2008). The evolution of these networks was likely driven by their primary roles in social cognition and community, language, and logical reasoning. Religious cognition likely emerged as a unique combination of these several evolutionarily important cognitive processes. Measurable individual differences in these core competencies (such as ToM and imagination) may predict specific patterns of brain activation in response to religious stimuli.

As with moral, legal, and political beliefs, religious beliefs also involve a complex neural network and are influenced by genetic factors. However, the neuroscience of religious beliefs is in its early days and many aspects of the religious brain need to be explored.

6 Conclusions

There is no single moral, legal, political or religious spot in the brain. The studies reviewed in this chapter conclude that there is no evidence of dedicated brain systems *uniquely* devoted to a specific kind of human social belief. Various regions within the prefrontal cortex in association with the anterior temporal lobe, reward networks, and limbic regions appear to critically mediate a variety of social belief systems in affiliation with other cortical regions. Are there general factors and dimensions important for evaluating belief systems? Yes. Such factors might include whether a presented statement constitutes a personal norm violation, the specific sentiments or dimensions that determine how people think about a belief, whether a subject has to decipher the intentions of an authority, whether agency is involved, whether the processing is explicit or implicit, and a person's emotional attachment to their beliefs. The potential for functional dissociations within and across such diverse and distributed social-cognitive brain networks using patients with focal brain lesions is great. Such knowledge about the functioning of social belief systems can help improve the management and treatment of patients with traumatic brain injury, stroke, and neural degenerations.

7 Future Directions/Main Outstanding Questions

Researchers have recently started to study the neural underpinning of human belief systems. Yet many questions need to be answered and investigated in future studies. Do most people, as opposed to a trusted/distrusted social or intellectual elite, only have a shallow level of knowledge about a belief system and instead rely on heuristics, advice, or stimulus surface features (e.g., faces) to form their own beliefs? In the studies reviewed in the present chapter we indicated that the belief system can be divided into moral, legal, political, and religious beliefs, but is there cross-priming across belief systems or do they retain some degree of cognitive segregation? Whether segregated or not, are human beliefs represented in some metric like frequency of use, similarity of actions or heuristics?

What negative or beneficial role do belief systems play in modulating ordinary cognitive processes?

Brain damage to the PFC is common in patients suffering from traumatic brain injury, stroke, and frontotemporal dementia. Can research on the cognitive and neural foundations of belief systems help us develop better ways to objectively assess patients with changes in social behavior after brain damage and potentially improve their functioning?

Human beliefs are very persistent, yet individuals may change their beliefs. What are the neural and cognitive processes that motivate and reflect belief conversion?

Do beliefs form an essential part of self and insure stability in our interactions with the world (social, natural, and supernatural)?

Does the intensity of emotion associated with certain beliefs confer special status and are potentially misleading cues about the grounding of such beliefs?

Future studies will be needed to explore the neural basis of how different individuals and social groups make use of strategies and heuristics to solve moral conflicts. The implications of this new knowledge for how societies conduct business, regulate social behavior, and plan for their futures remain to be investigated.

References

Baumeister RF, Masicampo EJ, Dewall CN (2009) Prosocial benefits of feeling free: disbelief in free will increases aggression and reduces helpfulness. Personal Soc Psychol Bull 35(2):260–268. doi:10.1177/0146167208327217

Boyer P (2008) Being human: religion: bound to believe? Nature 455(7216):1038–1039. doi:10.1038/4551038a

Casebeer WD (2003) Moral cognition and its neural constituents. Nat Rev Neurosci 4(10):840–846. doi:10.1038/nrn1223

Cristofori I, Viola V, Chau A, Zhong W, Krueger F, Zamboni G, Grafman J (2015) The neural bases for devaluing radical political statements revealed by penetrating traumatic brain injury. Soc Cogn Affect Neurosci. doi:10.1093/scan/nsu155

Cunningham WA, Raye CL, Johnson MK (2004) Implicit and explicit evaluation: FMRI correlates of valence, emotional intensity, and control in the processing of attitudes. J Cogn Neurosci 16(10):1717–1729. doi:10.1162/0898929042947919

Glass L, Moody L, Grafman J, Krueger F (2015) Neural signatures of third-party punishment: evidence from penetrating traumatic brain injury. Soc Cogn Affect Neurosci. doi:10.1093/scan/nsv105

Gozzi M, Zamboni G, Krueger F, Grafman J (2010) Interest in politics modulates neural activity in the amygdala and ventral striatum. Hum Brain Mapp 31(11):1763–1771. doi:10.1002/hbm.20976

Greenwald AG, McGhee DE, Schwartz JL (1998) Measuring individual differences in implicit cognition: the implicit association test. J Pers Soc Psychol 74(6):1464–1480

Just MA, Newman SD, Keller TA, McEleney A, Carpenter PA (2004) Imagery in sentence comprehension: an fMRI study. NeuroImage 21(1):112–124

Kapogiannis D, Barbey AK, Su M, Zamboni G, Krueger F, Grafman J (2009) Cognitive and neural foundations of religious belief. Proc Natl Acad Sci U S A 106(12):4876–4881. doi:10.1073/pnas.0811717106

Knutson KM et al (2006) Politics on the brain: an FMRI investigation. Soc Neurosci 1(1):25–40

Knutson KM, Krueger F, Koenigs M, Hawley A, Escobedo JR, Vasudeva V, Adolphs R, Grafman J (2010) Behavioral norms for condensed moral vignettes. Soc Cogn Affect Neurosci 5(4):378–384. doi:10.1093/scan/nsq005

Koenigs M et al (2007) Damage to the prefrontal cortex increases utilitarian moral judgements. Nature 446(7138):908–911

Krueger F, Parasuraman R, Moody L, Twieg P, de Visser E, McCabe K, O'Hara M, Lee MR (2013) Oxytocin selectively increases perceptions of harm for victims but not the desire to punish offenders of criminal offenses. Soc Cogn Affect Neurosci 8(5):494–498. doi:10.1093/scan/nss026

Krueger F, Hoffman M, Walter H, Grafman J (2014) An fMRI investigation of the effects of belief in free will on third-party punishment. Soc Cogn Affect Neurosci 9(8):1143–1149. doi:10.1093/scan/nst092

Liu W, Miller BL, Kramer JH, Rankin K, Wyss-Coray C, Gearhart R, Phengrasamy L, Weiner M, Rosen HJ (2004) Behavioral disorders in the frontal and temporal variants of frontotemporal dementia. Neurology 62(5):742–748

Mah L, Arnold MC, Grafman J (2004) Lesions of prefrontal cortex impair social perception. Am J Psychiatry 161:1247–1255

Mah L, Arnold MC, Grafman J (2005) Deficits in social knowledge following lesions of ventromedial prefrontal cortex. J Neuropsychiatry Clin Neurosci 17:66–74

Mitchell JP, Macrae CN, Banaji MR (2006) Dissociable medial prefrontal contributions to judgments of similar and dissimilar others. Neuron 50(4):655–663. doi:10.1016/j.neuron.2006.03.040

Moll J, Zahn R, de Oliveira-Souza R, Krueger F, Grafman J (2005) Opinion: the neural basis of human moral cognition. Nat Rev Neurosci 6(10):799–809. doi:10.1038/nrn1768

Moll J, Zahn R, de Oliveira-Souza R, Bramati IE, Krueger F, Tura B, Cavanagh AL, Grafman J (2011) Impairment of prosocial sentiments is associated with frontopolar and septal damage in frontotemporal dementia. NeuroImage 54(2):1735–1742. doi:10.1016/j.neuroimage.2010.08.026

Moretto G et al (2010) A psychophysiological investigation of moral judgment after ventromedial prefrontal damage. J Cogn Neurosci 22(8):1888–1899

Neary D, Snowden JS, Gustafson L, Passant U, Stuss D, Black S, Freedman M, Kertesz A, Robert PH, Albert M, Boone K, Miller BL, Cummings J, Benson DF (1998) Frontotemporal lobar degeneration: a consensus on clinical diagnostic criteria. Neurology 51(6):1546–1554

Paulhus DL, Carey JM (2011) The FAD-Plus: measuring lay beliefs regarding free will and related constructs. J Pers Assess 94:96–104

Robertson D, Snarey J, Ousley O, Harenski K, DuBois BF, Gilkey R, Kilts C (2007a) The neural processing of moral sensitivity to issues of justice and care. Neuropsychologia 45:755–766
Robertson D et al (2007b) The neural processing of moral sensitivity to issues of justice and care. Neuropsychologia 45(4):755–766
Robinson P, Kurzban R (2007) Concordance and conflict in intuitions of justice. Minnesota Law Rev 91:1829–1893
Rosen HJ, Allison SC, Schauer GF, Gorno-Tempini ML, Weiner MW, Miller BL (2005) Neuroanatomical correlates of behavioural disorders in dementia. Brain J Neurol 128(Pt 11):2612–2625. doi:10.1093/brain/awh628
Siegal M, Varley R (2002) Neural systems involved in "theory of mind". Nat Rev Neurosci 3(6):463–471. doi:10.1038/nrn844
Snowden JS, Bathgate D, Varma A, Blackshaw A, Gibbons ZC, Neary D (2001) Distinct behavioural profiles in frontotemporal dementia and semantic dementia. J Neurol Neurosurg Psychiatry 70(3):323–332
Takahashi H, Yahata N, Koeda M, Matsuda T, Asai K, Okubo Y (2004) Brain activation associated with evaluative processes of guilt and embarrassment: an fMRI study. NeuroImage 23(3):967–974. doi:10.1016/j.neuroimage.2004.07.054
Vohs KD, Schooler JW (2008) The value of believing in free will: encouraging a belief in determinism increases cheating. Psychol Sci 19(1):49–54. doi:10.1111/j.1467-9280.2008.02045.x
Zamboni G, Gozzi M, Krueger F, Duhamel JR, Sirigu A, Grafman J (2009) Individualism, conservatism, and radicalism as criteria for processing political beliefs: a parametric fMRI study. Soc Neurosci 4(5):367–383. doi:10.1080/17470910902860308
Zeelenberg M, Breugelmans SM (2008) The role of interpersonal harm in distinguishing regret from guilt. Emotion 8(5):589–596. doi:10.1037/a0012894

Believing in the Effectiveness of Treatment: From Placebo to Credition and Back

Karin Meissner

Abstract Recent placebo research has shown that the effectiveness of medical treatments depends not only on specific characteristics, such as pharmacological agents or physical properties, but also on contextual factors, including the patient's expectations, emotions, and beliefs. This explains why even inert treatments can lead to substantial symptom improvement. The chapter gives a brief overview of findings from placebo studies and discusses possible interrelations with the framework of 'credition'.

1 Introduction

'Credition' is a psychological term analogous to emotion and cognition denoting the mental activity related to the process of believing (Seitz and Angel 2012). Translating the process of believing into the context of placebo research involves considering all the processes that may play a role in the generation and maintenance of placebo effects: What are the psychological mechanisms that mediate placebo effects? What are the decisive factors/prerequisites for whether a patient will, or will not, believe in the success of a given treatment, and which factors can strengthen that belief? Furthermore, what happens in the brain if a patient believes that a treatment will help? Finally, which factors contribute to the stabilization of treatment expectations, and which situations lead to a change in these expectations? In this chapter, findings from placebo research related to these issues will be summarized, and possible interrelations with the framework of credition will be discussed.

K. Meissner (✉)
Institute of Medical Psychology, Ludwig Maximilian University of Munich, Munich, Germany

Division Health Promotion, University of Applied Sciences Coburg, Coburg, Germany
e-mail: karin.meissner@med.lmu.de

H.-F. Angel et al. (eds.), *Processes of Believing: The Acquisition, Maintenance, and Change in Creditions*, New Approaches to the Scientific Study of Religion 1,
DOI 10.1007/978-3-319-50924-2_9

1.1 What Is the Placebo Effect?

The placebo effect is defined as the effect of a placebo, i.e. an 'inert' therapy that lacks any pharmacological or otherwise 'specific' ingredients. The paradoxical outcome of a placebo as a successful treatment can be resolved best when considering that therapies are never performed in a vacuum but are embedded in a psychosocial context. This psychosocial context comprises characteristics of the patient (e.g., treatment expectations, prior experience with treatment, emotional state), characteristics of the doctor (e.g., status, attitude and belief toward therapy), characteristics of the treatment (e.g., mode of delivery, price), characteristics of the doctor-patient interaction (e.g., information about treatment, degree of trust and empathy), and characteristics of the medical setting (e.g., home or hospital) (Di Blasi et al. 2002). A favorable composition of these contextual factors will lead to health improvements even when only placebo treatment has been administered. However, placebo effects occur not only in response to inert therapies but can also significantly affect the outcomes of real treatments (Bingel et al. 2011; Colloca et al. 2004).

Thus far, placebo effects and the processes that produce them have not been conceptualized within the framework of credition. However, it is reasonable to assume that creditive processes play a central role whenever placebo effects occur. This is because placebo-inducing procedures involve the person's awareness of doing something (and therefore implicitly or explicitly believing something) to produce an outcome, even though the procedure may not include the known outcome-inducing agent or activity. In particular, the concept of credition not only offers a possible explanation but also provides a model of the ongoing process of believing. This yields an interesting bridge to mental processes that come into view in placebo research. The present chapter is a first step toward putting these two fields of research in relation to each other.

1.2 A Short History of Placebo Research

Henry Knowles Beecher (1904–1976), one of the first placebo researchers, noted that soldiers severely wounded in a World War II combat zone asked for analgesics to relieve their unbearable suffering much less frequently than patients with similar injuries in civilian hospitals (25% vs. 80%, respectively). Beecher reasoned that to the soldiers, being wounded meant that they had survived, whereas the civilians were more worried about their social and financial situation. Thus, the consequences anticipated by the patients may explain the difference in the demand for analgesics (Beecher 1956).

This interesting finding is the reason why Beecher became interested in exploring the power of placebos. His seminal paper, "The Powerful Placebo", in which he claimed that "placebos have a high degree of therapeutic effectiveness in treating subjective responses" and can also have "toxic effects" (Beecher 1955), has been cited more than 1800 times to date. Although his conclusions about the overall effect size and significance of placebo effects in clinical trials have been criticized (Kienle and Kiene 1997), his papers have nonetheless encouraged numerous medical doctors and scientists to study what we have come to know as 'placebo effects".

1.3 Motivations to Study the Placebo Effect

The aims of placebo researchers are versatile. Many placebo researchers in the field of basic sciences use placebo paradigms to learn more about innate mechanisms involved in the self-regulation of symptoms and organ functions, e.g. the central mechanisms of pain processing. More clinically-oriented placebo researchers aim to understand how the psychosocial context of treatments can be optimized in order to maximize the benefit for the patient. Finally, clinical-trial methodologists are most interested in factors that minimize placebo effects, since the effectiveness of new treatments is usually tested in comparison to placebo control groups.

2 Psychological and Neurobiological Mechanisms of Placebo Effects

Results from placebo research clearly indicate that the placebo effect is a real neurobiological phenomenon. Placebo interventions do not only alleviate symptoms, such as pain, nausea, itch and anxiety, but can also improve motor performance (e.g. in Parkinson's disease), immune functions (e.g. in allergic rhinitis), and the state of internal organs such as blood pressure, gastrointestinal activity, the diameter of cardiac vessels, and lung function. The psychological theories most accepted for explaining placebo effects are expectation and classical conditioning. Recent studies have additionally demonstrated that social observational learning represents another psychological mechanism for producing placebo responses. Further pieces of the placebo puzzle are integrated into the whole picture, for example, emotions, motivational aspects, and characteristics of the healing ritual itself. None of these mechanisms is strictly independent, however; instead, they interact with each other. In what follows, the most prominent mechanisms will be outlined and illustrated by examples.

2.1 Expectations

Expectations towards (placebo) treatment are typically induced by verbal suggestions in combination with the administration of a treatment. Placebo effects on acute pain, for example, can be evoked by the application of a placebo cream accompanied by information that the cream contains a potent painkiller. The greater the expectation of pain relief in such a setting, the greater the pain reduction. A similar association between positive expectations and symptom improvement has been shown for chronic pain conditions (Linde et al. 2007).

Expectation-induced placebo effects can display a high degree of specificity; according to the content of verbal suggestions, placebo effects can induce pain relief in a particular part of the body (Benedetti et al. 1999; Montgomery and Kirsch 1996) and can selectively affect inner organ functions (Meissner 2011, 2014). When the aim of a placebo intervention was to alter gastric activity, objective changes in gastric activity were measured while cardiovascular functions remained unchanged (Meissner 2009). In contrast, when the aim of a placebo intervention was the reduction in blood pressure, blood pressure decreased while gastric activity was not affected (Meissner and Ziep 2011). Even the diameter of coronary arteries has been selectively altered in response to a placebo injection said to be heart medication (Ronel et al. 2011).

Not surprisingly, expectation-induced placebo effects can be increased by enhancing treatment expectations. Several relevant factors that may increase treatment expectations have been identified, such as the price of a treatment. This seems to have an effect because the more we invest in a treatment, the more we expect from it. For example, 'cheap painkillers' induced smaller placebo effects than 'painkillers at a regular price', even though in reality placebo pills were administered to all participants (Waber et al. 2008). In addition, brand names can boost treatment expectations; placebo pills labeled as "aspirin", for example, were more effective in reducing pain than placebo pills labeled as a generic brand of aspirin (Fehse et al. 2015). Furthermore, there is increasing evidence that invasive placebo treatments, such as placebo injections, sham acupuncture, and sham surgery, are associated with larger placebo effects than oral placebo pills (Meissner et al. 2013), which is probably related to larger treatment expectations (Meissner and Linde 2013). Furthermore, side effects of placebo interventions, such as those induced by pepper ingredients in a nasal placebo spray, were shown to increase the effectiveness of the placebo, especially when subjects were informed that they could receive either a placebo spray or an active drug (Rief and Glombiewski 2012). Thus, in ambiguous situations, cues like side effects can strengthen the belief associated with an active treatment, which in turn will increase expectations, and thus the placebo effect.

2.2 *Learning Processes*

In addition to expectation, placebo effects can also be acquired via non-conscious learning processes such as classical conditioning. First described by Ivan Pavlov, classical conditioning refers to the phenomenon in which an intrinsic response to a novel stimulus comes to be elicited in response to a previously neutral stimulus via repeated pairings of the neutral stimulus with the novel stimulus. Not only can salivation be classically conditioned, as in Pavlov's dogs; drug responses can also be classically conditioned (Ader and Cohen 1975). After repeated pairings of immunosuppressive drugs with a novel saccharin-flavored drinking solution in rats, for example, the drug response can also be elicited by administration of a placebo drug in combination with the flavored drink. The therapeutic value of classical conditioning was first demonstrated in a patient with severe autoimmune disease. After repeated infusions with the immunosuppressive drug 'cyclophosphamide' in combination with cod liver oil and a strong scent of roses, the drug was added only every third time to the infusion. After 1 year, the patient showed the same clinical improvement as under the full dose of cyclophosphamide (Olness and Ader 1992). Meanwhile, classical conditioning paradigms have been successfully tested in clinical populations (Ader et al. 2010; Goebel et al. 2008). In patients with psoriasis, for example, the dose of corticosteroids could be reduced after classical conditioning by 50% without losing therapeutic efficacy. Conditioned placebo effects are not restricted to immunological functions; the pharmacological effects of painkillers, for example, can likewise be classically conditioned (Amanzio et al. 2001; Benedetti et al. 2011). Placebo effects acquired by classical conditioning could be experimentally enhanced by increasing the number of learning trials (Colloca et al. 2010). These findings suggest that repeated learning is important for producing robust placebo effects.

Interestingly, classical conditioning is also a means to enhance placebo effects that are induced by expectations. Typically, the following preconditioning procedure is used in experimental placebo studies: After applying the first series of pain stimuli, a 'potent painkiller' is administered, which in truth is a placebo. During the second series of pain stimulation and unbeknown to the participant, the stimulus intensity is reduced by 50% in order to strengthen the subject's belief in the effectiveness of the 'treatment'. During the last series of pain stimuli – the testing period – stimulus intensity is set back to 100%. By using such a preconditioning procedure, placebo effects on pain, itch and nausea could be effectively enhanced (Bartels et al. 2014; Geuter et al. 2013; Horing et al. 2013).

In addition to classical conditioning, other forms of learning processes can induce placebo effects as well. Placebo responses on pain, for example, can be triggered by instances of social observational learning. When participants observe the beneficial effects of a pain treatment in a demonstrator (actually a simulator) and then receive this treatment by themselves, they show comparable placebo analgesic responses as after a classical conditioning procedure (Colloca and Benedetti 2009). Most probably, placebo effects acquired by observational learning are mediated by the mirror neuron system, by which we can perceive the pain of others as if it was our own. In accord with this hypothesis, the placebo analgesic response induced by observational learning was largest in participants who showed the highest empathy scores in a validated questionnaire (Colloca and Benedetti 2009; Hunter et al. 2014).

2.3 Positive Shift in Emotions

There are several indications from experimental studies that placebo effects on pain are preceded by the reduction of negative emotional states, such as stress and anxiety (Aslaksen et al. 2011; Aslaksen and Flaten 2008), while positive emotions, such as excitement and hope, are increased (Petersen et al. 2014). The importance of a shift from negative to positive emotions is further corroborated by findings that a warm and trusting doctor-patient-relationship can enhance the efficacy of placebo interventions. In a clinical trial, for example, patients with irritable bowel syndrome were randomly assigned to either a waiting list (observation), placebo acupuncture, or placebo acupuncture with a patient-practitioner relationship augmented by warmth, attention, and confidence (Kaptchuk et al. 2008). At three weeks, the proportion of patients reporting adequate symptom relief was 28% on waiting list, 44% in the limited group, and 62% in the augmented group.

Oxytocin is a hormone that is known to reduce negative emotions, such as fear and anxiety, and to increase feelings of trust and confidence (Huber et al. 2005; Theodoridou et al. 2009; Viviani et al. 2011). It is released in both males and females during trustful social interactions. The hypothesis that administration of oxytocin by a nasal spray would increase placebo effects on pain has recently been tested in an experimental approach. Indeed, exogenous oxytocin increased the analgesic effect of an inert cream that supposedly contained a potent painkiller (Kessner et al. 2013). These findings suggest that the hormone oxytocin can enhance trust and belief in a doctor's words.

2.4 Is There a "Placebo Responder Personality"?

In addition to the psychological factors that are related to the therapeutic setting and how the placebo effects are initiated, personality factors also appear to play a role. While early attempts to define the typical 'placebo reactor' have failed (Shapiro and Morris 1978), certain personality traits associated with placebo effects have recently been identified. For example, traits related to reward and dopaminergic activation such as novelty-seeking and reward-responsiveness accounted for about 25–30% of the variance in placebo analgesic responses (Schweinhardt et al. 2009; Scott et al. 2008). Additionally, altruism (Mackenbach 2005), optimism (Geers et al. 2005, 2010; Morton et al. 2009), and spirituality (Hyland 2011; Kohls et al. 2011) have been found to modulate placebo responses. More recently, placebo researchers identified first-gene variants that are associated with larger placebo effects (Hall et al. 2015). On the whole, however, situational variables appear to be more important for the occurrence and size of placebo effects than personality traits and genetic variants.

2.5 *Neurobiological Mechanisms of Placebo Effects*

Placebo analgesia represents one of the best studied placebo responses. During the 1970s, it was proposed that expectation-induced placebo analgesia is mediated by the release of endogenous opioids, i.e. painkillers that are naturally produced in the body. In an early landmark study (Levine et al. 1978), after a tooth extraction, patients received first a placebo pill as a pain killer and one hour later either a placebo pill or the opiate antagonist naloxone. It was hypothesized that naloxone would antagonize the placebo response on pain by blocking the bodily response to endogenous opioids. In fact, patients who had responded to the first placebo treatment with pain relief again reported significant pain after the administration of naloxone. Neuroimaging studies provided even more convincing evidence that placebo analgesia is at least partly mediated by the release of endogenous opioids (Meissner et al. 2011).

Increased activation during placebo analgesia is found in a set of brain regions including the orbitofrontal cortex, the dorsolateral prefrontal cortex (DLPFC), the anterior cingulate cortex, and the periaqueductal grey. Several authors have suggested that these areas might reflect the expectation of pain relief or the maintenance of context representations that are mandatory to the creation of a placebo effect (Krummenacher et al. 2010; Lui et al. 2010; Petrovic et al. 2010; Wager et al. 2011). In fact, experimental disruption of the DLPFC by bilateral repetitive transcranial magnetic stimulation blocked the placebo analgesic response (Krummenacher et al. 2010). Increased activation during placebo analgesia is found in the classical pain-processing areas including the thalamus, the insula, and the somatosensory cortex (Meissner et al. 2011). However, the best predictors for the placebo effect on pain turned out to be activity changes in the lateral prefrontal cortex (and the pre- supplemental motor area) rather than changes in the classical pain-processing areas (Koban et al. 2013). These results raise the question of whether changes in frontal areas may represent a common mechanism of placebo interventions for different conditions. Indeed, studies investigating the placebo effect on unpleasant states such as disgust and anxiety could confirm the involvement of these frontal areas (Meyer et al. 2015; Petrovic et al. 2005; Schienle et al. 2014).

Research on the neurobiological mechanisms of placebo effects in conditions involving physical symptoms is still in its infancy. More than 10 years ago, de la Fuente-Fernandez et al. (2001) showed that placebo effects in patients with Parkinson's disease are associated with the release of dopamine in the striatum. Since the nigrostriatal dopaminergic system is damaged in patients with Parkinson's disease, these findings point again to the high specificity of placebo effects – there is not one placebo effect, but many. As mentioned above, placebo interventions can also modulate inner-organ functions. In a meta-analysis of placebo-controlled clinical trials, 'physical' parameters such as blood pressure, lung function and heart rate improved during placebo treatment, while biochemical parameters such as LDL cholesterol and glucose slightly deteriorated during placebo treatment (Meissner et al. 2007). In experimental studies parameters regulated by the autonomic nervous system such as blood pressure, stomach activity and coronary arteries were shown to be selectively affected by placebo administration in combination with specific verbal suggestions (Meissner 2009; Meissner and Ziep 2011; Ronel et al. 2011). Interestingly, the DLPFC is one of the key areas for central control of autonomic organ functions (Beissner et al. 2013). Further studies will have to evaluate whether the DLPFC is likewise involved in the initiation of placebo effects on inner-organ functions.

2.6 *The Dynamics of Treatment Expectations*

Recently, a framework of predictive coding has been applied to placebo research (Buchel et al. 2014). This framework allows not only the integration of the different neurobiological and psychological mechanisms of placebo effects, but also takes into account the dynamic nature of believing processes. Within this framework, expectations are viewed as the consequence of prior experience (including conditioning processes and social observational learning). Situation-specific expectations will lead to predictions, e.g. regarding the intensity of perceived pain after a (placebo) cream has been applied. These predictions result from higher-order brain processes and are compared with sensory input from lower brain processes, e.g. when pain stimuli are applied. As a result, the prediction on the basis of prior experience will either be confirmed or violated. While prediction confirmation will lead to stabilization of expectations, violation of the prediction (the 'prediction error') can be used for learning and updating of the internal model. However, people invest considerable resources into defending their belief systems before they update them (Rief et al. 2015). Accordingly, it has been proposed that incoming data are matched with predictions by 'explaining away the discrepancy', or prediction error" (Buchel et al. 2014). The larger the prediction error, the more likely expectations will change. That is, when the incoming data are too far away from the internal model, patients may question the efficacy of the (placebo) treatment and may update their expectations regarding this treatment.

An interesting assumption of the framework of predictive coding is that an expectation is not only characterized by its magnitude, but also by its precision or certainty: Telling patients that a cream contains a potent painkiller will lead to a more precise expectation/prediction, and thus to a more pronounced placebo effect than a less precise instruction, in which patients are told that the cream may be either a powerful painkiller or an inactive placebo. It has been suggested that modulatory neurotransmitters such as opioids, dopamine and oxytocin could signal the precision of predictions (Buchel et al. 2014). Experimental research is needed to test the feasibility and limitations of the predictive coding model within the context of placebo research.

3 Placebo Effects and the Framework of Credition

In the following paragraphs, three areas of placebo research will be exemplarily related to the framework of credition. There are, however, much more commonalities between these two lines of research, which should be addressed in further studies. For example, the predictive coding model fits nicely with current models of the believing process (Sugiura et al. 2015), as do findings related to oxytocin, empathy and mirror neurons (Seitz and Angel 2015; Sugiura et al. 2015).

3.1 Expectation

The term 'expectation' is central to placebo research. With regard to the framework of credition, the question arises as to whether expectation and credition refer to similar or different constructs. From the perspective of placebo research, both constructs appear to be rather similar. Thus, an important first step would be to elaborate on the commonalities and differences between these two constructs. This would pave the way for fruitful discussions regarding these two fields of research.

3.2 The Role of Consciousness

Results from placebo studies clearly indicate that by itself, conscious expectation of benefit is not sufficient to induce a placebo effect. For example, in a recent placebo study an inert nasal placebo spray successfully created the expectation that the treatment would lower blood pressure, while the placebo intervention did not decrease blood pressure (Zimmermann-Viehoff et al. 2013). It would be highly interesting to see how such a situation could be integrated into the framework of credition. In other words, what makes the difference between an effective expectation or belief, and an expectation that has no consequence for behavior?

A related but different question is whether conscious awareness is necessary in order to elicit a placebo response. Indeed, this has long been assumed by placebo and conditioning researchers. A recent study, however, provided initial evidence that demonstrated that placebo analgesia can also be activated by nonconscious cues (Jensen et al. 2012). This finding may be of special interest for the framework of credition, since it suggests that conscious stimuli are not necessary to activate beliefs. That is, under certain circumstances the converter function of the credition model may be activated by cues outside of conscious awareness.

3.3 *Neuroimaging Studies*

Interestingly, neuroimaging findings from both placebo and credition research point to the importance of frontal cortical areas regarding the process of believing. While placebo studies, however, suggest that changes in the DLPFC, the perigenual anterior cingulate cortex and the orbitofrontal cortex may represent expectation of improvement during placebo treatment, Seitz and Angel (2012) identified consistent activation of the medial frontal cortex (MFC) in studies addressing secular and religious belief processes. Further research is needed to disentangle the specific roles of these frontal areas for each component of credition. Research in this area appears very promising, since it could help to establish a neural map of the structure of credition and would allow further investigation into the commonalities and differences in the results from placebo research.

4 Conclusions

In this chapter, the most important findings from placebo research were summarized with the aim of building a bridge between this line of research and the framework of credition. Findings from placebo research indicate that believing processes in patients can have profound psychobiological consequences and that several conceptual approaches could be helpful in order to further elaborate and validate the concept of credition. In turn, placebo research could also benefit from a systematization of believing processes in order to better understand which factors contribute to the generation, maintenance and extinction of treatment expectations.

References

Ader R, Cohen N (1975) Behaviorally conditioned immunosuppression. Psychosom Med 37:333–340

Ader R, Mercurio MG, Walton J, James D, Davis M, Ojha V, Kimball AB, Fiorentino D (2010) Conditioned pharmacotherapeutic effects: a preliminary study. Psychosom Med 72:192–197

Amanzio M, Pollo A, Maggi G, Benedetti F (2001) Response variability to analgesics: a role for non-specific activation of endogenous opioids. Pain 90:205–215

Aslaksen PM, Flaten MA (2008) The roles of physiological and subjective stress in the effectiveness of a placebo on experimentally induced pain. Psychosom Med 70:811–818

Aslaksen PM, Bystad M, Vambheim SM, Flaten MA (2011) Gender differences in placebo analgesia: event-related potentials and emotional modulation. Psychosom Med 73:193–199

Bartels DJP, van Laarhoven AIM, Haverkamp EA, Wilder-Smith OH, Donders ART, van Middendorp H, van de Kerkhof PCM, Evers AWM (2014) Role of conditioning and verbal suggestion in placebo and nocebo effects on itch. PLoS One 9

Beecher HK (1955) The powerful placebo. J Am Med Assoc 159:1602–1606

Beecher HK (1956) Relationship of significance of wound to pain experienced. J Am Med Assoc 161:1609–1613

Beissner F, Meissner K, Bar KJ, Napadow V (2013) The autonomic brain: an activation likelihood estimation meta-analysis for central processing of autonomic function. J Neurosci 33:10503–10511
Benedetti F, Arduino C, Amanzio M (1999) Somatotopic activation of opioid systems by target-directed expectations of analgesia. J Neurosci 19:3639–3648
Benedetti F, Amanzio M, Rosato R, Blanchard C (2011) Nonopioid placebo analgesia is mediated by CB1 cannabinoid receptors. Nat Med 17:1228–1230
Bingel U, Wanigasekera V, Wiech K, Ni Mhuircheartaigh R, Lee MC, Ploner M, Tracey I (2011) The effect of treatment expectation on drug efficacy: imaging the analgesic benefit of the opioid remifentanil. Sci Transl Med 3:70ra14
Buchel C, Geuter S, Sprenger C, Eippert F (2014) Placebo analgesia: a predictive coding perspective. Neuron 81:1223–1239
Colloca L, Benedetti F (2009) Placebo analgesia induced by social observational learning. Pain 144:28–34
Colloca L, Lopiano L, Lanotte M, Benedetti F (2004) Overt versus covert treatment for pain, anxiety, and Parkinson's disease. Lancet Neurol 3:679–684
Colloca L, Petrovic P, Wager TD, Ingvar M, Benedetti F (2010) How the number of learning trials affects placebo and nocebo responses. Pain 151:430–439
de la Fuente-Fernandez R, Ruth TJ, Sossi V, Schulzer M, Calne DB, Stoessl AJ (2001) Expectation and dopamine release: mechanism of the placebo effect in Parkinson's disease. Science 293:1164–1166
Di Blasi Z, Kaptchuk TJ, Weinman J, Kleijnen J (2002) Informing participants of allocation to placebo at trial closure: postal survey. BMJ 325:1329
Fehse K, Maikowski L, Simmank F, Gutyrchik E, Meissner K (2015) Placebo responses to original vs generic ASA brands during exposure to noxious heat: a pilot fMRI study of neurofunctional correlates. Pain Med 6(10):1967–1974
Geers AL, Helfer SG, Kosbab K, Weiland PE, Landry SJ (2005) Reconsidering the role of personality in placebo effects: dispositional optimism, situational expectations, and the placebo response. J Psychosom Res 58:121–127
Geers AL, Wellman JA, Fowler SL, Helfer SG, France CR (2010) Dispositional optimism predicts placebo analgesia. J Pain 11:1165–1171
Geuter S, Eippert F, Attar CH, Buchel C (2013) Cortical and subcortical responses to high and low effective placebo treatments. NeuroImage 67:227–236
Goebel MU, Meykadeh N, Kou W, Schedlowski M, Hengge UR (2008) Behavioral conditioning of antihistamine effects in patients with allergic rhinitis. Psychother Psychosom 77:227–234
Hall KT, Loscalzo J, Kaptchuk TJ (2015) Genetics and the placebo effect: the placebome. Trends Mol Med 21:285–294
Horing B, Weimer K, Schrade D, Muth ER, Scisco JL, Enck P, Klosterhalfen S (2013) Reduction of motion sickness with an enhanced placebo instruction: an experimental study with healthy participants. Psychosom Med 75:497–504
Huber D, Veinante P, Stoop R (2005) Vasopressin and oxytocin excite distinct neuronal populations in the central amygdala. Science 308:245–248
Hunter T, Siess F, Colloca L (2014) Socially induced placebo analgesia: a comparison of a pre-recorded versus live face-to-face observation. Eur J Pain 18:914–922
Hyland M (2011) Motivation and placebos: do different mechanisms occur in different contexts? Philos Trans R Soc Lond Ser B Biol Sci 366:1828–1837
Jensen KB, Kaptchuk TJ, Kirsch I, Raicek J, Lindstrom KM, Berna C, Gollub RL, Ingvar M, Kong J (2012) Nonconscious activation of placebo and nocebo pain responses. Proc Natl Acad Sci U S A 109:15959–15964
Kaptchuk TJ, Kelley JM, Conboy LA, Davis RB, Kerr CE, Jacobson EE, Kirsch I, Schyner RN, Nam BH, Nguyen LT et al (2008) Components of placebo effect: randomised controlled trial in patients with irritable bowel syndrome. BMJ 336:999–1003

Kessner S, Sprenger C, Wrobel N, Wiech K, Bingel U (2013) Effect of oxytocin on placebo analgesia: a randomized study. JAMA 310:1733–1735
Kienle GS, Kiene H (1997) The powerful placebo effect: fact or fiction? J Clin Epidemiol 50:1311–1318
Koban L, Ruzic L, Wager TD (2013) Brain predictors of individual differences in placebo responding. In: Colloca L, Flaten MA, Meissner K (eds) Placebo and pain. Elsevier, Burlington, pp 89–101
Kohls N, Sauer S, Offenbächer M, Giordano J (2011) Spirituality – an overlooked predictor of placebo effects? Philos Trans R Soc Lond Ser B Biol Sci 366:1838–1848
Krummenacher P, Candia V, Folkers G, Schedlowski M, Schonbachler G (2010) Prefrontal cortex modulates placebo analgesia. Pain 148:368–374
Levine JD, Gordon NC, Fields HL (1978) The mechanism of placebo analgesia. Lancet 2:654–657
Linde K, Witt CM, Streng A, Weidenhammer W, Wagenpfeil S, Brinkhaus B, Willich SN, Melchart D (2007) The impact of patient expectations on outcomes in four randomized controlled trials of acupuncture in patients with chronic pain. Pain 128:264–271
Lui F, Colloca L, Duzzi D, Anchisi D, Benedetti F, Porro CA (2010) Neural bases of conditioned placebo analgesia. Pain 151:816–824
Mackenbach JP (2005) On the survival of the altruistic trait in medicine: is there a link with the placebo effect? J Clin Epidemiol 58:433–435
Meissner K (2009) Effects of placebo interventions on gastric motility and general autonomic activity. J Psychosom Res 66:391–398
Meissner K (2011) The placebo effect and the autonomic nervous system: evidence for an intimate relationship. Philos Trans R Soc Lond Ser B Biol Sci 366:1808–1817
Meissner K (2014) Placebo responses on cardiovascular, gastrointestinal, and respiratory organ functions. Handb Exp Pharmacol 225:183–203
Meissner K, Linde K (2013) What are the best placebos for the treatment of pain? In: Colloca L, Flaten MA, Meissner K (eds) Placebo and pain. Elsevier, Burlington, pp 235–242
Meissner K, Ziep D (2011) Organ-specificity of placebo effects on blood pressure. Auton Neurosci Basic Clin 164:62–66
Meissner K, Distel H, Mitzdorf U (2007) Evidence for placebo effects on physical but not on biochemical outcome parameters: a review of clinical trials. BMC Med 5:3
Meissner K, Bingel U, Colloca L, Wager TD, Watson A, Flaten MA (2011) The placebo effect: advances from different methodological approaches. J Neurosci 31:16117–16124
Meissner K, Fassler M, Rucker G, Kleijnen J, Hrobjartsson A, Schneider A, Antes G, Linde K (2013) Differential effectiveness of placebo treatments: a systematic review of migraine prophylaxis. JAMA Intern Med 173:1941–1951
Meyer B, Yuen KS, Ertl M, Polomac N, Mulert C, Buchel C, Kalisch R (2015) Neural mechanisms of placebo anxiolysis. J Neurosci 35:7365–7373
Montgomery G, Kirsch I (1996) Mechanisms of placebo pain reduction: an empirical investigation. Psychol Sci 7:174–176
Morton DL, Watson A, El-Deredy W, Jones AK (2009) Reproducibility of placebo analgesia: effect of dispositional optimism. Pain 146:194–198
Olness K, Ader R (1992) Conditioning as an adjunct in the pharmacotherapy of lupus-erythematosus. J Dev Behav Pediatr 13:124–125
Petersen GL, Finnerup NB, Grosen K, Pilegaard HK, Tracey I, Benedetti F, Price DD, Jensen TS, Vase L (2014) Expectations and positive emotional feelings accompany reductions in ongoing and evoked neuropathic pain following placebo interventions. Pain 155:2687–2698
Petrovic P, Dietrich T, Fransson P, Andersson J, Carlsson K, Ingvar M (2005) Placebo in emotional processing--induced expectations of anxiety relief activate a generalized modulatory network. Neuron 46:957–969
Petrovic P, Kalso E, Petersson KM, Andersson J, Fransson P, Ingvar M (2010) A prefrontal non-opioid mechanism in placebo analgesia. Pain 150:59–65

Rief W, Glombiewski JA (2012) The hidden effects of blinded, placebo-controlled randomized trials: an experimental investigation. Pain 153:2473–2477

Rief W, Glombiewski JA, Gollwitzer M, Schubo A, Schwarting R, Thorwart A (2015) Expectancies as core features of mental disorders. Curr Opin Psychiatry 28:378–385

Ronel J, Mehilli J, Ladwig KH, Blattler H, Oversohl N, Byrne RA, Bauer A, Schneider S, Linde K, Henningsen P (et al) (2011) Effects of verbal suggestion on coronary arteries: results of a randomized controlled experimental investigation during coronary angiography. Am Heart J 162:507–511

Schienle A, Ubel S, Schongassner F, Ille R, Scharmuller W (2014) Disgust regulation via placebo: an fMRI study. Soc Cogn Affect Neurosci 9:985–990

Schweinhardt P, Seminowicz DA, Jaeger E, Duncan GH, Bushnell MC (2009) The anatomy of the mesolimbic reward system: a link between personality and the placebo analgesic response. J Neurosci 29:4882–4887

Scott DJ, Stohler CS, Egnatuk CM, Wang H, Koeppe RA, Zubieta JK (2008) Placebo and nocebo effects are defined by opposite opioid and dopaminergic responses. Arch Gen Psychiatry 65:220–231

Seitz RJ, Angel HF (2012) Processes of believing – a review and conceptual account. Rev Neurosci 23:303–309

Seitz RJ, Angel HF (2015) Psychology of religion and spirituality: meaning-making and processes of believing. Relig Brain Behav 5:139–147

Shapiro AK, Morris LA (1978) The placebo effect in medical and psychological therapies. In: Garfield SL, Bergin AE (eds) Handbook of psychotherapy and behaviour change. Wiley, New York, pp 369–410

Sugiura M, Seitz RJ, Angel HF (2015) Models and neural bases of the believing process. J Behav Brain Sci 5:12

Theodoridou A, Rowe AC, Penton-Voak IS, Rogers PJ (2009) Oxytocin and social perception: oxytocin increases perceived facial trustworthiness and attractiveness. Horm Behav 56:128–132

Viviani D, Charlet A, van den Burg E, Robinet C, Hurni N, Abatis M, Magara F, Stoop R (2011) Oxytocin selectively gates fear responses through distinct outputs from the central amygdala. Science 333:104–107

Waber RL, Shiv B, Carmon Z, Ariely D (2008) Commercial features of placebo and therapeutic efficacy. JAMA 299:1016–1017

Wager TD, Atlas LY, Leotti LA, Rilling JK (2011) Predicting individual differences in placebo analgesia: contributions of brain activity during anticipation and pain experience. J Neurosci 31:439–452

Zimmermann-Viehoff F, Meissner K, Koch J, Weber CS, Richter S, Deter HC (2013) Autonomic effects of suggestive placebo interventions to increase or decrease blood pressure: a randomized controlled trial in healthy subjects. J Psychosom Res 75:32–35

The Power to Live with Disasters: Adaptive Believing Processes of the Self and World

Motoaki Sugiura

Abstract Eight factors have been identified in the personal characteristics that contribute to increased chances of survival in a disaster ("power to live"). To understand the role of the believing process during disasters, I will map these eight factors onto the two-dimensional matrix defined by the four credition functions crossed with three levels of internal schema of the self and world. In the face of adversity, the enclosure function seems to contribute the factors *problem solving* and *emotional regulation* by adaptive belief organization at the physical or interpersonal level and social-value level, respectively. For survival in the context of group dynamics, the converter function may facilitate the factors *altruism* and *leadership* by intimate association of the social situations with relevant interpersonal behaviors at the physical or interpersonal level and social-value level, respectively. In the face of confrontations with values, the stabilizer function can support the factors *stubbornness* and *self-transcendence* by protecting the values or beliefs in the physical level and interpersonal or social-value level, respectively. Finally, in the context of the optimization of the modulator function, the factor *active well-being* may facilitate the maintenance of the environment on the physical level and and *etiquette* do so on the interpersonal or social-value level. The mapping was in part validated from etiological perspectives. This map supports the comprehensiveness of the eight-factor model of the power to live and provides hypotheses of its neurocognitive underpinning. This, in turn, suggests the utility of the combined framework of the credition and the levels of internal schema.

1 Introduction

The cognitive process of believing, which involves having a specific belief in one's mind despite the ambiguity and uncertainty of the reality, is considered a highly sophisticated behavioral adaptive mechanism (Devinsky 2009; Festinger 1957; Friston 2010; Langdon and Coltheart 2000; Seitz and Angel 2012). This adaptive

M. Sugiura (✉)
IDAC, Tohoku University, Sendai, Japan

IRIDeS, Tohoku University, Sendai, Japan
e-mail: sugiura@tohoku.ac.jp

H.-F. Angel et al. (eds.), *Processes of Believing: The Acquisition, Maintenance, and Change in Creditions*, New Approaches to the Scientific Study of Religion 1,
DOI 10.1007/978-3-319-50924-2_10

nature is particularly evident in hazardous or adverse situations, including survival in the face of severe natural disasters. I came across plenty of such examples in interviews with survivors of the 2011 Great East Japan Earthquake disaster, as well as in my own experience as one of such survivors. The residents in the coastal areas who were able to escape from the massive tsunami were those individuals who believed in its arrival after experiencing the furious earthquake that preceded it, and were quick to immediately evacuate to higher ground. In the local community, which was isolated from the rest of the world for a few days due to the damage to the infrastructure in the area, belief in human nature enabled survivors to be willing to cooperate and share resources each other. In order for the long, difficult process of reconstructing life, community, and a city, a strong belief in the future must be maintained against the threat of desperation. In this chapter, I attempt to comprehend the mechanisms involved in the cognitive process of believing, and try to answer the question of how this process contributed to the different aspects of survival as represented in the now countless anecdotes.

This attempt is based on the integration of three conceptual frameworks. The first framework deals with the four important functional characteristics of the cognitive process of believing, namely, "credition" (Angel 2006). The second framework is concerned with the levels of hierarchical complexity in the contents of belief, namely, the layered structure of the "internal schemata" of the self and world (Sugiura 2013). Finally, the third framework addresses the eight major factors of the personal characteristics that prove advantageous for disaster survival, namely, the "power to live" (Sugiura et al. 2015a). In this chapter, I endeavor to explain each factor of the "power to live" as an adaptive believing process within the conceptual frameworks of credition and internal schema.

The concept of credition encompasses the different aspects of self-organizing characteristics of believing processes, which conceptually stem from an anthropological view on religious experiences; the term "credition" was coined to encompass both religious and secular beliefs. The characteristics of a credition were summarized into four functions: enclosure, converter, stabilizer, and modulator (Angel 2013). The enclosure function addresses the core self-organization process that integrates different knowledge items into a coherent knowledge set with a nested structure, often in a behaviorally adaptive way. The converter function denotes the intimate relationship between a specific belief and specific range of behavior. The stabilizer function is responsible for the stability of the belief despite the perpetual functioning of the enclosure function in a changing environment. The modulator function highlights the influence of the bodily state, particularly emotion, on the belief. In a recent conceptual development incorporating the cognitive neuroscience perspective, it is considered that a belief (i.e., knowledge set) is typically composed of the items not only in the perceptual or conceptual domain, but also in the value and action domains (i.e., perception-action-value triad). The inclusion of the action and value items may explain the converter and modulator functions, respectively (Seitz et al. 2009; Sugiura et al. 2015b).

The internal-schema framework outlines varying levels of complexity in the representation of the external world we interact with, as seen in the findings in neuroimaging research on different self-related cognitive processes (Sugiura 2013). In this model, the schema is conceptualized as the association between action and feedback perception acquired through the repeated experiences of interaction. The schema is assumed for three hierarchical levels: physical, interpersonal, and social value. At the physical level, the schema is relevant to our belief about the surrounding physical environment; the schema associates motor action and its feedback sensation (sensory-motor schema). The interpersonal schema associates one's action towards the other person and the perception of other's response on a conceptual level. This schema allows us to conceptualize the social relationship between the self and each person in the surrounding social environment. The social-value schema associates one's behavior in a specific context and the perception of the social evaluation on the behavior. This schema is concerned with the social self-concept, such as social role and identity integration. It is assumed that the maturation of the schema on a lower level is prerequisite to the development of the schema on a higher level.

The major factors of the power to live were identified by summarizing the opinions of survivors of the 2011 Great East Japan Earthquake disaster (Sugiura et al. 2015a). The authors conducted personal interviews with 78 survivors about their survival experiences and elicited their opinions about the power to live, such as the personality traits, attitudes, or daily habits that were relevant to those experiences. These opinions were then incorporated into a questionnaire that was completed by 1412 survivors. Factor analysis identified eight factors related to the power to live: leadership (F1), problem-solving (F2), altruism (F3), stubbornness (F4), etiquette (F5), emotional regulation (F6), self-transcendence (F7), and active well-being (F8). All factors showed significant associations with one or more measures of survival success in the disaster, including immediate tsunami evacuation, problem-solving in refugee situations, recovery during reconstruction, physical health, and mental health (in part based on unpublished data). Overall, the personal characteristics described by the eight factors largely overlap with similar concepts described in previous arbitrary models (Baltes and Smith 2008; Ministry of Education 2005; Siebert 2010).

From the perspective of cognitive science, the power to live concerns the individual differences in how one perceives, evaluates, and behaves in the context of adversity. Each factor of the power to live appears to address a specific aspect (i.e., function in the credition) of the adaptive believing process on specific levels of the representation of the self, world, and their interaction (i.e., internal schema). Therefore, it would be possible to map each factor of the power to live onto the two-dimensional matrix of the four functions of credition and three levels of internal schema (Fig. 1).

Due to the neurodevelopmental perspective of the internal-schema framework, this map may allow us to develop etiological and neurocognitive hypotheses of these factors.

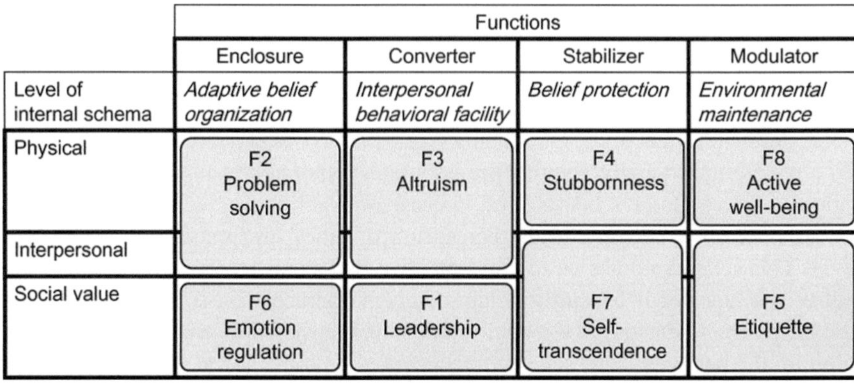

Fig. 1 Eight factors of the power to live are mapped onto the two-dimensional matrix of the four functions of credition (*columns*) and three levels of internal schema (*rows*). F1–F8 denote the identified order of the factor in the original inventory-construction study (Sugiura et al. 2015a). The factors problem-solving, altruism, self-transcendence, and etiquette was mapped over two neighboring levels of the internal schema. See text for the further details

2 The Factors of the Power to Live as Adaptive Believing Processes

2.1 Adaptive Belief Organization at the Face of Adversity (Enclosure Function)

I will first address two factors of the power to live, which I consider to represent adaptive "enclosure" functions. Although both factors are apparently unrelated to the believing process from their labels, I assume that both exert behavioral or health advantage through adaptive organization or reorganization of the belief representation about the adverse situation that one may face. The two factors differ in the domain or location of the situation, which is highlighted in the belief; that is, they differ in the levels of internal schema that are reorganized to construct an adaptive belief contents.

2.2 Problem-Solving

The factor problem-solving represents the attitude or habit of strategically tackling problems; its score was in fact associated with the rate of successful personal problem-solving in refugee situations in the 2011 Great East Japan Earthquake disaster. The questionnaire items for this factor include "When I am fretting about what I should do, I compare several alternative actions" and "When talking to someone, I think about that person's personality, wishes, and abilities, and choose the appropriate attitude and words accordingly." Reading through these items, the advantageous attitude or habit described in this factor seems to be essentially derived from the awareness of the factual and manipulative aspects of the situation. That is, the rich representations of such aspects of the situation in one's belief are the basis for the person who is high in this factor to be able to take the necessary actions to solve the problem. These aspects seem to correspond to the action domains of the internal schemata at the physical and interpersonal levels, which represent the external physical environment and relationship with relevant people, respectively.

2.3 Emotion Regulation

The factor emotion regulation represents the attitude or habit of endeavoring to stay calm in difficult or strained circumstances; its score was associated with several aspects of survival success in the disaster, including immediate tsunami evacuation and mental health. The items for this factor include "During difficult times, I endeavor to think positively, telling myself that this experience will benefit me in the future" and "During difficult times, I compare my circumstances to the situation around me and in society, and I think that matters cannot be helped." Thus, the endeavor typically exploits the reinterpretation of the event by reframing the situation, often expanding the scope of the situation to the time and social context in which one lives. That is, the ability to reframe or expand the scope of the situation allows the person who is high in this factor to confer positive evaluation to the event; this enables him or her to avoid psychological distress and to maintain the mental state for optimal decision-making. Such a reframing or expansion of the scope seems to correspond to the relocation of the event representation within the internal schema at the social-value level, in which a context where one's behavior and social value are associated can be adaptively determined.

These two factors of the power to live (problem solving and emotion regulation), therefore, appear to be highly relevant to the adaptive organization of the believing process. However, they seem to differ at the level of internal schemata where the organization process takes place, with the physical and interpersonal levels most relevant for the problem solving factor and the social-value level most relevant for the emotion regulation factor.

2.4 Interpersonal Behavioral Facility (Converter Function)

Some people are quick to perform adaptive interpersonal behaviors while others are hesitant to do so. During an emergency situation, such behaviors are often the determining factor for the survival of the group to which he or she belongs. Two factors in the power to live, altruism and leadership, appear to be involved in the different types of interpersonal behaviors exhibited in the social context in which such behaviors are beneficial. Both factors may be explained by the degree of intimacy in the relationship between the perceived situation and the desired behavior in that situation, that is, the quality of the "converter" function. Additionally, these two factors result in interpersonal behaviors that are associated with different types of social contexts and values; that is, they are converter functions at different levels of internal schema.

2.5 Altruism

The altruism factor represents the personality trait that causes people to care about and help others; its score was associated with the behavior of helping others during the emergency tsunami evacuation discussed earlier (unpublished data), which may have contributed to survival as a group. The items for this factor include "I like it when other people rely on me and are grateful to me" and "When I see someone having trouble, I have to help them." Here, the helping behavior is associated with the perception of feelings of distress in others, and the association is driven by the motivational value of empathy to that person. This perception-action-value triad may belong to either the automatic effortless domain or conscious elaborative domain of the human social-cognitive system (Frith and Frith 2006). The former domain may represent simple altruistic responses driven by the perception of another's distress, which is usually considered an extended form of sensory-motor associations supported by the internal schema at the physical level; the idea is exemplified by the expected role of the mirror neuron system (a network of the class of sensory-motor association neurons) in empathy (Iacoboni 2009). On the other hand, the latter domain may allow optimization of the altruistic behavior by utilizing information specific to the person and situation, which is represented in the internal schema at the interpersonal level.

2.6 Leadership

The factor leadership represents the attitude or habit of gathering and organizing people; its score was associated with the behavior of encouraging others to escape during the emergency tsunami evacuation (unpublished data), which may have contributed to survival as a group. The items for this factor include "To resolve problems, I gather together everyone involved to discuss the matter" and "Sophisticated words that move people's hearts come out of my mouth." Here, the problem seems to be relevant to the moral or collective values, rather than those in the personal or specific interpersonal context. To resolve the problem, it is necessary to clarify the context, including the problematic situation and goal, and to share the context with all the people involved in the situation, preferably using sophisticated words. Such interpersonal behavior is thus likely associated with moral or collective values or relevant situation perception, which is represented in the internal schema at the social-value level.

Thus, it appears reasonable to conceptualize these two factors of the power to live as representing the facility of interpersonal behavior as the intimacy in the relationship of the situational perception and relevant behavior; that is, the adaptive "converter" function. Between the two factors, however, the association of the perception and behavior, as well as the value facilitating this association, is represented in different levels of the internal schema; the factor altruism is in the physical and interpersonal levels and leadership in the social-value level.

2.7 Belief Protection Against the Value Disturbance (Stabilizer Function)

We live in world in which the values relevant to our physical desires, others around us, and social norms are subject to change. New values and beliefs appear around or within us and may make us feel that our values and beliefs are outdated or no longer situation-appropriate. It appears adaptive to conform to new values and beliefs at least for the moment. To gain long-term merit, however, such as to achieve a far-off goal or be consistent as a person across time, we must maintain our initial values and beliefs. Protecting beliefs and values may require one to reject consideration of levels of the information that disturbs them. Two factors of the power to live, stubbornness and self-transcendence, seem to represent this belief-stabilization process, protecting the values or beliefs on some levels of the internal schema while rejecting those on other levels.

2.8 Stubbornness

The stubbornness factor represents the personality trait, attitude, or habit of sticking to one's desires or beliefs; its score was associated with the maintenance of physical health in the disaster. The items for this factor include "I am stubborn and always get my own way" and "I clearly distinguish between black and white: what's good is good, and what's bad is bad." The key feature of this factor is the protection of the values that are relevant to the goal ("get my own way") and help quick decision-making ("good/bad"). The values are essentially materialistic or hedonistic desire represented at the physical level of internal schema. To protect these values and related beliefs, one decides against considering the interpersonal consequence of being stubborn or the potential context-dependency of such values, enduring the conflicts in the interpersonal and social-value schemata, respectively. While this aspect gives negative connotation to this factor, this stabilization process itself may be adaptive for achieving a specific goal.

2.9 Self-Transcendence

The self-transcendence factor represents awareness of the meaning of one's life from a spiritual perspective. The items for this factor include "I am aware that I am alive, and have a sense of responsibility in living" and "I am aware of the role I should play in society." This factor thus puts strong emphasis on one's social role or the merit of others, as well as the detachment from any egoistic or self-centered desire. In fact, the score of this factor was associated with the behavior of helping others during the emergency tsunami evacuation in the disaster (unpublished data). It is likely that this factor represents the protection of values at the interpersonal or social-value level of the internal schema while rejecting the consideration on the physical level under a devastating situation. Supporting this, an increased tendency for the personal characteristics similar to this factor was reported as one of the positive psychological outcomes after the experience of traumatic events (Tedeschi and Calhoun 1996); specifically, the "appreciation of life" factor in the Posttraumatic Growth Inventory (PTGI). In a neuropsychological study, conversely, an increase in the score of similar personality traits has been associated with a lesion in the parietal sensory-integration area, which is relevant to the physical-level internal schema (Urgesi et al. 2010).

These two factors thus appear to exert survival advantage through stabilizer function at the face of value disturbance. The two factors seem to be characterized by the levels of the internal schema where values or beliefs are either protected or rejected. For the factor of stubbornness, values or beliefs in the physical schema are protected at the expense of disregarding those in the interpersonal and social-value schema. For the factor of self-transcendence, those values or beliefs in the interpersonal or social-value schema are protected by discarding the consideration of these elements in the physical schema.

2.10 Environmental Maintenance (to Optimize the Modulator Function)

A proverb says, "A sound mind in a sound body." Any processes of believing, including the perception of the situation (i.e., enclosure function), belief-driven behavior (i.e., converter function), and resistance against the value disturbance (i.e., stabilizer function), are easily modulated by one's physiological and affective states, which are represented as the 'modulator' functions of the credition. The proper functioning of the believing processes, therefore, requires maintenance of such states; that is, an internal environment. Such an internal environment is also affected by an external environment. Two factors of the power to live, active well-being and etiquette, seem to represent the daily practice of such environmental maintenance activity.

2.11 Active Well-Being

The active well-being factor refers to the daily practice of maintaining or improving one's physical, mental, and intellectual status. Three items comprised this factor on the questionnaire given to the tsunami survivors, which describe the "habitual practice" for "relieving stress", the importance of "maintaining my physical health," and acquiring "new knowledge, skills, and attitudes." The score of this factor was, as expected, associated with the maintenance of physical and mental health in the disaster. One's status seemed to be maintained or improved, particularly its physical aspects, primarily due to the internal schema at the physical level. It is considered that mental status is also internally represented as the sensory-motor association, that is, the physical internal schema; the effect of one's behavior on one's own physiological and affective status is monitored through the interoceptive perception system (Craig 2002).

2.12 Etiquette

The factor etiquette represents the attitude or habit of conforming to social norms in daily behavior. The items for this factor include "On a daily basis, I take the initiative in greeting family members and people living in the neighborhood" and "In everyday life, I take care of myself as much as possible." The direct advantage of this factor in the disaster may be enhanced by one's social capital accumulated through daily practice of maintaining good relationships in the family and community. The score was in fact associated with a high chance of finding a person who could be relied on during the emergency tsunami evacuation in the disaster (unpublished data). In the context of the believing process, however, this factor may also exert advantage through an optimal modulator function, since a good social environment is considered the essential basis of mental well-being (Turner 1981). Irrespective of the path of the contribution to the survival advantage, the status maintained or improved in this factor seems to be represented the internal schema at the interpersonal and social-value levels.

The relevance of these factors to the believing process may appear subsidiary given that their direct advantage in disaster survival is attributed to the practice itself. It is, however, important to note that the appreciation of these factors parallels the deep understanding of the modulator function as a human nature. It is the wisdom of life that puts forth that the daily practice of maintaining good internal and external environment is only way to optimize the functioning of our believing process. Good physiological and affective states are warranted by good physical and mental conditions and good social relationships. The factors active well-being and etiquette seem to respectively support these two aspects, with the former being associated with the physical level and the latter with the interpersonal and social-value levels of the internal schema.

3 Discussion on the Map

It appears feasible to map all the factors of the power to live on the two-dimensional matrix of the credition functions and internal-schema levels. A few pieces of supporting data for this mapping are available in the original inventory-construction study of the power to live based on the data from 1412 survivors (Sugiura et al. 2015a). First, a significant age-dependency of the score, specifically the increase of the score along with the age within the age-range from 20s to 70s, was observed for the factors etiquette, emotion regulation, and self-transcendence. The factor leadership also had the same tendency. These factors are all assigned to the social-value level of the internal schema in the current mapping. The age-dependent facilitation of these factors is consistent with the suggested late development of this level of the internal schema, which continues after adolescence (Sugiura 2013). Second, a significant gender difference was observed for the five factors: males' scores were significantly higher in problem-solving, stubbornness, and active well-being, while females' scores were higher in etiquette and self-transcendence. Excluding problem-solving, these factors are all assigned to the belief stabilization or modulator-function optimizing practice; in addition, those that are assigned to the physiological level are higher in males and those to the interpersonal or social-value level are higher in females. There seem to be genetic or social backgrounds that cause gender difference in the functioning of these two aspects of believing process. These etiological issues are of tremendous importance for both understanding and applying the eight factor model of the power to live.

A single factor was mapped over two neighboring levels of the internal schema for four factors: problem-solving, altruism, self-transcendence, and etiquette. A question may arise here: Why did it occur over two lower levels (i.e., physical and interpersonal) for the adaptive belief organization or interpersonal behavioral facility, and why over higher two levels (i.e., interpersonal and social value) for the belief protection and environmental maintenance? It may be explained by the difference in the aspect of internal schemata that these believing processes primarily concern. For the adaptive belief organization or interpersonal behavioral facility, which concerns the organization of the belief representation per se, an important qualification is whether the representation is embodied (i.e., physical and interpersonal) or conceptual (i.e., social value), which are related to direct and indirect solutions of problems, respectively. On the other hand, for the belief protection or environmental maintenance, which concerns the selection of values in which one invests resources, a prominent individual difference exists in whether one places priority on social (i.e., interpersonal and social value) or non-social (physical) domains.

One may wonder why the "converter" function is focused on for non-egoistic interpersonal behaviors, that is, the factors altruism and leadership. This question may be associated with the more fundamental question of why simpler, more basic skills or intelligence are not included in the factors of the power to live. I consider such basic skills or intelligence factors to be more or less examples of converter functions, or perception-action associations, essential for survival, such as knowing not to cross the road when there is car traffic, not to eat a food that looks or smells strange, or the basic skills of reading, writing, and calculation. These critical skills or intelligence factors are, from the beginning, not included in the concept of the power to live, and thus were not mapped in the cells for the converter function. It is important to note this exclusion to understand the nature of the concept of the power to live. This concept does not deal with truly essential skills for literal biological survival, but with personal characteristics that may contribute to better living within a longer perspective aimed at not only the individual but also the social context. The original items for the construction of the power-to-live inventory were collected from the opinions of the survivors who not only survived the disaster but did better or more successfully than others in terms of the quality or context of survival (e.g., not only as an individual). Thus, the constellation of the factors extracted are likely to reflect the power to live beyond immediate biological survival, that is, to live as a human. This then explains why the converter function is focused on non-egoistic interpersonal behaviors.

The development of the concept of the power to live aims to widely cover the personal characteristics that are advantageous for better survival. The demonstrated coverage of all the matrix cells by the eight factors may suggest the fulfilment of this ambition.

4 Towards Neurocognitive Models

The mapping of the power-to-live factors within the two-dimensional matrix of the credition functions and internal-schema levels appears promising in paving the way to the cognitive neuroscience of the factors. The credition was proposed as the model of the cognitive process of believing (Angel 2013). The three levels of internal schema were proposed in association with different neuroanatomical structures (Sugiura 2013). It has been demonstrated that the combination of these two conceptual frameworks provides a comprehensive cognitive neuroscience view of our believing process on the self and world (Sugiura et al. 2015b). Due to the mapping, this comprehensive view is now also available for the eight factors of the power to live.

For the different columns of the matrix, that is, to the factors assigned to different credition functions, different hypotheses about the cognitive processes and relevant experimental designs are proposed. That is, we can predict the type of experimental setting where the individual difference in the power-to-live factors reflects the load of cognitive processing, then the amplitude of neural response. For the factors relevant to adaptive belief organization (i.e., enclosure function), a positive effect of the factor score on the cognitive-processing load is expected in experimental settings where original belief-representation is formed (i.e., everyday situation perception), as well as at those where its adaptive reorganization is necessary (i.e., at the face of adversity). A negative effect is also expected at the latter occasion due to some compensatory executive processes or affective responses in individuals with low factor scores. A similar pattern may be expected for the factors relevant to the interpersonal behavioral facility (i.e., converter function): a positive effect on the perception of relevant social context and both positive and negative effects on the need for relevant interpersonal behaviors. For the factors relevant to the belief protection (i.e., stabilizer function), both positive and negative effects are expected at the moment of value-disturbance: a negative effect on disturbance-relevant activation, and a positive effect on control processes of believing. Finally, for the factors relevant to the environmental maintenance (i.e., optimization of the modulation function), it is difficult to raise a possible hypothesis about the cognitive process at the moment. Although the previous section has discussed the effect of the practice on the environmental maintenance and then on modulator function, the discussion does not provide an explanation for the cognitive process that facilitates the practice per se. Considering the possible role of the daily concern for the well-being and resistance against the laziness in the maintenance of the habit, speculatively, the factors problem solving and stubbornness may share cognitive characteristics with the factors for the environmental maintenance.

For the different rows of the matrix, that is, to the factors assigned to different levels of internal schema, different hypotheses on the neuroanatomical correlates may be provided. It has been assumed that each level of the internal schema is represented in a set of cortical structures. For the factors assigned to a specific level, an increase in the activation of the structures for that level may be observed when increased cognitive load or reorganization of the belief representation is required during the task. It is highly likely that the physical schema is supported by the sensory and motor association cortices located primarily in the right hemisphere. The interpersonal schema is assumed to be represented by several amodal association cortices in the dorsomedial frontal and lateral posterior cortices. The social-value schema is considered relevant to the ventral aspect of the medial prefrontal cortex and the posterior cingulate cortex. It has also been suggested that the medial prefrontal (Seitz et al. 2009) and the right dorsolateral prefrontal (Coltheart 2010; Devinsky 2009) cortices may play a role in control processes of believing. The former may play a key role in belief generation within a specific internal-schema level, while the latter is assumed to coordinate potentially conflicting belief representations across the internal-schema levels (Sugiura et al. 2015b).

5 Conclusion

In this chapter, I have attempted to map the eight factors of the power to live on the two-dimensional matrix of the credition functions and internal-schema levels; it appears quite successful. The mapping enables us to explain the factors of the power to live as adaptive believing processes within the conceptual frameworks of the credition and internal schema. It expands our understanding of the mechanisms behind how the cognitive processes of believing contribute to the different aspects of survival. In addition, the map provides us with an important basis for developing etiological and neurocognitive hypotheses of the power-to-live factors.

The framework of credition, particularly when combined with the conceptual framework of the levels of internal schema, is a powerful tool for understanding and investigating the mechanism of the sophisticated minds and behaviors of humans.

Acknowledgments The preparation of this manuscript was in part supported by KAKENHI (26118702) from JSPS.

References

Angel HF (2006) Religiosität als menschliches Potential. Ein anthropologisches Modell im neurowissenschaftlichen Horizont. In: Angel HF, Broking-Bortfeldt M, Hemel U, Kunstmann J, Jakobs M, Pirner ML, Rothgangel M (eds) Religiosität. Kohlhammer, Stuttgart, pp 62–89

Angel HF (2013) Credition, the process of belief. In: Runehov A, Oviedo L (eds) Encyclopedia of sciences and religions. Springer, Dordrecht

Baltes PB, Smith J (2008) The fascination of wisdom: its nature, ontogeny, and function. Perspect Psychol Sci 3(1):56–64. doi:10.1111/j.1745-6916.2008.00062.x

Coltheart M (2010) The neuropsychology of delusions. Ann NY Acad Sci 1191:16–26. doi:10.1111/j.1749-6632.2010.05496.x

Craig AD (2002) How do you feel? Interoception: the sense of the physiological condition of the body. Nat Rev Neurosci 3(8):655–666

Devinsky O (2009) Delusional misidentifications and duplications right brain lesions, left brain delusions. Neurology 72(1):80–87. doi:10.1212/01.wnl.0000338625.47892.74

Festinger LA (1957) Theory of cognitive dissonance. Stanford University Press, Stanford

Friston K (2010) The free-energy principle: a unified brain theory? Nat Rev Neurosci 11(2):127–138. doi:10.1038/Nrn2787

Frith CD, Frith U (2006) The neural basis of mentalizing. Neuron 50(4):531–534. doi:10.1016/j.neuron.2006.05.001

Iacoboni M (2009) Imitation, empathy, and mirror neurons. Annu Rev Psychol 60:653–670. doi:10.1146/annurev.psych.60.110707.163604

Langdon R, Coltheart M (2000) The cognitive neuropsychology of delusions. Mind Lang 15(1):184–218. doi:10.1111/1468-0017.00129

Ministry of Education, Culture, Sports, Science and Technology, Japan (2005) A mind and body sustaining a "zest for living". National Printing Bureau, Tokyo

Seitz RJ, Angel HF (2012) Processes of believing – a review and conceptual account. Rev Neurosci 23(3):303–309. doi:10.1515/revneuro-2012-0034

Seitz RJ, Franz M, Azari NP (2009) Value judgments and self-control of action: the role of the medial frontal cortex. Brain Res Rev 60(2):368–378. doi:10.1016/j.brainresrev.2009.02.003

Siebert A (2010) Survivor personality: why some people are stronger, smarter, and more skillful at handling life's difficulties…and how you can be, too. Penguin, New York

Sugiura M (2013) Associative account of self-cognition: extended forward model and multi-layer structure. Front Hum Neurosci 7:535. doi:10.3389/Fnhum.2013.00535

Sugiura M, Sato S, Nouchi R, Honda A, Abe T, Muramoto T, Imamura F (2015a) Eight personal characteristics associated with the power to live with disasters as indicated by survivors of the 2011 Great East Japan Earthquake Disaster. PLoS One 10(7):e0130349. doi:10.1371/journal.pone.0130349

Sugiura M, Seitz RF, Angel HF (2015b) Models and neural bases of the believing process. J Behav Brain Sci 5(1):12–23. doi:10.4236/jbbs.2015.51002

Tedeschi RG, Calhoun LG (1996) The posttraumatic growth inventory: measuring the positive legacy of trauma. J Trauma Stress 9(3):455–471

Turner RJ (1981) Social support as a contingency in psychological well-being. J Health Soc Behav 22(4):357–367. doi:10.2307/2136677

Urgesi C, Aglioti SM, Skrap M, Fabbro F (2010) The spiritual brain: selective cortical lesions modulate human self-transcendence. Neuron 65(3):309–319. doi:10.1016/j.neuron.2010.01.026

Belief and Belief Formation: Insights from Delusions

Michael H. Connors and Peter W. Halligan

Abstract Beliefs are stable mental representations of reality that we accept as true. As such, they play a critical role in shaping our phenomenological experiences and determining the choices and actions we make. Despite their considerable importance, the cognitive nature of belief and the underlying processes involved in forming beliefs have received little formal investigation in their own right. This may be due, in part, to the challenges of operationalising intimately familiar, yet highly complex and distributed cognitive processes. One promising avenue, however, has come from cognitive neuropsychiatry and the investigation into delusions, considered by many as pathological forms of belief. Identifying the nature of the responsible causal pathologies can be used to reveal some of the cognitive processes likely to be present in non-pathological belief formation. In this chapter, we describe a tentative five-stage account of belief formation that accommodates some of the key features of both delusions and belief. We provide evidence for this account and discuss its implications for understanding belief.

1 Introduction

Beliefs, as veridical mental representations, provide the critical framework that allows us to navigate effortlessly in our phenomenological world (Connors and Halligan 2015; Frith 2007). Beliefs imbue our sensory experiences with meaning

M.H. Connors (✉)
ARC Centre of Excellence in Cognition and its Disorders, Department of Cognitive Science, Macquarie University, Sydney, NSW, Australia

Dementia Collaborative Research Centre, School of Psychiatry, University of New South Wales, Sydney, NSW, Australia

Sydney Medical School, University of Sydney, Sydney, NSW, Australia
e-mail: michael.connors@mq.edu.au

P.W. Halligan
School of Psychology, Cardiff University, Cardiff, Wales, UK
e-mail: HalliganPW@Cardiff.ac.uk

H.-F. Angel et al. (eds.), *Processes of Believing: The Acquisition, Maintenance, and Change in Creditions*, New Approaches to the Scientific Study of Religion 1,
DOI 10.1007/978-3-319-50924-2_11

and enable us to interact with our physical environment in a purposeful, goal-directed manner (Connors and Halligan 2015; Halligan Halligan 2006, 2007). To carry out even the most basic daily tasks, we rely on a wide array beliefs, including implicit beliefs about the physical world (Subbotsky 2004), beliefs about the properties of objects (which may be culturally or environmentally specific), and beliefs about the contingencies relating our actions to outcomes. Beliefs are also critical to defining our identity and perform many important social functions. As such, they are not simply reducible to what is rational or what has been acquired by direct experience, and instead may be modulated by emotion, motivation, and social forces. Regardless of their origin, once formed, beliefs change the way evidence is collected and evaluated (Barrett 2009; Reisberg et al. 2003; Vicente and Brewer 1993), thereby indelibly altering our experiences and perspective of the world.

Despite their considerable importance, the processes of forming new beliefs and believing have received little formal attention (Bell et al. 2006a). This neglect likely results from the challenges in operationalising such highly complex processes for empirical investigation. It may also stem from philosophical debates about the nature of belief and defining what can be seen as a nebulous concept (Bell et al. 2006a; Connors and Halligan 2015). One promising means of studying the nature of beliefs, however, is through investigating delusions, which are pathological beliefs that are strongly held and resistant to counter-evidence, despite often being relatively implausible. In this chapter, we discuss how delusions inform understanding of both belief formation and believing. In particular, we outline a general five-stage account of belief formation derived from studying clinical delusions.

2 Studying Delusions

The ability of delusions to provide insight into non-pathological beliefs has been previously highlighted by the discipline of cognitive neuropsychiatry (Halligan and David 2001), which seeks to explain psychopathology in terms of disruptions and alterations to normal cognitive processes. According to this general approach, identifying the causes of pathology can help reveal the processes underlying normal cognition, while theoretical accounts of normal cognition can, in turn, also be used to understand the pathology. As Marshall and Halligan (1996) note, this interrelationship between normal cognition and pathology is implicit in definitions of psychopathology as any conception of dysfunction presupposes a conception of normal function. A concept of delusion, for example, presupposes the existence of non-delusional belief and criteria by which the two can be distinguished.

It should be noted, however, that some philosophers question whether all delusions are pathological versions of belief, suggesting that they are instead “imaginings” (Currie 2000) or experiences (Parnas 2004). Such accounts, while possible for a subset of delusions, remain unconvincing as a general account of delusions because there is no empirical evidence to suggest that delusions are qualitatively different from the range of non-delusional beliefs (Bayne and Pacherie 2005;

Bortolotti 2009, 2013). Moreover, delusions show similar properties in terms of people's reported conviction and their effect on behaviour as non-delusional beliefs (Bortolotti 2009, 2013). Given this overlap, there is also considerable difficulty in providing a definition of delusions that distinguishes it from non-pathological belief in all cases (Coltheart 2007; David 1999; Spitzer 1990). Indeed, even if it were the case that some delusions were imaginings, patients believe in these imaginings, leaving it unclear whether there is any meaningful distinction between the two constructs from a practical perspective. Philosophical conundrums notwithstanding, the empirical study of delusions has shown that they are amenable to being investigated and understood as pathological beliefs (Bell et al. 2006b).

A number of different cognitive theories have been proposed to explain delusions. Common to many of these theories is the idea that delusions arise from the attempt to provide meaning for an unusual experience (Ellis and Young 1990; James 1890; Maher 1974, 1988; Reed 1972). Ellis and Young (1990), for example, noted that many misidentification delusions – including Capgras delusion, the belief that a familiar person has been replaced by an impostor – could arise from disruptions to normal face processing and person identification. In the case of Capgras delusion, damage to autonomic responsiveness in face processing could lead patients to encounter loved ones without the normal heightened arousal that they would expect to experience. As a result, these patients conclude that their loved one has been replaced by a look-alike impostor (Ellis and Young 1990; Stone and Young 1997). In support of this account, a number of studies have found that patients with Capgras delusion show reduced autonomic response (indexed by skin conductance recordings) to photographs of familiar faces and similar low levels of autonomic response to familiar and unfamiliar faces (Brighetti et al. 2007; Ellis et al. 1997; Hirstein and Ramachandran 1997). Across a wide range of other delusions, there are plausible deficits that can account for their content (Breen et al. 2000, 2001; Coltheart 2007; Connors et al. 2015a, b; Ellis and Young 1990; Maher 1974, 1988).

While such theories can explain the content of the delusions, they also need to explain why the delusion as an explanation is maintained over time and, in the case of Capgas delusion, why some patients with damage to autonomic responsiveness do not develop the delusion (Tranel et al. 1995). To account for this, Langdon and Coltheart (2000) proposed a two-factor theory of delusions. According to this, two independent factors come together to produce a delusion. The first factor (Factor 1) explains the delusion's content and typically involves a neuropsychological anomaly affecting perceptual, emotional, or autonomic processing. In the case of Capgras, this involves damage to autonomic responsiveness in face processing, as noted earlier. The second factor (Factor 2) explains the delusion's maintenance and involves a deficit in a belief evaluation process. As a result, patients fail to reject the delusional hypothesis as implausible, and so accept it as belief. Patients who have both Factors 1 and 2 are likely to develop a delusion (Coltheart 2007, 2010; Coltheart et al. 2011). This two-factor theory provides a compelling account of many bizarre monothematic delusions. It does not, however, fully explain why the delusional explanation for Factor 1 is selected when alternative explanations are possible. In addition, many people in the general population hold clinically similar unusual beliefs (Pechey and Halligan 2011), including beliefs akin to Capgras, and it is unlikely that all are due to neuropsychological damage.

A number of other theories have focused specifically on explaining persecutory delusions (the belief that others are conspiring to cause one harm), a common type of delusion. Such theories similarly invoke the notion that delusional ideation arises from attempts to explain an unusual experience. According to Freeman et al. (2002), persecutory delusions arise when individuals explain an anomalous experience, such as a hallucination or an unusual event in their environment, in terms of threat. In vulnerable individuals, a number of factors may foster such a persecutory explanation. These include emotions such as anxiety, anger, and depression; a cognitive bias to jump to conclusions on the basis of insufficient information; and pre-existing beliefs that consider the world as hostile. In support of this, research has identified varying levels of evidence for cognitive biases and emotional disturbances in individuals with persecutory delusions (Freeman 2007; Freeman and Garety 2014; Freeman et al. 2008; Garety and Freeman 1999, 2013).

Other deficits may contribute to persecutory delusions. Deficits in theory of mind (the ability to infer and reason about mental states in others) can lead patients to misinterpret the intentions and behaviours of others as hostile, and so generate persecutory ideation (Frith 1992). Alternatively, individuals with low self-esteem may develop attributional biases in order to compensate and avoid awareness of this. In particular, such individuals may come to attribute negative events to the harmful intentions of other people, rather than to themselves or the circumstance they are in, so that they avoid negative views of themselves (Bentall et al. 2001). While evidence for these two deficits remains equivocal (Freeman 2007; Garety and Freeman 1999, 2013), both can be incorporated into Freeman and colleagues' more general biopsychosocial account. Both accounts also similarly emphasise the importance of inferential reasoning in delusional ideation.

Another influential general theory of delusions is the "prediction error" account (Corlett et al. 2010; Fletcher and Frith 2009). According to this model, inappropriate "prediction error" – a mismatch between what is expected and what is experienced – can predispose patients to focus on and infer relationships between unrelated events. Such aberrant prediction error may explain why particular stimuli become salient to the individual and the focus of delusional beliefs. It may also explain the maintenance of the delusion. According to Corlett and colleagues, aberrant prediction errors can re-evoke the content of the delusion over time in a way that leads to reconsolidation of the delusion in the absence of any supporting evidence (Corlett et al. 2009). Thus, prediction error offers a parsimonious single-factor account of delusions and draws attention to possible mechanisms involved in belief formation. Importantly, however, this account does not yet explain the content of specific delusions – it does, for example, explain why particular hypotheses are selected over others. It also does not account for why some participants with aberrant experiences (and presumably aberrant prediction error) develop delusions and others do not.

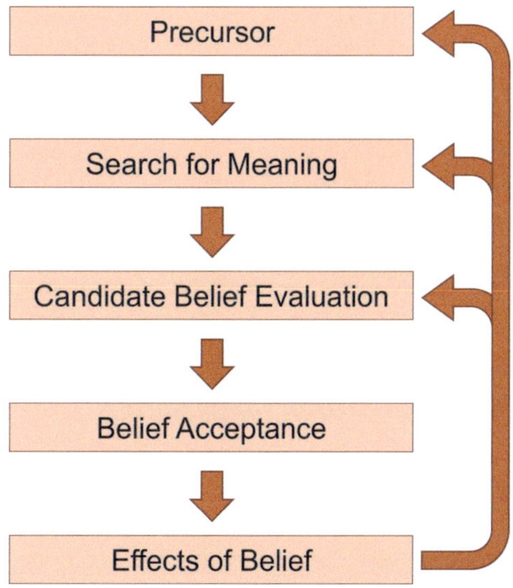

Fig. 1 A tentative five-stage model of belief formation

3 Stages of Belief Formation

Following these earlier theories of delusions, we recently proposed a tentative five-stage non-recursive account of belief formation (Connors and Halligan 2015). This model attempts to explain both delusions and ordinary belief. Drawing on evidence from clinical delusions and other research, we suggest that at least five stages are required to account for delusions and beliefs. The processes in each stage likely occur automatically and without explicit conscious awareness (Fig. 1).

3.1 Precursor

The first stage in belief formation is a precursor, a distal trigger that shapes the content of a future belief. This may involve direct experience. A sensory input, particularly if it is unexpected, emotionally salient, or self-relevant, may attract a subject's attention and initiate a search to explain it (Corlett et al. 2010; Fletcher and Frith 2009). In the case of delusions, a neuropsychological deficit – such as disrupted autonomic responsiveness in Capgras – can be a potent precursor for a delusion (Langdon and Coltheart 2000; Maher 1974). However, structural pathology may not be necessary. Unusual events in the environment can also provide a precursor for a delusion and lead to an inferentially incorrect explanation.

Not all beliefs, however, need to arise from direct experience (Sperber 2009; Sperber et al. 2010). Beliefs can be formed from interactions with other people or informational sources, such as books, television, or the internet. In these cases, the precursor is the verbal or written communication, which if trusted, provides the impetus for a new belief. This is apparent in delusions, for example, where two or more people in a close relationship come to accept the same delusional belief (Hughes and Sims 1997; Langdon 2013). Ideas specific to a certain culture or historical period can likewise influence delusional ideation (Cannon and Kramer 2011; Gold and Gold 2014; Škodlar et al. 2008; Speak 1990). Independent of social influences, a precursor can also involve a subject's own memories and pre-existing beliefs. Providing that these become salient, introspection or reappraisals of past events may initiate a search for meaning that provides the basis for a future belief.

3.2 The Search for Meaning

The second stage in the belief formation process is a search for meaning to account for the precursor. This draws upon both pre-existing beliefs and other relevant information in order to develop hypotheses to explain the precursor. This also includes ideas in the broader social environment that may influence the explanation offered. The resulting proto-beliefs provide candidate proposals to account for the perturbation and are the basis of future beliefs. The amount of inference required at this stage likely varies with the type of input. When an observation appears unambiguous or is highly consistent with pre-existing beliefs, it may simply be accepted as veridical without any further elaboration. Alternatively, if the observation is more ambiguous or inconsistent with pre-existing beliefs, a greater amount of inference and cognitive effort may be required to generate an explanation (Langdon and Bayne 2010).

As this search for meaning depends and builds upon pre-existing beliefs, the resulting proto-beliefs are likely to be both highly personal and idiosyncratic. Subjects, where possible, are likely to conserve existing beliefs to maintain consistent narratives. Subjects also inevitably adopt particular attributional styles – habitual tendencies to explain events in certain ways (Kelley and Michela 1980) – and rely on heuristics to reduce cognitive effort (Gigerenzer and Gaissmaier 2011; Kahneman 2011; Kahneman et al. 1982). Emotion is similarly a strong influence at this stage. Hypotheses may be generated because they are consistent with the subject's current emotion or mood (e.g., anxiety may lead to explanations involving threat) or because of their affective consequences. Explanations that offer comfort or certainty, or maintain self-esteem are more likely to be selected than equally plausible explanations that do not offer these benefits (Gilovich 1991; Helzer and Dunning 2012; Kunda 1990).

These processes are likely to occur in delusions. Pre-existing delusional beliefs, for example, may lead subjects to interpret innocuous stimuli in a delusional manner. Ideas from the subject's social environment may likewise influence how stimuli are interpreted and hence the content of the delusion (Cannon and Kramer 2011; Gold and Gold 2014; Škodlar et al. 2008; Speak 1990). Attributional style, heuristics, and cognitive biases that are present in the normal population may also lead subjects to form certain explanations over others when attempting to account for unusual events (Kihlstrom and Hoyt 1988). Some patients, however, may have cognitive deficits that restrict, limit or bias their search for meaning. This may lead subjects, for example, to prioritise emotion-driven explanations or initial hypotheses and ignore alternative explanations. Thus, when a delusional account is generated, it may be chosen because no alternative explanations are readily available, the delusional account is simply the most compelling (Freeman et al. 2004), or some form of dysfunction has produced a sub-optimal search for meaning.

3.3 Candidate Belief Evaluation

The third stage involves the evaluation of possible proto-beliefs. To be competitive, proto-beliefs need to be both observationally adequate (i.e., explain the precursor or reality change) and consistent with existing beliefs (McKay 2012; Stone and Young 1997). When there is tension between these two criteria, there is likely to be a predisposition towards conserving existing beliefs to maintain internal consistency. Indeed, observationally adequate proto-beliefs that are inconsistent with strongly held pre-existing beliefs may be subject to particularly intense scrutiny and eventually rejected, possibly even at a conscious level (Gilovich 1991; Halligan et al. 1993; Lord et al. 1979). As such, belief evaluation, like the search for meaning, is also concerned with satisfying meaning and is heavily influenced by pre-existing beliefs, often producing idiosyncratic results. If a subjects' pre-existing beliefs include some delusions, for example, belief evaluation may serve to reject non-delusional accounts that are inconsistent with these pre-existing beliefs, and instead select proto-beliefs that support the delusions.

In addition to this reliance on pre-existing beliefs, ordinary belief evaluation is likely to suffer from significant limitations. There are a number of well-known cognitive biases that can interfere with accurate reality testing. For example, people tend to seek confirmatory information that supports their hypothesis and become overly influenced by this, yet neglect information that is critical of it (Nickerson 1998, 2008). Likewise, people may focus on heuristics (Gigerenzer and Gaissmaier 2011; Gilovich et al. 2002; Kahneman 2011; Kahneman et al. 1982), use inefficient strategies that waste effort on non-diagnostic data (Fischoff and Beyth-Marom 1983), and ignore changes in evidence once they have selected a hypothesis (Anderson et al. 1980; Ross et al. 1975, 1977). Emotion can similarly have a powerful impact on belief evaluation and affect both the level of scrutiny and criteria used to evaluate proto-beliefs. Negative moods, for example, tend to cause subjects to scrutinise persuasive arguments more carefully than positive or neutral moods (Forgas 2000). Subjects are also more likely to recall memories congruent with their current emotions than memories that are incongruent (Kihlstrom et al. 2000). As a result of these various biases, people can accept beliefs without sufficient evidence and also retain incorrect beliefs longer than would be case if they sought out diagnostic information.

In the case of many delusions, these limitations of ordinary belief evaluation may be sufficient for subjects to accept a delusional account. Such biases may be particularly important in the genesis of delusions involving mundane content or delusions that are consistent with a subject's pre-existing beliefs. In the case of bizarre delusions, however, which involve highly implausible content, these limitations and biases may not be sufficient to explain why the delusional explanation is accepted. In such cases, a formal deficit in belief evaluation may be implicated (Coltheart et al. 2011; Langdon and Coltheart 2000; Turner and Coltheart 2010). This deficit in belief evaluation could result, for example, in a tendency to be overly influenced by current experience, which provides evidence for the delusion, and to ignore knowledge and past experience that is inconsistent with the delusional account (Hemsley 1993; McKay 2012). As a result, ideas that would otherwise be rejected may instead be accepted as belief.

3.4 Accepting or Holding the Belief

Proto-beliefs that survive evaluation become accepted as beliefs. Not all beliefs, however, are held with the same level of conviction. This conviction may depend on the similar criteria as those involved in belief evaluation, namely the extent to which the belief explains and predicts their experience of the world (i.e., its observational adequacy), and the degree to which the belief is congruent with other beliefs (i.e., conservation of pre-existing beliefs). As both criteria may vary across time and context, it is possible for some beliefs to vary in the conviction with which they are held (Bisiach et al. 1991; Connors and Coltheart 2011). Nevertheless, the majority of beliefs are likely to fit within a coherent, pre-existing web of other beliefs, thus remaining relatively stable over time.

3.5 Consequential Effects of Holding the Belief

Once accepted, and providing they are relevant to the current environment, beliefs can have immediate effects on a subject's other cognitive processes, emotions, and behaviours. At a cognitive level, new beliefs can help configure or even revise perception, attention, and memory. As a result, the subject will perceive and interpret the world in a way that is consistent with their new belief (Gilovich 1991; Hastorf and Cantril 1954; Jones and Russell 1980; Lord et al. 1979; Vallone et al. 1985; see also Connors 2015; Connors et al. 2015a). Ambiguous information may thus be perceived in a way that fits preconceptions, and so lead to the elaboration and extension of the existing beliefs. Paranormal beliefs, for example, predispose subjects to interpret new events as paranormal (Benassi et al. 1979; Irwin 2009; Singer and Benassi 1981).

In a similar way, beliefs also bias the encoding and retrieval of memories, such that they are consistent with the cognitive and emotional content of the beliefs (Berna et al. 2014; Conway 2005). Retrieved memories, for example, may be reinterpreted or distorted to fit new beliefs (Loftus 2004; Schacter et al. 2011). As a result of these processes, memories remain largely coherent with beliefs and serve to reinforce them. Furthermore, new beliefs influence a person's search for meaning in future events and their criteria for belief evaluation to ensure the overall coherence of beliefs (see Pechey and Halligan 2012). In the case of delusions, the net result of these processes may be a systematised delusional framework, particularly if the delusion affects appraisals of ongoing events.

Even at this stage, though, subjects can remain unaware that they hold a particular belief (that is, to be able to verbally articulate the substance of the belief). As a result of the belief's cognitive effects, the belief itself will instead simply be taken for granted and assumed to be an accurate view of reality. Many beliefs may be inferred from a subject's behaviour, but otherwise remain unconscious and acted upon involuntary. Indeed, subjects may only discover their beliefs when they reflect and consider what they are (Engel 2002). This variability in insight is also apparent in delusions. Those that express their delusions publically or act on them are likely to attract the attention of family members and health services. Other subjects may recognise that other people do not share their strongly held beliefs, so chose not to express them for fear of being marginalised. So while beliefs may guide behaviour, attention also needs to be given to the particular environment and social context in which they occur when interpreting them.

4 Conclusion

This five-stage account is underspecified and is in need of further research. Nevertheless, it offers a parsimonious framework with which to explore belief formation and guide investigation of both ordinary beliefs and clinical delusions. In the future, research from a number of areas of cognitive science will be required to test and extend this account. Particularly relevant areas of research include those that involve cognitive representations of the external environment, including, for example, social cognition, memory, attitudes, social influence, and top-down influences on attention and perception. Delusions, however, provide a unique window into how ordinary cognitive processes may be selectively compromised and the functional consequences of these disruptions. As such, delusions are likely to remain an important means of investigating belief and, in so doing, provide insight into how we understand ourselves and the world around us.

References

Anderson CA, Lepper MR, Ross L (1980) Perseverance of social theories: the role of explana-tion in the persistence of discredited information. J Pers Soc Psychol 39:1037–1049. doi:10.1037/h0077720

Barrett LF (2009) The future of psychology: connecting mind to brain. Perspect Psychol Sci 4:326–339. doi:10.1111/j.1745-6924.2009.01134.x

Bayne T, Pacherie E (2005) In defence of the doxastic conception of delusions. Mind Lang 20:163–188. doi:10.1111/j.0268-1064.2005.00281.x

Bell V, Halligan PW, Ellis HD (2006a) A cognitive neuroscience of belief. In: Halligan PW, Aylward M (eds) The power of belief: psychosocial influence on illness, disability and medicine. Oxford University Press, Oxford, pp 3–20

Bell V, Halligan PW, Ellis HD (2006b) Explaining delusions: a cognitive perspective. Trends Cogn Sci 10:219–226. doi:10.1016/j.tics.2006.03.004

Benassi VA, Sweeney PD, Drevno GE (1979) Mind over matter: perceived success at psychokinesis. J Pers Soc Psychol 37:1377–1386. doi:10.1037/0022-3514.37.8.1377

Bentall RP, Corcoran R, Howard R, Blackwood N, Kinderman P (2001) Persecutory delusions: a review and theoretical integration. Clin Psychol Rev 21:1143–1192. doi:10.1016/S0272-7358(01)00106-4

Berna F, Huron C, Kazès M, Offerlin-Meyer I, Willard D, Verry P, Danion JM (2014) Chronic persecutory delusion and autobiographical memories in patients with schizophrenia: a diary study. Isr J Psychiatry Relat Sci 51:25–33

Bisiach E, Rusconi ML, Vallar G (1991) Remission of somatoparaphrenic delusion through vestibular stimulation. Neuropsychologia 29:1029–1031. doi:10.1016/0028-3932(91)90066-H

Bortolotti L (2009) Delusions and other irrational beliefs. Oxford University Press, Oxford

Bortolotti L (2013) Delusion. In: Zalta EN (ed) Stanford Encyclopedia of philosophy. Stanford University Press, Stanford. Retrieved from http://plato.stanford.edu/entries/delusion/

Breen N, Caine D, Coltheart M, Hendy J, Roberts C (2000) Toward an understanding of delusions of misidentification: four case studies. Mind Lang 15:74–110. doi:10.1111/1468-0017.00124

Breen N, Caine D, Coltheart M (2001) Mirrored-self misidentification: two cases of focal onset dementia. Neurocase 7:239–254. doi:10.1093/neucas/7.3.239

Brighetti G, Bonifacci P, Borlimi R, Ottaviani C (2007) "Far from the heart far from the eye": evidence from the Capgras delusion. Cogn Neurodyn 12:189–197. doi:10.1080/13546800600892183

Cannon BJ, Kramer LM (2011) Delusion content across the 20th century in an American psychiatric hospital. Int J Soc Psychiatry. doi:10.1177/0020764010396413

Coltheart M (2007) The 33rd Bartlett Lecture: cognitive neuropsychiatry and delusional belief. Q J Exp Psychol 60:1041–1062. doi:10.1080/17470210701338071

Coltheart M (2010) The neuropsychology of delusions. Ann NY Acad Sci 1191:16–26. doi:10.1111/j.1749-6632.2010.05496.x

Coltheart M, Langdon R, McKay R (2011) Delusional belief. Annu Rev Psychol 62:271–298. doi:10.1146/annurev.psych.121208.131622

Connors MH (2015) Hypnosis and belief: a review of hypnotic delusions. Conscious Cogn 36:27–43. doi:10.1016/j.concog.2015.05.015

Connors MH, Coltheart M (2011) On the behaviour of senile dementia patients vis-à-vis the mirror: Ajuriaguerra, Strejilevitch and Tissot (1963). Neuropsychologia 49:1679–1692. doi:10.1016/j.neuropsychologia.2011.02.041

Connors MH, Halligan PW (2015) A cognitive account of belief: a tentative roadmap. Front Psychol 5:1588. doi:10.3389/fpsyg.2014.01588

Connors MH, Barnier AJ, Langdon R, Coltheart M (2015a) Hypnotic models of mirrored-self misidentification delusion: a review and an evaluation. Psychology of consciousness: theory, research, and practice 2:430–451. doi:10.1037/cns0000059

Connors MH, Langdon R, Coltheart M (2015b) Misidentification delusions. In: Bhugra D, Malhi GS (eds) Troublesome disguises: managing challenging disorders in psychiatry, 2nd edn. Wiley, Oxford, pp 169–185
Conway MA (2005) Memory and the self. J Mem Lang 53:594–628. doi:10.1016/j.jml.2005.08.005
Corlett PR, Simons JS, Pigott JS, Gardner JM, Murray GK, Krystal JH, Fletcher PC (2009) Illusions and delusions: relating experimentally-induced false memories to anomalous experiences and ideas. Front Behav Neurosci 3:1–9. doi:10.3389/neuro.08.053.2009
Corlett PR, Taylor AH, Wang XJ, Fletcher PC, Krystal JH (2010) Toward a neurobiology of delusions. Prog Neurobiol 92:345–369. doi:10.1016/j.pneurobio.2010.06.007
Currie G (2000) Imagination, delusion and hallucinations. In: Coltheart M, Davies M (eds) Pathologies of belief. Blackwell, Oxford, pp 167–182
David AS (1999) On the impossibility of defining delusions. Philos Psychiatry Psychol 6:17–20. doi:10.1353/ppp.1999.0006
Ellis HD, Young AW (1990) Accounting for delusional misidentifications. Br J Psychiatry 157:239–248. doi:10.1192/bjp.157.2.239
Ellis HD, Young AW, Quayle AH, de Pauw KW (1997) Reduced autonomic responses to faces in Capgras delusion. Proc R Soc B Biol Sci 264:1085–1092. doi:10.1098/rspb.1997.0150
Engel P (2002) Free believers. In: Pessoa J, Leclerc A, da Silva de Queiroz G, Wrigley MB (eds) Manuscrito XXV: proceedings of the third international colloquium in philosophy of mind, vol 15. Universidade Federal de Paraiba, Paraiba, pp 155–175
Fischoff B, Beyth-Marom R (1983) Hypothesis evaluation from a Bayesian perspective. Psychol Rev 90:239–260
Fletcher PC, Frith CD (2009) Perceiving is believing: a Bayesian approach to explaining the positive symptoms of schizophrenia. Nat Rev Neurosci 10:48–58. doi:10.1038/nrn2536
Forgas JP (2000) Feeling is believing? The role of processing strategies in mediating affective influences on beliefs. In: Frijda NH, Manstead ASR, Bem S (eds) Emotions and beliefs: How feelings influence thoughts. Cambridge University Press, Cambridge, pp 108–143
Freeman D (2007) Suspicious minds: the psychology of persecutory delusions. Clin Psychol Rev 27:425–457. doi:10.1016/j.cpr.2006.10.004
Freeman D, Garety P (2014) Advances in understanding and treating persecutory delusions: a review. Soc Psychiatry Psychiatr Epidemiol 49:1179–1189. doi:10.1007/s00127-014-0928-7
Freeman D, Garety PA, Kuipers E, Fowler D, Bebbington PE (2002) A cognitive model of persecutory delusions. Br J Clin Psychol 41:331–347. doi:10.1348/014466502760387461
Freeman D, Garety PA, Fowler D, Kuipers E, Bebbington PE, Dunn G (2004) Why do people with delusions fail to choose more realistic explanations for their experiences? An empirical investigation. J Consult Clin Psychol 72:671–680. doi:10.1037/0022-006X.72.4.671
Freeman D, Garety P, Fowler D (2008) The puzzle of paranoia. In: Freeman D, Bentall R, Garety P (eds) Persecutory delusions: assessment, theory, and treatment. Oxford University Press, Oxford, pp 121–142
Frith CD (1992) The cognitive neuropsychology of schizophrenia. Lawrence Erlbaum Associates Ltd., Hove
Frith CD (2007) Making up the mind: how the brain creates our mental world. Blackwell, Ox-ford
Garety PA, Freeman D (1999) Cognitive approaches to delusions: a critical review of theories and evidence. Br J Clin Psychol 38:113–154. doi:10.1348/014466599162700
Garety PA, Freeman D (2013) The past and future of delusions research: from the inexplicable to the treatable. Br J Psychiatry 203:327–333. doi:10.1192/bjp.bp.113.126953
Gigerenzer G, Gaissmaier W (2011) Heuristic decision making. Annu Rev Psychol 62:451–482. doi:10.1146/annurev-psych-120709-145346
Gilovich T (1991) How we know what isn't so: the fallibility of human reason in everyday life. The Free Press, New York
Gilovich T, Griffin D, Kahneman D (eds) (2002) Heuristics and biases: the psychology of intuitive judgment. Cambridge University Press, Cambridge
Gold J, Gold I (2014) Suspicious minds: how culture shapes madness. Free Press, New York

Halligan PW (2006) Beliefs: shaping experience and understanding illness. In: Halligan PW, Aylward M (eds) The power of belief: psychosocial influence on illness, disability and medicine. Oxford University Press, Oxford, pp xi–xxvi
Halligan PW (2007) Belief and illness. Psychol 20:358–361
Halligan PW, David AS (2001) Cognitive neuropsychiatry: towards a scientific psychopatholo-gy. Nat Rev Neurosci 2:209–215. doi:10.1038/35058586
Halligan PW, Marshall JC, Wade DT (1993) Three arms: a case study of supernumerary phantom limb after right hemisphere stroke. J Neurol Neurosurg Psychiatry 56:159–166
Hastorf AH, Cantril H (1954) They saw a game: a case study. J Abnorm Soc Psychol 49:129–134
Helzer EG, Dunning D (2012) On motivated reasoning and self-belief. In: Vazire S, Wilson TD (eds) Handbook of self-knowledge. Guilford, New York, pp 379–396
Hemsley DR (1993) A simple (or simplistic?) Cognitive model for schizophrenia. Behav Res Ther 31:633–645. doi:10.1016/0005-7967(93)90116-C
Hirstein W, Ramachandran VS (1997) Capgras syndrome: a novel probe for understanding the neural representation of the identity and familiarity of persons. Proc R Soc B Biol Sci 264:437–444. doi:10.1098/rspb.1997.0062
Hughes TA, Sims ACP (1997) Folie à deux. In: Bhugra D, Munro A (eds) Troublesome disguises: undiagnosed psychiatric syndromes. Blackwell, Oxford, pp 168–194
Irwin HJ (2009) The psychology of paranormal belief: a researcher's handbook. University of Hertfordshire Press, Hertfordshire
James W (1890) The principles of psychology, vol 2. Henry Holt and Company, New York
Jones WH, Russell D (1980) The selective processing of belief disconfirming information. Eur J Soc Psychol 10:309–312
Kahneman D (2011) Thinking, fast and slow. Farrar Straus and Giroux, New York
Kahneman D, Slovic P, Tversky A (1982) Judgment under uncertainty: Heuristics and biases. Cambridge University Press, New York
Kelley HH, Michela JL (1980) Attribution theory and research. Annu Rev Psychol 31:457–501. doi:10.1146/annurev.ps.31.020180.002325
Kihlstrom JF, Hoyt IP (1988) Hypnosis and the psychology of delusions. In: Oltmanns TM, Maher BA (eds) Delusional beliefs. Wiley, New York, pp 66–109
Kihlstrom JF, Eich E, Sandbrand D, Tobias BA (2000) Emotion and memory: implications for self-report. In: Stone A, Turkkan JS, Bachrach C, Jobe JB, Kurtzman HS, Cain VS (eds) The science of self-report: implications for research and practice. Erlbaum, Mahwah, pp 81–99
Kunda Z (1990) The case for motivated reasoning. Psychol Bull 108:480–498. doi:10.1037/0033-2909.108.3.480
Langdon R (2013) Folie à deux and its lessons for two-factor theorists. Mind Lang 28:72–82. doi:10.1111/mila.12009
Langdon R, Bayne T (2010) Delusion and confabulation: mistakes of perceiving, remembering and believing. Cogn Neurodyn 15:319–345. doi:10.1080/13546800903000229
Langdon R, Coltheart M (2000) The cognitive neuropsychology of delusions. Mind Lang 15:184–218. doi:10.1111/1468-0017.00129
Loftus EF (2004) Memories of things unseen. Curr Dir Psychol Sci 13:145–147. doi:10.1111/j.0963-7214.2004.00294.x
Lord CG, Ross L, Lepper MR (1979) Biased assimilation and attitude polarization: the effects of prior theories on subsequently considered evidence. J Pers Soc Psychol 37:2098–2109
Maher BA (1974) Delusional thinking and perceptual disorder. J Individ Psychol 30:98–113
Maher BA (1988) Anomalous experience and delusional thinking: the logic of explanations. In: Oltmanns TF, Maher BA (eds) Delusional beliefs. Wiley, New York, pp 15–33
Marshall JC, Halligan PW (1996) Towards a cognitive neuropsychiatry. In: Halligan PW, Marshall JC (eds) Method in madness: case studies in cognitive neuropsychiatry. Psychology Press, Hove, pp 3–12
McKayR(2012)Delusionalinference.MindLang27:330–355.doi:10.1111/j.1468-0017.2012.01447.x

Nickerson RS (1998) Confirmation bias: a ubitquitous phenomenon in many guises. Rev Gen Psychol 2:175–220
Nickerson RS (2008) Aspects of rationality: reflections on what it means to be rational and whether we are. Taylor & Francis, New York
Parnas J (2004) Belief and pathology of self-awareness. A phenomenological contribution to the classification of delusions. J Conscious Stud 11:148–161
Pechey R, Halligan P (2011) The prevalence of delusion-like beliefs relative to sociocultural beliefs in the general population. Psychopathology 44:106–115. doi:10.1159/000319788
Pechey R, Halligan P (2012) Using co-occurrence to evaluate belief coherence in a large non clinical sample. PLoS One 7:e48446. doi:10.1371/journal.pone.0048446
Reed G (1972) The psychology of anomalous experience: a cognitive approach. Hutchinson & Co, London
Reisberg D, Pearson DG, Kosslyn SM (2003) Intuitions and introspections about imagery: the role of imagery experience in shaping an investigator's theoretical views. Appl Cogn Psychol 17:147–160. doi:10.1002/acp.858
Ross L, Lepper MR, Hubbard M (1975) Perseverance in self-perception and social perception: biased attributional processes in the debriefing paradigm. J Pers Soc Psychol 32:880–892. doi:10.1037/0022-3514.32.5.880
Ross L, Lepper MR, Strack F, Steinmetz J (1977) Social explanation and social expectation: effects of real and hypothetical explanations on subjective likelihood. J Pers Soc Psychol 35:817–829. doi:10.1037/0022-3514.35.11.817
Schacter DL, Guerin SA, St. Jacques PL (2011) Memory distortion: an adaptive perspective. Trends Cogn Sci 15:467–474. doi:10.1016/j.tics.2011.08.004
Singer B, Benassi VA (1981) Occult beliefs. Am Sci 69:49–55
Škodlar B, Dernovšek MZ, Kocmur M (2008) Psychopathology of schizophrenia in Ljubljana (Slovenia) from 1881 to 2000: changes in the content of delusions in schizophrenia patients related to various sociopolitical, technical and scientific changes. Int J Soc Psychiatry 54:101–111. doi:10.1177/0020764007083875
Speak G (1990) An odd kind of melancholy: reflections on the glass delusion in Europe (1440–1680). Hist Psychol 1:191–206
Sperber D (2009) Culturally transmitted misbeliefs. [Commentary on McKay RT, Dennett DC, "The evolution of misbelief"]. Behav Brain Sci 32:534–535. doi:10.1017/S0140525X09991348
Sperber D, Clément F, Heintz C, Mascaro O, Mercier H, Origgi G, Wilson D (2010) Epistemic vigilance. Mind Lang 25:359–393. doi:10.1111/j.1468-0017.2010.01394.x
Spitzer M (1990) On defining delusions. Compr Psychiatry 31:377–397. doi:10.1016/0010-440X(90)90023-L
Stone T, Young AW (1997) Delusions and brain injury: the philosophy and psychology of belief. Mind Lang 12:327–364. doi:10.1111/j.1468-0017.1997.tb00077.x
Subbotsky E (2004) Magical thinking in judgments of causation: can anomalous phenomena affect ontological causal beliefs in children and adults? Br J Dev Psychol 22:123–152. doi:10.1348/026151004772901140
Tranel D, Damasio H, Damasio AR (1995) Double dissociation between overt and covert face recognition. J Cogn Neurosci 7:425–432. doi:10.1162/jocn.1995.7.4.425
Turner M, Coltheart M (2010) Confabulation and delusion: a common monitoring frame-work. Cogn Neurodyn 15:346–376. doi:10.1080/13546800903441902
Vallone RP, Ross L, Lepper MR (1985) The hostile media phenomenon: biased perception and perceptions of media bias in coverage of the Beirut massacre. J Pers Soc Psychol 49:577–585
Vicente KJ, Brewer WF (1993) Reconstructive remembering of the scientific literature. Cognition 46:101–128. doi:10.1016/0010-0277(93)90015-N

Functional and Dysfunctional Religious/ Spiritual Beliefs in Psychotic Disorders

Human-Friedrich Unterrainer

Abstract Many of religious/spiritual belief processes (as a possible form of "creditions") have been constantly demonstrated as being positively related to parameters of mental health, as well as to indicators of subjective well-being and personality factors. It has also been suggested that a religious/spiritual dimension might play an important role in coping with mental diseases. In particular, religion and spirituality were shown to be protective against addictive behaviours and suicide attempts. However, despite such findings, there have also been numerous instances of a religious person suffering from delusions and hallucinations. Furthermore, there is some evidence that dysfunctional religious/spiritual beliefs might have an aggravating effect, especially in neurotic, as well as psychotic, disorders. Currently, relevant empirical evidence is sparse and more research is needed in order to characterize the role of the religious/spiritual belief system more clearly as it may be part of the disease as well as part of the cure, or, indeed, simply irrelevant for its etiology. We aim to contribute to this ongoing discussion based on a synoptic review of recent findings, by focusing on the relationship between religious/spiritual belief processes and psychotic disorders.

This contribution is based on previously published work: Unterrainer HF (2014) Dimensions of Religious/Spiritual Well-Being and the Psychotic Experience: Empirical Results and Perspectives. In: Gale J, Robson M, Rapsomatioti G (eds) Insanity and Divinity: Studies in Psychosis and Spirituality. Routledge, East Soussex, pp. 177–193 Full permission for re-use of the material has been granted by Taylor & Francis Publishing Group UK.

H.-F. Unterrainer (✉)
Institute of Psychology, Karl-Franzens University of Graz, Graz, Austria

University Clinic of Psychiatry, Medical University of Graz, Graz, Austria

Center for Integrative Addiction Research (Grüner Kreis Society), Vienna, Austria
e-mail: human.unterrainer@uni-graz.at

H.-F. Angel et al. (eds.), *Processes of Believing: The Acquisition, Maintenance, and Change in Creditions*, New Approaches to the Scientific Study of Religion 1,
DOI 10.1007/978-3-319-50924-2_12

1 A Bio-Psycho-Socio-Spiritual Model of Health and Disease

The bio-psycho-social (BPS) model of health and disease, first proposed by Engel (1977) includes different dimensions of health and illness such as biological (e.g. cancer, heart attack), psycho-social (e.g. depressive/anxiety disorders) and socio-economic (e.g. financial problems, divorce). Following the basic idea of this model, it is proposed that there is an ongoing interaction between these dimensions within the process of health and disease (Engel 1981). Although to date, the bio-psycho-social model has been established on a theoretical level, there is still a lack of empirical research on this topic (Ghaemi 2009). In addition, after the evaluation of the relevant literature in this area, it can be concluded that the BPS model - though comprehensive in principle - disregards a variety of facets that might also become crucial in relation to physiological and psychological aspects of health and disease. In particular, the BPS model does not consider a spiritual dimension or religious/spiritual belief processes explicitly, which elsewhere has been documented as being important for health and subjective well-being (Mohr et al. 2006; Hill and Pargament 2008; Miller and Thoresen 2003). In response to this, it has to be clarified that in this chapter I focus on religious/spiritual belief processes, which have been discussed as being one possible kind of various belief processes, or so-called creditions (Angel 2013; Seitz and Angel 2015). Furthermore, there has been extensive research on whether religiosity/spirituality is an independent factor relative to those usually included in the BPS model. There have also been some attempts in personality research to enhance the "Big Five" model (Extraversion, Neuroticism, Agreeableness, Conscientiousness and Openness to Experience) by means of a sixth dimension, Spiritual Transcendence (Piedmont 2004; Saroglou 2002, 2009).

Furthermore, there is still no consensus on the questions, "How can spirituality/religiosity be best described?" or "What exactly can be understood by proclaiming a religious/spiritual belief system?" For more than 100 years, these questions have been a key problem for scholars coming from various disciplines who have tried to define religion or spirituality as an object of interest (James 1985; Pargament 1999; Wulff 1997; Zinnbauer et al. 1997), and there is still ongoing debate in the field. It is broadly accepted, at least, that both religiosity and spirituality relate to the realm of transcendence (as opposed to immanent).

In addition, there is still no consensus on the issues of how to define religion or spirituality, or what exactly should be understood by proclaiming a religious/spiritual belief system. It is broadly accepted that what is "religious" or "spiritual" to someone can vary greatly. However, scholars have recently tended to use the word "religion" as a complex cultural concept to refer to known faith traditions and institutions, whereas "spirituality" tends to be used in reference to individual life orientations, higher principles, purposes, and values, whether stated in other-worldly terms or not. Some regard a special thing or being as sacred, others emphasize whatever provides meaning in life. Thus, although religion has typically been described in terms of institutions and traditions, spirituality has been conceptualised as a broader construct, without confessional bonds. Religious/spiritual belief processes as a kind of meaning based coping strategy, for instance, have been found to play an important role in the process of dealing with a serious disease (Rosmarin et al. 2013; Folkman and Moskowitz 2004).

The spiritual dimension of human perception has also attracted a lot of interest from psychology and, in particular, psychoanalysis over its history. Beginning with Freud (1927), who became most famous because of his highly critical appraisal of religion, religious/spiritual beliefs have been addressed by highly established authors such as Erik Erikson, Donald W. Winnicott or Heinz Kohut, to name but a few (Kernberg 2000). More recently, Ana Maria Rizzuto (Rizzuto 1998) asked her self 'Why did Freud reject God?' and succeeded in giving an adequate answer from the very perspective of a psychoanalyst. Additionally, Shafranske (2009) proposed a psychodynamically-oriented psychotherapeutic approach: how to integrate the spiritual dimension into the therapeutic practice. Furthermore, religious/spiritual beliefs have also been discussed from an evolutionary-psychodynamic perspective, as being linked to different kinds of attachment styles (Kirkpatrick 1999).

In general, there is a large amount of research emphasising the beneficial effects of religiosity and spirituality on mental health and/or subjective well-being,; thus, religious/spiritual belief systems have also been found to play an important role in clinical settings (Smith et al. 2003; Miller and Thoresen 2003; Hook et al. 2010). There is substantial evidence for religiosity and spirituality being an efficient suicide buffer, especially among psychiatric patients, as Dervic et al. (2014) demonstrated that religious affiliation was substantially associated with less suicidal behaviour in depressed inpatients. After other factors were controlled, it was found that greater moral objections to suicide and lower aggression level in religiously affiliated subjects might function like protective factors against suicide attempts. This finding is in line with our own results consistently showing that an affiliation with a religious community was negatively related to suicide attempts or suicidal ideation (Unterrainer 2010).

Furthermore, there is also substantial evidence for a negative association between religiosity/spirituality and nearly all kinds of addictive diseases (Unterrainer et al. 2013, 2012a; Galanter et al. 2007). In a study by Kendler et al. (2003), different kinds of functional and dysfunctional religious/spiritual beliefs were found to be related to lifetime substance abuse disorders. Moreover, an extensive meta-analytical review of 263 papers supports this negative correlation between positive kinds of religious/spiritual beliefs and addictive disorders (Cook 2004). Although religion and spirituality are positively related with nearly every indicator of mental health (Dein et al. 2012), the working mechanisms behind these findings remain unexplained; this poses a challenge to neuroscientific brain research (Newberg and d'Aquili 2000; Fenwick 1996). Additionally, Sloan et al. (1999) criticised what they called a sometimes hasty over-interpretation of the positive connection between religiosity/spirituality and mental health. Additionally, as noted by Koenig (2008), there is still no clear conceptualisation of spirituality in the literature since parameters of subjective well-being are often mixed up with parameters of religiosity and spirituality. If this is so, then why does it still make sense to consider the religious/spiritual dimension as an important topic in clinical and health research?

As described by Ernest Becker (2007; McGregor et al. 1998) in *The Denial of Death* (1973), as human beings we confront our own mortality every second of our lives. Accordingly, religion and spirituality could be taken as an important means to transcend this kind of existential fear or dilemma of mortality through the facilitation of a feeling of heroism and, therefore, being part of something eternal. Along the lines of thought of Ernest Becker, mental illness is extrapolated as a failing in one's hero system(s) such as in depression. Depressed individuals are being consistently reminded of their mortality, resulting in a feeling of insignificance, without having any resources to counter-balance these feelings (Mikulincer and Florian 2000). Within this picture, schizophrenia might be taken as a step beyond depression, in which one's identity is falling apart, making it impossible to engender sufficient defence mechanisms against mortality. Thus, people diagnosed with a psychosis have to create their own reality or inner world in which they can continue to exist as heroes. However, as Julian Jaynes (1976:431) noted, we have to be careful in expanding our theories, especially in the field of schizophrenia research, as 'recent decades have watched with gratitude a strong and accelerating improvement in the way this illness [schizophrenia] is treated. But this has come about not under the banners of new and sometimes flamboyant theories… but rather in down-to-earth practical aspects of day-to-day therapy'.

2 Religious/Spiritual Beliefs and Psychosis – Two Sides of a Coin?

To begin with, we should clarify that psychosis is not considered necessarily the same as schizophrenia. Schizophrenia might be conceived as a specific form of psychiatric diagnosis (e. g. paranoid schizophrenia), while the term psychosis is used here to refer to a broader group of psychotic disorders, e. g. schizophreniform disorder, schizoaffective disorder, delusional disorder or brief psychotic disorder (Mohr et al. 2010). Furthermore, according to the *Diagnostic and Statistical Manual of Mental Disorders-IV* (DSM IV) (Sass et al. 1996), delusions can be described as false beliefs based on incorrect inferences about external reality that are firmly sustained and contrary to the normal beliefs of that person's culture and despite incontrovertible proof or evidence to the contrary of the belief. According to Peters (2001), there are several problems with this definition. These problems range from plainly false assumptions to points of vagueness and ambiguity, as well as several unjustified theoretical conjectures. Thus, several authors have pointed out that delusions need to be understood against a background of thorough knowledge of the psychology of beliefs (Freeman 2006). Hallucinations may manifest themselves in a variety of ways, since the *American Psychiatric Association's Psychiatric*

Glossary describes it simply as 'a sensory perception in the absence of an actual external stimulus' (Chen and Berrios 1996:54). Hallucinating comprises a common symptom in both medicine and psychiatry. According to Chiu (1989) the frequencies of auditory hallucinations in schizophrenia and acute organic brain syndrome are about 50% and 15% respectively, while the frequencies of visual hallucinations in these two disorders are about 10% and 30% respectively. Thus, doctors of any specialty are likely to encounter some patients exhibiting hallucinations in their practice. An alternative definition was given by Mullen (see Chiu 1989:293) who excluded dreams explicitly and argued that 'hallucinations are involuntary false perceptions occurring concurrently with real perceptions (thus excluding dreams), and having qualities of real perceptions, i.e. vividness, substantiality'(Chiu 1989). Furthermore, hallucinations might be taken as ordinary phenomena but can occur in neuropsychiatric disorders such as narcolepsy, chronic alcoholism and delirium. Unlike hallucinations, an illusion is a real (e.g. having an actual external stimulus) perception distorted in some way. It can be a normal (e.g. misperceiving the outline of a bush as that of a man at dusk) or a morbid phenomenon (e.g. a delirious patient mistaking inanimate objects for people). In the latter case, it frequently co-exists with hallucinations. According to S. Mohr et al. (2010), hallucinations and delusions with religious content are not restricted to schizophrenia, as they are described in nearly all kind of mental disorders (Siddle et al. 2002; Getz et al. 2001). Furthermore, the term "religious delusion" is often a confusing category for clinicians, as well as a stigmatising category for patients. However, there is evidence that religious delusions might be associated with a poorer prognosis, e.g. when they may lead to violent behaviour (Reeves and Liberto 2006). Generally, biological, psychological, sociological and spiritual factors are thought to account for schizophrenia and to mitigate the effects of various treatments (Mohr et al. 2010). Delusions, especially, have long been considered as a hallmark of psychotic disorders such as schizophrenia. However, it has to be noted that delusions may not only be observable in individuals with psychotic conditions but could also occur in nonclinical groups. There is clear evidence that the rate of delusional beliefs in the general population is higher than the rate of psychotic disorders. The frequency of delusional beliefs in non-clinical populations varies according to the content of the delusion and the characteristics of the sample/population. Approximately 1% to 3% of the non-clinical population has delusions of a level of severity comparable to clinical cases of psychosis. About 5% of the non-clinical population has a delusion but not of such severity. Although less severe, these beliefs are associated with a range of social and emotional difficulties. A further 10% to 15% of the non-clinical population has fairly regular delusional ideations. There is convincing evidence that delusions in clinical and nonclinical populations are related, and may lie on a continuum (Johns and Van Os 2001; Unterrainer and Lewis 2014; van Os et al. 2010). Therefore, it may be possible to obtain information about delusions seen in clinical settings by studying delusional ideation in nonclinical populations.

3 A Multidimensional Approach for the Assessment of Religious/Spiritual Beliefs

Based on varying theoretical backgrounds and different forms of religiosity/spirituality, some scales have been constructed or translated for German-speaking people (Unterrainer et al. 2010). The Spiritual Well-Being Scale (Ellison and Smith 1991) became particularly popular in this field. The instrument was originally developed by Ellison and Paloutzian and sought to measure the quality of one's spiritual health. In this context, spiritual well-being is conceptualised as a two-dimensional construct. First, religious well-being describes a vertical dimension of well-being as it relates to God or a transcendent dimension. Second, existential well-being describes a horizontal dimension of well-being as it relates to a sense of life purpose and life satisfaction, without any specific reference to a higher power (Ledbetter et al. 1991). Motivated by our positive experience with these scales in several research projects, we developed a multi-dimensional version by adding a new concept of religious/spiritual well-being covering several aspects of psychological well-being concerning an immanent/transcendent area of perception (Unterrainer and Lewis 2014).[1] Religious/spiritual well-being is defined as the 'ability to experience and integrate meaning and purpose in existence through a connectedness with self, others or a power greater than oneself'. In the following paragraph, different dimensions of religious/spiritual well-being are discussed on a theoretical level in order to explain the meaning of the whole scale more thoroughly. Furthermore, item examples are given for each sub-scale to explain each dimension more precisely. The scale measures six dimensions of religious wellbeing are General Religiosity, Forgiveness, Hope-immanent, Hope-transcendent, Connectedness, and Experience of Sense and Meaning. Each dimension comprises eight items creating a total of 48 items for each scale. These dimensions could be broadly described as follows:

General Religiosity This dimension includes the belief in God, who is merciful, with whom one is able to converse with a feeling of closeness, and thus experience contentment, security and trust in God's help. It also presupposes attendance in communitarian religious events and the recognition of the presence of God in nature. Item example: 'My faith gives me a feeling of security'.

Forgiveness The items here measure the willingness to forgive, absence of hate, avoidance of revenge and wishing well of enemies (for an enhanced discussion of the Forgiveness concept see McCullough 2000). Item example: 'There are things which I cannot forgive' (coded reversely).

Hope-Immanent Being optimistic that the future is going to be exciting. This dimension includes a sense that life is moving in the right direction or certain that things will improve in the future, at least. Hope-immanent also implies having a

[1] For details about the items of the English version of the scale, together with a short manual, please contact the author of this chapter or refer to Unterrainer et al. (2012b).

clear picture of the future and expecting positive experiences and the possibility to live as one envisages life. Item example: 'I view the future with optimism'.

Hope-Transcendent While hope-immanent is focused on this life even if it is about the future, hope-transcendent is about the afterlife. It consists of the recognition that this life is transient, together with the hopeful acceptance of a life after death as well as an experience of hope that emerges from the possibility of being remembered after death. Item example: 'I often think about the fact that I will have to leave behind my loved ones' (coded reversely).

Connectedness This dimension refers to the experience of the feeling of being absorbed into something greater. For instance, being reborn after death, a feeling of supernatural connection with some people, the experience of the ineffable, and a strong belief in an existence after death. Item example: 'I have experienced the feeling of being absorbed into something greater'.

Experiences of Sense and Meaning This dimension is about the experience of authentic feelings, including deep affection and true friendship. It takes into account a sufficient comprehension of the meaning of life. This also includes meaningful experiences of openness and honesty as well as occasions of getting absorbed into something to the point of forgetting everything around. Item example: 'I have experienced true (authentic) feelings'.

The MI-RSWB has been employed in several research projects concerning the role of religiosity and spirituality in the process of mental health and illness. Dimensions of religious/spiritual well-being (RSWB) were found to be substantially associated with indicators of subjective well-being and personality, like a sense of coherence, as the core concept in the *salutogenesis* approach (Antonovsky 1996). Dimensions of RSWB have also been discussed in the context of varying indicators of psychiatric illness. Unterrainer (2010) reports substantial negative correlations with e.g. depression and anxiety as well as with psychoticism. Furthermore, dimensions of RSWB have been linked, especially in German regions, with the very established concept of the structure and centrality of religiosity (Huber and Huber 2012). Different profiles of RSWB were found depending on the amount of centrality of religiosity. A more in-depth analysis showed positive and negative god representations to be substantially connected to different indicators of mental health and mental illness, even after controlling for the general amount of religiosity (Unterrainer 2010).

4 Magical Thinking as an Indicator of Schizotypy

According to Paul Meehl (1990), magical ideation might be described as 'belief, quasi-belief, or semi-serious entertainment of the possibility that events which, according to the causal concept of this culture, cannot have a causal relation with each other, might somehow nevertheless do so'. An increased amount of magical ideation was found among persons prone to schizophrenia or schizotypy (Eckblad and Chapman 1983). The term schizotypy (as a short form of schizophreny phenotype) was first coined by Rado (1953) to characterise persons showing eccentric personality traits, similar to symptoms of schizophrenia. Meanwhile, there is substantial evidence that schizotypy might be best described as a multifactorial continuous construct, of three or even four factors (paranormal experiences and beliefs, cognitive failures, introvertive anhedonia, asocial behaviour) that can be identified consistently in this context (Goulding 2004). Along with this, numerous scales have been developed to assess the various aspects of the schizotypy concept and its multifactorial structure (Farias et al. 2005; Feldman and Rust 1989; Fisher et al. 2004; Vollema and van den Bosch 1995; White et al. 1995). Accordingly, there might be a neuronal or biochemical defect – namely schizotaxy, which was found to be increased among family members of people suffering from schizophrenia and might lead to schizotypy depending on specific developmental circumstances (Faraone et al. 2001). More recently, Raballo and Parnas (2011) reported anomalous subjective experiences as an expression of schizotaxic vulnerability. According to the DSM-IV (Sass et al. 1996), personality disorders are pervasive, inflexible, maladaptive collections of traits that impair individuals and interfere with their ability to function productively. Correspondingly, Raine and Benishay (1995) describe schizotypal personality disorder as representing a serious personality disturbance that borders on the major psychoses and might be closely related to schizophrenia. Based on the International Classification of Diseases (ICD 10, see Dilling et al. 1994) a 'schizotypal disorder' is characterised by eccentric behaviour, anomalies of thinking and affect which resemble those seen in schizophrenia, though no definite and characteristic schizophrenic anomalies have occurred at any stage. No dominant or typical disturbance can be described, but odd communication, paranoid ideation and social isolation might be taken as the core symptoms (McGlashan 1987).

5 The Relationship between Religious/Spiritual Beliefs, Magical Thinking and Personality Functioning

Eysenck's model of personality (Eysenck 1968) consists of three factors: psychoticism (solitary, troublesome, cruel, inhumane personality traits), extraversion (sociable, carefree, optimistic, sensation seeking personality traits) and neuroticism (anxious, worrying, moody and depressive personality traits). There is a large body of evidence that higher religiosity scores are associated with lower psychoticism scores in adults (Francis 1993; Kay 1981; Smith et al. 2009; White et al. 1995) as well as in children and adolescents (Francis 1993), whereas no relevant associations were found with neuroticism or extraversion. According to H. J. Eysenck (1992) this association might be taken as a function of conditioning, as religiosity belongs to the domain of tender-minded attitudes. People who score low on psychoticism are known to condition more readily. Furthermore, Eysenck described psychoticism as representing a dimension of aggressiveness defined at the far ends of schizophrenia. Thus, higher scores on religiosity should be linked to lower levels on schizophrenic-relevant measures (Corr 2010). Moreover, Maltby and Day (2001) noted that a 'wealth of information … suggests that low psychoticism is fundamental to religiosity across a number of cultures' (p. 187). However, there are conflicting results: Caird (1987) found no significant relationship between mystical experiences and the three personality dimensions, whereas Eckblad and Chapman (1983) reported magical thinking to be substantially associated with the Eysenck Psychoticism Scale. More recently, we were able to characterize a more complex relationship between religious/spiritual beliefs and schizotypy (Unterrainer and Lewis 2014). The Multidimensional Inventory for Religious/Spiritual Well-Being and the Schizotypal Personality Questionnaire-Brief Version were applied together for this study. The use of Canonical Correlational Analysis suggested that two distinct relationships exist between schizotypy and spirituality. First, a positive association between cognitive/perceptual features of schizotypy and spiritual connectedness emerged. Second, a more global negative relationship between feelings of spiritual isolation and despair was found for all aspects of schizotypy. These results challenge the previous literature based on one-dimensional measures of subjective well-being, where only a negative relationship was observed. We concluded for this study that the positive association between connectedness and cognitive-perceptual aspects of schizotypy raises important questions about the possible benefit of certain types of schizotypal experience. In line with this assumption, we also found dimensions of creative thinking as being linked with certain facets of positive schizotypy (Fink et al. 2012; Mohr and Claridge 2015), which in turn supports the notion of the "happy schizotype" as a highly gifted person, who exhibits a high amount of creativity, along with a high amount of spirituality. Moreover, there is a large body of research confirming the idea of an underlying trait which might be responsible for a higher amount of religious/spiritual beliefs in individuals who score high on schizotypy scales; for instance, Day and Peters (1999) reported an increased amount of schizotypy in members of new religious movements. These findings stand rather in contrast to evidence which is based on a single case study. In this study, a 19-year-old college student, who was suffering from anxious/depressive symptoms mainly caused by severe multi-drug abuse, was successfully treated with a combined approach of neurofeedback and psychodynamic psychotherapy (Gruzelier 2014). Notably, while being severely depressed at the beginning of the psychotherapy sessions, the student also exhibited an excessively high amount of religious/spiritual well-being in combination with increased schizotypal symptoms. In this particular case, his religious/spiritual beliefs seemed to be detached from these co-existing feelings of anxiety and depression. However, these findings might underline the former notion by Unterrainer and Lewis (2014) that the relationship between spirituality and schizophrenia proneness might be best conceptualized in a multidimensional manner.

6 The Function of Religious/Spiritual Beliefs in Psychotic Patients

Menezes Jr. and Moreira-Almeida (2010) discuss the relationships between religion, spirituality and psychosis. Here they argue that although religious/spiritual problems may appear to be synonymous with psychotic problems, this might also be taken to be a manifestation of non-pathological religious/spiritual experiences. This was based on the result of empirical evidence demonstrating that hallucinations also occur in non-clinical populations, and thus are not exclusive to psychotic/schizophrenic patients. Other studies point out the strong presence of religious content in psychotic patients, as spirituality and religiousness have been shown to be highly prevalent in this patient group (Revheim et al. 2010). Furthermore, several questions arise concerning the relationship between religion and mental illness among patients with psychotic disorders. The first question asks whether religion affects the development of psychosis and whether it could have a harmful influence for psychotic/schizophrenic patients. According to S. Mohr et al. (2010) there is some evidence that religion and spirituality can be harmful for patients with psychosis; for example, patients who have delusions with religious content may experience a worse long-term prognosis. Are patients more prone to engage in religious activities and is there a positive effect of religious coping? Mohr et al. (2006) studied the function of religious coping among 115 stabilised patients with schizophrenia or schizoaffective disorder. It was found that for 45% of the patients, religion was an important part of their lives. Furthermore, 71 of the patients used positive religious coping strategies (e.g. meaning, purpose, hope) to deal with their illness, and only 14% reported negative religious coping strategies (guilt, shame). In addition, the authors of this study were able to replicate these findings in 123 patients living in Quebec (Huguelet et al. 2010).

The last question (also from the perspective of a clinician) might reference how to deal with delusions with religious content presented by psychotic patients. S. Mohr et al. (2011) list three ways in which religiosity/spirituality might help psychotic patients in a way that could be addressed by the clinician: (1) religion and spirituality could be used to cope with current symptoms as well as social and interpersonal problems; (2) religion and spirituality might help to prevent potentially harmful behaviours, including substance abuse as well as suicide and suicide attempts; and (3) religion and spirituality might even allow patients with severe forms of schizophrenia to experience personal growth. Thus, we conclude that religious delusions, as an expression of a psychiatric disorder on the one hand, and religious/spiritual belief processes, especially when being applied as religious coping strategies, on the other hand, may interact in a very complex manner among psychotic patients. Consequently, it is a challenging task for the clinician to differentiate between them, as religion and spirituality might, at the same time, be part of the cure as well as part of the disease. Accordingly, it might also be a challenging task for credition research to focus on the role of religious/spiritual belief processes as being related to various parameters of mental health and illness for the future.

References

Angel HF (2013) Credition, the process of belief. In: Encyclopedia of sciences and religions. Springer, Dordrecht, pp 536–539

Antonovsky A (1996) The salutogenic model as a theory to guide health promotion. Health Promot Int 11(1):11–18

Becker E (2007) The denial of death: Simon and Schuster. Simon & Schuster, New York

Caird D (1987) Religiosity and personality: are mystics introverted, neurotic, or psychotic? Br J Soc Psychol 26(4):345–346

Chen E, Berrios G (1996) Recognition of hallucinations: a new multidimensional model methodology. Psychopathology 29(1):54–63

Chiu LP (1989) Differential diagnosis and management of hallucinations. J Hong Kong Med Assoc 41(3):292–297

Cook CC (2004) Addiction and spirituality. Addiction 99(5):539–551

Corr PJ (2010) The psychoticism–psychopathy continuum: a neuropsychological model of core deficits. Personal Individ Differ 48(6):695–703

Day S, Peters E (1999) The incidence of schizotypy in new religious movements. Personal Individ Differ 27(1):55–67

Dein S, Cook CC, Koenig H (2012) Religion, spirituality, and mental health: current controversies and future directions. J Nerv Ment Dis 200(10):852–855

Dervic K, Oquendo MA, Grunebaum MF, Ellis S, Burke AK, Mann JJ (2014) Religious affiliation and suicide attempt. Am J Psychiatry

Eckblad M, Chapman LJ (1983) Magical ideation as an indicator of schizotypy. J Consult Clin Psychol 51(2):215

Dilling H, Mombour W, Schmidt MH, World Health Organization (1991) Internationale Klassifikation psychischer Störungen: ICD-10, Kapitel V (F, klinisch-diagnostische Leitlinien)

Ellison CW, Smith J (1991) Toward an integrative measure of health and well-being. J Psychol Theol 19(1):35–48

Engel GL (1977) The need for a new medical model: a challenge for biomedicine. Science 196(4286):129–136

Engel GL (1981) The clinical application of the biopsychosocial model. J Med Philos 6(2):101–124

Eysenck H (1968) Eysenck personality inventory manual. Educational and Industrial Testing Service, San Diego

Eysenck HJ (1992) The definition and measurement of psychoticism. Personal Individ Differ 13(7):757–785

Faraone SV, Green AI, Seidman LJ, Tsuang MT (2001) Schizotaxia: clinical implications and new directions for research. Schizophr Bull 27(1):1–18

Farias M, Claridge G, Lalljee M (2005) Personality and cognitive predictors of new age practices and beliefs. Personal Individ Differ 39(5):979–989

Feldman J, Rust J (1989) Religiosity, schizotypal thinking and schizophrenia. Psychol Rep 65(2):587–593

Fenwick P (1996) The neurophysiology of religious experiences. Psychiatry Relig Context, Consens Controversies:167–177

Fink A, Slamar-Halbedl M, Unterrainer HF, Weiss EM (2012) Creativity: genius, madness, or a combination of both? Psychol Aesthet Creat Arts 6(1):11

Fisher JE, Mohanty A, Herrington JD, Koven NS, Miller GA, Heller W (2004) Neuropsychological evidence for dimensional schizotypy: implications for creativity and psychopathology. J Res Pers 38(1):24–31

Folkman S, Moskowitz JT (2004) Coping: pitfalls and promise. Annu Rev Psychol 55:745–774

Francis LJ (1993) Personality and religion among college students in the UK. Personal Individ Differ 14(4):619–622

Freeman D (2006) Delusions in the nonclinical population. Curr Psychiatry Rep 8(3):191–204

Freud S (1927/2012) The future of an illusion. Broadview Press, Peterborough
Galanter M, Dermatis H, Bunt G, Williams C, Trujillo M, Steinke P (2007) Assessment of spirituality and its relevance to addiction treatment. J Subst Abus Treat 33(3):257–264
Getz GE, Fleck DE, Strakowski SM (2001) Frequency and severity of religious delusions in Christian patients with psychosis. Psychiatry Res 103(1):87–91
Ghaemi SN (2009) The rise and fall of the biopsychosocial model. Br J Psychiatry 195(1):3–4
Goulding A (2004) Schizotypy models in relation to subjective health and paranormal beliefs and experiences. Personal Individ Differ 37(1):157–167
Gruzelier JH (2014) EEG-neurofeedback for optimising performance. III: a review of methodological and theoretical considerations. Neurosci Biobehav Rev 44:159–182
Hill PC, Pargament KI (2008) Advances in the conceptualization and measurement of religion and spirituality: implications for physical and mental health research
Hook JN, Worthington EL, Davis DE, Jennings DJ, Gartner AL, Hook JP (2010) Empirically supported religious and spiritual therapies. J Clin Psychol 66(1):46–72
Huber S, Huber OW (2012) The Centrality of Religiosity Scale (CRS). Religion 3(3):710–724
Huguelet P, Mohr S, Gillieron C, Brandt PY, Borras L (2010) Religious explanatory models in patients with psychosis: a three-year follow-up study. Psychopathology 43(4):230–239
James W (1985) The varieties of religious experience, vol 13. Harvard University Press, Cambridge
Jaynes J (1976) The origin of consciousness in the breakdown of the bicameral brain. Houghton-Mifflin, Boston
Johns LC, Van Os J (2001) The continuity of psychotic experiences in the general population. Clin Psychol Rev 21(8):1125–1141
Kay WK (1981) Psychoticism and attitude to religion. Personal Individ Differ 2(3):249–252
Kendler KS, Liu XQ, Gardner CO, McCullough ME, Larson D, Prescott CA (2003) Dimensions of religiosity and their relationship to lifetime psychiatric and substance use disorders. Am J Psychiatry 160(3):496–503
Kernberg OF (2000) Psychoanalytic perspectives on the religious experience. Am J Psychother 54(4):452–476
Kirkpatrick LA (1999) Toward an evolutionary psychology of religion and personality. J Pers 67(6):921–952
Koenig HG (2008) Concerns about measuring "spirituality" in research. J Nerv Ment Dis 196(5):349–355
Ledbetter MF, Smith LA, Vosler-Hunter WL, Fischer JD (1991) An evaluation of the research and clinical usefulness of the spiritual well-being scale. J Psychol Theol 19:49–55
Maltby J, Day L (2001) Spiritual involvement and belief: the relationship between spirituality and Eysenck's personality dimensions. Personal Individ Differ 30(2):187–192
McCullough ME (2000) Forgiveness as human strength: theory, measurement, and links to well-being. J Soc Clin Psychol 19(1):43–55
McGlashan TH (1987) Testing DSM-III symptom criteria for schizotypal and borderline personality disorders. Arch Gen Psychiatry 44(2):143–148
McGregor HA, Lieberman JD, Greenberg J, Solomon S, Arndt J, Simon L et al (1998) Terror management and aggression: evidence that mortality salience motivates aggression against worldview-threatening others. J Pers Soc Psychol 74(3):590
Meehl PE (1990) Toward an integrated theory of schizotaxia, schizotypy, and schizophrenia. J Personal Disord 4(1):1–99
Menezes A Jr, Moreira-Almeida A (2010) Religion, spirituality, and psychosis. Cur Psychiatry Rep 12(3):174–179
Mikulincer M, Florian V (2000) Exploring individual differences in reactions to mortality salience: does attachment style regulate terror management mechanisms? J Pers Soc Psychol 79(2):260
Miller WR, Thoresen CE (2003) Spirituality, religion, and health: an emerging research field. Am Psychol 58(1):24
Mohr C, Claridge G (2015) Schizotypy—do not worry, it is not all worrisome. Schizophr Bull 41(suppl 2):S436–S443

Mohr S, Brandt PY, Borras L, Gilliéron C, Huguelet P (2006) Toward an integration of spirituality and religiousness into the psychosocial dimension of schizophrenia. Am J Psychiatr 163(11):1952–1959
Mohr S, Borras L, Betrisey C, Pierre-Yves B, Gilliéron C, Huguelet P (2010) Delusions with religious content in patients with psychosis: how they interact with spiritual coping. Psychiatry 73(2):158–172
Mohr S, Perroud N, Gillieron C, Brandt PY, Rieben I, Borras L et al (2011) Spirituality and religiousness as predictive factors of outcome in schizophrenia and schizo-affective disorders. Psychiatry Res 186(2):177–182
Newberg AB, d'Aquili EG (2000) The neuropsychology of religious and spiritual experience. J Conscious Stud 7(11–12):251–266
Pargament KI (1999) The psychology of religion and spirituality? Yes and no. Int J Psychol Relig 9(1):3–16
Peters E (2001) Are delusions on a continuum? The case of religious and delusional beliefs. Psychosis Spiritual Explor New Front:191–207
Piedmont RL (2004) Spiritual transcendence as a predictor of psychosocial outcome from an outpatient substance abuse program. Psychol Addict Behav 18(3):213
Raballo A, Parnas J (2011) The silent side of the spectrum: schizotypy and the schizotaxic self. Schizophr Bull 37(5):1017–1026
Rado S (1953) Dynamics and classification of disordered behavior. Am J Psychiatr 110(6):406–416
Raine A, Benishay D (1995) The SPQ-B: a brief screening instrument for schizotypal personality disorder. J Personal Disord 9(4):346–355
Reeves RR, Liberto V (2006) Suicide associated with the Antichrist delusion. J Forensic Sci 51(2):411–412
Revheim N, Greenberg WM, Citrome L (2010) Spirituality, schizophrenia, and state hospitals: program description and characteristics of self-selected attendees of a spirituality therapeutic group. Psychiatry Q 81(4):285–292
Rizzuto AM (1998) Why did Freud reject God? A psychodynamic interpretation. Yale University Press, New Haven
Rosmarin DH, Bigda-Peyton JS, Öngur D, Pargament KI, Björgvinsson T (2013) Religious coping among psychotic patients: relevance to suicidality and treatment outcomes. Psychiatry Res 210(1):182–187
Saroglou V (2002) Religion and the five factors of personality: a meta-analytic review. Personal Individ Differ 32(1):15–25
Saroglou V (2009) Religiousness as a cultural adaptation of basic traits: a five-factor model perspective. Per Soc Psychol Rev
Sass H, Wittchen H, Zaudig M (1996) DSM-IV, Diagnostisches und Statistisches Manual psychischer Störung. Hogrefe, Göttingen
Seitz RJ, Angel HF (2015) Psychology of religion and spirituality: meaning-making and processes of believing. Relig Brain Behav 5(2):139–147
Shafranske EP (2009) Spiritually oriented psychodynamic psychotherapy. J Clin Psychol 65(2):147–157
Siddle R, Haddock G, Tarrier N, Faragher EB (2002) Religious delusions in patients admitted to hospital with schizophrenia. Soc Psychiatry Psychiatr Epidemiol 37(3):130–138
Sloan RP, Bagiella E, Powell T (1999) Religion, spirituality, and medicine. Lancet 353(9153):664–667
Smith TB, McCullough ME, Poll J (2003) Religiousness and depression: evidence for a main effect and the moderating influence of stressful life events. Psychol Bull 129(4):614
Smith L, Riley S, Peters E (2009) Schizotypy, delusional ideation and well-being in an American new religious movement population. Clin Psychol Psychother 16(6):479–484
Unterrainer HF (2010) Seelenfinsternis? Struktur und Inhalt der Gottesbeziehung im klinisch-psychiatrischen Feld, Waxmann

Unterrainer HF, Lewis AJ (2014) The Janus face of schizotypy: enhanced spiritual connection or existential despair? Psychiatry Res 220(1):233–236
Unterrainer HF, Huber HP, Ladenhauf KH, Wallner-Liebmann SJ, Liebmann PM (2010) Die Entwicklung eines multidimensionalen Inventars zum religiös-spirituellen Befinden
Unterrainer HF, Huber HP, Stelzer K, Fink A (2012a) Spiritus contra spiritum?: spiritual well-being and depression among male alcohol dependents in treatment. Alcohol Treat Q 30(1):67–77
Unterrainer HF, Nelson O, Collicutt J, Fink A (2012b) The English version of the Multidimensional Inventory for Religious/Spiritual Well-being (MI-RSWB-E): first results from British college students. Religion 3(3):588–599
Unterrainer HF, Lewis A, Collicutt J, Fink A (2013) Religious/spiritual well-being, coping styles, and personality dimensions in people with substance use disorders. Int J Psychol Relig 23(3):204–213
van Os J, Kenis G, Rutten BP (2010) The environment and schizophrenia. Nature 468(7321):203–212
Vollema MG, van den Bosch RJ (1995) The multidimensionality of schizotypy. Schizophr Bull 21(1):19
White J, Joseph S, Neil A (1995) Religiosity, psychoticism, and schizotypal traits. Personal Individ Differ 19(6):847–851
Wulff DM (1997) Psychology of religion: classic and contemporary. Wiley, New York
Zinnbauer BJ, Pargament KI, Cole B, Rye MS, Butter EM, Belavich TG et al (1997) Religion and spirituality: unfuzzying the fuzzy. J Sci Study Relig:549–564

Part III
Philosophy

The Theory of Credition and Philosophical Accounts of Belief: Looking for Common Ground

Aku Visala and Hans-Ferdinand Angel

Abstract The nature and function of belief and the goal of believing have been central topics in Western philosophical and theological traditions since Antiquity. Basic questions have been asked, for instance, about the relationship between belief and knowledge, belief in God or gods, and the nature of believing itself. Is belief somehow inferior to knowledge, and how is it related to evidence? In this chapter, we introduce some historical and contemporary philosophical discussions about these issues and explore a number of ways in which the theory of credition could benefit from engaging with the philosophical literature on belief. We begin by looking at some historical and contemporary accounts of the relationship between belief and knowledge. After that, we address the perennial association of religion with belief. Finally, we conclude the chapter by making some preliminary suggestions as to how we could relate philosophical debates and discussions to the theory of creditions. We suggest that philosophy has much to give to the theory of credition and vice versa.

1 Belief and Knowledge

Since the founding positions of Plato (428/27–348/347 B.C.) and Aristotle (384–322 B.C.), the relation between belief and knowledge [Politeia, esp. 477–478] has been debated and discussed extensively (cf. Weber in this volume). The distinction between knowledge (ἐπιστήμη/episteme) and belief (δόξα/doxa), which Plato developed in his dialogues Gorgias and Theaitetos, became highly influential. The basic idea was to distinguish popularly held opinions, which Plato called beliefs,

A. Visala (✉)
Faculty of Theology, University of Helsinki, Helsinki, Finland
e-mail: aku.visala@helsinki.fi

H.-F. Angel
Institute of Catechetics and Religious Education, Karl-Franzens University of Graz, Graz, Austria
e-mail: ferdinand.angel@uni-graz.at

H.-F. Angel et al. (eds.), *Processes of Believing: The Acquisition, Maintenance, and Change in Creditions*, New Approaches to the Scientific Study of Religion 1,
DOI 10.1007/978-3-319-50924-2_13

from true knowledge. Whereas the Sophists would manipulate or influence popular opinions, a true philosopher would strive for knowledge. Knowledge, in turn, was defined as justified (reasoned), true belief.

Although Aristotle's criticisms of Plato are well known, both agreed on a fundamental point about knowledge (Miller 2014, 285): "Aristotle agrees with Plato that knowledge is superior to belief: "He who has beliefs is, in comparison with the man who knows, not in a healthy state as far as the truth is concerned" (*Met* Γ.4 1008b27–31; cf. Plato *Rep.* VI 508d4–9). Despite this agreement, Aristotle disagreed with Plato's view of the objects of knowledge. For Plato, "knowledge has its own special object, such as the Form of Beauty, and belief has its own special object, such as a particular beautiful thing. There is therefore an unbridgeable divide between knowledge and belief. The attempt to grasp knowable objects such as the Forms by means of belief would be futile and fundamentally misguided, because belief is prone to error and falsehood in a way that knowledge is not. Aristotle cannot of course accept Plato's solution, insofar as it presupposes the theory of Forms rejected by Aristotle" (Miller 2014, 286).

Aristotle's rejection of the Platonic theory had the unfortunate consequence that Aristotle failed to supply a coherent concept or a theory of belief: his "remarks concerning belief are scattered throughout his works, none of which contains a systematic discussion of this topic" (Miller 2014, 285).

Fast forwarding to contemporary philosophy the concepts of "belief" and "believing" are very much back on the agenda. What beliefs are and how they are related to knowledge, language, thought, rationality, and justification are hotly debated in many areas of analytic philosophy. Epistemology, which is the study of knowledge, belief, justification and other such notions, is where the concept of belief is most often found. However, the nature of beliefs is a prominent topic in other fields of philosophy as well, like philosophy of mind, philosophy of psychology and philosophy of language. Despite the almost infinite diversity of theories and accounts of beliefs, certain basic assumptions about beliefs and believing are rather common among contemporary analytic philosophers (Schwitzgebel 2015).

Let us begin from the link between belief and knowledge. Based on the traditional Platonic definition of knowledge, for one to have knowledge that p (any proposition), (a) one has to believe that p is true, (b) p has to be true and (c) one has to have good reasons to believe that p (for an overview, see Ichikawa and Steup 2014). This last condition is often called the justification condition, and whatever it is that bridges the gap between true belief and knowledge is, thus, often called justification (or warrant). The need for such a condition was already implicit in Plato's discussion in Theaitetos: knowledge requires something more than just true opinion or belief and this something is what guarantees or makes sure that the correct relationship exists between the knower and the known. As we can see from this definition, belief is a necessary condition for knowledge: in order to know a proposition p, I must also believe it. Conversely, I cannot know that p, if I either lack the attitude that p is true or believe that p is false. I cannot know that it is raining outside, if I do not believe that it is raining outside, for instance.

Until the 1960s, most philosophers were content to operate with the standard definition of knowledge as justified, true belief. However, after the famous article by Edmund Gettier (1963), the standard definition became somewhat problematic. In an unusually short paper, Gettier presented a number of cases, in which individuals fulfilled the standard conditions for knowledge, but it nevertheless seemed that the required connection between the knower and the known was lacking or in some other way problematic. Without going into the cases themselves, we think it is fair to say that Gettier's examples launched an avalanche of reflection and debate on how the traditional definition of knowledge should be developed or what conditions should be added (safety, virtue or sensitivity, for instance). Fortunately for our topic, the link between belief and knowledge, for the most part, remained as a basic condition for knowledge (for an overview, see Ichikawa and Steup 2014).

Although the link between knowledge and belief is quite uncontroversial among contemporary philosophers, the issue of justification or warrant is not. Especially after Gettier's cases, debates about this aspect of knowledge have been fierce. Most philosophers agree that having true beliefs is necessary for knowledge but not enough: something more is required and accounts of justification seek to describe what this "extra bit" is.

Accounts of justification come in many different flavors. Some philosophers (e.g., Kornblith 2008) even deny the need for justification altogether. Two approaches to justification and warrant have been dominant in recent debates. Traditionally, evidentialists have maintained that a belief is justified by other beliefs that provide as reasons or evidence for the truth of the belief (e.g., Dougherty 2011). So, when we want to find out whether a belief is justified or not we look at whether the belief has adequate evidence for its favor. If I want to know whether my belief that there is a computer screen in front of me is justified, I need to tend to the evidence I have for this belief.

Opposed to evidentialism are reliabilists, who focus on the actual psychological processes through which beliefs come about. For the reliabilist, basic beliefs do not require evidence or consciously accessible reasons in order to be justified. Instead, the reliabilist maintains that a basic belief owns its warrant to the reliability and trustworthiness of the cognitive process that produced it (for an overview, see Goldman and Beddor 2015). A perceptual belief, such as there is a computer screen in front of me, does not require reasons to be justified. What is required is that visual perception under normal conditions is a reliable source of beliefs about how things are in my office. I am, thus, in my epistemic rights to take the belief that there is a computer screen in front of me to be true without considering evidence. And if it is the case that there is indeed a computer screen in front of me, I am in the state of knowing this fact.

Now that we have a basic grasp of the link between belief, knowledge, and justification, let us return to the exact nature of belief. We think it is rather uncontroversial to maintain that most contemporary philosophers analyse the notion of belief in the same way (Schwitzgebel 2015). In the most general sense, beliefs are understood as epistemic attitudes towards certain propositions or content. For instance, my belief that it is raining outside includes two components: the proposition "it is raining outside" and my attitude towards it, that is, taking it to be true. The proposition or content is here understood as representing reality to be in a certain way and not some other way. In other words, propositions represent or signify how things are. When we believe something, we take a specific proposition to represent the world correctly, that is, to be true. In this sense, a person who takes proposition p to be true (or probably true) is in the state of believing that p.

Most philosophers agree that belief attitudes are to be distinguished from other types of epistemic attitudes by examining the attitude involved. Robert Audi, for instance, carefully distinguishes a number of different kinds of hope, acceptance, faith, and belief (2011, 51–88). So, I can hope that it is raining outside or trust that it is raining outside but these are acts of hoping or trusting, not believing. Moreover, it is very common to take both the attitude of taking something to be true and the proposition or content of the belief as mental states of some kind or another. Accounts of belief and believing are, in this sense, basic building blocks for philosophical theories of our cognitive, mental lives.

Most philosophers draw a distinction between occurrent beliefs and dispositional beliefs (e.g. Audi 2015, 11–27). Occurrent beliefs are mental states that the person has just now and are, for the most part, consciously accessible. For instance, I currently believe that there is a computer screen in front of me and that I am at work. Contrary to this, dispositional beliefs need not be mental states that the person has just now but have the tendency to be reflectively formed under certain circumstances, for instance, when I am asked to reflect on something. So I can dispositionally believe that my mother's name is Eva and sugar dissolves in water even when I am asleep, while not thinking of anything and no sugar is just now dissolving in water. The distinction between occurrent and dispositional beliefs is meant to highlight the diversity of our believing. We can have beliefs that come about through reflection and of which we are very conscious. Opposed to this, we often have extremely mundane, implicit beliefs that we are very seldom aware of or consciously reflect upon.

Why do we have this interest in knowing and believing in the first place? The reason why philosophers are so interested in beliefs and believing is that they are taken to be constitutive of knowledge, which is for many the aim of our epistemic lives. Knowing is a value in itself and also instrumentally valuable for the way we live our lives (for an overview, see Pritchard and Turri 2014). In order to live good and valuable lives we need to know things. We need to know whether our friends can be trusted, where we are right now, how we can distinguish false statements from true ones, and what the causes are of our not getting a specific job, for instance. Because knowledge is so important and beliefs are constitutive of knowledge, beliefs and believing have always been central in philosophy.

There are also a number of other reasons to be interested in beliefs. In philosophy of mind beliefs and believing are central because of their role in understanding and explaining human action. Even in everyday life, we explain the actions of persons on the basis of their beliefs and other mental states. When we want to explain why Sally went to the supermarket, for instance, we invoke Sally's belief that she must prepare the dinner for the whole family and that the supermarket does have the kind of meat that her children love. Indeed, without positing beliefs and processes of believing to Sally, her actions would become unintelligible to us. Unsurprisingly, philosophers hotly debate how explanations that invoke beliefs work and how to understand beliefs and other kinds of mental states in this context. These debates are closely linked to debates about cognition and mentality as a whole (for an overview, see Bermudez 2005).

Finally, we want to highlight that philosophers often debate the nature of their own theories. In the case of belief, issues revolve around what philosophical accounts of belief are supposed to do. Are they descriptions of what actually happens when people believe, in which case philosophical accounts would be like scientific theories? Or are philosophical accounts of belief something else, like normative accounts of how we should form beliefs in order to get to truth and how we should ascribe beliefs to others in order to rationally explain their actions? For example, the aforementioned reliabilists, often motivated by naturalism, seek to integrate their account of believing and knowing with cognitive science, psychology and neuroscience. Some reliablists, like Alvin Goldman (2000), have even suggested that we should develop a non-epistemic account of justification and completely avoid such terms as "justification", "warrant", "has reason to believe" and so on. The idea is to replace these with terms that have scientifically describable content, like "believes that", "cause" and so on (Runehov and Angel 2013). Nevertheless, we think it is fair to say that most philosophers, including many reliabilists, are in the business of offering something like normative theories of belief and rationality. The central aim of these theories is not simply to describe our actual belief-forming processes, but to offer an account of how we should acquire beliefs and rationally conduct our epistemic lives.

2 Belief and Religion

What we want to address next is the common thought that belief is intrinsically linked with religion. This association is encouraged by a long tradition of Western thinking (Smith 1987). Though in Antiquity (of the Western and Oriental world) the Greek verb "to believe" (Greek: πιστεύειν/pisteuein, Latin: credere) was used in a secular as well as religious manner (Seidl 1952), the meaning of the term has since moved towards being associated with religion more than anything else. This change of meaning was partly caused by Christianity itself. In the Bible, the use of the stem "belief/to believe" is overwhelming: It appears 243 times. In his letters, apostle Paul makes use of the noun 91 times and of the verb 42 times. Interestingly, the Gospel of St. John uses the verb "πιστεύειν" (pisteuein/to believe) 96 times, while not using the noun "πίστις" (pistis/faith) at all. Furthermore, the New Testament provides a number of different accounts of what it means to believe in God (Matthew 9:22; Luke 17:5f; Hebrews 11:1). In Hebrews 11:1, for instance, faith is taken to be a kind of trust in God's promise of future salvation and living according to that trust at the present moment.

Apostle Paul's teaching on justification and faith (e.g., Galatians 2:16; Romans 3:28) also contributed to the association between belief, faith, and religion. For Paul, it is not fulfilment of the law (Torah), but only faith in Christ that can lead to a communion with God (Aune 2013; Marguerat 2013). "To believe in Christ" became the most significant feature of being a Christian. Thus, Christian religion became almost intrinsically linked with the notion of faith (Greek: πίστις/pistis, Latin: fides).

Later theological developments also contributed heavily on this link between faith and Christianity. During the third and fourth Christian centuries, the church went through a number of internal and external theological battles. During these battles, basic doctrines, like the Trinity and the doctrine of incarnation, were formulated. This period changed the focus from the affective processes of believing towards the more dogmatic aspects of belief (Theobald 2012). Many Christian thinkers worked out a deeper understanding of belief, for example St. Augustine ("De fide et operibus"), John of Damascus ("Ékdosis akribès tē̄s Orthodóxou Pisteos"), or Clemens of Alexandria ("Stromateis"). Importantly, Greek philosophy was seen as a helpful, if not necessary precondition to understand the role of belief.

Medieval thought expanded greatly on the received notions of belief and faith by emphasizing their interdependence and close links with other emotional and cognitive states. Anselm of Canterbury's famous dictum "credo ut intelligam" ("I believe so that I may understand), became the starting point of a theological and philosophical program that, one the on hand, made a distinction between religious faith and knowledge, but on the other hand, linked them closely together. The relation between fides and ratio remained the subject of vivid discussions. Duns Scotus and Thomas Aquinas stressed the importance of love, which was to be integrated closely with faith, or as Aquinas put it, faith is "*fides caritate formata*" ("faith formed by love"). During the Reformation period, Martin Luther argued for a clear distinction between faith and love. Among many other theologians, Luther was worried that by linking faith with love would lead to a situation in which by engaging in "works of love (caritas)", one could accrue merits and earn salvation for oneself. Against this, Luther maintained that one is saved "through faith alone" and faith itself is a gift from God. Acts of love are consequences of God's work in humans, not means by which individuals reach salvation.

During the Enlightenment period, the medieval model of relating faith to knowledge began to break down. Philosophers like Voltaire, Kant, and Hume argued that faith was unduly respectful of traditions and authorities. Instead, we should base our beliefs on pure reason alone. The foundation of our self-understanding should be located in our unique faculty to think. The famous sentence "cogito ergo sum", which was coined by Descartes, highlights the centrality of thinking for the Enlightenment project. This new and euphoric vision of human rationality had a profound effect both in philosophy and the emerging natural sciences.

At this point, it should be noted that we have been using the terms "belief in God" and "faith" interchangeably. It is a peculiar feature of the English language to have two distinct words "belief" and "faith". Many other European languages, like German and Finnish, for instance, lack such a distinction and have just one word for religious belief/faith and belief in general. Nevertheless, this does not mean that we cannot distinguish between having faith in the religious sense and believing in the general sense. Indeed, theologians of all traditions and languages have made such a distinction. Given what was said before about how beliefs should be understood (as taking something to be true), most theologians think that there is a considerable difference between believing in God and having faith in God or religious faith. Believing in God, in the strict sense of the word, only refers to the epistemic attitude towards the proposition "God exists". But this kind of attitude is not the full picture of what the relationship between God and humans is supposed to be according to the Christian tradition (or any theistic tradition, for that matter). On the contrary, a believer is supposed to not just believe in the existence of God, but trust God, have hope that God will fix things in the future, display positive affective attitudes towards God, and so on (e.g., Swinburne 2005, 137–158).

Coming finally to our contemporary situation, the philosophical debate about belief and faith is as diverse and extensive as ever. Most epistemologists and theologians agree that religious life involves many different kinds of attitudes, such as hoping, trusting, and having faith. Nevertheless, many philosophers think that religious life also includes belief in the very basic sense (holding a proposition true) or something like it (e.g., Audi 2011). Of course there are some who disagree and maintain that religious people do not believe, for instance, that God loves them, but simply hope or have faith that this is so. They often emphasize the number of other functions that faith offers: it gives moral motivation and provides orientation for our life projects. Against this, many philosophers maintain that such functions would be difficult to understand were it not for at least some degree of believing (e.g., Swinburne 2005, 83–136). We will put this debate aside here and focus on those for whom beliefs in a fairly straightforward sense are indeed involved in religious life.

One of the main topics in religious epistemology has been the question of how religious beliefs should be justified and whether they are indeed justified. The evidentialist-reliabilist divide is observed here as well. Some philosophers think that religious beliefs should be justified on the basis of evidence, reasons that can be given for or against them (e.g., Swinburne 2004). Many opponents of religion take this line and argue that religious beliefs are irrational or fail to achieve high epistemic standard, because they lack sufficient evidential support (e.g., Phillipse 2012). Others examine religious beliefs from the perspective of the cognitive mechanisms that produce them. If religious beliefs are products of mechanisms that we usually consider reliable under suitable circumstances, it seems that basic religious beliefs could be rational even without evidential support (that is, other beliefs), at least when there is no evidence against them (e.g., Plantinga 2000, Plantinga & Wolterstorff 1983). Here the focus of the debate is more on the mechanisms of believing than on the evidence marshaled in support or against religious beliefs.

3 From Belief to Believing: The Theory of Credition and Philosophical Accounts of Belief

What we aimed to do in this chapter was to provide a brief overview of two basic and overlapping issues. First, we examined the concepts of belief and believing and how they are linked knowledge. We made some basic distinctions between different aspects of knowledge (belief, truth, and justification) and gave some examples as to how these aspects have been understood. Second, we also examined the link between belief, faith, and religion. We pointed out that this link has gone through a number of changes in the history of Western philosophy and theology. We concluded with some points about contemporary philosophical debates on the topic.

In this final section, we want to draw the reader's attention to some points and issues that emerge when the previous discussion is examined from the point of view of credition project. What the credition project aims at is a workable theory of the process of believing (Angel 2016). So far, we maintain, such a unified theory has been lacking. Currently, we only have inklings of what such a theory might look like, but we nevertheless maintain that such a theory should include the fluidity of belief processes. A model of credition should include answers to following questions:

- What is the starting point of a process of believing?
- What is the end point of a process of believing?
- On which level can the process be described?
- What terms are used to describe the process?
- How can time be integrated in the model of belief process.

As we can see from these basic questions, one of the main convictions behind the credition project has been to translate static definitions and concepts of belief into the language of "belief or believing processes". Beliefs, according to this view, are not simply states of the mind, but are acquired and maintained by complex cognitive and affective processes (Angel 2013). In order to move from the static notion of belief to that of fluid believing and see it as a fundamental brain function, we need an interdisciplinary conversation that will include philosophical epistemology, philosophy of mind, cognitive science, and neuroscience (Angel and Seitz 2016). It is clear that the move from belief to the process of believing will not be easy. It will require multilevel data mapping and two-directional translation of concepts, theories, and data from different disciplines. In other words, it will be an enormous hermeneutical challenge that will involve transformation and translation from level of analysis to adjacent levels in order to see the degree to which they correspond. With this goal in mind, we will now draw some morals from the philosophical discussions.

First of all, credition refers to processes that underlie all belief-formation and maintaining processes. In other words, we are interested in normal and healthy, not just pathological, belief processes. Of course, one must work towards an analysis of what healthy and normal (rational) belief processes in fact are. Here normative approaches, like philosophical epistemology, can be of much help. In addition to examining and debating about various aspects of rational and justified belief processes, philosophers maintain that belief and believing are very central for our mental and everyday lives. Beliefs are neither pathological nor irrational, but normal components of our lives, irrespective of whether we are religious, irreligious, agnostic, mentally healthy, or mentally disturbed. Indeed, our actions and mental lives would be totally incomprehensible if we would not ascribe beliefs or belief-like states to one another. Therefore, we emphasize that there is no reason to restrict our examination of beliefs and believing to religious or pathological beliefs only. The acquisition and maintenance beliefs are normal human cognitive functions that operate in all domains of life.

Second, we want to make it clear that philosophers, unlike many laypeople, do not completely disassociate belief and knowledge (or scientific fact). Beliefs and believing are not opposite of knowing, but are instead central components of it. Similarly, justified beliefs are needed for establishing scientific facts and scientific knowledge. In this way, a theory about the processes of credition would have a very large scope. It would not simply be a theory of religious beliefs, but a account that would help us to examine belief-forming and maintaining processes in all domains of life, including everyday life and even the sciences.

Third, we must be careful not to unreflectively mix normative accounts of rational believing and descriptive accounts of how beliefs are acquired and maintained. As philosophers are fond of pointing out, there is no straightforward way to drawn conclusions about the epistemic status of a belief (whether it is true or justified or rational) on the basis of how that belief comes about or how it is maintained cognitively This is because there are different accounts of what the relationship between the cognitive process of believing that p and the epistemic status of the belief that p is. According to some views, the underlying cognitive process is very important, and according to others it is not (Jong and Visala 2014).

Fourth, we want to highlight an empirical fact about believing that is well known to all psychologists but is often neglected by philosophers, namely, that believing processes undergo many changes in the ontogenetic development of individuals (Boutilier 1995). For example, it is normal that processes of believing change, even quite radically, when an individual moves from childhood to adolescence and then to adulthood (Langdon and Connaughton 2013).

Fifth, philosophers sometimes have a tendency to see believing as insulated from other kinds of cognitive and affective processes. Against this, a theory of credition emphasises the interconnectedness of emotion and cognition. Indeed, the theoretical term "bab" was coined just for this purpose. Propositions and other kinds of representations are, when viewed at the level of the brain, not static entities but processes that are maintained by many different sub-systems (Connors and Halligan 2015).

Sixth, it is clear that translating philosophical and normative notions of belief, knowledge, and justification to a more process-oriented language will be a very difficult task. Nevertheless, there are already a number of points from which to begin this process. Can we, for instance, understand justification as a kind of process? We maintain that we can, and many philosophers already agree: reliabilists and other externalists have long emphasised that the cognitive processes that actually produce them warrant beliefs. There is a clear connection here between the credition model and contemporary philosophy (for an extended discussion of this point, see Runehov's chapter in the present volume). Furthermore, we can ask the same question about knowledge. How can we see knowledge as a process rather than a state? Is there are difference between knowing and believing on the level of the brain? There are many such debates in contemporary philosophy of mind and epistemology that could function as meeting points with the theory of credition. These include, for example, Robert Audi's discussion (2005) on intuitions and belief dispositions, reliabilist accounts of warrant, and the debates about the mechanisms of believing and how folk psychological notions work in general.

We maintain that the move from belief to the process of believing opens up new spaces for interdisciplinary reflection and encounter. This is, and will be, a fascinating prospect: finding out similarities and dissimilarities between approaches and finding a shared way towards a tentative roadmap of the process of credition. We believe that such a way can be found and look forward to this work with enthusiasm.

References

Angel HF (2013) Credition. In: Runehov A, Oviedo L (eds) Encyclopedia of sciences and religion, vol 1. Springer, Dordrecht, pp 536–539 (= Angel 2013a) http://www.springerreference.com/docs/html/chapterdbid/357430.html

Angel HF (2016) A process of merging interior and exterior reality: a short view on the structure of credition. In: Teixeira MT (ed) Mind in nature. European Studies in Process Thought. Cambridge Scholars Publishing. [in press]

Angel HF, Seitz RJ (2016) Processes of believing as fundamental brain function: the concept of credition. SFU Res Bull 1:1–20. doi:10.15135/16.4.1.1-20

Audi R (2005) The good in the right: a theory of intuition and intrinsic value. Princetown University Press, Princeton

Audi R (2011) Rationality and religious commitment. Oxford University Press, New York

Audi R (2015) Rational belief: structure, grounds, and intellectual virtue. Oxford University Press, New York

Aune DE (2013) Recent readings of Paul relating to justification by faith. In: Aune D (ed) Jesus, Gospel tradition and Paul in the context of Jewish and Greco-Roman antiquity. Mohr, Tübingen, pp 472–523

Bermudez J (2005) Philosophy of psychology. Routledge, London

Boutilier C (1995) Generalized update: belief change in dynamic settings. In: Proceedings of the fourteenth International Joint Conference on Artificial Intelligence (IJCAI'95), pp 1550–1556

Connors MH, Halligan PW (2015) A cognitive account of belief: a tentative roadmap. Front Psychol 5:1588. doi:10.3389/fpsyg.2014.01588

Dougherty T (ed) (2011) Evidentialism and its discontents. Oxford University Press, New York

Gettier E (1963) Is justified true belief knowledge? Analysis 23:121–123

Goldman A (2000) What is justified belief. In: Sosa E, Jaegwon K (eds) Epistemology. An antology. Blackwell Publishers, Oxford, pp 89–104

Goldman A, Beddor B (2015) Reliabilist epistemology. In: Zalta EN (ed) The Stanford encyclopedia of philosophy. http://plato.stanford.edu/archives/win2015/entries/reliabilism/

Ichikawa JJ, Steup M (2014) The analysis of knowledge. In: Zalta EN (ed) The Stanford encyclopedia of philosophy. http://plato.stanford.edu/archives/spr2014/entries/knowledge-analysis/
Jong J, Visala A (2014) Evolutionary debunking arguments against theism, reconsidered. Int J Philos Relig 76(3):243–258
Kornblith H (2008) Knowledge needs no justification. In: Smith Q (ed) Epistemology: new essays. Oxford University Press, New York, pp 5–24
Langdon R, Connaughton E (2013) The neuropsychology of belief formation. In: Krueger F, Grafman J (eds) The neural basis of human belief systems. Psychology Press, Hove, pp 19–42
Marguerat D (2013) The Pauline Gospel of justification of faith. In: Marguerat D (ed) Paul in acts and Paul in his letters. Mohr, Tübingen, pp 179–219
Miller FD Jr (2014) Aristotle on belief and knowledge. In: Anagnostopoulos G, Miller Jr FD (eds) Reason and analysis in ancient Greek philosophy. Springer, Dorderecht, pp 285–307
Phillipse H (2012) God in an age of science: a critique of religious reason. Oxford University Press, Oxford
Plantinga A (2000) Warranted Christian belief. Oxford University Press, Oxford
Plantinga A, Wolterstorff N (1983) Faith & rationality. Reason & belief in God. University of Notre Dame Press, Notre Dame
Pritchard D, Turri J (2014) The value of knowledge. In: Zalta EN (ed) The Stanford encyclopedia of philosophy. http://plato.stanford.edu/archives/spr2014/entries/knowledge-value/
Runehov ALC, Angel HF (2013) The process of believing: revisiting the problem of justifying beliefs. Stud Sci Theol 14:205–218
Schwitzgebel E (2015) Belief. In: Zalta EN (ed) The Stanford encyclopedia of philosophy. http://plato.stanford.edu/archives/sum2015/entries/belief/
Seidl E (1952) Pistis in der griechischen Literatur bis zur Zeit des Peripatos. Innsbruck. Microfiche OCLC-number 153944003
Smith WC (1987) Faith and belief. Princeton University Press, New York
Swinburne R (2004) The existence of God. Clarendon Press, Oxford
Swinburne R (2005) Faith and reason. Clarendon Press, Oxford
Theobald C (2012) Le christianisme comme style. Cerf, Paris

Credition and Justification

Anne L.C. Runehov

Abstract When it comes to subjective beliefs (including religious ones), we tend to be interested in or even skeptical about what others believe. We may ask, "what makes you believe this or that?" What we ask is "how did you come to believe this or that; can you justify your belief?" Differently it is with scientific beliefs, which are considered to be real due to the sensations external objects bring about are consistent. Hence, such beliefs do not need to be justified by the believing person. For example, the belief that particles are real is justified, because, in Henri Poincaré's words, regardless of there being scientific paradigm shifts or competitive theories, there is always some-thing essential that remained and will remain through time. It is assumed that subjective beliefs do not possess or seldom possess such consistency. Indeed, analytic philosophers have been concerned mostly with processes of knowing, "how do we know?", which may include belief but only in the sense of "justified belief". For instance, René Descartes (1596–650) (2008) and John Locke's (1632–1704) (1836) aim was to provide a secure foundation for knowledge, which implied that since then we have tend to conceive knowledge and belief as two antithetic poles. Furthermore, a distinction was made between faith and belief in the sense that faith might include knowledge when it is based on empirical experiences. For example, take the postulation "having faith that the sun will rise tomorrow", which is based on the experience that the sun actually rises every morning. Belief, on the other hand, has been seen as something that is personal, subjective, and in need of justification. One problem is that knowledge, faith and belief are nouns. Focusing on nouns has the consequence that important aspects of the mental status of belief are lost, for example, the aspect concerned with what happens when one believes, knows, has faith? In this chapter, the verbal brother of the noun belief, namely, to believe is studied. In other words, the *processes of believing*, or the *processes' character* is put on a philosophical table of research. In order to do so, the problematic static notions such as belief and knowledge are avoided. Instead the focus lies on a novel understanding using the dynamic term coined by Hans-Ferdinand Angel, *credition* (the processes of believing) (Angel et al. 2006). The aim is to show that the argument given by Poincaré can be challenged. This means,

A.L.C. Runehov (✉)
Department of Theology, University of Uppsala, Uppsala, Sweden
e-mail: annerunehov@gmail.com

H.-F. Angel et al. (eds.), *Processes of Believing: The Acquisition, Maintenance, and Change in Creditions*, New Approaches to the Scientific Study of Religion 1,
DOI 10.1007/978-3-319-50924-2_14

however, having to depart from the traditional epistemic way of thinking. This can be done because, when focusing on the processes of believing rather than on the noun "belief", it could be argued that "there always will be something essential" in that process of believing that remains and probably will do so over time, even if the whole of the process of believing may and most probably will, include changes due to the different functions of the processes involved. This means that, regardless of the type of process of believing (credition), religious, secular or scientific, it might be justified, not on the basis of its epistemic value but on the basis of its process.

1 Introduction

A lot of research has been performed on the process of knowing, "how do we know?" and to some extent this process includes belief, in the sense of "justified belief". Within philosophy, the study of knowledge and justified belief is known as epistemology. Questions are raised about the necessary and sufficient conditions of knowledge. The question "how do we know" looks for its answers within the sources of knowledge. Another important question within epistemology is the question of justification. In other words, what makes justified beliefs justified? Observe that epistemology concerns "knowledge" and "belief", (as nouns) and their relationship. The relationship between knowledge and belief has been discussed since the ancient Greece. Also, Descartes and Locke's aim was to provide a secure foundation for knowledge. Since then we have tend to conceive knowledge and belief as two antithetic poles. Hence, the question *what happens when* someone is doing what we call "he/she believes" remains unanswered, because the answer cannot be found within the "source" of a particular belief.[1] However, the answer can be found in the processes of believing, i.e. in its "credition".

For example, the seed to Albert Einstein's (1837–1955) Special Theory of Relativity (1905) was formed in a paradox which, he experienced at the age of 16. He tried to imagine how a ray of light would look like for an observer traveling parallel with it, with the speed of light. He came to the conclusion that such an observer would see an electromagnetic field oscillating there and back, with-out ever moving itself, in other words, without building a wave. This result was contrary to the laws of physics of that time. But Einstein believed in his intuition and hence he could later assert that the Theory of Relativity can be carried out when describing electromagnetic phenomena, on condition that all space-and time regulations are relative. Einstein put his ideas into practice. Years of intellectual as well as personal

[1] How interesting the topic of epistemology, traditionally understood, is. It is not the topic of this chapter, because the goal of this chapter is to depart from traditional epistemology and look at the possibility of non-epistemic methods in order to give the process of believing justice. While it could be interesting to compare epistemic and non-epistemic analyses in length, doing so within the frame of this chapter would firstly, take me to far away from the aim of the chapter and secondly, would take time not available at present.

experiencing followed. That this transformation is complex can be illustrated by the mix of abilities Einstein possessed to put his ideas in action. Firstly, he had a profound knowledge of theoretical physics. Secondly, he had the mental gift to visualize thought experiments. Thirdly, he was educated in philosophy from which he developed a sceptical attitude towards things that could not be observed. Fourthly and related to the last ability, he questioned authority (Isaacson 2008:113). In addition, Einstein's social conditions were fruitful for his thinking process since he lived and studied in Zurich at the turn of the former century, something that liberated his mind (Feuer 1989:4). Nevertheless, he struggled with what he came to believe, even to a point he wanted to leave the whole idea behind. However when he spook about his dilemma with his best friend Michelle Besso, something happened; suddenly he understood the key of the problem. Einstein's insight was that "Maxwell's theory [of electrodynamics] employed an ether state of rest; but that state of rest could not be revealed by observation. So somehow the principle of relativity needed to be upheld" (Norton 2007).[2]

His idea was stabilized and after 5 weeks, he sent off his famous paper, "On the Electrodynamics of Moving Bodies" (Isaacson 2008:122–123).

In the following sections I will analyse the concepts of belief, faith and justified belief, where after a final conclusion will be drawn.

2 What Is Belief?

It is not always clear what we mean by belief. Neither is it common to distinguish between belief and faith. Nevertheless, our language provides such opportunity. Richard Swinburne (1837–1909) distinguishes between belief and faith in *Faith and Reason* (Swinburne 1984). To him, belief means that one proposition is preferable over another. For example, to believe so-and-so is more probable than to believe such-and-such (Swinburne 1984:4). However, this means that belief is relative due to there being plenty of alternatives available for what to believe. The most obvious alternative to belief is, according to him its negation. For example, "there is a God versus there is no God" (Swinburne 1984). Relying on the comprehension of the concept of belief by the early Christians, he makes the distinction between belief and faith in the sense that faith (or trust) involves acting on assumptions (Swinburne 1984:121).[3] In a similar manner I want to make a distinction between belief and faith in the sense that I also regard believe to be relative and faith to be something "to act upon"; faith, I argue is basic to belief. However, since the purpose is to investigate the processes of believing, this distinction has to be understood in accordance to credition. In other words, while faith is basic, and perhaps instant and static, it can lead to dynamic processes of believing. Let us now regard the distinction made between faith and belief.

---

[2] http://www.pitt.edu/~jdnorton/teaching/HPS_0410/chapters_2015_Jan_1/origins_pathway/index.html Accessed 10-27-2015.

[3] In his view the biblical translations should have been "trust" instead for faith, and "put trust in" instead of believe in.

Faith is not relative; indeed, to have faith that the sun will rise again tomorrow is not relative. The sun rises every morning; we can trust this process and act upon it (e.g. putting our alarm clock on 6 a.m.) Of course when you for example live in the North of Sweden during wintertime, the sun will not rise for some months. You will experience less and less sun for every day that passes until you trust that the sun will not rise the next morning, which it will not. However, the fact that you do not experience a rising sun during some winter months in polar environments, is not the same as that the sun does not rise at all. This means that you still can have faith that the sun will rise tomorrow, only not where you live.

It is different with belief. Belief is relative and is in need for justification. As far as it concerns beliefs based upon scientific ideas, we are inclined to accept them as justified. However, are we as inclined to accept this when the beliefs are based on (subjective) religious ideas or (subjective) religious experiences? Regard the following beliefs:

1. The world as we know it is a process of evolution put in action by God
2. The world as we know it is a process of evolution put in action by a Big Bang

The first belief is typically a religious one; the second is a scientific one. The first belief is mostly considered as a private, subjective belief, and hence seldom receives the status of being justified. Different it is with the second type of belief, which in most cases receives the status of being justified due to the consistency of essential elements in the scientific theories of evolution and the Big Bang theory through time. Indeed, the Big Bang theory has formed the basis of our understanding of the origin of the universe since it was first suggested by George Lemaitre in 1927, even if it lately has been revised.[4] The theory is also based on Einstein's theory of general relativity.

In my opinion, one reason for why these two types of belief are placed in different classes of justifiability is due to the fact that we focus on evidence for or against the beliefs in question rather than on whether the belief in question is rational, desirable or useful. Often, religion is seen as the most irrational and un-useful type of belief. Even belief in processes of nature as well as in divine processes, are seen through sceptic spectacles. The question is; can private-subjective beliefs be ignored that easily? I think it depends on how belief is defined.

The *Merriam-Webster* provides two explanations of the concept of belief. Firstly, belief is explained as a state or habit of mind in which trust or confidence is placed in some person or thing. Take as an example, the sentence, "I believe my brother is telling the truth". My belief is based on my experience that my brother always tells the truth no matter the consequences and that he did this since our childhood. Hence, my belief that my brother is telling the truth is very close to faith or trust, I can act upon it. Secondly, belief is understood as a conviction of the truth of some statement or the reality of some being or phenomenon especially when based on examination

[4] Nevertheless, the theory of the Big Bang has been revised lately which amounted into some alternatives for understanding the origin of the universe. See Physics: from Quarks to Quasars, http://www.fromquarkstoquasars.com/revising-the-big-bang-new-theory-on-creation/

of evidence. For example, I believe spring has arrived. I base this belief on the fact that I saw several swallows and also saw some wood anemones. Hence, my belief is fairly justified, due to the evidence I can put forward. However, what does it mean when I say that I believe in God? Is my belief in God a belief along the first explanation, i.e. a state or habit of mind in which trust or confidence is placed in some person or thing? I do not think this is the case, because even if one trusts or has confidence in God, God cannot be described as a person or a thing. Neither is the second explanation of the term sufficient, i.e. a conviction of the truth of some statement or the reality of some being or phenomenon especially when based on examination of evidence. This is so because, even if one is convinced of the existence of God, one is not able to justify it by way of examination or evidence, as in the case of believing that spring has arrived. This means that when it comes to religious beliefs or other subjective beliefs, we need to think differently. It will become clear that skipping the noun belief and accepting the dynamic term credition will proof to be fruitful.

3 What Is Faith?

As mentioned above, faith is something that allows for action. According to *Merriam-Webster*, faith implies loyalty (to a person or duty), fidelity (to one's promises) and sincerity (of intentions). However, I would rather call this "being faithful to" than "faith or have faith". Furthermore and importantly, faith is also explained as trust in something for which there is no proof. Hence, instead of evidence and examination, conviction is given as a necessary parameter. However, another term that can be used instead or in line with conviction is intuition. With intuition I do not intend a hunch, or feeling, rather the synonyms for intuition I want to use is insight and awareness, which imply a kind of primary conviction. There is no doubt involved; one wants to act upon one's insight, more or less like Archimedes did when he uttered eureka. As such one can have faith in God in the sense that one is convinced or has the intuition that God exists, or to take the example of Einstein's idea of relativity, in the sense that he had a clear intuition that the physical world was not exactly as it was described thus far. This means that faith and belief are not synonyms, something several philosophers have already emphasized. Nevertheless, they are related. The question is how are they related? I suggest that faith is the basis of belief. In other words, faith could be seen as an a-priori state of mind, implying that one does not necessarily need to have experiences in order to have faith or trust, while belief then could be seen as an aposteriori state of mind, developed from the initial state of faith.[5] Referring to the eleventh chapter of the Letter to the Hebrews,

[5] One might ask why we do not also explain the concept of knowledge. The reason is firstly the present manuscript paper focuses on processes of believing (credition). Secondly, if I would do so I first would have to face the problem, named when introducing "process of believing": knowledge is a noun. To relate creditions to "knowledge" it would be necessary to refer to the "process of

also Fritz Marti argues that faith is the basis for belief. He writes, "faith is the ground for (our belief regarding) things to be hoped for, it (takes the place of) a proof for what has no appearance" (1946:31). Taking faith as the ground of belief gives us some advantages.

1. Faith might be the starting point of the process of believing, i.e. of credition.
2. Where belief is connected to the apparent, faith is connected to both the apparent and the non-apparent.
3. It concerns both secular and religious beliefs.

The essential point is that faith refers to future beliefs. Turning this argument around, there are no beliefs without ground, even if beliefs can be proved to be erroneous. In this sense, and only in this sense, beliefs are real. Marti writes, "[f]aith is an attitude, not a profession; it is an alignment, not an assertion; it is real, not yet rational" (Marti 1946:33). I found this description of faith quite attractive and useful for my purpose, i.e. to investigate the credibility of the concept of credition for justification. Faith could be seen as the neural/mental process creating vague ideas, intuitions, values, hopes, etc. However, before continuing with this analysis, another concept needs some clarification, namely, process.

4 What Is a Process?

From a more systematic point of view, five types of processes can be presented and tested on their validity for the process of believing. These types are natural processes, processes of change, structural processes, mental or psychological processes and project processes.

1. A clear example of what I call *a natural process* is the process of **life** itself. Life has a typical beginning: it starts with fertilization and ends with death, ceteris paribus of course. This type of process has a continuing natural or biological/chemical activity or function.
2. However, the process of life includes other processes as for example, the process of growth, which is explained as a natural phenomenon marked by gradual changes that lead toward a particular result. Therefore, I call this type of process, processes of change.
3. The process of life also includes structural processes, i.e. biological, neurological, chemical and physical processes, for example, neural processes, but also gravidity, quantum jumps, etc.

knowing". The "process of knowing" is a complex as the process of believing and to step into this discussion would take me away from the main focus which is on processes of believing. However, that I cannot analyze something for the time being does not mean that I refrain from doing so all together.

4. Furthermore, the process of life obviously also includes mental or psychological processes. Thinking, dreaming, hoping, desiring, etc. belong to this type.
5. A different type of process is what I chose to call, project processes. This type includes all from research projects, manufacturing, building advanced societies and institutions, cleaning the garden, house or taking a bath. They all begin with an idea and/or design and end with a concrete result: a book, published paper, towns, churches, schools, a clean gar-den, house or body.

The question raised now is, which of these types of processes would be applicable to the process(es) of believing, to credition?

The term *credition* was coined by Hans-Ferdinand Angel (2006) and is to be understood as a neologism, which denotes the "process of believing" as it might appear in a religious or secular manner. In this sense, credition is conceived as a psychological term in the sense that credition is tightly related to cognition and emotion (Angel et al. 2006; Angel 2009, 2011).

Processes are usually top-down and bottom-up processes. With this I mean that the parts affect the whole as well as the whole effects the parts. Since the process of believing is a mental process. It is linked to a structure process since the mental and the neurological cannot be separated. I argue that the brain correlates to the mind and is essential for (human) being (*esse*), which includes processes of believing amongst other things[6]. I argue that neither by themselves postulate the essence for human sein. The sine qua non of (human) existence or being (sein) is to be an experiencer. Experiences are what constitute our reality. (Walach and Runehov 2010:158; Runehov 2014:299–300). According to Alfred North Whitehead (1861–1947), there is no such thing as mind-matter dualism. The mind, he argues is an abstraction from an occasion of experience but it also has a material aspect, which in turn is yet another abstraction from it. (Griffin et al. 1978) Logically then, the mental and the material aspects are abstractions from one and the same concrete occasion of experience. Thinking along these lines implies that the process of believing necessarily includes a process of change, not least due to the plasticity of the brain. However, one could also argue that the process of believing is also a project process. It is a process from "idea" to "result or production", as the Einstein example shows. Furthermore, processes of believing, or Credition is proposed to be characterized by four interdependent bio-psychological functions: The enclosure-function, the converter-function, the stabilizer-function and the modulator-function.[7]

If we return to the example of Einstein we observe that all functions are included in his process of believing in, what would come to be, his theories of relativity.

Let us begin with describing the bab that reached Einstein. The proposition can be described as "let all space and time regulations be relative". This thought must have been an exciting experience, perhaps an experience of awe. We can accept this suggestion because his idea was contrary to the laws of physics of that time (the

---

[6] In a previous article I made a distinction between being as sein and being as ein Wesen – a being (Runehov 2006:62).

[7] For the complete description of credition see the introductory chapter by Hans-Ferdinand Angel.

blobs). Due to this, he probably also felt insecure, in need for more nour-ishment for his idea. He probably find himself a bit irritated which let him to start to take action, he needed to talk to someone he could trust, which he did. Looking at the functions of credition we can establish that *the enclosure-function* was responsible for Einstein's intuition that the world was not really as it was described thus far, which led to his revolutionary idea. Secondly, that *the converter-function* of credition was activated when bab-configurations (Einstein's idea or intuition) was transformed into action, (his thought experiment at the age of 16, 1896), which is a complex transformation. Hence, this is the stage of credition when Einstein puts his idea into practice. Thirdly, *the stabilizer-function* of credition is in-evitable and brings creditions into touch with attitudes and mindsets. This was the period of struggling for Einstein, even to the point he wanted to leave the whole idea behind. However, during a conversation with his best friend Michelle Besso, something happened; the little bab became a mega one, suddenly making him understanding the key of the problem. His idea was *stabilized* and after 5 weeks, he sent off his famous paper, "On the Electrodynamics of Moving Bodies" 1905. (Isaacson 2008:122–123; Norton 2007:chap 2). *The modulator-function* highlights in a specific way the differences of individuals and the differences of situations, in which creditive process can occur. Credition is interrelated to body, individual memory, gender, the state of cognitive and/or emotional development, health, disability or psychic integrity, environmental -, cultural -, social – and religious factors. Referring to Einstein, Lewis Feuer writes,

To understand the social setting that gave sustenance to Einstein's revolutionary mode of thought, we must first recapture the spirit of Zurich, Switzerland, as it was at the turn of the [former] century. For Zurich molded Einstein as Athens shaped Socrates. It liberated his mind. (Feuer 1989:4).

5 What Is Rationality?

We can argue that Einstein was rational in believing in relativity, in believing that there was more to physics that hitherto discovered. That did not mean that Newtonian physics were abundant. On the contrary. As Einstein put it:

> [...] to create a new theory is not to destroy an old barn and to build a skyscraper instead. Rather it is to climb a mountain, get broader views, discover unexpected connections between our starting place and its comprehensive surroundings. But our starting place still exists and it is still visible only it has become smaller and builds a little part in the wide view which we achieved through conquering the obstacles on our adventurous way to the top of the mountain (Zukav 1981:45).

Climbing such a mountain is exactly what processes of believing, credition, including its functions, are all about. However, why was Einstein's belief in relativity rational? Without digging deeper into the philosophical problem of rationality, I want to present a distinction provided by Mikael Stenmark that might be fruitful to credition (Stenmark 1994). Usually, rationality is defined as being the quality or state of being reasonable, based on *facts* or *reason*. It implies the conformity of one's beliefs with one's reasons to believe, or of one's actions with one's reasons for actions. One way to have these facts or reasons is searching for scientific evidence, which is based on good reasons and subject to good peer review. However, that restricts rationality to the fields of science (including social sciences). Beliefs what are not based on (empirical) evidence might be seen as lacking reason for being regarded as rational. Stenmark makes a distinction between deontological and means-end rationalities. With deontological rationality he intends having certain epistemic responsibilities to search for the truth for its own sake and therefore to adhere to rational standards. However, that type of rationality is not very helpful for subjective/religious beliefs. The problem is that beliefs are regarded as static states of being, some-thing which our project wants to refrain from. What is meant by searching for the truth for its own sake? And what are the rational standards in order to do so when it comes to subjective and religious beliefs? The other type of rationality he suggests is called means-end rationality and here he intends that whatever helps us to achieve our goals is rational. But, as he admits himself, this type of rationality is not without problems. Because, suppose your goal is to feel good and in order to achieve feeling good you take some cocaine. Obviously, that is not a rational thing to do. Hence, a third type suggested is holistic rationality. The aim is to search to seek to articulate basic human interests and need beyond mere desires. Stenmark frequently turns to his example that his is rational in believing that his wife loves him. Similarly I could say the same referring to my husband. Our beliefs are based on facts, experience, emotions, feelings, cognitive activity, etc. None of these can stand alone to guarantee that it is rational to belief that such is the case though.

Take for example the fact that we are married for 25 years does not by itself make it rational for me to believe that my husband loves me. Many couples are married for many years, even for life-time, but is there always love involved? Experiences by themselves alone do not give you a guarantee either. You might have a lovely time together but, to play the devils lawyer, that does not exclude that the lovely times are merely or often part of playing the good husband or wife. When it comes to feeling and emotions, we need to ask how much we can trust them, again taken by themselves alone. The list can be made much longer. One point I want to make is that why we come to believe something is based on many factors, and these need not always to be coherent. In other words, a belief-system might include one or more disturbing babs. In this sense Stenmark's holistic rationality is fruitful.

However, it is limited because, as other philosophers, he also sees belief as a noun and therefore it becomes difficult to claim that one's beliefs are rational. One needs to refer to facts, etc. and there is the claim of coherency in order to make a belief rational. Especially when it comes to subjective and religious beliefs, philosophers would argue that there are limited (or not) facts and the belief is incoherence with for example other parts of one's world-view. Again, I think the solution is to refrain from belief but to turn to be-lieving, to its processes, to credition. To return to Einstein once more, his believing in relativity, is rational, not on the basis of facts (he had none to begin with except for the fact that he felt that the classical laws of physics did not tell the whole truth), not on the ba-sis of good reasoning (he struggled and doubted for many years), but on the basis of the process leading him to this belief in relativity, in this lies the rationality. Holistic rationality indeed, but we should reframe it to be holistic-process-rationality.

The question we now have to raise is how then is it possible to justify credition? Is there anything we can be sure of?

6 What Is Justified Belief?

Justified belief is necessary for and closely linked to knowledge (Goldman 2000). However, his idea of justification is compared to act-utilitarianism in ethics, meaning that "an action is right if and only if it produces, or would produce, at least as much net happiness as any alternative open to the agent" (Goldman 2000:340). Hence, similarly to act-utilitarianism being a non-ethical theory, he wants a theory of justification that is non-epistemic. Examples of terms that are epistemic and need to be avoided are "'justified', 'warranted', 'has (good) grounds', 'has reason (to believe) ', 'knows that', 'sees that', 'apprehends that', 'is probable' (in an epistemic or inductive sense), 'shows that', 'establishes that', and 'ascertains that'" (Goldman 2000:340). I found this a very fruitful and promising insight. The non-epistemic terms are, "'believes that', 'is true', 'causes', 'it is necessary that', 'implies', 'is deducible from', and is 'probable' (either in the frequency sense or the propensity sense)" (Goldman 2000:340). Goldman thus departs from traditional epistemic theories of justified beliefs. In other words, he is not interested in whether the believer knows that his belief is justified, or whether he can provide a range with evidence or arguments for his belief. Tout court, he is not interested in the justification by the person. What he argues for is a justified belief gets its status of being justified from "*some processes or properties*", which according to him does not need to have an argument or reason (Goldman 2000:340). What does he mean? What is the difference between an epistemic theory of justified belief and a non-epistemic one? The difference lies in the modus operandi.

6.1 *Modus Operandi for an Epistemic Theory of Justified Belief*

If S feels p at t and S believes he feels p at t, than his belief of p is justified. In plain words, if you feel hungry at, say seven o clock and you believe you feel hungry at seven o clock then your belief that you are hungry is justified: i.e. you are hungry! Unfortunately, this way of justifying beliefs is not adaptable to the notion of credition, because there is no process, no dynamics, merely an observation, and a state of affairs. Now let us take a closer look at the modus operandi for a non-epistemic theory of justified belief.

6.2 *Modus Operandi for a Non-epistemic Theory of Justified Belief*

S is *ex-ante* justified in believing *p* at *t* if and only if there is a reliable belief-forming operation (process) available to S, which is such that if S applied that operation to his total cognitive state at *t*, S would believe *p* at *t*-plus Δ" (for a suitably small Δ") and that belief would be *ex-past* justified. (Goldman 2000:342). The interesting point here is that Goldman's non-epistemic theory of justified belief is firstly, adaptable to both scientific and non-scientific beliefs and secondly, the distinction between exante and pastante and because of the addition of Δ" data it is adaptable to the process of believing, i.e. credition. I think we can agree that Einstein's process of believing in relativity, even though it was a long process involving several types of processes and functions of credition can be justified. How-ever, can Goldman's protocol for belief justification be applied to a *process of religious believing?* I think that might be the case.

Suppose you believe in God. Within your mental state U then, let S be you, *p* be God and *t* be 9 am. This means that you are ex-ante justified in believing in God at 9 am. if and only if you have a reliable belief-forming process available to you (e.g. a revelation during a meditation session), which is such that if you applied that process to your total cognitive state at 9 am., you would believe in God at 9 am. plus Δ" (whatever happens during the day) and that belief would then be ex-past justified. It seems like, because the process of your believing in God is applied to your total cognitive state (including Δ) you have a reliable belief-forming process available and hence your belief in God is justified in a non-epistemic manner. However your belief in God would not be justified in the classical epistemic way. Still, I believe Goldman's idea of non-epistemic justification can be fruitful for justifying processes of believing that have limited or even lack evidence. At least the argument given by Poincaré is challenged because, (1902) when focusing on the processes of believing rather than on the mental state "I believe", it can be argued that "there always will be something essential" in that process of believing that remaines and probably will do so over time, even if the whole of the process of believing may and most probably will, include changes due to the different functions of creditions. This means that regardless of the type of the process of believing, religious, secular or scientific, it might be justified, not on the basis of its epistemic value but on the basis of its process. (Runehov and Angel 2013–2014)

7 In Conclusion

It has been shown that it is more fruitful to think in terms of processes of believing, which are dynamic, than thinking in terms of the noun belief, which is a static term, in order to understand what makes one believe what one believes. In other words, in order to understand the character of the processes of believing. Processes are usually both top down and bottom up processes. To put it differently, the parts effect the whole as well as the whole effects the parts. Credition is a mental process that involves both cognition and emotion and is linked to a structure process but also to a project process. Credition has four functions, the encloser -, the converter -, the stabilizer -, and the modulator function. What "belief" and "credition" have in common is that when it comed to religious or other subjective (private) beliefs or processes of believing it seems that they fall into a different class of justification compared to scientific (intersubjective) beliefs or processes. On way to try to solve the problem of justified belief is to distinguish between faith and belief. However, this philosophical strategy has not been that successful when it comes to the matter of justification. What has been more fruitful, in my opinion, is what I, inspired by Goldman, suggested above, namely to skip the epistemic theory of justified belief and to turn to a non-epistemic one. This strategy does not look for evidence or arguments. Rather it concentrates on processes or properties which do not need to have an argument or reason for its justification. Hence thinking in terms of credition is a fruitful strategy for justifying what one believes.

References

Angel H-F (2009) Man glaubt mehr als man glaubt. Themenzentrierte Interaktion 1:57-67
Angel H-F (2011) Ist das Konzept der Creditionen für die Religionspsychologie brauchbar? Wege zum Menschen 63:4–26
Angel H-F, Bröking-Bortfeldt M, Hemel U, Jakobs M, Kunstmann J, Pirner ML, Rothgangel M (2006) Religiosität. Kohlhammer, Stuttgart
Descartes R (2008) Meditations. Cosimo Classicsm, New York
Feuer LS (1989) Einstein and the generations of science. Transaction Publications, New York
Goldman A (2000) What is justified belief. In: Sosa E, Jaegwon K (eds) Epistemology. An Antology. Blackwell Publishers, Maldern/Oxford, pp 89–104
Griffin D, Sherburne R, Sherburne DW (eds) (1978) Alfred North Whitehead: process and reality. Corrected version. Free Press, New York
Isaacson W (2008) Einstein: his life and universe. Simon & Schluster, London
Locke J (1836) An essay concerning human understanding. Free EBook. https://books.google.se/books?id=vjYIAAAAQAAJ&printsec=frontcover&dq=Locke+Essay+I&hl=en&sa=X&ved=0CCwQ6wEwAmoVChMIn8y_h7WFxgIVQrxyCh2Z_wAf#v=onepage&q=Locke%20Essay%20I&f=false
Marti F (1946) Faith versus Belief. J Relig 26(1):30–41
Merriam-Webster. http://www.merriam-webster.com/
Norton JD (2007) Einstein for everyone. Nullarbor Press, Pittsburgh. http://www.pitt.edu/~jdnorton/teaching/HPS_0410/chapters/

Poincaré H (1902) Sur la ValeurObjective de la Science. Revue Métaphysique et de Morale 10(3):263–293
Runehov ALC (2006) A being or to be. Eur J Sci Theol 2(1):55–66
Runehov ALC (2014) God or ultimate reality in theory and practice. In: Schmidt S, Walach H (eds) Meditation – neuroscinetific approaches and philosophical implications. Springer, Heidelberg, pp 297–316
Runehov ALC, Angel HF (2013-2014) The processes of believing: revisiting the problem of justifying beliefs. Stud Sci Theol 14:205–219
Runehov ALC (2016) The human being, the world and God: studies at the interface of philosophy of religion, philosophy of mind and neuroscience. Springer, Switzerland
Stenmark M (1994) Rationality in science, religion and everyday life: a critical evaluation of four models of rationality. Uppsala University, Uppsala
Swinburne R (1984) Faith and reason. Oxford University Press, Oxford
Walach H, Runehov ALC (2010) The epistemological status of transpersonal psychology: the database argument revisited. J Conscious Stud 17(1–2):145–166
Zukav G (1981) The Dancing Wu Li Masters. Askild & Kärnekull Förlag, Stockholm Physics: from Quarks to Quasars. http://www.fromquarkstoquasars.com/revising-the-big-bang-new-theory-on-creation/

Hume on the Origins of Religious Belief

Anders Kraal

Abstract This paper is concerned with the bearings of recent neuroscientific credition research on David Hume's influential idea in *The Natural History of Religion* (1757) that religious belief originates in and is sustained by a fear of misery coupled with mistaken beliefs as to the true causes of happiness. I argue that neuroscientific credition research, in particular of the sort associated with the work of Rüdiger Seitz, Hans-Ferdinand Angel and their colleagues, makes it possible, in principle, to provide some degree of empirical confirmation or disconfirmation for Hume's idea. However, I also argue that this research is incapable of confirming or disconfirming Hume's idea conclusively. The upshot of this is that Hume-style accounts of the grounds of religious belief would do well to take this sort of research into account.

1 *Hume's* The Natural History of Religion *and the Modern Study of Religion*

I begin with some words on the importance of David Hume's work for the development of the modern study of religion. In the modern era, Hume's *Natural History of Religion* has often been characterized (perhaps with some exaggeration) as "the origin of the modern science of religion" (Thomsen 1909:269), "the beginning of the modern socio-anthropological approach to the study of religion" (Bender 1968:60), "essentially modern" (Mossner 1980:333), "the first move in what might now be called the sociology of religion" (Gaskin 1988:145), and the like.

To understand why the *Natural History of Religion* has come to be viewed in this way, we need to take into account that prior to its publication, the standard view among European intellectuals of the originating and sustaining causes of religious belief was, by and large, the Biblical view. According to this view, God created the first human beings, Adam and Eve, in his image, and this image caused them to possess knowledge of God. But following the fall, the human race drifted further and further away from God and from the knowledge of God, ending up, for the most

A. Kraal (✉)
Department of Philosophy, University of British Columbia, Vancouver, BC, Canada
e-mail: anders.kraal@ubc.ca; akraal@ucalgary.ca

H.-F. Angel et al. (eds.), *Processes of Believing: The Acquisition, Maintenance, and Change in Creditions*, New Approaches to the Scientific Study of Religion 1,
DOI 10.1007/978-3-319-50924-2_15

part, as gross idolaters. But even in this fallen state, human beings maintained a certain knowledge of God (albeit confused and distorted), for "the heavens declare the glory of God; and the firmament sheweth his handiwork" (*Psalm* 19:1 [KJV]), and "the invisible things of him from the creation of the world are clearly seen, being understood by the things that are made" (*Romans* 1:20 [KJV]).

This, then, was the standard view among European intellectuals. Then came the Radical Enlightenment of the eighteenth century, and a growing number of intellectuals came to view the Biblical narrative as (in Hume's provocative but representative words) the product of "a barbarous and ignorant people, written in an age when they were still more barbarous, and in all probability long after the facts which it relates, corroborated by no concurring testimony, and resembling those fabulous accounts, which every nation gives of its origin," and which, on account of its many miracle reports, could only be believed by a person "conscious of a continued miracle in his own person, which subverts all the principles of his understanding, and gives him a determination to believe what is most contrary to custom and experience" (Hume 2000 [1748]:99).[1]

With the rejection of the Biblical narrative came a desire for alternative explanatory models of the phenomena that had earlier been taken care of by the Biblical narrative, models that were founded not on religious authority but on empirical research and reasoned judgment. Out of this endeavour came a number of secular accounts of the originating and sustaining causes of religious belief, the most well-known account being that found in Hume's *Natural History of Religion*, which, in brief, takes religious belief to be the product of cognitive and emotional states that can be explained in wholly naturalistic terms, i.e. without the need to invoke supernatural agency. And this naturalistic approach has become, in our day, the standard approach in Western academia.

Whether Hume's naturalistic approach, and the specific account that he offers of the originating and sustaining causes of religious belief, constitute real progress in our understanding of religion, is, of course, a matter of continued debate. With regard to Hume's naturalistic approach, there have appeared a series of serious attempts during the last few decades to show that it betrays at the outset a deep-rooted bias towards an irreligious epistemology, and so in effect prejudges many of the crucial issues (Johnson 1999; Earman 2000). And with regard to Hume's account of the originating and sustaining causes of religious belief, it has been urged, in particular by proponents of so-called Reformed Epistemology, that there are alternative accounts of the causes of religious belief that are equally legitimate, and which might even do a better job of explaining the relevant phenomena (Plantinga 2000, 2011).

[1] For a discussion of the historical influence of Hume's biblical criticism, see Addinall (2001). For a general survey of the Radical Enlightenment critique of Biblical Christianity, see Israel (2001).

2 An Overview of Hume's Account of the Causes of Religious Belief

It has become increasingly clear in modern Hume scholarship that Hume's views on the originating and sustaining causes of religious belief are heavily indebted to Thomas Hobbes's *Leviathan* (Russell 2008:47–69). In *Leviathan*, Hobbes argues that human beings have a natural tendency to develop "fear" or "anxiety" in view of their deep interest in securing their own welfare and avoiding misery, coupled with their ignorance of the true causes of welfare or misery (Hobbes 2012 [1651]:164). This particular form of fear or anxiety, Hobbes goes on to say, "must needs have for object something," and so is externalized and projected onto an imaginary "*Power*, or Agent *Invisible*," and in this way gives rise to "the many Gods of the Gentiles" (Hobbes 2012 [1651]:166). Hume's account of the originating and sustaining causes of religious belief follows this Hobbesian account to a considerable extent.

The idea that the relevant sort of fear or anxiety is produced by a concern with securing our welfare and avoiding misery, coupled with ignorance of the true causes of our welfare and misery, is expressed by Hume as follows:

> We are placed in a world, as in a great theatre, where the true springs and causes of very event are entirely concealed from us [...] We hang in perpetual suspense between life and death, health and sickness, plenty and want; which are distributed among the human species by secret and unknown causes, whose operation is oft unexpected, and always unaccountable. [...] These *unknown causes*, then, become the constant object of our hope and fear; and while the passions are kept in perpetual alarm by an anxious expectation of the events, the imagination is equally employed in forming ideas of these powers, on which we have so entire a dependence. (Hume 2007 [1757]:40)

Hume expresses the idea that this fear or anxiety is externalized and projected onto an imagined supernatural being in such passages as these:

> Agitated by hopes and fears of this nature, especially the latter, men scrutinize, with a trembling curiosity, the course of future causes, and examine the various and contrary events of human life. And in this disordered scene, with eyes still more disordered and astonished, they see the first obscure traces of divinity. (Hume 2007 [1757]:38–39)
>
> There is an universal tendency among mankind to conceive all beings like themselves, and to transfer to every object, those qualities, with which they are familiarly acquainted, and of which they are intimately conscious. (Hume 2007 [1757]:40)
>
> Any of the human affections may lead us into the notion of invisible, intelligent power; hope as well as fear, gratitude as well as affliction: But if we examine our own hearts, or observe what passes around us, we shall find, that men are much oftener thrown on their knees by the melancholy than by the agreeable passions. (Hume 2007 [1757]:42)

Hume thinks that by externalizing the causes of welfare and misery as invisible and intelligent powers, human beings acquire a sense of the ability to influence their fortune for the better, and so are naturally led to resort to a multiplicity of "method[s] of appeasing those secret intelligent powers, on whom are fortune is supposed entirely to depend" (Hume 2007 [1757]:42). Hume posits that out of this striving have risen the multiplicity of religious ritual and worship found throughout the world.

The above, then, is Hume's basic picture of the originating and sustaining causes of religious belief. When it comes to the details of the picture, Hume has very little to say. In this respect, *Natural History of Religion* is a programmatic piece; it offers a general outline of the way in which religious belief arises, but leaves it to others to fill in the details.

To get a more concrete picture of how Hume understands the mechanisms behind religious belief, we could construct the following imaginary scenarios. I begin by constructing a scenario in which Hume would want to say that the relevant sort of fear functions as an originating cause of religious belief, and then a further scenario in which he would want to say that it functions as a sustaining cause of religious belief.

Scenario I Imagine a time when human beings lived in small tribes scattered across the earth, a time when a human being was little more than – in Hume's phrase – "a barbarous, necessitous animal" (Hume 2007 [1757]:35), devoid of any religious belief or worldview. Suppose that at such a time there was a small tribe in the Amazon jungle, whose tribesmen had learned from experience that life could be both pleasurable and painful, since there were times when there was plenty of food and few attacks from vicious animals, and times when there was not much food and many attacks from animals. The tribesmen had come to desire the pleasurable times and to fear the painful ones, and out of this desire grew a wish to secure the pleasurable times and avoid the painful ones. This wish naturally led the tribesmen to form ideas about the causes of the pleasurable and the painful times, and it made sense to them to think that there was a class of invisible beings – spirits, gods – which sometimes provided them with the pleasurable things, and sometimes withheld these things. In this scenario, Hume would want to say that the desire for welfare, the fear of misery, and an ignorance of the true causes of these things, have all come together as an originating cause of religious belief.

Scenario II Imagine next a scenario in which someone, in our day and age, grows up in a Christian household, learns about God, the Bible and the Church, and acquires by this means a real, but somewhat unreflective, religious belief. Suppose that this person often goes for long periods of time without praying or giving much thought to God, and sometimes even entertains the thought that religion is just a fairytale. But every now and then, the person is confronted with a sudden danger, – a near car crash on the way to work, say – and is then led to call upon God, and to believe that God is the one who averted the sudden danger. In this scenario, Hume would have us think that a fear of misery, a desire for welfare, and an ignorance of the true causes of these things, have all converged as a sustaining cause of religious belief.

Suppose that Hume's view of the originating and sustaining causes of religious belief is (on the whole) correct. What was Hume's aim in putting forth this view?

One of Hume's foremost eighteenth century critics, the Anglican Bishop Richard Hurd, took Hume's account to aim at undermining belief in the Biblical narrative. To support this, he noted that in one passage of *Natural History of Religion,* Hume identifies the true causes of human welfare and misery with "the particular fabric and structure of the minute parts of… bodies and of external objects" (Hume 2007 [1757]:40), which clearly conflicts with the Biblical view of a providential governance of the world (Hurd 1757:11, 25–27).

Contemporary commentators typically agree with Hurd that Hume intended his account to be subversive of religious belief, but understand its subversive thrust a bit differently. According to J.C.A. Gaskin, Hume's aim was to undermine the so-called Argument from General Consent, i.e. the argument that one can rationally believe that God exists since all human beings naturally believe this, by showing how the naturalness of such belief can be explained in a way that lends no support to its credibility (Gaskin 1988:143). According to an alternative view proposed by P.J.E. Kail, Hume's aim was to destabilize the rationality of religious belief by arguing that religious belief is sustained by fear and ignorance while assuming that a person is not rationally entitled to a belief that is formed on the basis of what one wants to be true, provided that there is no independent justification for it (Kail 2007:194–195, 199). Regardless of which of these views one ends up favouring, the more general point that Hume intended his account to be subversive of religious belief seems to be fairly obvious, and widely conceded.[2]

3 The Bearings of Neuroscientific Credition Research on Hume's Account

It is apparent that recent developments in neuroscience have remarkable *prima facie* relevance for the assessment of Hume's account of the originating and sustaining causes of religious belief, for some of these developments have been concerned specifically with explaining the very phenomena that Hume is concerned with explaining.

A first neurophysiological development of relevance to the assessment of Hume's account pertains to findings relating to the neural correlates of fear. In a study conducted by Feinstein et al. (2011), a subject whose amygdala has been seen to be severely damaged via neuroimaging methods, was exposed to various fear-inducing phenomena, such as snakes, spiders, a haunted house tour, horror movies, and the like. Interestingly, none of these things evoked any experience of fear in the subject, nor did she manifest any of the usual behavioural manifestations that go along with fear, such as withdrawal behaviour, increased heartbeat frequency, and so on. These findings lead Feinstein et al. to conclude that "the human amygdala plays a pivotal role in triggering a state of fear and that the absence of such a state precludes the experience of fear itself" (Feinstein et al. 2011:38).

The relevance of this finding for Hume's account of the causes of religious belief is that it gives reason to believe that, if the idea that fear is an important cause of religious belief is correct, the process of religious believing ought presumably to be

[2] For a very different take on Hume's aim in the *Natural History*, see Falkenstein (2003).

associated with some corresponding activity in the amygdala. The next question to ask, then, is whether any association of this sort can be established, or at least detected.

But before we raise this question, we presumably ought to know a bit more about the brain areas associated with processes of religious believing.

There are a number of well-known neurophysiological studies concerned with identifying neural correlates of religious experience.[3] These sorts of findings are not quite what we are looking for at present, however, as we are presently concerned with identifying neural correlates not of *religious experience* but of *processes of religious believing*.

What we need, then, is a neurophysiological study concerned specifically with neural correlates of the processes of believing (and preferably with the processes of religious believing). For some pioneering studies in this direction, the best place to turn is to the work of Hans-Ferdinand Angel, Rüdiger Seitz, and their collaborators.

Angel and Seitz note that the term "belief" is ambiguous in terms of being able to differentiate between the content of belief and the mental act of believing, and so introduce the term "credition" to denote the latter phenomena. Creditions, they argue, involve "subjective perspective taking, valuation of internal states and external events, perceptive reinforcement learning, and selection and preparation of action" (Seitz and Angel 2012: 306; see also Angel 2013:536–537). With the notion of credition in hand, they have conducted pioneering studies seeking to identify neural correlates of creditions in general and of religious creditions in particular, relying chiefly on familiar neuroimaging methods. A main outcome of this research has been the finding that "in processes of believing, the medial frontal cortex plays a critical role" (Seitz and Angel 2012:303).

Relying on the above findings, we may at this point note that neurophysiological studies suggest that the emotion of fear is correlated with the amygdala, and that processes of believing are correlated with the medial frontal cortex. A next question to ask, accordingly, is whether any studies have been conducted which seek to determine whether, in processes of religious believing, any simultaneous activity can be detected in the amygdala and in the medial frontal cortex. If this is detectable, it would seem that we have some neurophysiological evidence for the idea that there is a causal connection between religious belief and the emotion of fear, in line with Hume's account of the causes of religious belief.

The closest we get to a neurophysiological study addressing this question is a study conducted by Seitz and his collaborators at Düsseldorf in the late 1990s, reported in their paper "Neural correlates of religious experience" (Azari et al. 2001).

[3] For example, in a study conducted by Beauregard and Paquette (2006), fifteen Carmelite nuns were asked to recall their strongest experiences of union with God, and in so doing Beauregard and Paquette were able to detect "[s]ignificant loci of activation" in several brain areas, including the left medial prefrontal cortex, the right medial orbitofrontal cortex, and the right middle temporal cortex (Beauregard and Paquette 2006:188). For more on this, see Runehov (2007): 143–151, 173–174, and 2010: 214–215.

In the relevant study, a number of German Evangelicals were asked to meditate on one of their central religious beliefs, namely that expressed in Psalm 23:1, "The LORD is my shepherd; I shall not want," and while they did this their brains were monitored for any heightened activities in specific brain areas. The research team reported that although heightened activities were detected in the areas associated with processes of believing, they didn't detect any changes in the activity of the amygdala (Azari et al. 2001:1651). We are thus led to conclude that one of the neurophysiological studies that appears to have a direct bearing on Hume's account of the causes of religious belief does not provide any evidence for this account.

Of course, none of this comes close to *disconfirming* Hume's account. All it shows is that the neurophysiological study that has the strongest relevance to an assessment of Hume's account of the causes of religious belief does not provide confirming evidence for the account.

At this point, it would seem worthwhile to point out that neurophysiological studies of the sort mentioned above could never *conclusively* confirm or disconfirm Hume's account of the originating and sustaining and causes of religious belief. That is the case tor at least two reasons.

A first reason is that neurophysiological studies are concerned with identifying neural correlates, and, as Deborah Lowe and Steven Rogers have pointed out, identifying correlations between brain areas and religious experiences (and, we might add, beliefs) does not show that these experiences (and beliefs) are *caused* by the relevant brain areas, only that there *is* a correlation between them (Lowe and Rogers 2013:1504). Hume's account, on the other hand, is concerned with the causes of religious belief. So it would seem that the relevant neurophysiological studies are not capable, even in principle, of confirming or disconfirming Hume's account in any conclusive way.

A second reason is as follows. According to Hume's account of the causes of religious belief, religious belief is not simply the product of fear, but of fear coupled with ignorance of the true causes of human welfare and misery. Hence, a strong correlation between fear and religious belief will not, by itself, suffice to confirm Hume's account; what also needs to be shown is that the relevant sort of fear is in fact tied to ignorance of the true causes of human welfare and misery. Moreover, what Hume clearly implies, in speaking of ignorance of the true causes of human welfare and misery, is that these things are *not* brought about by supernatural agency, but by quite natural causes, namely, and as was noted above, "the particular fabric and structure of the minute parts of… bodies and of external objects" (Hume 2007 [1757]:40). And this, of course, is a metaphysical claim, and not something that can be settled by neuroscience.

It would seem, then, that although contemporary neuroscientific credition research is of clear relevance to the assessment of Hume's account of the causes of religious belief, we should beware of rushing to the conclusion that this sort of research could do more than provide partial empirical evidence for or against Hume's account.

References

Addinall P (2001) Philosophy and biblical interpretation. Cambridge University Press, Cambridge
Angel HF (2013) Credition, the process of belief. In: Azari N, Oviedo L, Runehov A (eds) Encyclopedia of sciences and religions, vol 1. Springer, Dordrecht/New York, pp 536–539
Azari N, Nickel J, Wunderlich G, Niedeggen M, Hefter H, Tellmann L, Herzog H, Stoerig P, Birnbacher D, Seitz RJ (2001) Neural correlates of religious experience. Eur J Neurosci 13:1649–1652
Beauregard M, Paquette V (2006) Neural correlates of a mystical experience in Carmelite nuns. Neurosci Lett 405:186–190
Bender F (1968) The natural history of religion by David Hume. Rev Relig Res 10:60–61
Earman D (2000) Hume's abject failure. Oxford University Press, Oxford
Falkenstein L (2003) Hume's project in the 'natural history of religion'. Relig Stud 39:1–21
Feinstein J, Adolphs R, Damasio A, Tranel D (2011) The human amygdala and the induction and experience of fear. Curr Biol 21:34–38
Gaskin JCA (1988) Hume's philosophy of religion, 2nd edn. Macmillan, London
Hobbes T (2012) Leviathan, vol 2. Clarendon Press, Oxford
Hume D (2000 [1748]) An enquiry concerning human understanding. Clarendon Press, Oxford
Hume D (2007 [1759]) The natural history of religion. A dissertation on the passions. Clarendon Press, Oxford
Hurd R (1757) Remarks on David Hume's essay on the natural history of religion. Cadell, London
Israel J (2001) Radical enlightenment: philosophy and the making of modernity 1650–1750. Oxford University Press, Oxford
Johnson D (1999) Hume, holism and miracles. Cornell University Press, Ithaca
Kail PJE (2007) Understanding Hume's natural history of religion. Philos Q 57:190–211
Lowe D, Rogers S (2013) Neuropschology. In: Azari N, Oviedo L, Runehov A (eds) Encyclopedia of sciences and religions, vol 3. Springer, Dordrecht/New York, pp 1500–1508
Mossner E (1980) The life of David Hume, 2nd edn. Oxford University Press, Oxford
Plantinga A (2000) Warranted Christian belief. Oxford University Press, Oxford
Plantinga A (2011) Where the conflict really lies. Oxford University Press, Oxford
Runehov A (2007) Sacred or neural? The potential of neuroscience to explain religious experience. Vandenhoeck & Ruprect, Göttingen
Runehov A (2010) Naturalistic understandings of religious experiences. In: Engberg-Pedersen T, Henrik Gregersen N (eds) Essays in naturalism and Christian semantics. Publications from the Faculty of Theology, Copenhagen, no. 18, pp 201–222
Russell P (2008) The riddle of Hume's treatise: skepticism, naturalism, and irreligion. Oxford University Press, Oxford
Seitz R, Angel HF (2012) Processes of believing – a review and conceptual account. Rev Neurosci 23:303–309
Thomsen A (1909) David Hume's natural history of religion. Monist 19:269–288

The Structure of Credition in Whitehead's Metaphysics of Experience

Helmut Maaßen

Abstract The locus of credition in Whitehead's *Process and Reality: An Essay in Cosmology* (PR) would clearly be the section "Higher Phases of Experience," which has rarely been analysed in detail. Whitehead refers to belief at one point of his analysis of feeling, claiming that "the final real things of which this world is made up" (18) are actual occasions or momentary self-constituting actual occasions. To understand social and historical phenomena, it is necessary to look at 'societies' in which actual entities are embedded. This is because, as Whitehead states, an "actual occasion has no history. It never changes. It only becomes and perishes" Whitehead (Adventures of Ideas. Free Press, New York, 1933/1967, 204). Therefore, it follows that one should analyse one such embedding phenomena, namely religion.

1 Credition and Proposition

The Credition Research Project is the attempt to analyze the process of believing and to synthesize it into a convincing model. A major metaphysical concepts of process in the twentieth century has been developed by Alfred North Whitehead. In his opus magnum *Process and Reality* he develops a relational metaphysics. Reality is conceived as a process, a structured multitude of ‚subject processes'. These ‚subject processes' he calls actual entities. A grounding of the Credition Research Project in Whiteheads process-metaphysic should be welcomed. The following article explores the significance of these aspects.

Whitehead's metaphysics has been described as a metaphysics of experience (e.g. Hampe 1990). A closer examination of *Process and Reality, An Essay in Cosmology* (PR) demonstrates this. One way of getting around a frustrating attempt to study this publication from the beginning to the end is to start with Part I ("The Speculative Scheme") and then go on to Part III ("The Theory of Prehension"), which deals with experience in Whitehead's terminology, with feelings and

H. Maaßen (✉)
Heinrich-Heine-University Düsseldorf, Düsseldorf, Germany
e-mail: h.maassen@uni-duesseldorf.de

H.-F. Angel et al. (eds.), *Processes of Believing: The Acquisition, Maintenance, and Change in Creditions*, New Approaches to the Scientific Study of Religion 1,
DOI 10.1007/978-3-319-50924-2_16

propositions. When doing so, one should take note of Whitehead's special coinage of these terms and their philosophical presuppositions.

Peter Strawson (1959) distinguishes between descriptive and revisionary metaphysics. Whitehead's views clearly belong to both forms of metaphysics, which a short look at Part I of PR shows:

> *Speculative Philosophy is the endeavour to frame a coherent, logical, necessary system of general ideas in terms of which every element of our experience can be interpreted. By this notion of 'interpretation' I mean that everything of which we are conscious, as enjoyed, perceived, willed, or thought, shall have the character of a particular instance of the general scheme. Thus the philosophical scheme should be coherent, logical, and in respect to its interpretation, applicable and adequate.* (PR, 3)

Whitehead also states that the ideal of speculative philosophy "has its rational side and its empirical side" (1978/1929: 3) A wide range of philosophers share this interpretation of Whitehead's metaphysics as both descriptive and revisionary. (e.g. Kann 2001; Poser 1986)

Whitehead calls the basic elements or units in his metaphysics actual occasions or actual entities. The term "actual occasion" stresses the process character of the elements and prevents a substantialist interpretation of an actual entity (for information concerning why Whitehead still uses both terms see e.g. Maaßen 1987). The forms each occasion gains are called eternal objects, similar to the Platonic forms.[1]

These elementary entities are bipolar; they have a physical and a mental pole.

> *In each concrescence there is a twofold aspect of the creative urge. In one aspect there is the origination of simple causal feelings; and in the other aspect there is the origination of conceptual feelings. These contrasted aspects will be called the physical and the mental poles of an actual entity. No actual entity is devoid of either pole; though their relative importance differs in different actual entities.* (Whitehead 1978/1929: 239)

Concrescence describes the process of becoming of an actual entity.

What does Part III ("The Theory of Prehension") deal with? What are prehensions?

You will look for "prehension" or "to prehend" in vain in the Oxford English Dictionary, since they are inventions by Alfred North Whitehead. "Prehendere" in Latin means:

> I lay hold of, seize, grasp, grab, snatch, take, catch.
> I detain someone in order to speak with him, accost, lay or catch hold of.
> I take by surprise, catch in the act.
> (*of trees*) I take root.
> (*poetic*) I reach, arrive at, attain.
> (*poetic*) I take in, reach or embrace with the eye.
> (*figuratively, rare, of the mind*) I seize, apprehend, comprehend, grasp. (Wiktionary)

Whitehead introduces a principle by which he wants to describe his metaphysical endeavour: the ontological principle. He writes, "According to the ontological

---

[1] For a short overview of the similarities in Plato and Whitehead concerning forms see my article Revelation, Myth And Metaphysics: Three Traditional Concepts Of God And Whitehead's Dipolar God. (Maaßen 1994)

principle there is nothing which floats into the world from nowhere" (1978/1929: 244). This principle of rationality, if you like, corresponds to a causal principle: "this ontological principle means that actual entities are the only reasons; so that to search for a reason is to search for one or more actual entities" (1978/1929: 24). The dominance of the ontological principle becomes clearer in several other ways. It explains the emotional value implication of each process of prehension. Each genetic process of an actual entity involves a value judgment. Whitehead explains this, saying, "The ontological principle asserts the relativity of decision; whereby every decision expresses the relation of the actual thing, for which a decision is made, to an actual thing by which that decision is made" (1978/1929: 43). Whitehead even goes further, when he claims that "the ontological principle declares that every decision is referred to one or more actual entities, because in separation from actual entities there's nothing, merely nonentity – the rest is silence" (1978/1929: 43). It follows that, for Whitehead, metaphysics has to refer to the here and now, to the actual, not to generalities, abstractions, to something which is beyond the world.

As I mentioned earlier, the key section in the understanding of the internal process of the becoming of an actual entity is Part III of *Process and Reality*. Although the third part is called the Theory of Prehensions, the first four chapters explicitly deal with feelings and only the fifth chapter is called the Higher Phases of Experience. The fifth chapter first deals with feelings and then with the more complex ones, which lead to consciousness. I will not go into the details of this section, but I can outline Whitehead's argument for his philosophy of organism.

> *The philosophy of organism is a cell theory of actuality. Each ultimate unit of fact is a cell complex, not analysable into components with equivalent completeness of actuality. The cell can be considered genetically and morphologically. The genetic theory is considered in this part; [335] the morphological theory is considered in Part IV, under the title of the 'extensive analysis' of an actual entity.* (1978/1929: 219)

After this outline of Whitehead's metaphysics, there is still the question of where one can place the concept of credition and which status it should have, a revisionary or a descriptive one. The locus of credition in *Process and Reality* would be clearly the Higher Phases of Experience, a section in PR which rarely has been analyzed in detail.[2] At one point of his analysis of feeling, Whitehead refers to belief:

> *A feeling is termed a 'belief,' or is said to include an element of 'belief,' when its datum is a proposition, and its subjective form includes, as the defining element in its emotional pattern, a certain form, or eternal object, associated with some gradation of intensity. This eternal object is 'belief character.' When this character enters into the emotional pattern, then, according to the intensity involved, the feeling, whatever else it be, is to some degree a belief."* (1978/1929: 267)

In these higher forms of experience, Whitehead introduces a new term, proposition. He ascribes a special meaning to it:

> *A proposition is the potentiality of the objectification of certain presupposed actual entities via certain qualities and relations, the objectification being for some unspecified subject for*

[2]There is a very early and clear analysis by Hooper (1945) and a recent one by Berve (2015).

which the presupposition has meaning in direct experience. The judgment is the conscious affirmation by a particular subject for which the presupposition holds that this potentiality is, or is not, realized for it. It must be noticed that 'realized' does not mean 'realized in direct conscious experience,' but does mean 'realized as being contributory to the datum out of which that judging subject originates." (1978/1929: 196–197)

Whitehead explains in detail what this definition of a proposition would mean for the statement "Caesar crossed the Rubicon" (1978/1929: 196). Major points are the potentiality character of a proposition and its relation to a nexus, complex societies of actual occasions. Since each process involves feeling as well as physical data, the bifurcation of nature, as Whitehead calls it, is avoided.[3]

John Cobb provides a further helpful explanation:

"The dog is brown." "The dog" refers us to what Whitehead would describe as a very complex "society" of "actual occasions." "Brown" refers us to an "eternal object." The statement brings these together. Now we note that, for Whitehead, the statement points us to a potential. The potential is not the statement but the dog itself as brown. Propositions exist in the real world as what Whitehead describes as "lures for feeling." Some of the propositions are realized in the world, some are not. The latter may be called false, but "false" propositions may be more important than true ones. For example, they may describe the way things should be and move us to action. (Cobb 1998: 47–48)

The unusual usage of feelings in Whitehead's metaphysics needs further explanation as well. The shortest definition is given in *Process and Reality*:

A feeling i.e., a positive prehension is essentially a transition effecting a con-crescence. Its complex constitution is analysable into five factors which express what that transition consists of, and effects. The factors are: (i) the 'subject' which feels, (ii) the 'initial [338] data' which are to be felt, (iii) the 'elimination' in virtue of negative prehensions, (iv) the 'objective datum' which is felt, (v) the 'subjective form' which is how that subject feels that objective datum. (1978/1929: 223)

There are, of course, too numerous possible interactions of prehensions, propositions and feelings in the concrescence of societies and nexus. It may suffice for the present to consider a graph by Elizabeth Kraus in her book *The Metapysics of Experience – A Companion to Whitehead's Process and Reality* (Kraus 1998: 125) (Fig. 1).

A possible clearer elucidation may be provided by an example, with which many of us are familiar. If one proposes marriage to another person, this could shed some light on the intricate structure of a proposition. To propose marriage clearly has a highly emotional content as much as it involves physical, legal and logical aspects. Thus for Whitehead, the act of believing, and not just in religious terms, is a propositional feeling. Whitehead avoids the above mentioned bifurcation of nature through the overlapping of emotional and physical factors.

Whitehead's notion of a proposition seems close to what Angel and others define as bab. Angel states why a bab is so important for credition:

the term "bab" does not only name a content or a proposition – for these there would not have arisen the need for a new term. A "bab" is in fact characterized by four different aspects. Every single "bab" is characterized by

[3] For an overview on overcoming the bifurcation of nature, i.e. the split of nature into primary and secondary qualities see Maaßen (2012).

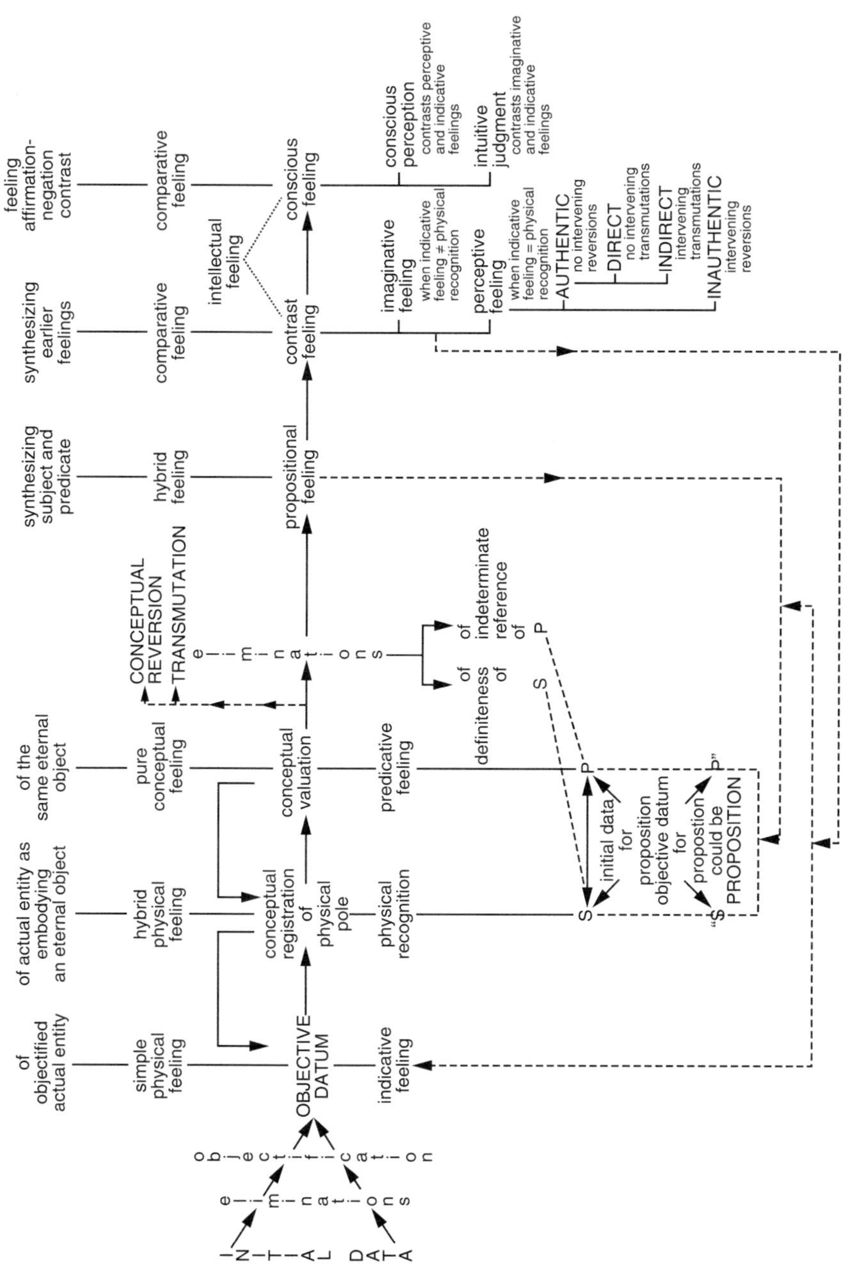

Fig. 1 Concrescence of an actual entity

- a propositional aspect
- the emotional loading of its content
- the sense of mightiness for the individual meaning-making
- the degree of certainty which is [merely subjectively] attributed to the content. (Angel 2015: 266)

One could therefore rephrase Angels' general description in the following 'Whiteheadian' way:

> *The introduction of "bab"* (instead Whitehead's term proposition H.M.) *into the scientific discussion reflects recent discoveries in brain function, which will modify a long debate concerning the primacy of cognition or emotion which is well known in the history of psychology because it has led to the building of its own scientific camp. It had started as a result of the presentation of the so called "two factor theory of emotion"* (Schachter 1964) *and was pushed by the protagonists Richard Lazarus and Robert Zajonc. This debate meanwhile gets a new (unifying) dimension by recent discoveries in neuroscience* (Gray et al. 2002; cf. for the following also Seitz and Angel 2014; Angel 2015: 266).

After placing the concept of credition in the framework of Whitehead's metaphysics, it will be possible to relate the intricate interconnection of a Whiteheadian position to the theological-psychological-neurological findings of the credition project. It may result in a revision of Whitehead's concept or could prove to be descriptive and adequate and. As far as Whitehead is concerned, the individual fact of 'belief' or credition is embedded in a society, either in the most general sense as culture or in the more specific one, which is religion.

To relate credition to a community of creditioners seems to me to be required and promising. Therefore, as a possible and may be necessary supplement, we should consider how Whitehead embeds the evolution of "belief" in history and society.

2 Proposition and Religion

Whitehead's famous definition states that "Religion is what the individual does with his own solitariness" (1926/2011: 6). At the same time, "the topic of religion is individuality in community (1926/2011: 88). In an interesting comparison between arithmetic and religion, Whitehead shows their similarities and differences. Truth in mathematics arises when, in history, simple doctrines dawned in the human mind, for instance, that two and three make five. In religion we not only do not know similar truths, but even a widely accepted definition of religion is lacking. Despite these differences, the most important one describes a specific attitude towards these different areas of mankind: "You *use* arithmetic, but you *are* religious (1926/2011: 4–5)

This implies that religion not only deals with truths, but that it has an effect on behavior. In Whitehead's words: "*A religion, on its doctrinal side, can thus be defined as a system of general truths which have the effect of transforming character when they are sincerely held and vividly apprehended*" (1926/2011: 15).

In Whitehead's "theory of religion," the development of religion leads in his later work to a *rationalization* of religious experience (1926/2011: 20–36; cf. Lowe

1966: 79–116; Wilmot 1979: 19–29; cf. for Whitehead's theory of the four steps of the development of religion see Welker 1965: 287–291). Although religious concerns were initially preoccupied with rituals, partial myths, and emotional stabilization, later religious consciousness evolved increasingly towards the recognition of universal connectivity, leaving behind provincial rituals and social bonds (1926/2011: 28). For Whitehead, this process of the "rationalization" of religion occurs within reciprocal movements towards *solitariness* and *solidarity*. These opposite features reveal the meaning of "religious intuition," namely, to be the *universal mediation of uniquely experienced events.*

In Whitehead's (1926/2011: 58) words: "The contrast of *singularity* and *universality*, *solitariness* and *solidarity*, illuminates "the origin of rational religion". "Religion is what the individual does with his own solitariness" (16) *and* "religion is world-loyalty" (59). Thus, the religious experience of uniqueness is both the experience of "solitariness" and that of "loyalty" to the world (1926/2011: 86). It is this dual structure that expresses Whitehead's theory of "religious intuition": "Rational religion appeals to the direct intuition of special occasions and to the elucidatory power of its concepts for all occasions. It arises from that which is special, but it extends to what is general. The doctrines of rational religion aim at being that metaphysics which can be derived from the super-normal experience of mankind in its moments of finest insight" (31).

"Religious intuition," as analyzed, has two aspects, or directions of motion:

1. *Singularity*: religious intuition is a "*direct* intuition" which cannot be resolved by general terms (such as rationality, metaphysics), but may only be *experienced.* Hence, religious intuition cannot be conceptualized completely, but is bound to the *uniqueness* of the experienced over against all conceptual generality (cf. Whitehead 1926/2011: 65).[4] In this *unpronounceable* uniqueness, religious intuition constitutes "the ultimate religious evidence, beyond which there is no appeal" (Whitehead 1926/2011: 65);
2. *Rationality*: although "intuitions" occur as events under *unique* conditions, they must, due to their accessibility for others, be subject to a process of communicability by theoretical transformation, i.e., the process of their "*rationalization*" (cf. Whitehead 1926/2011: 63)[5] "Intuitions," as it were, introduce the uniquely new into the world. However, at the same time, they must be generalized to be accessible for others' experience.[6] Or, as Whitehead says, the relevance of its

[4]Whitehead (1926/2011: 65) compares this experience of the unpronounceable, that is nevertheless known, with the knowledge of the mothers, who "can ponder many things in their hearts which their lips cannot express."

[5]Cf. RM, 63: "But reason is the safeguard of the objectivity of religion: it secures for it the general coherence denied to hysteria."

[6]This applies in particular to the religious experience, in which "novelty" cannot be expressed by any "formula." Nevertheless, religious experience becomes (and remains) accessible by its rational generalization (RM, 129ff). Cf. a quite similar description of "intuition" in Lachmann (1994: 84–88).

concepts can only be distinctly discerned in moments of insight, and then, for many of us, only after suggestion from without.

It is important to realize that, in Whitehead's view, "religious intuition" has *irreplaceable* meaning for any general "theory of the world." On the one hand, it allows for a unique base of experience, or "one select field of interest" (1926/2011: 86).[7] On the other hand, it maintains that concepts of religion, "though derived primarily from special experiences, are yet of universal validity" (1926/2011: 31). For a general theory of the world, the *irreplaceable* contribution of *religious* experience consists in the fact that it proceeds from the "super-normal experience of mankind in its moment of finest insight" (1926/2011: 31). "Religion starts from the generalization of final truths first perceived as exemplified in particular instances. These truths are amplified into a coherent system and applied to the interpretation of life. They stand or fall, like other truths, by their success in this interpretation. The peculiar character of religious truth is that it explicitly deals with values" (Whitehead 1926/2011: 110).

What follows is a stimulating evaluation of dogmata,[8] their truth and their limitations, how much they can stimulate and express experience as well as in what way and in which circumstances they can cause the opposite effect: "a one-sized formulation may be true, but may have the effect of a lie by its distortion of emphasis" (Whitehead 1926/2011: 127). Coming back to the pragmatic evaluation of religious experience, Whitehead (1926/2011) relates it to the evaluation of scientific development: "Progress in truth – truth of science and truth of religion – is mainly a progress in the framing of concepts, in discarding artificial abstractions or partial metaphors, and in evolving notions which strike more deeply into the root of reality" (131).

2.1 Symbolization of Religious Experience

If religion for Whitehead is primarily individual,[9] it inevitably entails the problem of expression. This would involve "individual expression" and rituals, which are communal forms of expression.[10] In my view, the surprising statement concerning

[7] Cf. RM, 31: "a small selection from the common experience," or "one among other specialized interests of mankind whose truths are of limited validity."

[8] "The dogmas, however true, are only bits of the truth, expressed in terms which in some ways are over-assertive and in other ways lose the essence of truth. When exactly understood in relation to an exact system of philosophic thought, they may – or may not – be exactly true." (RM, 129/130)

[9] "Thus religion is primarily individual, and the dogmas of religion are clarifying modes of external expression. The intolerant use of religious dogmas has practically destroyed their unity for a great, if not the greater part, of the civilized world." (RM, 122)

[10] "The later phases of the antecedent communal type of religion are dominated by the conscious reaction of human nature to the social organization in which it finds itself. Such reaction is partly emotion clothing itself in belief and ritual, and partly reason justifying practice by the test of social preservation. Rational religion is the wider conscious reaction of men to the universe in which they find themselves." (RM, 30/31)

religion in Whitehead is his insistence on "every day experience" as its basis, although there can be extraordinary experiences as well.

> *The final principle of religion is that there is wisdom in the nature of things, from which flow our direction of practice, and our possibility of the theoretical analysis of fact. It grounds this principle upon two sources of evidence, first upon our success in various special theoretical sciences, physical and otherwise; and secondly, upon our knowledge of a discernment of ordered relationships, especially in aesthetic valuations, which stretches far beyond anything which has been expressed systematically in words.* (1926/2011: 143)

Truth claims play an important role in religious discussion. At the same time, one should keep Whitehead's famous statement concerning any scheme of philosophy in mind: "If we consider any scheme of philosophic categories as one complex assertion, and apply to it the logician's alternative, true or false, the answer must be that the scheme is false. The same answer must be given to a like question respecting the existing formulated principles of any science" (1978/1929: 8). In a similar fashion: "Philosophers can never hope to formulate these metaphysical first principles…" (1978/1929: 4); "There is not even the language in which to frame them" (1978/1929: 13). These are distinct statements regarding relationalism as suitable forms of philosophizing, to avoid the Scylla of absolutism and the Charybdis of relativism.

Thus, the major problem for philosophy and theology is dealing with symbols concerning experience.

> *So much of human experience is bound up with symbolic reference, that it is hardly an exaggeration to say that the very meaning of truth is pragmatic. But though this statement is hardly an exaggeration, still it is an exaggeration, for the pragmatic test can never work, unless on some occasion in the future, or in the present there is a definite determination of what is true on that occasion. Otherwise the poor pragmatist remains an intellectual Hamlet, perpetually ad-journing decision of judgment to some later date.* (1926/2011: 181)

3 Conclusion

Religious experience seeks expression. Whitehead describes the different stages of expression which finally step beyond themselves and become dogma. This process "is the return from solitariness to society" (1926/2011: 137); at the same time, there is the danger of dogmatism by losing the vividness and openness of solitary, individual religious experience. Another danger which can lead to dogmatism concerning religious experiences is the necessary use of symbols. Indeed, dogma "is the precise enunciation of a general truth" (1926/2011: 126), but taken as expressing these experiences "without a context," taken as absolute truth it becomes a *contradictio in adjecto*: it contradicts its own individual origin and it contradicts the social and historical context of every symbol (e.g. 1926/2011: 129–130).

How this concept of religion could be reformulated in the credition concept has to be left to future research.

References

Angel HF (2015) How to understand the process of believing? In: Lamza JDL (ed) Advances in process thought: society, education, and God. Cambridge Scholars, Newcastle upon Tyne, pp 265–280
Berve A (2015) Spekulative Vernunft, symbolische Wahrnehmung, intuitive Urteile. Höhere Formen der Erfahrung bei A.N.Whitehead. Karl Alber, Freiburg/München
Cobb J (1998) Whitehead word book. P&F Press, Claremont
Emmet D (1966) Whitehead's philosphy of Organism. Macmillan, New York
Gray JR (et al.) (2002) Integration of emotion and cognition in the lateral prefrontal cortex. Proc Natl Acad Sci USA 99(6):4115–4120
Hampe M (1990) Die Wahrnehmungen der Organismen: Über die Voraussetzung einer naturalistischen Theorie der Erfahrung in der Metaphysik Whiteheads, Göttingen
Hooper SE (1945) Whitehead's philosophy: the higher phases of experience. Philosophy 20:57–78
Kann C (2001) Fußnoten zu Platon. Philosophiegeschichte bei A.N. Whitehead, Hamburg
Kraus E (1998) The metapysics of experience. A companion to Whitehead's Process and Reality (2 Rev ed.). Fordham University Press, New York
Lachmann R (1994) Ehtik und Identität. Der ethische Ansatz der Prozessphilosophie A.N. Whiteheads und seine Bedeutung für die gegenwärtige Ethik. Freiburg
Lazarus RS (1982) Thoughts on the relation between emotion and cognition. Am Psychol 37:1019–1024
Lowe V (1966) Understanding Whitehead. Johns Hopkins Press, Baltimore
Maaßen H (1987) Gott, das Gute und das Böse in der Philosophie A.N. Whiteheads. Peter Lang, Frankfurt
Maaßen H (1994) Revelation, myth and metaphysics: three traditional concepts of God and Whitehead's dipolar God. Process Stud 23:1–9
Maaßen H (2012) Alfred North Whitehead: categoreal scheme, modes of existence, types of orders, nexus, values. In: Ogrodnik B, Grodek K (eds) Studia Whiteheadiana, Krakau, pp 11–27
Poser H (1986) Whiteheads Kosmologie als revidierbare Metaphysik. In: Rapp F (ed) Whiteheads Metaphysik der Kreativität. Internationales Whitehead-Symposium Bad Homburg 1983, Freiburg, pp 105–126
Schachter S (1964) The interaction of cognitive and physiological determinants of emotional states. Berkowitz
Schaefer A, Gray JR (2007) A role for the human amygdala in higher cognition. Rev Neurosci 18(5):355–363
Seitz RJ, Angel HF (2014) Psychology of religion and spirituality. Meaning making and processes of believing. Relig, Brain Behav 22–30. doi:10.1080/2153599X.2014.891249
Strawson P (1959) Individuals: an essay in descriptive metaphysics. London
Whitehead AN (1926/2011) Religion in the making. Fordham, New York
Whitehead AN (1933/1967) Adventures of Ideas. Free Press, New York
Whitehead AN (1978/1929) Process and Reality: an essay in cosmology. The Free Press, New York (ed. by Griffin DR, Sherburne DB)
Wiktionary. The free dictionary (2012) prehendo. http://en.wiktionary.org/w/index.php?title=prehendo&oldid=16631091. Accessed 7 Apr 2012
Zajonc RB (1984) On the primacy of affect. Am Psychol 39:117–124

Brain and Self – A Neurophilosophical Account

Georg Northoff

Abstract We have experience and are conscious of the world. Who, though, is conscious? This is the subject, or self, of experience. While in the past the concept of self has been a matter of philosophical discussion, psychoanalysis shifted it into the domain of psychology where it surfaced as ego. More recently, brain imaging allows researchers to investigate the neural mechanisms underlying our subjective experience of a self. This chapter focuses on discussing the different concepts of self as based on philosophical accounts. These are then complemented by neuroscientific data on the self and self-reference. Finally, both philosophical and neuroscientific accounts are directly compared to each other while at the same time their relevance for psychoanalysis of self and ego are pointed out.

Summary

The present chapter aims to target yet another central feature of the mind, the self, which is the subject of all our experience and hence of consciousness. More specifically, the focus is on different concepts of the self and how they are related to recent findings about neural mechanisms involved in the self-reference of stimuli. I will first introduce different basic concepts of the self as they are currently discussed in philosophy. The first concept of self is the self as mental substance, which was originally introduced by Descartes. This is rejected by current and more empirically-oriented concepts of the self where the idea of a mental substance is replaced by assumptions of specific self-representational capacities. These self-representational capacities illustrate the physical, neuronal states of the body and brain in a summarized, coordinated, and integrated way. As such, the self-representational concept of the self must be distinguished from the phenomenological concept of self that is supposed to be an integral part of the experience and thus of consciousness. This phenomenal self resurfaces in the current debate as the 'minimal self'—a basic sense of self in our experience that is supposed to be closely related to both brain

G. Northoff (✉)
Mind, Brain Imaging and Neuroethics Research Unit, Institute of Mental Health Research, Royal Ottawa Mental Health Centre, Ottawa, Canada
e-mail: Georg.Northoff@theroyal.ca

H.-F. Angel et al. (eds.), *Processes of Believing: The Acquisition, Maintenance, and Change in Creditions*, New Approaches to the Scientific Study of Religion 1,
DOI 10.1007/978-3-319-50924-2_17

and body. Current neuroscience investigates the spatial and temporal neural mechanisms underlying those stimuli that are closely related to the self when compared to stimuli that show no relation or reference to the self. This is described as the self-reference effect. When comparing self- versus non-self-specific stimuli, neural activity in the middle regions of the brain, the so-called cortical midline structures, is increased. Moreover, increased neuronal synchronization in the gamma frequency domain can be observed. The question is how specific these findings are for the concept of self as discussed in philosophy. Neuronal specificity describes the particular and exclusive association of the midline regions with the self. This is not the case since the same regions are also associated with a variety of other functions. This goes along with the quest for the psychological and experimental specificity of psychological functions and experimental paradigms and measures used to test for the self. One may also raise the issue of phenomenal specificity, which refers to whether the phenomenal features of the self that is mindness and belongingness are distinguishable from other phenomenal features like intentionality or qualia. Finally, one may discuss the question of conceptual specificity that targets the distinction between the concepts of self-reference and self.

1 Background: Conceptual Determination of the Self in Philosophy

You're winning a game of tennis while your partner is watching. You feel pride. Who experiences that pride? You. Without you as subject of this experience, you could not experience anything at all, not even boredom. This subject of experience has been described as the 'self'. Your 'self' makes it possible for you to experience things. In other words, it is a necessary condition for experience and thus also for consciousness. It is clear, therefore, that there is much at stake when it comes to the self.

The concept of self has been subject to intense philosophical discussion over the centuries. Different philosophers have suggested different concepts of self. Recent conceptual issues that have been discussed in the philosophical literature range from discussions of self-consciousness (Peacocke 2014), the certainty of self-existence (Campbell 2004), to questions of self-knowledge (Burge 2013) and self-constitution (Velleman 2006). Because of time and space constraints, we will only focus on those that are relevant in the attempt to map the interface between philosophical and neuroscientific accounts of the self. In the model of credition, the concept of self plays a central role (Sugiura et al. 2015).

There are four main concepts of self that are discussed in current philosophy. First is 'the mental self,' which is based on our thoughts and a specific mental substance. Second is the 'empirical self'— this concept of the self represents and reflects the biological processes in one's body and brain.

Third is the 'phenomenal self,' from which our experience in consciousness originates. Our consciousness is accompanied by an awareness of our self, referred to as pre-reflective self-awareness or phenomenal self. Finally, and most recently, philosophers speak of a 'minimal self'. This concept of the self is based on our body and its physiological processes. I will discuss each of these different concepts and how they relate to the brain in this chapter.

Before we do this, I will shed some light on several related concepts. We experience our self in daily life during, for example, the act of perceiving certain objects, persons, or events in our environment. For example, while making a list of all the things you have to do today, you experience not only the act of thinking and writing, but an awareness and experience of your own self. Hence, your self as the very subject of experience seems to be part of that experience. In other words, your self is a content of your consciousness. This is described as self-consciousness. The concept of self-consciousness will be the focus of the next chapter.

However, there is more to the self than the self itself and our experience of it in self-consciousness. You wake up every morning. Every day. Every week, every year. Your body changes. You become older. You get wrinkled and your hair turns white. Despite all these bodily changes, you nevertheless have the feeling that you are the same self. You still experience your self as being the same self of 20 years ago.

You are one and the same person. Thus, there is a temporal dimension to your self that seems to be coherent and persistent across time. The temporal dimension of your self has consequently been discussed under the umbrella of what is called 'personal identity' in philosophy. While our discussion will touch upon the temporal dimension of the self and thus upon personal identity, we will not explicitly discuss it.

In a world of over seven billion people, there are many, many selves: you, your friends, your family, etc. Most interestingly, you can relate to them – you can communicate with other selves and sometimes even feel their emotions as in, for instance, the grief someone might feel when they lose a loved one. Or you might experience pain when your boyfriend's arm is broken. How is this possible? In philosophy, this is called 'intersubjectivity'. Intersubjectivity shall be discussed in Chap. 19.

Finally, your self is not isolated from the rest of the world. You can share others' experiences and feel connected to the world. The world, with its specific objects, persons, and events, has meaning to you—you can relate to it more or less and can appropriate it for your own self. How is such basic integration of your own self within the world possible? And how is that related to your brain and its neuronal mechanisms? This will be the focus in the fourth chapter in this part.

2 Background: Empirical Investigation of the Self in Neuroscience

How can we investigate the self? In order to experimentally address the self, we need some quantifiable and objective measures that can be observed from a third-person perspective. How can we obtain such measures? Psychologists focusing on memory observed that items related to ourselves were better remembered than those unrelated (Northoff et al. 2006). For example, as a resident of Ottawa, I recall the recent thunderstorm that wiped away several houses locally much better than a person who, perhaps living in Germany, just heard about it in the news.

Thus, there is superiority in the recollections of those items and stimuli that are related to one's self. This is described as the self-reference effect (SRE). The SRE has been well validated in several psychological studies. Most interestingly, it has been shown to operate in different domains; not only in respect to memory, but also in relation to emotions, sensorimotor functions, faces, words, etc. In all these different domains (see below for details), stimuli related to one's own self, known as self-specific stimuli, are recalled much better than those that are unrelated to one's own self, known as non-self-specific stimuli.

How is the SRE possible? Numerous investigations (Klein 2012; Klein and Gangi 2010 for summaries) show that the SRE is mediated by different psychological functions. These range from personal memories including autobiographical memories, memories of facts (semantic memories), to those cognitive capacities that allow for self-reflection and self-representation. Hence, the SRE by itself is not a solitary function, but rather a complex multifaceted psychological composite of functions and processes.

How can we link the SRE to the brain? Before the introduction of functional imaging techniques such as fMRI in the early 1990s, most studies focused on the effect of dysfunction or lesions in specific brain regions caused by brain tumours or stroke. These revealed that lesions in medial temporal regions that are central in memory recall, such as the hippocampus, change and ultimately abolish the SRE effect.

With the introduction of brain imaging techniques such as fMRI, we could then transfer the experimental paradigms of comparing self- and non-self-specific stimuli to the scanner and investigate the underlying brain regions. The basic premise here is that if self-specific stimuli are recalled better than non-self-specific stimuli, they must be processed by the brain in a different way. This might be, for instance, by higher degrees of neural activity and/or different regions.

This led to the investigation of numerous experimental designs of SRE-like paradigms in the fMRI scanner. For example, subjects were presented trait adjectives that were either related to themselves (such as for me, my hometown, Ottawa) as opposed to (Sydney, an unrelated city for me). In other tests, the participant was presented with images of his or her own face and these were compared with faces of other people. Also, autobiographical events from the subject's past were compared with those from other people. One's own movements and actions could also be compared with those of other people, implying what is called ownership (e.g., my movements) and agency ('I myself caused that action').

The stimuli belonged to different domains such as memory, faces, emotions, verbal, spatial, motor, or social. Most of the stimuli were presented either visually or auditorily and the presentation of these stimuli was usually accompanied by an on-line judgment about whether the stimuli are related and personally meaningful or not to the research subject.

On the whole, we can see that current neuroscience can investigate the self in various experimental ways using mainly functional brain imaging. However, any empirical research relies on certain presuppositions. This also holds true for current neuroscientific research on the self, which aims to reveal the neuronal mechanisms underlying our experience, or sense of self. However, before examining the neuroscientific findings, we need to briefly shed some light on the concept of the self and how it has been defined in philosophical discussions.

3 Philosophical Concepts: Mental Self

What is the self? What must it look like in order to presuppose experience and be the subject of our experience? The self has often been viewed as a specific 'thing'. Stones are things, and the table on which your laptop stands is a thing. And in the same way the table makes it possible for the laptop to stand on it, the self may be a thing that makes experience and consciousness possible. In other words, metaphorically speaking, experience and consciousness stand on the shoulders of the self.

However, another question is whether the self is a thing or, as philosophers such as Rene Descartes suggest, a substance? A substance is a specific entity or material that serves as a basis for something like a self. For instance, the body can be considered a physical substance, while the self is can be associated with a mental substance.

Is our self real and thus does it exist? Or is it just an illusion? Let us compare the situation to perception. When we perceive something in our environment, we sometimes perceive it not as a real thing, but as an illusion that in reality does not exist. The question of what exists and what is real is what philosophers call a metaphysical question. Earlier philosophers, such as Rene Descartes, assumed that the self is real and exists.

However, Descartes also assumed that the self is different from the body. Hence, self and body exist, but differ in their existence and reality. Thus, from this perspective, the self cannot be a physical substance and is a mental substance instead. It is a feature not of the body, but of the mind.

However, the characterization of the self as a mental entity has been questioned. For example, the Scottish philosopher David Hume argued that there is no such thing as self as a mental entity. There is only a complex set or 'bundle' of perceptions of interrelated events that reflect the world in its entirety. There is no additional self in the world; instead, there is nothing but the events we perceive. Everything else, such as the assumption of a self as a mental entity, is an illusion. The self as a mental entity, and thus, as a mental substance, does not exist and is therefore not real.

To reject the idea of self as a mental substance and to dismiss it as a mere illusion is currently popular. One major proponent of this view today is the German philosopher Thomas Metzinger (2004). In a nutshell, he argues that through our experience, we develop models of the self, so-called 'self-models'. These self-models are nothing but information processes in our brain. However, since we do not have direct access to these neuronal processes (e.g., those processes and activities of the cells,

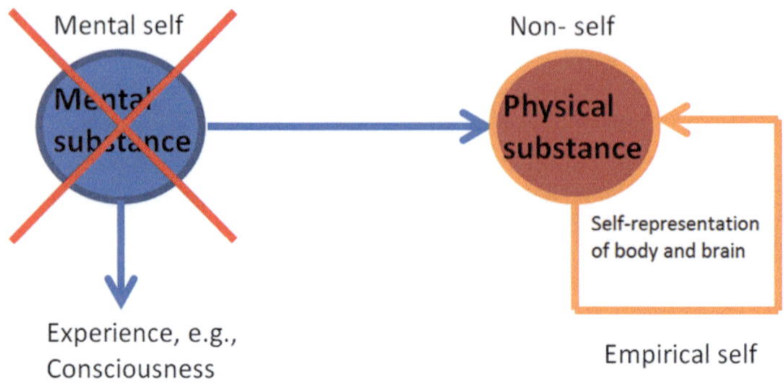

Fig. 1 The figure shows the concepts of empirical (**a**) and phenomenal (**b**) self. (**a**) The empirical self replaces the mental self (*left*) by physical features while the self is then accounted for by self-representation (*right part*) (**b**) The phenomenal self can be characterized by continuous experience of a stream of time, the stream of consciousness

neurons, in the brain), we tend to assume the presence of an entity that must underlie our own self-model. This entity is then characterized as the self (Fig. 1).

According to Metzinger, the assumption of the self as a mental entity results from an erroneous inference based on our experience. We cannot experience the neuronal processes in our brain as such; nobody has ever experienced their own brain and its neuronal processes. Therefore, the outcome of our brain's neuronal processes, the self, cannot be traced back to its original basis (the brain) in our experience.

Where then does the self come from? We assume that it must be traced back to a special instance that is different from the brain. This leads us to assume that the mind and the self are mental entities rather than physical, neuronal entities originating in the brain itself. Metzinger argues that the self as a mental entity simply does not exist. Therefore, Metzinger (2004) concludes, selves do not really exist. Hence, the title of his book: *"Being No One"*.

4 Philosophical Concepts: From the Metaphysical to the Empirical Self

What is the self, if not a mental entity? Current authors, such as Metzinger (2004) and Churchland (2002), argue that the self as a mental substance or entity does not exist. How do we come up with the idea of a self or the self-model as Metzinger calls it? The model of our own self is based on summarizing, integrating, and coordinating all the information from our own body and brain.

What does such integration look like? Take all that information together, coordinate and integrate it, and then you have a self-model of your own brain and body and their respective processes. In more technical terms, our own brain and body are represented in the neuronal activity of the brain. Such representation of the own brain and body amounts then to a model of your self. The self-model is therefore nothing but an inner model of the integrated and summarised version of your own brain and body's information processing. The self is thus a mere model of one's own body's and brain's processes.

The original mental self, the self as mental substance or entity, in this line of thinking is replaced by a self-model. This implies a shift from a metaphysical discussion of the existence and reality of self, to the processes that underlie the representation of body and brain as a self-model. Since this representation is based on the coordination and integration of the various ongoing processes in brain and body, it is associated with specific higher-order cognitive functions such as working memory, attention, executive function, and memory, amongst others.

What does this imply for the characterization of the self (presupposing a broader concept of self beyond the self as mental substance)? The self is no longer characterized as a mental substance, but as a cognitive function. Methodologically, this implies that the self should be investigated empirically rather than metaphysically.

We therefore need to search for the cognitive processes underlying the special self-representation. The self is consequently no longer an issue of philosophy, but rather one of cognitive psychology and ultimately of cognitive neuroscience. According to this model, the self is no longer a metaphysical matter, but a possible subject of empirical investigation. Metzinger's critique of the self is directed towards the assumption of a metaphysical self as mental entity or substance. In contrast, he does not deny the experience or sense of self. Therefore, the title of his book "Being No One" is somewhat misleading – there is one being that we continuously experience, but it is not a mental substance or entity.

5 Philosophical Concepts: Minimal Self

How can we describe the pre-reflective self-consciousness in more detail? It is always already there in every experience, so that we cannot avoid it or separate it from the experience. The self is always present in our consciousness and thus in our subjective experience. Even if we do not focus on the self as such, we cannot avoid or remove its presence. Hence, the term pre-reflective self-conscious describes an implicit or tacit experience of our self in our consciousness.

Since the self as pre-reflectively experienced is the basis of all phenomenal features of our experience, it must be considered as essential for any subsequent cognitive activity. Such a basic and fundamental self occurs in our experience before any reflection. For instance, when reading the lines of this book, you experience the contents and, in addition, you also experience your self as reading these lines.

Hence, your immediate experience and consciousness comes with both the content and your own self. Since the experience of such self occurs prior to any reflection and recruitment of higher-order cognitive functions, the concept of self is sort of a minimal version of the self. Current phenomenological philosophers such as Gallagher (2000) and Zahavi (2005) speak therefore of a 'minimal self' when referring to the self as implicitly, tacitly, and immediately experienced in consciousness.

How can we describe the concept of the 'minimal self'? The minimal self refers to a basic form of self that is part of any experience. As such, it is not extended across time like it is in the experience of the self that has continuity across time in personal identity. Instead, the minimal self describes a basic sense of self at any particular given moment in time, but does not yet provide a link between different moments in time and thus continuity across time.

How can such continuity across time be constituted? Cognitive functions such as memories and autobiographical memories in particular may be central. In this model, the self may become more complex. One might speak of a cognitive, extended or autobiographical self, as does, for example, the Portuguese-American neuroscientist, Damasio (1999, 2010).

Another important feature of the minimal self is that although we experience it, we may not be aware of it as such. This means that we might not be able to reflect upon it in order to gain knowledge of it. We are, to put it in technical terms, only pre-reflectively aware of the minimal self. In contrast to such pre-reflective awareness, there is no reflective awareness of the minimal self. How can we become reflectively aware of the minimal self? For that to be possible, the different moments or points in time need to be integrated and, as philosophers say, represented. For such representation to occur, cognitive functions are needed which make it possible to link together the different time points.

Finally, the minimal self may also occur prior to verbalization and thus linguistic expression. Rather than being tied to specific linguistic concepts, as is the case with more cognitive concepts of the self, the minimal self must be considered pre-linguistic. It is an experience, a sense of self that can barely be put into concepts. We can experience the self but are not really able to describe these experiences in terms of concepts and articulate them in a linguistic way.

Thus, the minimal self is pre-linguistic and pre-conceptual and will therefore, speculatively, not be affected by second language acquisition. It is the kind of experience, an implicit sense of self, which most likely subjects will take with them as more or less stable when moving to a new country where they have to acquire a new language. However, at the same time, the minimal self provides the essential basis upon which more cognitive forms of self are developed. These are then central and instrumental in providing the ability to learn a second language.

6 Philosophical Concepts: Social Self

How does the self interact with other selves? So far we described the self in an isolated and purely intra-individual way. However, in daily life, the self is not isolated from others, but always related to other selves. This is called inter-individualism rather than intra-individualism. This raises questions about what is described as the 'problem of other minds' or, more generally, questions concerning intersubjectivity. Here we will here give a brief description of the problem of intersubjectivity.

How can we make the assumption of attributing mental states, and thus self and mind, to other people? Philosophy has long relied on what is called the 'inference by analogy'. What is the 'inference by analogy'? 'Inference by analogy' goes like this. We observe person A to show the behavior of type X. And we know that in our own case, the same behavior X goes along with the mental state type M. Since our own behavior and that of person A are similar, we assume that the other person A to show the same mental state type M we experience when exhibiting behavior X.

What kind of inference do we draw here? There is similar or analogous behavior between ourselves and the other person. In addition, my own behavior is associated with a particular mental state. Since now the other person shows the same behavior, I infer that she also experiences the same mental state that is associated with my own behavior. Hence, by indirect inference and analogy via our own case, we claim to obtain knowledge of the other person's mental state. How can we make such an inference? We may make it on the basis of our own mental states and their associated behavior. And what we do may also hold true for the other person who in the same way attributes mental states to us by inferring them from the comparison between our behavior and their own mental states.

Why do we make such inferences? Because it seems to be the easiest and best way for us to explain other people's behavior. The assumption of mental states thus seems to be the best explanation for your behavior. The 'inference by analogy' may thus be considered an inference to the best possible explanation.

The inference by analogy describes intersubjectivity in a very cognitive and ultimately linguistic way when attributing mental states and a self to other persons. There might be, however, a deeper level of intersubjectivity. We also feel the other persons' mental states when sharing the emotional pain, for example, that one's spouse experiences when her father died. Such sharing of feeling is described as empathy and sheds light on a deeper pre-cognitive and pre-verbal dimension of intersubjectivity. This has been emphasized especially in phenomenological philosophy (see for instance Zahavi 2005; Metzinger 2004).

However, both empathy and the attribution of mental states to another person are puzzling: despite that the fact that we do not experience the other's mental states and consciousness, we nevertheless either share them (as in empathy) or infer them (as in inference by analogy). We have no direct access to other persons' experience of a self and its mental states in first-person perspective, yet nevertheless share their mental states and assume that they have a self. How is that possible?

This is where we need to introduce yet another perspective. There is first-person perspective – tied to the self itself and its experience or consciousness of objects, events, or persons in the environment. Then there is the third-person perspective—this perspective allows us to observe the objects, events, or persons in the environment from the outside, rather than from the inside. The picture is not complete.

What is second-person perspective? Second-person perspective has initially been associated in philosophy with the introspection of one's own mental states. Rather than actually experiencing one's own mental states in first-person perspective, second-person perspective makes it possible to reflect on and introspect about one's own mental states. An example of this is when you ask yourself whether the voice you heard was really the voice of your good friend (see also Schilbach et al. 2013).

The second-person perspective thus allows us to put the contents of our consciousness as experienced in first-person perspective into a wider context, the context of oneself as related to the environment. In other words, the second-person perspective makes it possible to situate and integrate the purely intra-individual self with its first-person perspective into a social context. This transforms the intra-individual self into an inter-individual self. Another way of thinking of second-person perspective is to call this concept of the self, the 'social self'.

How can we define the concept of the social self? The concept of the social self describes the linkage and integration of the self into the social context of other selves. This shifts the focus from experience or consciousness in the first-person perspective to the various kinds of interactions between different selves as associated with the second-person perspective. As we already indicated, there may be different kinds of social interactions, including affective pre-cognitive and more cognitive ones, that involve meta-representation as described above.

7 Neuroscientific Findings: Spatial Patterns of Neural Activity During Self-Specific Stimuli

How can we relate the various philosophical concepts of the self to the neuroscientific findings of self-reference? Above, we discussed that psychology, and later neuroscience, quantified the self in terms of the self-reference effect (SRE). The SRE describes the different impact of self-referential and non-self-referential stimuli on psychological (e.g., reaction time, recall, etc., see above) and neural (e.g., degree of activity, regions, etc. see below) measures. Below, we want to briefly highlight some of the main findings of recent imaging studies on the self-reference effect.

What results did the various imaging studies yield in the fMRI? Two different kinds of regions showed up. First, one could see that the regions specific for respective domains like emotions or faces were recruited. For instance, there is a region in the back of the brain that specifically processes faces (as distinguished from, say, houses); this is called the fusiform face area. This region is obviously active during the presentation of faces, no matter whether it is one's own face or another person's face. Importantly, clear differences between self- and non-self-specific stimuli could not be observed in these domain-specific regions in most studies (see Northoff et al. 2006).

What about other regions that are not specific to particular domains (also known as domain-independent regions) involved in the neural processing of the self? Meta-analyses of the various studies demonstrated the involvement of a particular set of regions in the middle of the brain. These regions include the perigenual anterior cingulate cortex (PACC), the ventro- and dorsomedial prefrontal cortex (VMPFC, DMPFC), the supragenual anterior cingulate cortex (SACC), the posterior cingulate cortex (PCC) and the precuneus. Since they are all located in the midline of the brain, they have been coined 'cortical midline structures' (CMS).

The self-specific stimuli—those that were personally relevant for the subjects—induced higher neural activity in these regions than non-self-specific stimuli, or those that remained irrelevant und unrelated to the person. This was observed in the various domains for faces, trait adjectives, movements/actions, memories, and social communication. Therefore, the CMS seem to show a special significance to the self and self-reference.

However, there is also some differentiation within the CMS. The self-specific stimuli may be presented in different ways to the subject in the scanner. If subjects have to make judgments requiring cognitive involvement, the dorsal and posterior regions such as the SACC, DMPFC and PCC are recruited to a stronger degree. If, in contrast, stimuli are merely perceived without any judgment, and thus without any cognitive component, the ventral and anterior regions such as the VMPFC and PACC were highly involved (Fig. 2).

This led to the assumption that the different regions mediate different aspects of self-reference. The ventral and anterior regions, such as the PACC and VMPFC, may be more involved in the representation of the degree of self-reference in the stimulus. However, dorsal regions, such as the SACC and the DMPFC, may be related to monitoring and reflection of the stimulus and its self-reference when we become aware of the stimulus as self-specific.

Finally, the posterior regions, such as the PCC, may be implicated in integrating the stimulus and its degree of self-reference into the autobiographical memory of the respective person. These regions seem to be implicated in the recall and retrieval of especially personally relevant and autobiographical information from the past of that person. Thus, it can be concluded that specific regions in the midline of the brain, the cortical midline structures, seem to be involved in the neural processing of self-reference or attributing personal relevance or self-relevance to stimuli.

8 Neuroscientific Findings: Temporal Patterns of Neural Activity During Self-Specific Stimuli

In addition to the spatial patterns of self-reference, its temporal patterns have also been investigated using EEG. Again, self- specific and non-self-specific stimuli have been compared to each other while the subjects undergo EEG measurement. This revealed early changes during self-specific stimuli at around 100–150 ms after stimulus onset.

More specifically, self-specific stimuli induced different electrical activity changes already at 130–200 ms after their onset when compared to non-self-specific stimuli. This was accompanied by later changes around 300–500 ms. Hence, the temporal pattern between self- and non-self-specific stimuli shows both early and late differences.

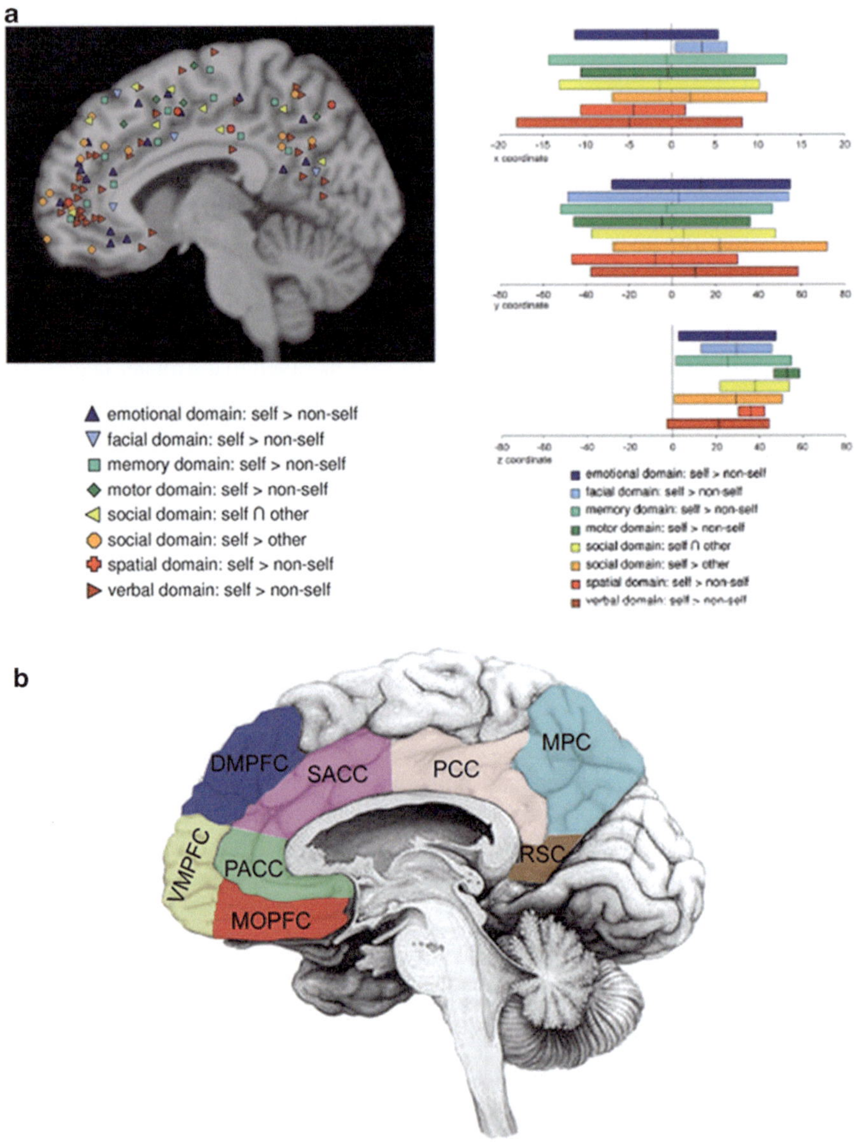

Fig. 2 The figure illustrates findings about the neural localization of self in the cortical midline structures (**a**) The figures shows on the left an overview of all different studies on self-relatedness and their location in the cortical midline structures; on the right one sees the coordinates, x, y, and z for the location of the activation (**b**) the different regions in the cortical midline structures are illustrated (see text for abbreviations)

In addition, different frequencies of neural activity were investigated. The neural activity oscillates rhythmically in different frequency ranges in the fluctuations of the neuronal activity.

One frequency often induced by stimuli are gamma frequencies in the range of 30–40 Hz. Interestingly, some EEG (and MEG) studies observed higher power in the gamma range in anterior and posterior midline regions during self-specific stimuli than non-self-specific stimuli. The question though is whether such increases in gamma power is specific to self-specific stimuli since it can also be observed in other functions independent of self-reference (see below).

8.1 Neuroscientific Findings Ic: Social Patterns of Neural Activity During Self-Reference

How can we investigate the social nature of the self described earlier? Various studies have been conducted to investigate different kinds of interaction between different selves. Pfeiffer et al. (2013) and Schilbach et al. (2012) distinguish two different methodological approaches. One investigates social cognition, the cognition of mental states in other people, from a third-person perspective. Here, social cognition is investigated in an "offline" mode. More recently, this "offline" methodological strategy has been complemented by an "online" mode. In the "online mode," social interaction is investigated from the "inside," by taking on the perspective of the interacting selves (rather than the observer's point of view).

Besides conducting several studies, the same group has recently investigated the neural overlap between emotional processing, resting state activity, and social-cognitive processing (Schilbach et al. 2012). They conducted a meta-analysis including imaging studies from all three kinds of investigations: resting state, emotional, and social-cognitive. First, they analysed the regions implicated in each of the three tasks. This yielded significant recruitment of neural activity, especially in the midline regions like the ventro and dorsomedial prefrontal cortex and the posterior cingulate cortex (bordering to the precuneus). In addition, neural activity in the temporo-parietal junction and the middle temporal gyrus was observed.

In the second step, they overlaid the three tasks, emotional, social-cognitive, and resting state, in order to detect commonly underlying areas. This indeed revealed the midline regions, the dorsomedial prefrontal cortex and the posterior cingulate cortex, to be commonly shared among emotional and social-cognitive tasks and resting state activity. Based on this neural overlap, the authors concluded that there may be an intrinsically social dimension in our neural activity which might be essential for consciousness of both our own self and other selves. If this is true, it will have radical consequences, not only for the concept of the self, but also for consciousness in general.

9 Neurophilosophical Discussion: Different Forms of Specificity

So far we have covered philosophical approaches to the concept of the self. We also discussed neuroscientific findings about self-reference. Now, the question is how both philosophical concepts and neuroscientific findings are related to each other. *This requires what one may describe as a neurophilosophical discussion. A neurophilosophical discussion directly relates empirical findings in neuroscience to concepts in philosophy.*

How are the neuroscientific findings about self-reference related to the philosophical concepts of self? Are the philosophical concepts of self empirically plausible and thus compatible with the neuroscientific findings of self-reference? In order to address these questions, one should start by investigating the degree of specificity for the self demonstrated by neuroscientific findings. One can thus speak of neuronal specificity of the cortical midline structure for the self. The concept of neuronal specificity describes the quest for the exclusive association of a particular neuronal measure, like the activity of a certain region or network, with exclusively one specific function.

And they may also be discussed in the context of psychological functions associated with the self and thus psychological specificity. Furthermore, one may question the ability of the experimental designs and measures to really tap into the self. This is called experimental specificity (Fig. 3).

One may also raise the question of whether the results really reflect the experiential, and thus phenomenal features, related to the self. For instance, experience may

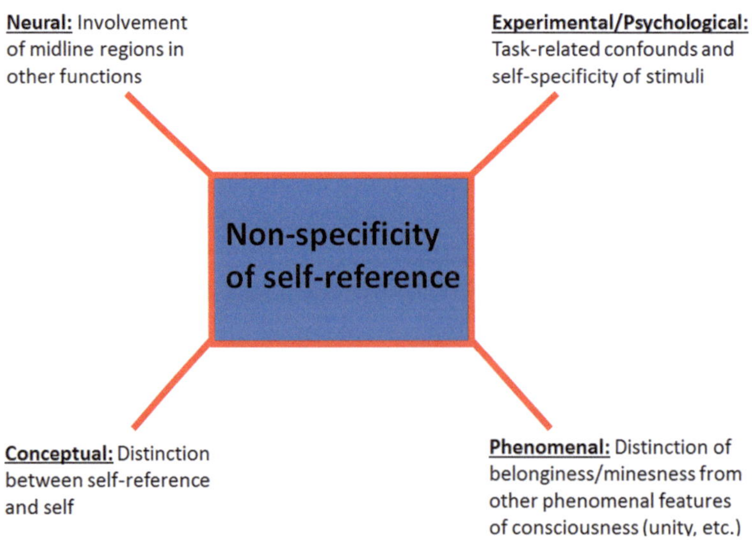

Fig. 3 The figure illustrates the different problems with regard to self-specificity; this includes neural, conceptual, phenomenal, and experimental issues

be confounded by features that are not directly related to the self. One may thus want to speak of phenomenal specificity. Finally, one may want to discuss how the results relate to the different concepts of the self and whether they correspond exclusively to one specific concept. If done, this would imply conceptual specificity.

10 Neurophilosophical Discussion: Neuronal Specificity of Midline Regions

Let's start with neuronal specificity. The concept of neuronal specificity describes whether the spatial and temporal patterns of neural activity observed in studies about self-specificity are really specific to the self. We roughly distinguished between two kinds of different regions, the domain-specific regions and the domain-independent regions.

Domain-specific regions are those that are related to the processing of content in a specific modality (e.g., sensory) or domain (e.g., verbal, sensory, motor, etc.). Depending on the stimuli and/or the task, domain-specific regions were activated in the above-described imaging data.

Are these domain-specific regions specific for the self? No, because the imaging data show that the very same regions are also recruited when applying stimuli that are not related to the self at all. For example, you are shown a house in Brazil. For you, a resident of Canada (with no connection to Brazil), this image has no degree of self-specificity or self-relatedness to you. It nevertheless activates your fusiform face area.

The self-specialist may now want to argue that at least the degree of neural activity in the fusiform face area or other domain-specific areas may be different between self- and non-self-specific stimuli. However, empirical data are not clear. While some studies report some difference, though small, in sensory regions, the majority of studies apparently did not observe differences between self- and non-self-specific stimuli in these domain- specific regions. Hence, it seems as if the domain-specific regions like the sensory and motor cortex remain unspecific for the self. This implies neuronal unspecificity.

What about the domain-independent regions like the cortical midline structures? There has been much discussion about whether these regions are specific for self-specific stimuli as distinguished from non-self-specific stimuli. Is the self 'located' in the midline regions? Initial enthusiasm was in support of the theory that the midline regions are specific for the self, recent investigations implicated the same set of regions in a variety of different functions.

Let me be more specific. Tasks requiring the need to understand other people and their mental states – mind-reading as described in theory of mind in psychology—strongly recruit the midline regions. Emotional stimuli and emotional tasks also led to strong activation in the midline regions. In addition, various kinds of social tasks that require social exchange and reciprocity also recruit these regions. Finally, daydreaming or mind-wandering and other forms of introspection also recruit these regions.

The involvement of the midline regions in various functions other than self-reference sheds some doubt on the neuronal specificity of the midline structure for the self. Hence, even the domain-independent regions like the midline regions do not seem to show any specificity for the self.

The same diagnosis of neuronal unspecificity also is true of the reported gamma synchronizations. Gamma synchronization is not specific to the self but has been observed in a variety of different functions including sensorimotor, working memory, attention, and episodic memory retrieval. Hence, there is neuronal non-specificity in both a temporal and spatial sense with regard to the self.

11 Neurophilosophical Discussion: Psychological and Experimental Specificity

Most of the fMRI studies discussed above compared self- versus non-self-specific stimuli, such as a grand piano for a professional pianist compared to a saw for a carpenter. In addition to the mere perception, subjects were required to make a judgment after each stimulus about whether it was self- or non-self-specific. This raises questions about what exactly the study is measuring - the perception or the judgment of the stimulus? Is it capturing the effect of the stimulus itself, or the task related to that stimulus?

Most likely the results reflect a mixture between stimulus- and task-related effects. This, therefore, casts some doubt on whether the midline regions show psychological specificity for the self. The judgment about self-specificity requires various cognitive functions such as attention, working memory, and autobiographical memory retrieval. Some authors, such as the French neuroscientist D. Legrand, argue that the midline regions may be more related to what she describes as 'general evaluation function', than being specific to the self and self-specific stimuli.

What about when research investigates the self in relation to more basic functions, such as movements and actions? Even when subjects perform some motor tasks, we face the same confusion related to different functions: the self's components, such as ownership (my own movement), as well as agency (whether I am the agent of the movement), may be confounded by the neural mechanisms underlying the execution of the movement/action by the person.

Such psychological non-specificity highlights the need in neuroscience to specify the experimental design and measures. We need measures that are specific to the self as distinguished from the various associated sensorimotor, affective, and cognitive functions. We also need experimental designs to segregate stimulus-related effects and task-related effects. For example, we might do this by spacing perception and judgment temporally apart from each other.

12 Neurophilosophical Discussion: Self-Specificity and Other Functions

We also need to discuss the relationship between the self and other functions. Recent imaging studies demonstrated a strong neural overlap between the self and reward, the self and emotions, and the self and decision-making. For example, when receiving a reward in relation to a specific stimuli, such as money, regions of the reward system like the ventral striatum (VS) and the ventromedial prefrontal cortex (VMPFC) become active (Northoff 2012). These same regions are also active when the same stimulus is conceived of as self-specific, rather than non-self-specific by the respective subject.

The same effects can be observed in emotions where emotional and self-specific stimuli have been shown to overlap in the anterior midline regions especially. Finally, the same effect can be observed in decision-making: if external cues are provided when making a decision (such as a higher or lower price of the same kind of apples), lateral cortical regions become active. If, in contrast, no such external cues are provided, we need to come up with some internal criterion to guide our decision about which apples to purchase (Nakao et al. 2012). Such internal criterion can only stem from our self. Studies comparing both kinds of decision-making show predominant involvement of the midline regions in internally-guided when compared to externally-guided decision-making (Nakao et al. 2012).

Together, this neural overlap between the self and other functions, such as reward, emotions, and decision-making, raises questions about the relationship between them. Different models could be imagined. Self- and self-specificity could be an independent function just like attention, working memory, emotion, sensorimotor, etc. However, in that case, one would expect specific regions in the brain and specific psychological functions to sub-serve specifically, and exclusively, self-specificity. However, at this point in time, this cannot be supported empirically.

Finally, one could also suggest that self and self-specificity are basic functions that underlie and provide the basis for all other functions—sensorimotor, affective, cognitive and social. In this sense, self and self-specificity would occur prior to the recruitment of the other functions. Self-specificity would then always be present, making its involvement and manifestation in the various functions unavoidable. Rather than searching for self-specificity in relation to specific functions, such as language, one would need to look for more basic functions that must occur prior to sensorimotor, affective, or cognitive functions.

One could, for instance, imagine that the strong involvement of the self in language acquisition requires the recruitment of midline regions. Such involvement of midline structures may be implicitly presupposed in many of the tasks or paradigms described above when presenting self- and non-self-relevant words, known as trait adjectives. While the linguistic tasks themselves seem to involve the lateral cortical regions more, their degree of activity may nevertheless be dependent upon the midline regions and their high resting state activity. Hence, future studies should investigate the relationship between midline regions and the lateral networks implicated in language, which psychologically may correspond to the relationship between self and language.

13 Neurophilosphical Discussion: Self, Belief and Valuation

The chapter so far has focused mainly on the self itself and its nature and structure and how it is distinguished from self-reference. Self-reference concerns the operational-mechanistic process that supposedly constitutes the contents that we associate with our self. In contrast, I have left open the capacities of the self. One such capacity of the self is to belief and value. Valuation is a central component in our life. Normative judgment, moral attitudes, and ultimately many decisions we make in daily life rely and are based on valuation and belief. Psychologically, valuation is closely related to reward, namely to assign reward value to otherwise neutral or value-less stimuli, events, and persons.

Where, though, does the value come from? It may be closely related to the self that links and relates the seemingly neutral and valueless stimuli to itself and makes possible thereby the attribution of value to the stimuli. If so, one would expect a close relationship between self and reward, including their underlying neural correlates. Indeed, researchers have conducted imaging studies that directly compared self and reward. Subjects were presented with stimuli upon which they had either to gamble obtaining reward or to judge their degree of self-relatedness (de Greck et al. 2008).

What were the results? First, de Greck et al. (2008) analysed those regions related to the gambling, and thus the reward. This yielded activity in, as expected, the ventral tegmental area (VTA), the ventral striatum (VS), and the ventromedial prefrontal cortex (VMPFC); all well-known to typically mediate reward. In a second step, the neural activity changes in exactly these reward-related regions during the presentation of the same stimuli when they had to be judged with regard to their self-relatedness were investigated. Most interestingly, high self-related stimuli induced high activity in all three, VTA, VS, and VMPFC whereas those stimuli judged by the subjects as low self-related did not induce any activity change in these regions at all. These data illustrate the close relationship between reward and self-relatedness in that the former's regions, VTA, VS, and VMPFC, also mediate self-relatedness.

Are reward and self-relatedness identical? DeGreck et al. (2009, 2010) conducted the same paradigm in patients with alcohol and pathological gambling. These results showed normal reward-related activity in VTA, VS, and VMPFC whereas neither high nor low self-related stimuli induced activity changes. This suggests that self and reward, though being closely related, are not identical since otherwise they could not dissociate from each other in their neural activities in VTA, VS and VMPFC.

What do these data tell us about the relationship between self and valuation? One essential capacity of the self is to give and assign value to otherwise value-less stimuli, etc. Though preliminary, the data suggests that this capacity may be closely related to the reward system and its close relationship with self, the neural overlap between both in typical reward regions like VTA, VS, and VMPFC. However, neural overlap is not to be confused with the neural identity between reward and self, since empirical evidence does not support such a conclusion. Hence, the self seems to utilize reward-related regions, though apparently in a slightly different yet unclear way when compared to reward. This is compatible with the fact that self and valuation are not identical but closely related as we experience almost on a daily basis. Our self is more than just belief and valuation to which the neuroscientist may add that neurally, our self is more than just the reward system.

References

Burge T (2013) Cognition through understanding: self-knowledge, interlocution, reasoning, reflection: philosophical essays, vol 3. OUP, Oxford

Campbell J (2004) The first person, embodiment, and the certainty that one exists. Monist 87(4):475–488

Churchland PS (2002) Self-representation in nervous systems. Science 296(5566):308–310. doi:10.1126/science.1070564

Damasio AR (1999) How the brain creates the mind. Sci Am 281(6):112–117

Damasio A (2010) Self comes to mind: constructing the conscious mind. Pantheon, New York

de Greck M, Rotte M, Paus R, Moritz D, Thiemann R, Proesch U, Bruer U, Moerth S, Tempelmann C, Bogerts B, Northoff G (2008) Is our self based on reward? Self-relatedness recruits neural activity in the reward system. NeuroImage 39(4):2066–2075. doi:10.1016/j.neuroimage.2007.11.006

de Greck M, Supady A, Thiemann R, Tempelmann C, Bogerts B, Forschner L, Ploetz KV, Northoff G (2009) Decreased neural activity in reward circuitry during personal reference in abstinent alcoholics – a fMRI study. Hum Brain Mapp 30(5):1691–1704

de Greck M, Enzi B, Prosch U, Gantman A, Tempelmann C, Northoff G (2010) Decreased neuronal activity in reward circuitry of pathological gamblers during processing of personal relevant stimuli. Hum Brain Mapp 31(11):1802–1812

Gallagher II (2000) Philosophical conceptions of the self: implications for cognitive science. Trends Cogn Sci 4(1):14–21

Klein SB (2012) Self, memory, and the self-reference effect: an examination of conceptual and methodological issues. Personal Soc Psychol Rev 16(3):283–300. doi:10.1177/1088868311434214

Klein SB, Gangi CE (2010) The multiplicity of self: neuropsychological evidence and its implications for the self as a construct in psychological research. Ann N Y Acad Sci 1191:–15. doi:10.1111/j.1749-6632.2010.05441.x

Metzinger T (2004) Being no one: the self-model theory of subjectivity. MIT Press, Cambridge

Nakao T, Ohira H, Northoff G (2012) Distinction between externally vs. internally guided decision-making: operational differences, meta-analytical comparisons and their theoretical implications. Front Neurosci 6:31. doi:10.3389/fnins.2012.00031

Northoff G (2012) Immanuel Kant's mind and the brain's resting state. Trends Cogn Sci 16(7):356–359. doi:10.1016/j.tics.2012.06.001

Northoff G, Heinzel A, de Greck M, Bermpohl F, Dobrowolny H, Panksepp J (2006) Self-referential processing in our brain – a meta-analysis of imaging studies on the self. NeuroImage 31(1):440–457

Peacocke C (2014) The mirror of the world: subjects, consciousness, and self-consciousness. OUP, Oxford

Pfeiffer UJ, Timmermans B, Vogeley K, Frith CD, Schilbach L (2013) Towards a neuroscience of social interaction. Front Hum Neurosci 7:22. doi:10.3389/fnhum.2013.00022

Schilbach L, Bzdok D, Timmermans B, Fox PT, Laird AR, Vogeley K, Eickhoff SB (2012) Introspective minds: using ALE meta-analyses to study commonalities in the neural correlates of emotional processing, social & unconstrained cognition. PLoS One 7(2):e30920. doi:10.1371/journal.pone.0030920

Schilbach L, Eickhoff SB, Schultze T, Mojzisch A, Vogeley K (2013) To you I am listening: perceived competence of advisors influences judgment and decision-making via recruitment of the amygdala. Soc Neurosci 8(3):189–202. doi:10.1080/17470919.2013.775967

Sugiura M, Seitz RF, Angel HF (2015) Models and neural bases of the believing process. Behav Brain Sci 5(1):12–23. doi:10.4236/jbbs.2015.51002

Velleman J (2006) So it goes. Stud Soc Justice:1–23

Zahavi D (2005) Subjectivity and selfhood: investigating the first-person perspective. MIT press, Cambridge

Creditions and Self-Identity: Embodiment Between Actions and (Life) Decisions

Ivan Colagè and Nicola Gobbi

Abstract In this chapter, we will draw some connections between the theory of creditions and other recent neuroscientific and philosophical topics. In particular, we will focus on those developments that lend insights into the issue of self-identity and consciousness. We will not only show how the theory of creditions is interestingly connected with other scientific and philosophical research lines, but we will provide insights about future research perspectives that may profit from such connections. We will begin with a brief summary and review of key aspects of the theory of credition. Then, we will suggest how recent developments in the neuroscience of voluntary actions may tell something interesting about the issue of beliefs. Subsequently, also with the help of some philosophical insights, we will expand from the issue of "actions and beliefs" to that of "beliefs and self-identity". Here, we will suggest that self-identity is strictly linked to a person's system of beliefs, and that, in turn, the system of beliefs depends on the experiences and life-story of the person, according to an embodied perspective. Finally, in the conclusion, we will briefly mention some explicit connection of what we will address in the following with religion.

1 Introduction

In this paper, we will draw some connections between the theory of creditions and other recent neuroscientific and philosophical topics. In particular, we will focus on those developments that lend insights into the issue of self-identity. Cognitive neuroscience is now providing insightful evidence as to the brain regions more active during self-related processes (i.e. those processes that require more or less explicit reference to the subject's own state, personal experience and life-trajectory) or

---

I. Colagè (✉)
Pontifical University Antonianum, Rome, Italy
e-mail: i.colage@antonianum.eu

N. Gobbi
Pontifical Gregorian University, Rome, Italy
e-mail: nicolagobbi@virgilio.it

H.-F. Angel et al. (eds.), *Processes of Believing: The Acquisition, Maintenance, and Change in Creditions*, New Approaches to the Scientific Study of Religion 1,
DOI 10.1007/978-3-319-50924-2_18

consciousness. Moreover, in recent years, philosophy has enquired into the topic of self-identity also in the light of new scientific findings and perspectives. This is relevant also from the methodological viewpoint, as it testifies that topics as complex as the self require a wide interdisciplinary approach, i.e. an approach that involves not only adjacent scientific disciplines but also more distant fields (up to the rich philosophical, and even theological, traditions).

The theory of creditions represents, in our view, a valuable occasion to practice such an interdisciplinary approach. We will not only show how the theory of creditions is interestingly connected with other scientific and philosophical research lines, but we will provide insights about future research perspectives that may profit from such connections.

We will begin with a brief summary and review of key aspects of the theory of credition. Then, we will suggest how recent developments in the neuroscience of voluntary actions may tell something interesting about the issue of beliefs. Subsequently, also with the help of some philosophical insights, we will expand from the issue of "actions and beliefs" to that of "beliefs and self-identity". Here, we will suggest that self-identity is strictly linked to a person's system of beliefs, and that in turn the system of beliefs depends on the experiences and life-story of the person, according to an embodied perspective. Finally, in the conclusion, we will briefly mention some explicit connection of what we will address in the following with religion.

2 Elements of a Credition Theory

The term "credition" points to the process of believing, and has been introduced as analogous with the terms "emotion" and "cognition", as the belief-related counterpart of affect-related and knowledge-related mental processes (Angel 2006, 2013). The process character of believing should therefore be contrasted with a static, mental-construct view of beliefs (Sugiura et al. 2015). Creditions are certainly related to religion and religious faith. However, credition theory tends to incorporate religious as well as secular beliefs, and we will see that the theory is proposed as a rather general way for understanding the process of believing in connection with several other psychological and neuro-cognitive topics.

At the conceptual level, two other aspects of credition theory should be mentioned. The first one concerns the basic, postulated elements: "babs" and "blobs". These may be conceived as the nodes of a network (or of a "bab/blob-configuration") that constitute a belief or, more precisely, a credition. Any internal or external perception, even "vague or doubtful", may count as a bab. Blobs would be "non-conscious babs", and are subliminal in kind though effective in bab/blob-configurations.

The second aspect has to do with the four functions defined by the theory and that act on bab/blob-configurations: enclosure function, converter function, stabilizer function, and modulator function (See also Angel's contribution in this volume). The enclosure function assembles or enriches a bab/blob-configuration by clustering and framing together several babs/blobs. The converter function translates a bab/blob-configuration into a course of action that is consistent with the belief (credition) represented in the configuration. The stabilizer function tends to maintain and preserve a given configuration against abrupt fluctuation in the current situation or in the (emotional) state of the subject; it transforms unstable bab/blob-configurations in stable attitudes and mindsets. The modulator function "highlights in a specific way the differences of individuals and the differences of situations" (Angel 2013: 538), and may influence the working of the other three functions.

It is relevant that babs and blobs may be connected with a variety of cognitive processes, such as perception, memory, action control, emotion, empathy and the self-concept. Therefore, in their being networks or configurations of babs/blobs, creditions allow for understanding the integration of the disparate elements involved in the process of belief formation, change, and effectiveness upon human choices and behaviour.

More recent work in credition theory (Seitz and Angel 2012; Sugiura et al. 2015) has tried to propose initial insights into the neural bases of the process of believing. Seitz and Angel (2012) performed a meta-analysis of eleven studies addressing religious or secular beliefs. The analysis unveiled that the process of believing involves a widespread network of brain areas encompassing the medial and lateral frontal cortex, the precuneus, the temporo-parietal junction, the cingulate and the cerebellum. The authors highlighted that the medial frontal cortex may play a key role, especially as far as the integration of emotion-based and cognition-based perspective-taking is involved in the process of believing.

Following these preliminary results, the authors (Sugiura et al. 2015) also proposed a comprehensive model proposing that specific brain areas might be particularly responsible for the four functions of creditions. In this model, the medial frontal cortex is still regarded as a key hub integrating perception-related information mainly represented in posterior cortices, action-related information mainly coming from frontal regions, and emotion/value-related information in the (para-) limbic system. Due to its integrative role, the medial frontal cortex is the best candidate to be the substrate for the enclosure function (i.e. the functions that generates bab/blob-configurations and thus beliefs). Indeed, in the framework of credition theory, the representation of beliefs must recruit elements of perception, action, and emotion/value, which is exactly the kind of information that medial frontal cortex integrates. Moreover, as the medial frontal cortex displays motor aspects and is strongly connected with motor and pre-motor cortices, it is also a good candidate for the converter function (i.e. the function that translates a belief into an action or action plan). Finally, as it integrates emotion- and value-related information, the medial frontal cortex may also represent the brain substrate for the modulator function (which is the function that adjusts, so to speak, the process of believing to the actual bodily, emotional and situational states of the subject).

The model by Sugiura, Seitz and Angel (Sugiura et al. 2015) also attributes a role to the dorsolateral prefrontal cortex: this brain region seems to be crucially involved in the belief evaluation process and may thus underpin the stabilizer function, that is, the function that tends to maintain beliefs against the fluctuations induced by the changing environment and experience of the subject. It is worth stressing that the stabilizer function "brings creditions into touch with attitudes and mind-sets" (Angel 2013: 538); we will see the relevance of this in a following section.

With this brief sketch of some relevant features of credition theory in mind, we can now see how this theory is fruitfully and prospectively linked to other recent philosophical and neuro-scientific tenets.

3 From Actions to Beliefs

The first features of credition theory which we would like to focus on are its process character, and its understanding of the process of believing in a way that integrates cognition, action and emotion/value (the authors speak of the "perception-action-value triad" – Sugiura et al. 2015; see also Seitz et al. 2009).

To begin with, the process character of credition theory finds an interesting analogy with key elements of C. S. Peirce's philosophy (see, e.g., Peirce 1878a, b, 1903, 1905; see also Colagè 2010, 2013, 2014). In Peirce's opinion, any process of research starts with a doubt (i.e. something that surprises us and to which we do not know how to respond) and finds a provisional end in the establishment of a belief (i.e. in finding out an opinion or conviction that solves the original doubt). Moreover, on the background of his overall philosophy, it is clear that the process from doubts to the establishment of beliefs is a highly dynamic one, essentially characterizing the whole "cognitive" life of individuals (indeed, the examples he cites span from simple, daily-life choices to scientific or moral issues). Peirce's philosophy is relevant to another aspect as well: the link between beliefs and actions. The fundamental proposition of his pragmatism recites: "a conception, that is, the rational purport of a word or other expression, lies exclusively in its conceivable bearing upon the conduct of life" (Peirce 1905: 162). Such a statement, if understood within Peirce's overall thought, strongly links the cognitive aspect of the believing process with actual and concrete actions. This is in line with the idea implicated by credition theory that the selection of beliefs is equivalent to the selection of actions and that beliefs, life-conduct and personal valuation processes are strictly interconnected (Seitz and Angel 2014; Sugiura et al. 2015).

In the last decades, research in cognitive neuroscience has unveiled several aspects of the action-related brain processes. Interestingly, this research discovered that the motor cortex performs complex cognitive processes and its role is not limited to execute commands coming from elsewhere in the brain. The discovery of the mirror neurons in the macaque brain (Rizzolatti et al. 1996a; Gallese et al. 1996), and of a mirror system in the human brain (Rizzolatti et al. 1996b), certainly represents a notable instance of these advancements. Here, we will focus on the perspective undertaken by Marc Jeannerod (2001, 2006, 2009), as it shows how the domain of actions is tightly related to the issues of beliefs and of self-identity.

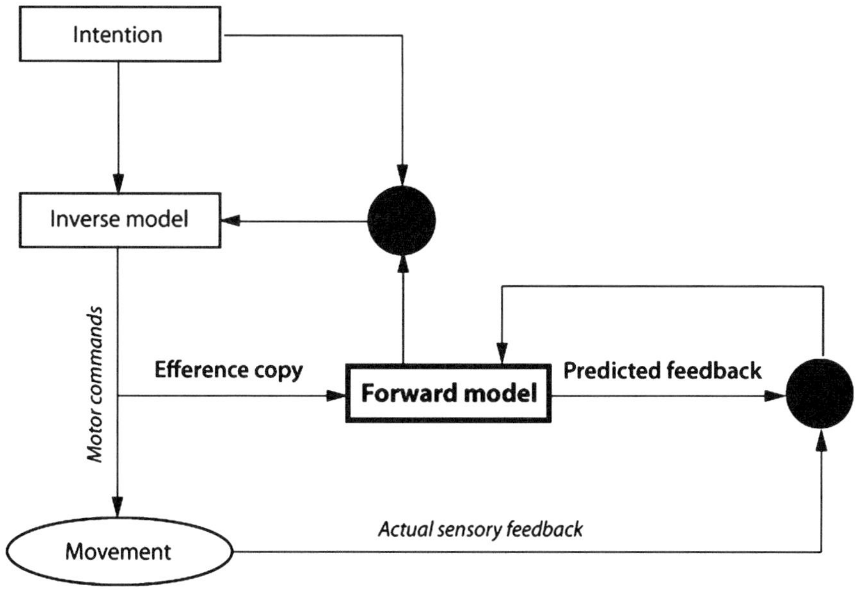

Fig. 1 Graphical representation of the internal forward model. The motor commands are also used to produce an efferent copy of the action. The forward model predicts the sensory feedback of the movements on the basis of the efferent copy. Then, the predicted feedback are compared with the actual sensory feedback. The possible mismatch between actual and predicted feedback is then used to correct the motor strategy (Adapted from Jeannerod 2006: 21)

The core of Jeannerod's theory of "motor cognition" may be found in the notion of "internal forward model" for action control (Fig. 1 – Jeannerod 2006: 20–21; see also Wolpert et al. 1995; Wolpert and Ghahramani 2000). The point is that the brain motor system not only produces motor commands (which eventually determine muscle contraction and actual movements of the limbs or other biological effectors), but also a so-called "efference copy" of such commands. The efference copy is used by the motor system to produce an internal forward model of the planned (and/or ongoing) action. The internal forward model has the key role of predicting the sensory feedbacks that the actual execution of the action will produce at the visual, proprioceptive and kinesthetic levels (see Fig. 1). Such predictions are then compared with the actual feedback inputs. Therefore, thanks to the internal forward model, the correct unfolding of an action can be constantly monitored, and it can also be corrected on-line if the actual feedback of the ongoing action deviate from the feedback predicted by the internal forward model. It is important to note that all this happens at the implicit, automatic and unconscious level, so that the acting subject is unaware both of the ongoing motor details and of the possible corrections triggered by the mismatch between the actual and the predicted feedback.

However (and this is a fundamental point for what follows), the mismatch between actual and predicted feedback may also trigger a "*prise de conscience*" (cf. Jeannerod 2006: 54) of the ongoing action. Experimental and clinical observations show that this happens when the mismatch between the actual and the predicted feedback increases and exceeds a certain threshold (Fourneret and Jeannerod 1998; Fourneret et al. 2002; Slachewsky et al. 2001; Knoblich and Kircher 2004; see also Jeannerod 2006: 45–58). When this happens, the subject engages consciously in the reconsideration and revision of the (motor) strategy deployed for reaching the action's goal. This amounts to say that, when the mismatch increases, the needed corrections cannot be performed in a totally automatic and implicit way, but require the contribution of more explicit and reflective processes. In other words, "as a consequence of the mismatch between the desired motor output and its observed results, the action is de-automatized, delayed, and will continue under conscious control" (Jeannerod 2013: 107).

Now, the reconsideration of strategies and the conscious control of actions imply at least three things: a) the awareness of the goal of the action, b) the awareness of the intention to act, and c) the selection of alternative action-segments. At this point, it is important to note that the main brain region that seemingly underlies the processing of the mismatch between actual and predicted outcomes is the posterior parietal lobe, specifically including Brodmann areas 7 and 40 (cf. Jeanerod 2006: 15, 55 and 83–85; Fink et al. 1999). Processing of the mismatch in this areas is also crucial for self-attributing one's actions to oneself (a point whose relevance will appear below). Moreover, there is evidence of the involvement of the dorsolateral prefrontal cortex (Brodmann area 46) in conscious perception of intentions, selection and choice of appropriate actions, and suppression of inappropriate actions (Jeannerod 2006: 39–40, 62 and 66–69; see also Spence and Frith 1999). The relevance of these neuro-anatomical details will become clear below. By now, let us stress two points. First, the importance of a parietofrontal network for conscious elaboration of new (cognitive) strategies has been emphasized by another research line explicitly concerned with the issue of consciousness and "conscious access", i.e. the transition from implicit and unconscious processing of information to conscious processing characterized by the reportability of one's own "internal world" (Dehaene et al. 1998; Dehaene and Changeux 2011). This approach (which integrates computational models and neuro-imaging data) suggests that when new strategies have to be searched for, excogitated and deployed, an intense activation of dorsolateral prefrontal and posterior parietal cortices occurs (Changeux and Dehaene 2008, especially p. 747; see also Frith et al. 1999). Second, as we have seen above, both posterior parietal cortices (specifically the medial portion of Brodmann area 7 – the so-called precuneus) and the dorsolateral prefrontal cortex are key regions for the process of believing, and thus for credition theory.

According to Jeannerod's approach, the framework outlined thus far implies that the role of conscious will cannot be that of causing actions and movements (Jeannerod 2006: 63–64; Jeannerod 2009: 244 and 250; Jeannerod 2013: 103–104, 107 and 110). Indeed, we have seen that consciousness appears after the action has already begun and is connected with the processing of the results of the action. This position is obviously against the subjective and intuitive experience that our conscious events are the causes of our actions, and thus prompts the question about the role of volition and conscious will.

The actions addressed in the experimental studies mentioned throughout this section, the ones to which the internal forward model can be immediately applied (like pressing a button, moving a finger, reaching and grasping a rod, and pronouncing a syllable or word), are very simple actions, lasting short amounts of time, and having an immediately present and accessible goal. Obviously, human behaviour consists of actions that are much more complex, with distant and absent goals, and extended timeframes. To grasp the distinction between these two kinds of actions, Jeannerod resorts to the distinction between prior intentions and intentions-in-action (or "motor intentions", in Jeannerod's vocabulary) drawn by John Searle (Searle 1983; see also Jeannerod 2006: 1–4). Prior intentions are about complex courses of actions and are formed consciously and voluntarily. In some cases, the very formation of the prior intention (i.e. the process of deliberation and choice) requires extended time and intensive reflection: think to such life-choices like becoming a marathon runner, an academician, or a priest. Once such a prior intention has been formed, an entire and hierarchically structured course of actions must be unrolled, each action having its own specific proximate goal and motor intention.

Jeannerod's approach proposes a model according to which the degree of awareness during the enacting of such complex actions changes in time (see Fig. 2). Specifically, consciousness is high when the prior intention is elaborated and fixed, decreases during the actual execution of the concrete action segments, and increases again when the results of the action segments have to be evaluated in view of the prior intention framing the simple and concrete action segments (Jeannerod 2009, Chapter 10; Jeannerod 2013). This model implies: 1) that consciousness has no causal role in the execution of the single action segments, and 2) that the sense of being the cause of the action sequences is just an inference (with internal, subjective import) from the comparison between the results of the actual action segments and the elements of the prior intention. The prior intention and the recognition of the actual results of the action are the only conscious elements of the whole process (the former preceding, and the latter following, the action realization). Therefore, "conscious knowledge about willing an action should essentially be a post-hoc phenomenon" (Jeannerod 2013: 109), and cannot be considered as the (direct) cause of actions. Nonetheless, Jeannerod's approach attributes an important role to consciousness (although, to repeat, not that of motorically causing actions). In a word, it might be said that the role of consciousness is that of building up a "narrative self" (Gallegher 2000). The notion of narrative self has to do with the temporal continuity of the subject who identifies itself as the author of its own actions; this process of self-recognition and self-attribution relies upon the comparison between the intention elaborated prior to the action and the evaluation of the eventual results of the actions.

Jeannerod describes the dynamics of this process in analogy with the internal forward model presented above (see Fig. 3). Now, in the forward model for simple actions regulated by motor intentions (depicted in Fig. 1 above), the mismatch between actual and predicted feedback determines an automatic correction of the motor strategy and, in some cases, the ignition of conscious processes to revise the

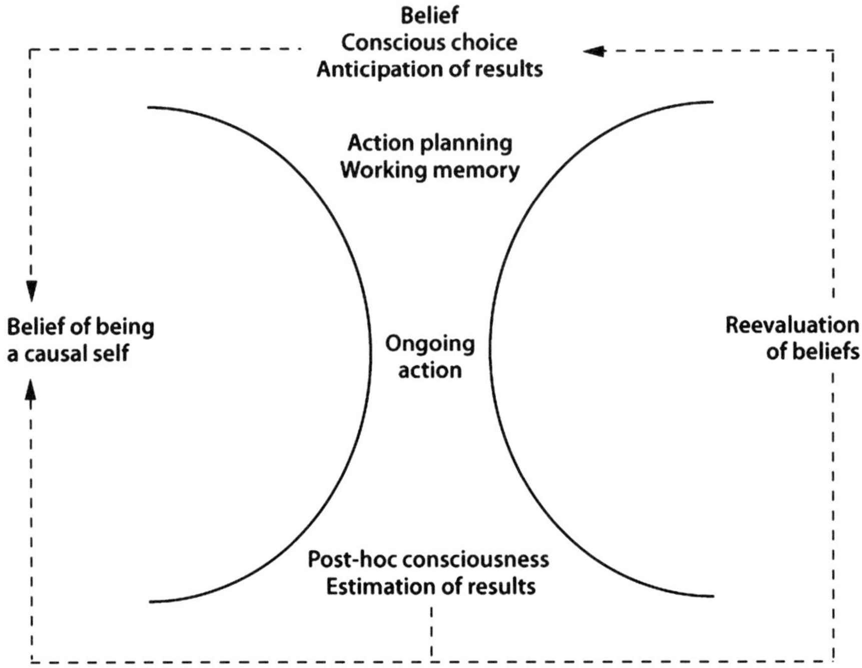

Fig. 2 Schematic representation of the cycle of consciousness along action development. Curved lines represent consciousness: when the distance between them is larger consciousness is higher. Before the action, consciousness may by high (e.g. in elaborating prior intentions). During the action execution, the level of consciousness falls. After the action, the results are evaluated consciously (Adapted from Jeannerod 2009: 254)

motor strategy. On the contrary, at the level of complex, long-term and voluntary actions (where prior intentions come in), the mismatch between the general result (explicitly) anticipated in the prior intention at an abstract/conceptual level and the actual results of a concrete course of action (meant to achieve the general goal) determines not only a motor revision, but also a revision of beliefs (Figs. 2 and 3), and thus some modifications in the subject's "system of beliefs" from which prior intentions are built up (Jeannerod 2009: 163–166; Jeannerod 2013: 110–112).

In this section we have reached the level of beliefs starting from simple, unconscious actions (and this may already anticipate the relevance of all this for the theory of credition). At this point in our discussion, we have acknowledged a post-hoc role for consciousness. However, note that this role is crucial for linking consciousness to self-identity (as stressed by the notion of narrative self). In the next section, we will see how the issue of the "system of beliefs" and that of self-identity may come in very close contact. This will also allow us to retrieve a genuinely causal role of consciousness for our actions and behaviours. The relevant point is that this will be made possible by some elements and implications of the theory of creditions.

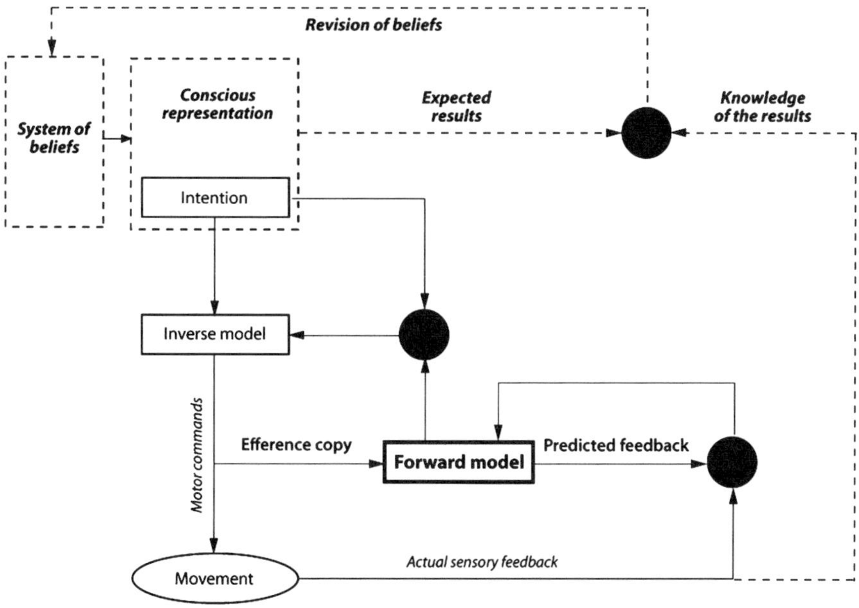

Fig. 3 The implicit internal forward model (solid lines) represented within the larger conscious process (dashed lines). The conscious appraisal of the results of the action may trigger a revision of the beliefs that affected the conscious representation of the action, which in turn generated the intention triggering the internal forward model (Adapted from Jeannerod 2009: 265)

3.1 Beliefs and Self-Identity

Let us begin by noting a fundamental tension within Jeannerod's approach to motor cognition and consciousness. On the one hand, he repeatedly stresses that the manifestation of consciousness is essentially post-hoc (as it relates to what follows actions) and cannot be the direct cause for the initiation of our actions and behaviour. On the other hand, he states that processing at the conscious level may induce revision of belief and modification of the subject's system of beliefs. If one looks at Fig. 3 (which is redrawn after Jeannerod 2009: 265; Jeannerod 2013: 111), it appears clearly that the system of beliefs affects the conscious representation of actions and the formation of intentions (from which actual actions eventually stem). Regarded from this viewpoint, it seems plausible to acknowledge an effective causal role of conscious processes for actions. How can we reconcile these two sides of the approach?

Looking at a single action-segment, the array of empirical evidence gathered in the lab indeed speaks against a causal role of conscious processes for the initiation and management of ongoing actions. This also follows from the path-breaking results by Benjamin Libet (Libet et al. 1983; Libet 1985; Libet 2011; Haggard et al. 2002; Wegner 2002), which are extensively quoted by Jeannerod. However, if we look at more realistic situations (clearly less amenable to experimental enquiry), our behaviour is composed of cycles of actions (both simple actions segments and more complex processes regulated by prior intentions). From this point of view, the conscious processes following a certain action may well influence, in a truly causal although not direct manner, the course of future actions.

In other words, we are here proposing that the cognitive re-arrangement stemming from the conscious processes that follow an action or an entire course of actions actually set the foundation upon which future actions will be planned and executed. This background is also the one against which future actions will be controlled and their results evaluated. It is here that the issue of beliefs and the issue of self-identity significantly merge. Self-identity is the narrative continuity of the subject's awareness of being the author of past actions and of the coherence of his/her life-story, with the array of actions and experiences, choices and decisions, changes of mind, blame or appreciation for his/her own conduct, etc. Therefore, the system of beliefs is both the root of narrative self-identity and its outcome. If we take a genuinely dynamic and diachronic stance, at each moment of our life our system of beliefs is both the fruit of our past experience and the starting-point for our future conduct. Obviously, this system is never completely and entirely conscious, nor one's entire narrative identity always conscious; only specific portions of our system of beliefs and self-narrative have access to consciousness, depending on what engages us from time to time – being it the evaluation of the results of our actions or the elaboration of decisions and action plans (see Fig. 2). The key point here is that the conscious processing (both the one the precedes and plans actions and the one that follows and evaluates the outcomes) *must leave neural traces in our brains*, and such traces affect the entire process; both the conscious, explicit and reflective part and the unconscious, implicit and automatic one. According to this systemic standpoint, it is easy to acknowledge a causal, although indirect, role of consciousness upon action, behaviour and conduct; consciousness affects future behaviour by modifying (or strengthening) elements of the neural network underlying the subject's system of beliefs, upon which one's self-identity is rooted. This follows from a rather embodied perspective of all these topics, which directly connects consciousness to one's system of beliefs and self-identity, and indirectly to one's future action precisely via his/her system of beliefs.

We may offer a two-step argument in support of our proposal. The first one follows from an attempt to integrate three influential research lines in recent cognitive neuroscience that explicitly deal with the issues of consciousness, narrative self and self-identity (see Auletta and Colagè 2013a for a first move in this direction). The second step explicitly deals with the theory of credition and its linkages with all what we have seen so far and what we will see now.

Let us develop the first step of our argument. We have mentioned that the model for access to consciousness developed by Changeux and Dehaene postulates that conscious processing in a distributed parietofrontal network is ignited in effortful cognitive tasks when a novel solution to a problem must be searched, elaborated and chosen. The model also states that once a new and appropriate solution has been found, the activation of the conscious network decreases and the new solution is applied automatically (Changeux and Dehaene 2008). This is a way to understand our proposal that conscious processing is able to affect behaviour even when no actual conscious processing is going on.

Moreover, at the anatomical level, the parietal activation in the conscious search for a new solution (see Figure 8 in Changeux and Dehaene 2008) largely coincides with what Antonio Damasio calls the postero-medial cortices (PMC), encompassing Brodman areas 7, 23, 29, 30 and 31 (Parvizi et al. 2006; see also Auletta and Colagè 2013b). The PMC seems to be a key region for consciousness and self-identity. Indeed, Alzheimer's disease mainly affects the PMC, and lesions in these regions cause states similar to those of patients with advanced Alzheimer's disease. In addition, anaesthesia (i.e. lack of consciousness) determines a remarkable reduction of blood flow in the PMC. The PMC is also one of the regions where patients in a vegetative state display diminished metabolism, and these very same regions are among the first to regain activity in those patients recovering from a vegetative state. It should also be noted that the PMC has strong and often bi-directional connectivity with a large amount of cortical and sub-cortical areas, thus being able to gather and process information coming from the rest of the brain, the body, and the environment. On the basis of these data, Damasio proposed that the PMC could be one of the main brain structures underlying what he calls the "autobiographical self", which means something quite close to the narrative self mentioned above.

The PMC is also a key hub in what has become known as the default or resting-state brain network (Raichle et al. 2001). The default network is a set of brain areas that show sustained activation in resting-state, i.e. when a subject lies calmly awake but without being involved in any goal-directed task. The areas composing the default network are those in the medial surface of the brain, especially the medial prefrontal cortex, the posterior cingulate and the precuneus along with other medial parietal cortices. These areas have been identified as task-negative regions, i.e. regions that decrease their activity when the subject engages in externally directed tasks and are more active in the resting state. The functional significance of the default network has not yet been conclusively established. However, key indications come from the behaviour of the medial prefrontal cortex, specifically Brodmann areas 8, 9, and 10 (Gusnard and Raichle 2001). These regions are part of the default network; indeed they display decreased activation when the subject engages in externally directed tasks and increased activity in the resting state. The interesting point is that the very same regions further increase their activation when the subject is engaged in self-related processes, i.e. processes where the attention is turned towards oneself (see also Gusnard et al. 2001; McGuire et al. 1996). The activity of the medial prefrontal cortex therefore seems involved in explicit representations of the states of the self, and may be attenuated by goal-directed behaviour only if the latter are non-self-referential (see also Frith and Frith 1999). By extrapolation, one of the main functions of the entire default network might be that of sustaining "the continuity of a stable, unified perspective of the organism relative to its environment (a 'self')" (Gusnard and Raichle 2001: 692). This suggestion receives further support form what we have seen just above about the PMC.

Let us now turn to the second step of our argument. We should note that, according to what we have seen so far, there seems to be significant overlapping between brain regions involved in action-control and choice, consciousness, self-related processes, and the default network. In particular:

(A) The parietal cortices, and especially Brodmann area 7, seem involved (i) in processing the mismatch between actual and predicted feedback of actions, (ii) in the parietofrontal network active in conscious access and excogitation, (iii) in the autobiographical self underpinned by PMC, as well as (iv) in the default network (and its probable self-related function);
(B) The dorsolateral prefrontal cortex (Brodmann area 46) appears to be involved (i) in conscious perception of intentions, (ii) in choice of appropriate actions and suppression of inappropriate actions, as well as (iii) in conscious elaboration of new strategies.
(C) The medial frontal cortex (Brodmann areas 8, 9, 10) seems implicated (i) in self-referential processes and (ii) in the default network.

As we have seen at the beginning of the paper, the precuneus (Brodmann area 7), the dorsolateral prefrontal cortex, and the medial frontal cortex are among the regions found to be involved in the believing process (Seitz and Angel 2012). Specifically, according to the credition model (Sugiura et al. 2015), the parietal cortex is implicated in the representation of beliefs, the dorsolateral prefrontal cortex serves belief evaluation processes (the stabilizer function in the theory of credition), and the medial frontal cortex is responsible for integration of perception-related, action-related, and emotion/value-related information (the enclosure function).

This is an important observation, not only because it brings together action, belief, consciousness and self-identity, but also because of some relevant aspects of the theory of credition. The enclosure function forms bab/blob-configurations (i.e. creditions). As babs are conscious and blobs are not, the enclosure function may work both at the subliminal level and at the supraliminal one; however, once the bab/blob configuration has been formed or modified by the enclosure function, its structure should be taken as affecting the process both at the conscious and at the unconscious level (this follows form the assumption that the modification leaves an embodied neural trace). The converter function manages the passage from the bab/blob-configuration to actions. Again, this may happen at the subliminal or supraliminal level. The action may give results in agreement with the predictions or not (note that also this may concern the automatic, implicit level or the reflective, explicit one as well). If there is not agreement, a process of correcting the strategy begins and modifies the course of action. When this happens at the implicit level, this may result in automatic refinement of the bab/blob-configuration (most likely the changes would concern the unconscious part: the blobs). When the correction reaches the explicit level, then a modification of the system of beliefs occurs (and this likely affects the conscious level of babs). If there is agreement between the expectations and the obtained outcomes, the bab/blob-configuration is evaluated positively (note that it is the entire configuration – both conscious babs and unconscious blobs – to be evaluated). This would be the role of the stabilizer function.

"Creditions theorists" have often stressed the connection of the stabilizer function with the issue of attitudes and mindsets. Angel's contribution to this volume insists on this point to emphasize the process character of creditions (i.e., the process of believing). We think that the notion of attitude is crucial to understanding the causal role of consciousness for our actions, behaviour and conduct. According to what we have seen so far throughout this chapter, establishment of attitudes is affected by conscious processing. In turn, attitudes affect future behaviour. We think that this point is elegantly stressed by Seitz's contribution to this volume, where he speaks of the role of beliefs in decision-making and to cope with the future. One could easily agree that the system of beliefs, attitudes and mindsets are central elements in one's own self-identity. Regarded from this standpoint, therefore, self-identity is not just a matter of building up a coherent narrative of our past experiences; it is also, and perhaps mainly, a matter of our future conduct.

4 Conclusion: Credition Theory and Its Promise

We have tried to suggest that the theory of credition may indeed be helpful in prompting a comprehensive model for integrating several research lines in contemporary neuroscience, especially those related to the difficult problems about the real complexity of the human life-form, which is de facto concerned with issues like consciousness and self-identity, and with a level of enquiry extremely difficult to be comprehensively addressed within the laboratory. Of course, empirical data remain indispensable, but addressing these issues seems to necessarily require fine work even at the theoretical and interdisciplinary level.

In concluding this chapter, we would like to mention a topic related to the religious dimension. What we have seen so far is not directly conceived of for religious beliefs; the theory of creditions, as well, is not restricted to religion and has a more general scope. However, religion is an important field to which the theory of creditions is intended to apply.

Religion is intrinsically social; myths and rites (which are essential elements of any religion) require a living social dimension. The social dimension is explicitly taken into consideration by the theory of creditions since the system of beliefs, as well as narrative self-identity, has undeniable social connotations. We suggest the idea that religious narratives imply social interactions where each participant has a role related to his/her own self-narrative, which, in turn, rests upon his/her system of beliefs. Religious narratives, then, are sustained by underlying personal systems of beliefs, reflected in personal narratives. Moreover, it is to be taken into account that religious narratives are "ergo-logical" (i.e. related to and aimed at concrete actions), and tend to prompt the integration of physical and social-cultural dimensions of human life (Durkheim 1915; Turner 1986). Now, in our view, sacred religious narrations (such as, e.g., the Last Supper narrative) affect action production twofold. First, they can affect common actions, and this is evident when sacred narratives are re-enacted during collective ritual actions (as in the taking of the

Eucharist in the Roman Catholic tradition). Second, they can contribute to the construction of one's system of beliefs and individual self-narratives and, consequently, have an impact on one's attitudes, mindsets and future conduct – consider, for example, the immense moral implications of the acknowledgment of Jesus' sacrifice for humanity (Gobbi and Bonaccorso 2015). We think that the way in which this happens has substantial analogies with the process of modifying and stabilizing our creditions, attitudes, systems of belief and, eventually, our self-identity.

Acknowledgments Many thanks to the Editors of this volume for their propulsive and patient work in assembling the chapters. Special thanks to Prof. Hans-Ferdinand Angel for organizing beautiful meetings in Graz (Austria): this work has profited significantly from these events. The research presented here has been in part supported by a now-closed grant from the John Templeton Foundation; the opinions expressed here are those of the authors and do not necessarily reflect those of the Foundation.

References

Angel HF (2006) Religiosität als menschliches Potential. Ein anthropologisches Modell im neurowissenschaftlichen Horizont. In: Angel HF, Broking-Bortfeldt M, Hemel U, Kunstmann J, Jakobs M, Pirner ML, Rothgangel M (eds) Religiosität. Kohlhammer, Stuttgart, pp 62–89

Angel HF (2013) Credition, the process of belief. In: Runehov ALC, Oviedo L (eds) Encyclopedia of sciences and religions. Springer, Dordrecht, pp 536–539

Auletta G, Colagè I (2013a) Consciousness and the global neural workspace hypothesis: from bottom-up to top-doan causation and vice versa. In: Auletta A, Colagè I, Jeannerod M (eds) Brains top down: is top-down causation challenging neuroscience? World Scientific, Singapore, pp 235–272

Auletta G, Colagè I (2013b) The neural basis of consciousness and the issue of downward causation. Notes by Gennaro Auletta and Ivan Colagè on Antonio Damasio's contribution. In: Auletta A, Colagè I, Jeannerod M (eds) Brains top down: is top-down causation challenging neuroscience? World Scientific, Singapore, pp 89–101

Changeux JP, Dehaene S (2008) The neuronal workspace model: conscious processing and learning. In: Menzel R (ed) Learning theory and behavior, Learning and memory: a comprehensive reference, vol 1. Elsevier, Oxford, pp 729–758

Colagè I (2010) Interazione e inferenza. Epistemologia scientifica ispirata al pensiero di Ch. S. Peirce. Gregorian & Biblical Press, Rome

Colagè I (2013) Le scienze naturali e la filosofia della natura: alcune riflessioni epistemologiche. In: Auletta G, Pons JS (eds) Si può parlare oggi di una finalità dell'evoluzione? Gregorian & Biblical Press, Rome, pp 59–79

Colagè I (2014) Prospective Fruitfulness as a criterion for theory-change and research-strategy option. Comprendre, revista catalana de filosofia 16(1):61–86

Dehaene S, Changeux JP (2011) Experimental and theoretical approaches to conscious processing. Neuron 70:200–227

Dehaene S, Kerszberg M, Changeux JP (1998) A neuronal model of a global workspace in effortful cognitive tasks. Proc Natl Acad Sci USA 95:14529–14553

Durkheim É (1915) The elementary forms of the religious life. George Allen & Unwin Ltd, London

Fink GR, Marshall JC, Halligan PW, Frith CD, Driver J, Frackowwiack RSJ, Dolan RJ (1999) The neural consequences of conflict between intention and the senses. Brain 122:497–512

Fourneret P, Jaennerod M (1998) Limited conscious monitoring of motor performance in normal subjects. Neuropsychologia 36:1133–1140

Fourneret P, Paillard J, Lamarre Y, Cole J, Jeannerod m (2002) Lack of conscious recognition of one's own actions in haptically deafferented patiens. Neuroreport 13:541–547
Frith CD, Frith U (1999) Interacting minds – a biological basis. Science 286:1692–1695
Frith CD, Perry R, Lumer E (1999) The neural correlates of conscious experience:an experimental framework. Trends Cogn Sci 3:105–114
Gallagher S (2000) Philosophical conceptions of the self: implications for cognitive sciences. Trends Cogn Sci 4:14–21
Gallese V, Fadiga L, Fogassi L, Rizzolatti G (1996) Action recognition in the premotor cortex. Brain 119:593–609
Gobbi N, Bonaccorso G (2015) Action and narrativeness: a serlian account for individual and social-religious identity. To be published in Antonianum periodicum trimester (December 2015)
Gusnard DA, Raichle ME (2001) Searching for a baseline: functional imaging and the resting human state. Nat Rev Neurosci 2:685–694
Gusnard DA, Akbudak E, Shulman GL, Raichle ME (2001) Medial prefrontal cortex and self-referential mental activity: relation to a default mode of brain function. Proc Natl Acad Sci U S A 98:4259–4264
Haggard P, Clark S, Kalogeras J (2002) Voluntary action and conscious awareness. Nat Neurosci 5:282–285
Koblich G, Kircher TTJ (2004) Deceiving oneself about being in control: conscious detection of changing in visuomotor coupling. J Exp Psychol Hum Percept Perform 30:467–472
Jeannerod M (2001) Neural simulation of actions: a unifying mechanism for motor cognition. NeuroImage 14:103–109
Jeannerod M (2006) Motor cognition: what actions tell the self. Oxford University Press, Oxford
Jeannerod M (2009) Le cerveau volontaire. Odile Jacob, Paris
Jeannerod M (2013) The functional role of conscious will in voluntary action: cause or consequence? A position paper. In: Auletta A, Colagè I, Jeannerod M (eds) Brains top down: is top-down causation challenging neuroscience? World Scientific, Singapore, pp 103–120
Libet B (1985) Unconscious cerebral initiative and the role of conscious will in voluntary action. Behav Brain Sci 6:529–566
Libet B (2011) Do we have free will? In: Nadel L, Sinnott-Armstring W (eds) Libet, free will and responsibility. Oxford University Press, Oxford
Libet B, Gleason CA, Wright EW, Pearl DK (1983) Time of conscious intention to act in relation to onset of cerebral activity (readiness potential). The unconscious initiation of a freely voluntary act. Brain 106:623–642
McGuire PK, Paulesu E, Frackowiak RSJ, Frith CD (1996) Brain activity during stimulus independent thought. Neuroreport 7:2095–2099
Parvizi J, Van Hoesen GW, Buckwalter J, Damasco A (2006) Neural connections of the posteromedial cortex in the macaque. Proc Natl Acad Sci U S A 103:1563–1568
Peirce CS (1878a) How to make our ideas clear. Popul Sci Mon 12:286–302 (Reprinted in Peirce 1931–1958, 5.388–410)
Peirce CS (1878b) Deduction, induction, and hypothesis. Pop Sci Mon 13:470–482
Peirce CS (1903) Lecture VII on pragmatism (delivered in Cambridge in 1903) (Reprinted in Peirce 1931–1958, 5.180–212)
Peirce CS (1905) What pragmatism is. Monist 15:161–181 (Reprinted in Peirce 1931–1958, 5.411–437)
Peirce CS (1931–1958) Collected papers of Charles Sanders Peirce, vols I–VI: Hartshorne C, Weiss P (eds) Cambridge (1931–35), vols. VII–VIII: Burks A (ed), Cambridge (1958)
Raichel ME, MacLeod AM, Snider AZ, Powers WJ, Gusnard DA, Shulman GL (2001) A default mode of brain function. Proc Natl Acad Sci U S A 98:676–682
Rizzolatti G, Fadiga L, Gallese V, Fogassi L (1996a) Premotor cortex and the recognition of motor actions. Cogn Brain Res 3:131–141

Rizzolatti G, Fadiga L, Matelli M, Bettinardi V, Paulesu E, Perani D, Fazio F (1996b) Localization of grasp representations in humans by PET: 1. Observation versus execution. Exp Brain Res 111:246–252

Searle JR (1983) Intentionality: an essay in the philosophy of mind. Cambridge University Press, Cambridge, 2nd ed. 1997

Seitz RJ, Angel HF (2012) Processes of believing – a review and conceptual account. Rev Neurosci 23(3):303–309

Seitz RJ, Angel HF (2014) Psychology of religion and spirituality: meaning-making and processes of believing. Relig Brain Behav 22–30

Seitz RJ, Franz M, Azari NP (2009) Value judgments and self-control of action: the role of the medial frontal cortex. Brain Res Rev 60:368–378

Slachewski A, Pillon B, Fourneret P, Pradat-Diehl A, Jeannerod M, Dubois B (2001) Preserved adjustment but impaired awareness in a sensory-motor conflict following prefrontal lesions. J Cogn Neurosci 13:332–340

Spence SA, Frith CD (1999) Towards a functional anatomy of volition. J Conscious Stud 6:11–29

Sugiura M, Seitz RJ, Angel HF (2015) Models and neural bases of the believing process. J Behav Brain Sci 5:12–23

Turner VW (1986) The anthropology of performance. Paj Publications, New York

Wegner D (2002) The illusion of conscious will. MIT press, Cambridge

Wolpert DM, Ghahramani Z, Jordan MI (1995) An internal model for sensorimotor integration. Science 269:1880–1882

Wolpert DM, Ghahramani Z (2000) Computational principles of movement neuroscience. Nat Neurosci 3:1212–1217

A Process Pragmatist Heuristics of Believing

Michel Weber

Abstract In order to sketch a process pragmatist heuristics of believing, one needs, first, to set the stage of the discussion in classical Greece and especially to introduce the "gnôsis/pistis" contrast. It is then possible to show how Plato provides useful concepts to understand the history of that contrast. Eventually, James and Whitehead are brought in to specify the process nature of the religious phenomena and to bring the debate up to date.

1 Introduction

The concept of credition rejuvenates a discussion of the relationship between religiosity and faith (Angel 2013), and it inevitably refers to a few long lasting debates in philosophy. The putative theory of credition brings several different but interdependent issues to the surface. One predominant issue is the relation between religion and faith; another of equal importance is how to correctly understand belief as a noun, in comparison to understanding believing as a verb with its accent on the process. Both issues are embedded in a long history of philosophical thinking.

The paper will highlight some traditional discussions in these fields, which may help expand our framework for understanding creditions. When philosophy addresses the issue of believing, somehow it always relies on the antique bipolar juxtaposition of "gnôsis/pistis," that beautifully captures all the major stakes. The exact origin of the contrast is unclear, just as the cradle of the sects that are brought together under the umbrella term "Gnostics." However, a remarkable first instantiation has (nearly) taken place in the works of Plato, who browsed, and sometimes systematized, all the concepts he encountered in his inquiries. Plato, however, "is never entirely self-consistent, and rarely explicit and devoid of ambiguity. He feels the difficulties, and expresses his perplexities. No one could be perplexed over

M. Weber (✉)
Centre for Philosophical Practice, Brussels & Department of Educational Foundations, University of Saskatchewan, Saskatoon, SK S7N 5C5, Canada
e-mail: weber@chromatika.org

H.-F. Angel et al. (eds.), *Processes of Believing: The Acquisition, Maintenance, and Change in Creditions*, New Approaches to the Scientific Study of Religion 1,
DOI 10.1007/978-3-319-50924-2_19

Aristotle classifications; whereas Plato moves about amid a fragmentary system like a man dazed by his own penetration" (Whitehead 1969:146–147).

On the other hand, contemporary philosophy of religion arguably still relies upon such a contrast, expressed through the prism of Schleiermacher and James. Let us specify the issue and precise the step of our argument.

From a philosophical perspective, it does make sense to heuristically work with a generalized version of the "gnôsis/pistis" contrast. As Whitehead wrote, we should seek simplicity, but not trust it (Whitehead 1964:163). *Gnôsis* refers to knowledge, and more precisely to a radical religious form of knowledge by acquaintance; according to William James's lexicon, it constitutes a first-hand experience, not without epistemological consequences. What I have experienced has been—as a matter of fact—experienced, even if it does not make sense to me and makes even less sense to my community. This is especially important in the gnostic context *per se*, because in this case we are dealing with an experience of the Ultimate (Whitehead), with the *Ganz Andere* (Otto). *Pistis* refers to faith or belief; it is a knowledge that is gained thanks to a third party and brings paradoxical results. *Stricto sensu*, the faithful does not necessarily believe anymore in what s/he has personally experienced. Heteronomy was substituted for autonomy. In other words, when a religion is institutionalized, we promptly obtain a three-layered structure: at the top—or at the edges—there is the founder of the religious group and the ones who seek through *askesis* to live and experience the divine; then come the priests who claim to obtain, through certain rituals and practices, a significant proximity with the founder and beyond with the divine. They are the pure, the unsullied, the *catharoi* who are in charge of those who do not have access to such knowledge. Now, the structure cannot be absolutely waterproof, as some social capillarity has to be provided; however, this may not necessarily happen during the lifetime of a given individual, who can, for instance, obtain salvation only after a life in the lower religious caste… It goes without saying that all this has nothing to do with the contemporary science and religion debate—unless you argue that techno-science still includes some traces of the antique *theoria* and of philosophy *qua askesis*.

The following three steps are expedient to sketch a process pragmatist heuristics of believing. Firstly, in order to introduce the "gnôsis/pistis" contrast it is important to set the stage of the discussion in classical Greece. Secondly, we see how Plato provides useful concepts to understand the history of that divergence. Thirdly, James and Whitehead are brought in, in order to specify the process nature of the religious phenomena and to bring the debate up to date.

2 Religion in Classical Greece

First of all, since our argument takes place in a European cultural atmosphere, one should remember the Greek religious state of affairs. This does not mean that the "gnôsis/pistis" bipolar is not active, in one way or another, in other traditions, past or present, or that these traditions do actually matter less than the European one—we simply have to start somewhere and one's own experience and background constitute an obvious choice. Four complementary religious phenomena should be distinguished in Classical Greece, each one balancing the "gnôsis/pistis" in its own way (Vernant 1990: 827).

First, the civil religion *per se:* The religion of the Athenian *polis* was a political issue. Its secular polytheism was celebrated in civic ceremonies and festivals dedicated to Athena, Adonis, Aphrodite and their kin. Although rituals always bring forward emotions and personal experiences, these civic ceremonies clearly belonged to the sphere of *pistis*. The political and the religious organization of the City were fully intermingled.

Second, let us consider the Dionysian Mysteries, which consisted of rituals using intoxicants and other trance-inducing techniques (such as dance and music) to remove social inhibitions and to allow a return to a natural state akin to the Saturnalia and the Bacchanalia to occur. A closer look reveals that the first-hand experiences facilitated by the Dionysia did not belong either to *gnôsis* (consciousness is obliterated, not elevated) or to *pistis* (the citizen is personally active during the entire festival).

Third, the Mystery religions (sometimes called "sacred mysteries") were, so to speak, at the edge of the civil religion. The famous, but not well-known, Eleusinian Mysteries were secret initiation ceremonies held every year for the cult of Demeter and Persephone/Kore. Aristotle underlines that the Mysteries did not teach anything (ontological, theological, ethical…), but rather stimulated the emotions in order to obtain a certain state of mind. The experience was a vision whereby the pilgrim became "someone who saw," an "epoptes." We have here conceivably a full-fledged gnostic experience.

Fourth, in the margins of the religious life of the City, one found the Orphic mysteries, that provided both esoterical religious practices and exoterical beliefs. We can only speculate about the exact nature of the healing ceremonies and the actual usage of sacred plants to obtain physical and emotional purge. The first-hand experiences aided by the Orphic mysteries belonged to *gnôsis* (contact was made with the Ultimate) and to *pistis* (a dogmatic context was provided a priori and a symbolic interpretation was available a posteriori).

3 Plato's Divided Line

There is an essential question that is altogether seldom asked in philosophy: from what experience exactly did a given philosophical system spring? In the case of Plato, it is now clear that he was influenced by Orphism, both directly, through his personal involvement in rituals including Eleusinian ceremonies, and indirectly, through fellow philosophers such as Pythagoras and Socrates. In other words, Plato's world of ideas is the conceptual outcome of his own Orphic initiation.

Plato notoriously experienced many intuitions, but he did not always provide the necessary systematization. An important exception is the *Republic's* analogy of the

Divided Line, immediately followed by the Allegory of the Cave. The question is onto-epistemological: does the human mind have access to Truth? If yes: under what circumstances? If no: because of what predicament? For the purpose of the present argument, it is sufficient to keep the following hierarchy in mind: two kinds of knowledge and two kinds of opinion. These states of consciousness are said to be as clear as their objects are true.

On the one hand, (some) humans can enjoy some knowledge ("episteme") of the intelligible world. Its highest form is a direct intuition ("noêsis") of the Idea of the Good; its lowest is a discursive reasoning ("dianoia") about the intelligible forms themselves. On the other hand, (most) humans are crippled with opinions ("doxa") about the visible world. Sometimes we nurture belief or confidence ("pistis") about the perceptible things around us (common sense). Other times we only conjecture ("eikasia") about likenesses (images, shadows, reflections…) or imagine such realities.

In sum, Plato gives a particular twist to the contrast between *gnôsis* and *pistis*. *Gnôsis* is the common Greek noun for knowledge, *noêsis* is Plato's concept (Liddell and Scott 1987:167). The realm of knowledge is disclosed in *noêsis*, which means that a vision of particular objects—of Ideas dwelling in the noetic sphere—is required. For its part, the realm of beliefs is purely mundane: *pistis*, *genesis* and *aisthesis* go hand in hand. Here one finds Plato's heavy debt to Parmenides, who designed the "Way of Truth" and "Way of Seeming" as incommensurable.

The same pattern defines the Gnostic worldview (Jonas 1934; Weber 2011a). *Stricto sensu*, Gnosticism fosters a heterodoxical interpretation of the meaning and significance of Jesus's life and works. *Lato sensu*, Gnosticism is a deep religious trend entrenched by a long mystical tradition, such as the one evoked in our first section. The Gnostics were "the Knowing ones," which means that they had had a personal encounter with the divine. To a certain extent, one can claim that the Gnostics obtained, or extracted from their epiphany, a theology of sorts, or at least elements of understanding of that ineffable experience. These elements could then be weaved and submitted to the benevolent attention of the faithful, who were deprived of *gnôsis* but endowed with *pistis*. The said epiphany makes faith contingent, whereas the absence of vision makes it necessary for salvation. According to Valentinius (c.100–c.160), a third category is expedient: the chosen ones are ruled by the Spirit (they are the "pneumatic" or "spiritual" ones), the faithful are ruled by the soul ("psychic" or "mental"), and the pagans, so to speak, are under the spell of the body alone ("hylics" or "terrestrial").

4 William James' Process Pragmatism[1]

The Reformation had many complementary sources, such as the justification by faith alone (together with the other "solas"), the large-scale corruption in the Roman Catholic Church (and especially the sale of indulgences), and the inconsistencies in the biblical text (that will later spring the "documentary hypothesis" and the Modernist movement). If the historical roots of the true Christian life as well as its contemporary institutions appear quite problematic, the sharpest answer is to re-center the life of the believer upon his/her own faith and religious emotions. It is really a bottom-up dialectic that was developed against Rome; it started with the insistence upon *pistis* and hermeneutics to the detriment of a hierarchical church, and it slowly and gently ended with the return to a mild form of *gnôsis*. Schleiermacher's account of religion with intuition and feeling ("Anschauung" and "Gefühl") goes clearly in this direction (Schleiermacher 1799; Otto 1899). The individual religiosity creates the collective religion; and religion is the process of the socialization of a certain type of feeling.

In the pragmatist and process traditions, the common sense approach of James and Whitehead is taken as a landmark (Weber 2011b). It is now easy to understand why. James argues for two kinds of knowledge that are broadly and practically distinguishable (James 1950: I, 221)

Knowledge of acquaintance knows things "together"; it copes with the full thickness of our variegated experience and brings events, relations, harmony, discord and meaning in the discussion. But the immediate experience of these fringes and overtones are not fully rational—to which any gnostic experience amply testifies. *Knowledge-about* deals with the nucleus of our experience and it constitutes thus a very important part of any epistemological debate, but at the same time, it deals only with experiential thinness or quantities. As such, it can also refer to more or less sophisticated beliefs. When we pay attention to the fringes of our experience, we realize that we never experience the same event twice; when we live according to concepts, we think we grasp the same objects twice… but "there is no proof that the same bodily sensation is ever got by us twice." (James 1890:231). Those who doubt their own experience are either on the verge of psychosis or hardened philosophers. It can be wise, on the other hand, to doubt the interpretation of one's experiences.

In *Varieties of Religious Experience*, the "Knowledge of acquaintance"/" Knowledge-about" distinction illustrates the contrast between "first-hand and original forms of (religious) experience"—or (individual) religiousness on the one side and (collective) religion *qua* "second-hand religious life" on the other side. The book's working hypotheses are stated clearly and early: it would profit us very little to study "second-hand religious life," i.e., the life of an "ordinary religious believer," who follows the conventional observances imposed upon him/her by local social contingencies, says James: "His religion has been made for him by others, commu-

[1] With regard to the contemporary criticisms of James' theory of religion, see the approaches outlined in Oviedo's chapter in this book.

nicated to him by tradition, determined to fixed forms by imitation, and retained by habit" (James 1902:6). He knows as much of religion as a Welsh farmer knows of the tigers in India. On the contrary, we need to focus on "exceptional and eccentric" personalities who replace that conceptual and representative knowledge by an intuitive one:

> We must make search rather for the original experiences which were the pattern-setters to all this mass of suggested feeling and imitated conduct. These experiences we can only find in individuals for whom religion exists not as a dull habit, but as an acute fever rather. But such individuals are "geniuses" in the religious line; and like many other geniuses who have brought forth fruits effective enough for commemoration in the pages of biography, such religious geniuses have often shown symptoms of nervous instability. Even more perhaps than other kinds of genius, religious leaders have been subject to abnormal psychical visitations. Invariably they have been creatures of exalted emotional sensibility. Often they have led a discordant inner life, and had melancholy during a part of their career. They have known no measure, been liable to obsessions and fixed ideas; and frequently they have fallen into trances, heard voices, seen visions, and presented all sorts of peculiarities which are ordinarily classed as pathological. (James 1902:334–335, 337)

Interestingly enough, when James writes that the second-hand religious life is designed by others, communicated by tradition, determined by imitation, and retained by habit (1902:6 quoted supra), he reminds us of the Aristotelian characterization of tragedy; here is Kerenyi's synthetic overview:

> Aristotle investigated both what happened in the minds of the audience at a tragedy and the experience offered by the annually recurring venture of Eleusis. The spectator at the tragedy had no need to build up a state of concentration by ritual preparations; he had no need to fast, to drink the *kykeon*, and to march in a procession. He did not attain a state of *epopteia*, of "having seen," by his own inner resources. The poet, the chorus, the actors created a vision, the *theama*, for him at the place designed for it, the theatron. Without effort on his part, the spectator was transported into what he saw. What he saw and heard was made easy for him and became irresistibly his. He came to believe in it, but this belief was very different from that aroused by the *epopteia*. He entered into other people's sufferings, forgot himself and—as Aristotle stressed—was purified. In the Mysteries, a purification—*katharmos*—had to take effect long before the *epopteia*. The theater audience achieved katharsis only at the end. "Through pity and terror," wrote Aristotle in his *Poetics* VI 2 (1449b), "tragedy brought purification from all of these passions." (Kerenyi 1967:113, cf. 144)

There is a price to pay to live religiously: discipline and purification ("katharsis") makes it possible to go through initiation proper ("telete"), and this process is crowned by a contact with the Ultimate ("epopteia"). The fact that the entire ceremony is culturally determined is irrelevant. On the other hand, the believer is like a member of the audience who is passively going through a *katharsis* of sorts whose effects are a posteriori. Imitation has been substituted for action. This is, at best, a vicarious life.

But what is James himself really talking *about*? After having climbed Mount Marcy in his beloved Adirondack forest, in quest of his primeval sanity, James wrote the following to his spouse, on July 9, 1898:

> I got into a state of spiritual alertness of the most vital description. The influences of Nature, the wholesomeness of the people round me, especially the good Pauline, the thought of you

and the children, dear Harry on the wave, the problem of the Edinburgh lectures, all fermented within me till it became a regular Walpurgis Nacht. (James 1920: II, 26–27)

This tentative articulation of first-hand and second-hand experiences is not without ontological consequences; our acquaintance with reality "grows literally by buds or drops of perception. Intellectually and on reflection you can divide these into components, but as immediately given, they come totally or not at all." (James 1911/1996:155) Reality grows thus by "abrupt increments of novelty" (James 1911/1996:187): these increments, drops, buds, or steps, are characterized by some (microscopic) duration and extension; they are the "building blocks" of our (macroscopic) world.

The same argument basically holds in Whitehead's late philosophy: only actual experience fleshes out the perennial claims made by religious traditions. The validity of monotheism is, for instance, left pending. In support of his contention that there is a "becoming of continuity"—and no "continuity of becoming" (Whitehead 1978:35)—Whitehead also refers to James (Whitehead 1978:68). But Whitehead resumes the discussion of *Varieties* at the level of the distinction between first-hand and second-hand experiences. Whereas James did not want to deal with the dogmatic sedimentation of epiphanies, Whitehead urges us to think anew about the necessary dialectic that unites them: first-hand experiences always occur within a given cultural space that provides its general atmosphere (the set and setting) and the experience usually brings clues that deserve to be shared. So we have hyperdialectics between first-hand and second-hand experiences: first-hand experiences lead to second-hand experiences that, in turn, supply the background for new first-hand encounters, and so forth (Weber 2006:115–136). Notice that religious institutions can feel uncomfortable with the new encounters with the divine because, by definition, they never fit perfectly with the dogmatic expression of the founder's experience. This is how and why religions are always in danger of sclerosis—just like science. As a result, Whitehead actually demands that we understand the development of religious dogma in the same way we envisage the revolutions in scientific theories, and vice-versa. Negatively, this means that "dogma" can be indeed a derogative term in science; and, positively, that the doctrinal development in religion should be praised.

Now, to foster a process pragmatist heuristics of believing means three things. First, speculative philosophy can provide only an *attempt*, the *best shot possible*. Whitehead often uses Plato to exemplify his thesis: humans "should be satisfied to ask for no more than the likely story"[2]; we should accept that we will be able to reach only "the most likely tale" (Whitehead 1969:147).

Second, *process* means that religiosity is *becoming* and that religion is in the making. On the one hand, when the *homo religiosus* is enjoying a first-hand experience, s/he is at one with the creative advance of nature. On the other hand, religion,

[2] "The true method of philosophical construction is to frame a scheme of ideas, the best that one can, and unflinchingly to explore the interpretation of experience in terms of that scheme." (*Timæus* at Whitehead 1933)

like any other field, is always benefiting (and sometimes suffering) from the contingencies of its epoch.

Third, *pragmatism* stands here for a method foreign to utilitarian dogmatism: in an argument, one should take into account only the *consequential fruits for life* of a given experience or of a given concept, without worrying excessively about the exact causes and reasons.[3] There are many intricate claims behind this simple motto; the main one is the fact that, in an ever-evolving universe, it no longer makes sense to attempt to discover the everlasting "principle," since this "principle," if it exists, is itself susceptible to significant fluctuations… Remember that James argues that an Absolute would give us "moral holidays." (James 1907: 73–74)

4.1 A Summary of Contingent Claims

First, the "gnôsis/pistis" contrast is plausibly at work in all religious manifestations and it constitutes a precious tool with which to understand the dialectic that exists between the religious experience, its social expression and its dogmatic sediment. To review the variegated forms of the Greek religious life brings important exemplifications to the fore. A typology of religious groups could be extracted from these historical tokens.

Second, Plato provides useful concepts with which to understand the history and the uses of that contrast within philosophy. Their evocation summons furthermore the question of Plato's own epiphany and of his involvement in Mystery religions. In more concise terms: Plato apparently provided the systematization of visions gathered during a certain late (hence sophisticated) form of shamanic ritual.

Third, James and Whitehead are relevant to specify the process nature of the religious phenomena. A process pragmatist heuristics of believing involves three things: first, speculative philosophy can only provide the *best shot possible* … and has to continue trying. Second, process means that religiosity is *becoming* and that religion is in the making. The *homo religiosus*, just like the institutions that crystallizes from its experiences, are fleeting. Third, pragmatism adopts the standpoint of the outcome of the process, not of its source. Speculation about the source is however still welcome, provided that it is bridled by a concern for the assessment of the consequences involved.

The past is an important place to look when discussing a process pragmatist heuristics of believing, and the future is equally important to help us consider the research and outcomes that will help us to expand upon this.

First, one should focus on religion in the making rather than on religion made. The meaning and significance of the bipolar "gnôsis/pistis" are better assessed when we focus on "gignôsko/pisteuo," i.e., when the verbs are preferred to the nouns or when propositions substitute for terms. Knowledge and faith are no doubt abstractions from acts such as "I know" and "I believe." What do such acts involve?

[3] "There is no difference of truth that does not make a difference of fact." (Peirce 1878:286–302)

This is one question that obviously preoccupied Whitehead, and his most complete answer is to be found in *Process and Reality* (1929). A sharp ontological distinction is required between events in the making and events made, and at least three processes are intertwined: the *eventing* of the event that Whitehead calls "concrescence," the *evented* event, i.e., the efficacy of the past event, aka "transition" in the Whiteheadian lexicon, and the passage from one to the other: "perishing." And then we "should balance Aristotle's—or, more rightly, Plato's—doctrine of becoming by a doctrine of perishing. When they perish, occasions pass from the immediacy of being into the not-being of immediacy. But that does not mean that they are nothing. They remain 'stubborn fact':—Pereunt et imputantur" (Whitehead 1933:237). If we could processualize our language, it would be easier to dynamize our epistemology of religion, but perhaps that language is hindered by grammar and that only symbols allow us to go further.

Second, the relevance of science for religious studies has to be relativized. Science, as it was defined by the obliteration of the Florentine *Quattrocento* by the Northern Classics, guided a sharp political turn. For Ficino, Pico, Agrippa, Bruno and Campanella, science was basically alchemical: what you do transforms you, your community, and the world itself, including god. This is "gignôsko" in practice: I do what is meaningful to me; by doing it I grow in my mind and in my soul; and such a growth has necessarily strong (and hopefully positive) consequences for my community, for nature, and for god. The problem is, of course, that such an understanding of the scientific quest is nothing less than revolutionary, as it clearly endangers the existing social, political, and religious establishment(s). Once put steadfastly to work, reason leads to pantheism and republicanism—and if the universe does not need a divine monarch, a country has certainly no use for a king (and vice versa). Hence what some scholars have named the second Renaissance, that substituted mechanicism for animism, transcendentalism for pantheism, and staunch monarchy for democratic utopias. The empowerment of individuals was not welcome anymore. With Galilée, Descartes, Mersenne, Gassendi and Hobbes we discover that, *volens nolens*, science has actually a very limited scope in which you do what you are doing, and nothing more. Since such "doing" involves quantification, without quantification, even only a statistical one, there is no science. There is however a price to be paid: part of the experienced data is always ignored. More precisely, the problem is that amongst these data you find the subject having the experiences! If the experiencing subject is mentioned, a case in point being of course the relativity theories, it is an *objective* subject, a subject that has lost any form of subjectivity; in short, a scientific subject. Science requires speaking in a purely impersonal mode; the scientist is, by definition, not involved in the experience, s/he is solely instrumental in an experiment. This has proven quite problematic with quantum science (this is already plain in the works of Bohr, Heisenberg, Schrödinger) but the basic dogma of objectivity has remained overall.

Third, it is no surprise that the humanities or liberal arts ("Geisteswissenschaft") should be assessed differently than the so-called hard science ("Naturwissenschaft"). It is not just a matter of the selection of the data and of the nature of the consequential theoretical body, but also of the involvement of the scholar in the epistemic process. Under the cover of objective science, a Catholic priest can be acknowledged as a renowned Buddhist scholar whereas he has no first-hand knowledge of the discipline and certainly no intention to gain one; or a historian can become an acclaimed authority on the Hermetic tradition without showing any sign of interest other than academic; or an anthropologist, pretending to be a specialist of shamanism, can actually boast that, of course, he wishes to have no personal encounter whatsoever with the matter of his "expertise"—and even less with a practitioner.

On the contrary, one should expect those who speak, write, teach or even preach about any topic, and all the more so when dealing with the Ultimate, to have had some direct experience of it, and to speak accordingly. On the one hand, it is not wise to speak about realities that are unknown to us (in the gnostic sense, not the pistic one). On the other hand, if our experience does not match the dogmatic framework that is traditionally adopted in our culture, it means that we need to advocate an improvement. Such an experiential anchor and sense of urgency is blatant in the work of the philosophers evoked here: William James, of course, but also Whitehead, Bergson, Dewey, Wittgenstein, even Russell, in his own way.

References

Angel HF (2013) Credition, the process of belief. In: Encyclopedia of sciences and religions. Springer, Dordrecht, pp 536–539

Friedrich Daniel Ernst Schleiermacher, Über die Religion. Reden an die Gebildeten unter ihren Verächteren (1799), neu herausgegeben von Rudolf Otto, Göttingen, Vandenhoeck und Ruprecht, 1899.

James W (1890) The principles of psychology. Dover Publications, New York. [1950], p 221

James W (1902) The varieties of religious experience. A study in human nature. Being the Gifford lectures on natural religion delivered at Edinburgh in 1901–1902. Longman, Green, and Co., New York

James W (1907) Pragmatism. A new name for some old ways of thinking. Longman, Green and Co, New York, pp 73–74

James W (1911/1996) Some problems of philosophy. A beginning of an introduction to philosophy [Posthumously published by Horace M. Kallen with the assistance from Ralph Barton Perry and Henry James, Jr.], New York, London, Bombay, and Calcutta, Longmans, Green, and Co., 1911. Bison Edition, Lincoln and London, University of Nebraska Press, 1996

James W (1920) The letters of William James. Edited by his son Henry James. The Atlantic Monthly Press, Boston, pp 76–77

James W (1950) The principles of psychology [1890]. Authorized Edition in two volumes, Dover Publications, New York

Jonas H (1934) Gnosis und späntantiker Geist. Die mythologische Gnosis, mit Einer Einleitung zur Geschichte und Methodologie der Forschung, vol 1. Vandenhoeck & Ruprecht, Göttingen

Kerenyi K (1967) Eleusis: Archetypal image of mother and daughter. Translated from the German by Ralph Manheim. Princeton University Press, Princeton, 1967 [German Original: Die Mysterien von Eleusis, Zürich, Rein-Verlag, 1962]

Liddell HG, Scott R (eds) (1987) Gnôsis. In: A Greek-English Lexicon. Clarendon Press, Oxford

Peirce CS (1878) How to make our ideas clear. Popular Science Monthly:286–302

Schleiermacher FDE (1799) Über die Religion. Reden an die Gebildeten unter ihren Verächteren. Vandenhoeck & Ruprecht, Göttingen

Vernant JP (1990) Mythe et religion en Grèce ancienne. In: Œuvres complètes, vol I. Éditions du Seuil, Paris [2007], p 827
Weber M (2006) The hyperdialectics of religiousness and religion. In: Weber M, Rouvillois S (eds) L'Expérience de Dieu. Lectures de religion in the making, Aletheia. Revue de formation philosophique, théologique et spirituelle, pp 115–136
Weber M (2011a) Essai sur la gnose de Harvard. Whitehead apocryphe. Éditions Chromatika, Louvain-la-Neuve
Weber M (2011b) Whitehead's pancreativism. Jamesian Applications. Ontos Verlag, Frankfurt/Paris
Whitehead AN (1929) Process and reality. An essay in cosmology. Gifford Lectures delivered in the University of Edinburgh during the session 1927–28. Corrected Edition. Edited by David Ray Griffin and Donald W. Sherburne The Free Press New York, 1978
Whitehead AN (1933) Adventures of ideas. The Free Press, New York [1969], pp 146–147
Whitehead AN (1964) The concept of nature [1920]. Cambridge University Press, Cambridge
Whitehead AN (1969) Adventures of ideas [1933]. The Free Press, New York
Whitehead AN (1978) Process and reality. An essay in cosmology [1929]. The Free Press, New York/London

Part IV
Theology, Religious Studies, and Anthropology

Cognition, Emotion, and the Ethics of Authenticity

Oliver Davies

Abstract In this chapter, I argue for a connection between religions, with their emphasis upon the unity of reason and emotion, and our everyday beliefs, developing an argument from neuroscience on the observable character of this unity. I will suggest that this unity is brought about through a process of convergence, between our linguistic consciousness and pre-thematic social cognition, and that this convergence is already encoded in the work of a medieval theologian such as John Duns Scotus, where Scotus poses questions about the structure of cognition in the beatific vision.

1 Introduction

The concept of 'creditions' fosters an interesting new perspective on the extent to which emotion and reason combine to shape our beliefs. This raises the possibility of a link between religions, in which cognition and emotions characteristically combine, with everyday instances of believing, though perhaps most directly where our beliefs are responses to challenges or to significant change. Cognitions in this instance signal discrete cognitive activity while emotions are more reflective of 'a change in the feelings perceived as well as bodily reactions, conditions or expressions'.[1] As the interdependence of cognitions, emotions, and creditions is central for the concept of credition (Seitz and Angel 2012, 2013), this chapter offers an analysis of this interdependence from a theological, or rather anthropological, perspective. It will enlarge this interdependence by highlighting important contributions to this topic such as the role of knowledge and love in medieval thought (Duns Scotus). The overall method applied here sits within the framework of 'neuroanthropology' (Lende and Downey 2012), which seeks to introduce a decisively and generously interdisciplinary approach to understandings of scientific knowledge in engagement with culture. Both body and mind are concerned here then in our changing reactions to the world around us. Hans-Ferdinand Angel, who created the term 'credition,' is

[1] http://credition.at/en/modell/ (accessed 11/7/15).

O. Davies (✉)
Department of Theology and Religious Studies, King's College London, London, UK
e-mail: oliver.davies@kcl.ac.uk

H.-F. Angel et al. (eds.), *Processes of Believing: The Acquisition, Maintenance, and Change in Creditions*, New Approaches to the Scientific Study of Religion 1,
DOI 10.1007/978-3-319-50924-2_20

implicitly arguing that there is a greater continuity to be observed between the motivations of religious believing and our 'beliefs' more generally, where these in fact reflect a greater fullness of the human person, as including both feeling and emotion and the more abstract aspects of rational cognition. In the following pages, I wish to explore one way in which this statement or proposal can be nuanced in terms of contemporary neuroscience. My approach to neuroscience will be generic and will find its focus in a tendency which has been described as 'neuroanthropology'.[2] I will be concerned less with specific areas of brain activity than with the overarching conceptualization of the human person in the light of the new self-knowledge that comes to us from contemporary neuroscience.

2 Beliefs and Judgments

In the first place, we need to recall that beliefs are not entirely fluid entities but that they presuppose and recur to specific reflective judgments. A belief that has never been defended is arguably not yet fully a belief. Emotions in this sense cannot be considered to be beliefs, since they do not rest on reflective judgments, but rather they incorporate forms of believing in sustained and dynamic ways. In fact, we can perhaps describe emotions metonymically as the body's 'beliefs'. In any case, we need to mark a difference between those beliefs which rest on reflective judgments, and so are defensible, and those beliefs which are implicit within emotional dispositions and which represent a spontaneous self-positioning with respect to states of affairs encountered in the world (Solomon 1988:183–191; for a view of emotions specifically as judgments of values, see Nussbaum 2001:19–88).

The first point of nuance here then is to mark a separation between emotions as evaluative in non-reflective ways and beliefs as evaluative in reflective ways. The binary 'reflective/non-reflective' requires a further explanation and points in fact to the role of language as organizing data and allowing the objectification of processes of believing in such a way as to make possible a moment of reflexivity within the evaluation. Effectively, this is to point to a kind of internal space or ground of possibility for the considered rejection of the belief or its affirmation, *even in the process of arriving at, or determining the belief in the first place*. The reflexivity, which is internal to advanced human language, is well-captured by Kant in his work *Anthropology from a Pragmatic Perspective*, where Kant points out that it depends on the alien character of the oral sign (Kant 2006:47). What we *see* physically or noetically is translated into a contrary sensory medium, thus making possible our distancing from the content of the sign, which is the ground of reflective evaluation. Kant links language, with its semiotic alienation-representation, with the principle of judgment itself. We can only come to judgment about what we believe and do because we have human language. Language objectifies belief and creates the pos-

[2] A general overview of this new field can be found in Wikipedia (https://en.wikipedia.org/wiki/Neuroanthropology) (accessed 11/7/15).

sibility of our reflexive capacity to adjust, renounce or consolidate the beliefs we hold (Kant 2006:15–6).

The role of language in consciousness is key to our understanding of the relation between the non-reflective evaluations of emotions and the reflective character of our higher-order 'rational' deliberations. 'Judgment', properly used, implies deliberation predicated upon the objectification of thought through language. These do not, arguably, constitute a separate dimension of the human that is forever set apart from, or indeed placed above, the emotional realities of the body's own self-communicating evaluative processes. Deliberation, which is grounded in the linguistic objectification of mental processes that include emotional information, can be thought of rather as a moment *within* the body's own evaluation. It is the thinking we do in our advanced linguistic consciousness that arises from the body's life as a moment of reflexivity within it. Here, mental processes, which can be associated with interconnectivity of the brain, or with Bernard Baar's 'global workspace theory', may function as a 'trigger' or 'valve' which is the source of decision-making in the fluid and rapidly developing activity of the brain (Baars 1997). If our first point of nuance concerns the *separation* of the reflective judgment of our linguistically-founded, rational power of decision from the non-reflective evaluation of our non-reflective emotional states, then our second point concerns their unity. How might we envisage the *unity* of this rational 'trigger' or 'valve' with the emotional flows which it governs? Even if this trigger, or our power of reflective reasoning, is embedded *within* the self-communicating emotional states of our body's life, it clearly represents a distinction within it, to the extent that this is a decisively linguistic, self-objectifying dimension which is *a posteriori* with respect to the emotional life of the body. Through language, the prior power of our emotional evaluation is taken up into a higher-order capacity for reflective judgment, which grants us a potentially high degree of circumspection and discrimination within the very life of the body as evaluative. While embedded within our emotional states, this reflexivity nevertheless also represents a reflexive power that acts upon the emotional evaluation, endorsing it or restraining it. Reason is a trigger or valve that controls the directionality of the emotional flows. We need to consider then why this does not in fact constitute a definitive separation of reason from emotion in belief, but rather identifies a structure that allows us properly to inquire into the potential unity of reason and emotion in our beliefs, in accordance with 'creditions' theory.

3 Reason (Cognition) and Flow (Emotion)

But in order to approach the question of the potential unity of the reflective and non-reflective levels, of reason and emotion, we first need to be more clear about the nature of linguistic consciousness. Both studies of the origins of language and of what we might call the 'ontology' of language (Hurford 2007) emphasize the materiality of language. In the first place, evolutionary biology shows a connection between language development and use and the development and use of tools

(Steele et al. 2012). Andy Clark describes words as 'material objects' which are 'amodal' to the extent that they can be 'carried' (like Levallois tools) between different contexts (Clark 2011:44–60). An important article on the theme of the relation between 'action', 'gesture' and meaning as 'representation', bears the title 'A Word in the Hand' (Cartmill et al. 2012). Comparative work with other higher primates suggests that human language may have initially developed from facial expressions or rhythms (Ghazanfar et al. 2012). Language appears as a performative, tool-like product of the body then which extends the body's communicative rhythms and gestures into new modes of expressivity. This relation to tool use also underlines the relatively late development of human language and especially advanced language in our human evolutionary history (Hurford 2007).

But there is also a neurological perspective on language use which in a parallel way suggests that words are 'potent real-world structures' which ground the 'neural wet-ware' of the fluid processes of our consciousness and cognition, helping us to consolidate and objectify through material form what it is that we think (Clark 2011:56). An artificial intelligence specialist, Clark associates the materiality of words with the capacity of the human mind to recruit elements within the environment that will allow the generation of higher levels of awareness, through forms of objectification. Arguably, it is these processes which led to the extension of human subjectivity in time, with memory and projection beyond the immediacy of the present and with a capacity to tell stories about different places and different times (Clark 2011:44–60). In Clark's phrase, words 'press minds like ours from the biological flux' in our own immediate environment (Clark 2011:60). Therefore, we can critically identify a two-way movement in language here: one of the mind away from immediacy and into temporal distention, involving memory and futurity and an increasing power of narrative, while the other is a movement of the speaker back into the embedded 'here and now', and into the heuristics of complex interrelationality and communicative embodiment.

In addition, we have to consider the elective character of language. As Ferdinand de Saussure shows us, it is part of the very nature of language as a communicative system that our meaning is determined also by the words we choose *not* to use. 'Parole' always presupposes a moment of selection within 'langue', so that the lexical item we choose entails the non-selection of others (de Saussure 1986:9–10, 15). We cannot use language as such without in some degree *choosing* the words we speak. This means that human language use already presupposes that we can be asked: 'Why did you say that?', or 'Why did you say it that way?'. This evocation of choice has further implications for the structures of responsibility and judgment which attend our acts (as Kant noted). A creature that can choose words can also choose whether or not to act, and how to act: this, then, is a creature who can assume some degree of responsibility.

But responsibility for what? What is it we are doing, for instance, when we speak? Finally, then, we have to consider the *personal* dimension of language. Let us recall that the structure of consciousness presupposes the co-positing of consciousness and perception: to be self-aware is to possess an awareness of the world. Although these two are co-positing, this is nevertheless a dynamic relation since mind itself is immaterial. Mind is a reflexivity that turns back upon the materiality from which it arises, as a power that can observe, understand and – through technology – can even shape its own material ground. The exercise of that power is itself already a form of responsibility because language, which is elective in the way that de Saussure outlines, is also communitarian, presupposing a shared set of signs. How we exercise that freedom, or selection, will have implications, whether positive or negative, for our social relations.

We are in life, dynamically, therefore in the ways that we speak. Speech reproduces the mind-body relation or our state of being co-posited with the world that we know through the senses, but does so personally and responsibly, at a higher level of reflexivity. Communication is the dynamic energy of the mind-body relation finding traction in life: it is our self-reproduction as concrete forms of expression in the flow of history. In language, the structure of our consciousness as co-posited with the world becomes dynamic and *historic*. In Rowan Williams' words, it is through language that we can definitively position ourselves as subjects in time: as persons who can be held to account for what we say and do (Williams 2014: loc. 1532).

3.1 Reason and Complexity

What then do we do with this responsibility for our speech? And how might this cast light on how reason (which reflectively discriminates) and emotion (which shows non-reflective evaluation) can be unified in us? Here we need to recall that, as 'trigger' or 'valve', consciousness – the consciousness of an advanced higher primate – is fundamentally the way in which we manage the complexity of the real. Human social complexity and the development of the human brain go hand-in-hand in the archaeological record. We reason in ways that reduce complexity and make the world manageable. When we ask scientific questions about the nature of the world around us, i.e., when we reason as an observer, we can then cope with the world's complexity by refining the questions we ask and extending the deadlines of their asking. We seek irrefutability, or reliable knowledge. Alternatively, when we function as agents in the world, seeking to act effectively in pursuit of our own self-interests, then we do so as a participant in the world who reduces its complexity simply by filtering the events through the lens of our own needs and perspectives. By simplifying our agenda, we can obviate the intractable complexity of real life.

But there is a third mode of reasoning with which we must be concerned, which Paul Janz has called 'finality of non-resolution' (Janz 2009). This is distinctive in that we cannot reduce the complexity of the world as it comes to meet us in the human other, simply because we need to accommodate the perspective of the other on the world – a perspective unavoidably different from my own. Here we have to come to judgment without the certainty of knowing we are doing the right thing. Indeed, because complex decision-making in fluid situations involves the interests of others, it is inevitable that we will have to make the best of what are incommensurable sources of knowledge, in the accommodation of what will always remain the different *perspective* of each and every human other, for whom we choose to accept some degree of responsibility. This will inevitably be a form of reasoning which is contextualized through an affective and empathetic bond with those others who may be impacted by the decision we make. This burden of responsibility marks our 'finality of non-resolution' as a kind of *ethical* or *social* reasoning, which characteristically combines elements of both cognition and affectivity, or empathy, in our concern for the other.

3.2 The Pre-thematic and the Linguistic: Towards a Structure of Convergence

It is to this social or ethical reasoning that we must now look for the mutual implication of reason and emotion in belief proposed by the theory of creditions. Such reasoning represents a unity of the person as willing, feeling, and evaluating, in the face of the complex other. It is precisely in our social or ethical reasoning for and with the human other that the deeply embedded and ancient systems of social cognition within us combine with the much more recently evolved powers of high-level and instrumentalising language. For an explication of that structure and what we shall call its 'convergence' or realized unity, we shall need to look to evolutionary biology.

We need to note the relative lateness of our advanced, reflective, linguistic consciousness with respect to the origins of our affective and empathetic sociality. Strong, cooperative forms of sociality are already apparent in Homo erectus, about two million years ago. In a parallel way, other higher primates show ample evidence of altruism in their social behaviour without sharing our advanced linguistic capacities. This underlines in fact the 'trigger' or 'valve' nature of consciousness in modern *Homo sapiens*. We can surmise that our advanced linguisticality sits as a recently formed membrane, as it were, around the ancient core of our primitive, primate sociality. It is this ancient socio-biological inheritance which generates the bio-energy of intense community. But we know how focused and constrained that intensity can be, confined in discrete, related groups. In the more extended contexts of our modern social forms of life, we can imagine that culture, or language, continues to operate as a control mechanism, as we sometimes choose to extend the bio-energy of our proximate relationships into more remote social horizons (e.g., through cultural mechanisms of religious, national, ethnic, or generational identities).

And it is here that we encounter a factor of very considerable significance. We have noted above the question of the separation of our linguistic consciousness, with its reflective deliberation, from our emotional non-reflective evaluation, and we have considered the question of their potential unity. We have noted that the very distinctive place of freedom, or election, which is operative in linguistic consciousness, can seem to mark an inseparable divide between the two 'levels' of the self. This divide has been all the more pronounced in the light of our relative unawareness, as conscious, reflexive, self-aware self, of the 'deeper', non-reflective and feeling-centred nature of our biological inheritance. In recent centuries, there has been a strong cultural preference for the self-transparency and self-groundedness of rationalism, which has flourished in analytical philosophy and in phenomenology alike. In short, we have been unaware of our ancient, pre-linguistic inheritance, which is in fact no less constitutive of who we are. One of the functions of the neurological revolution of recent years has been laying bare the richness of our non-linguistic or non-self-aware life and indeed showing the extent to which consciousness is itself organically grounded in pre-thematic interactions with the environment (Noë 2006).

But at the core of this discovery there lies one significant theme. While at a cultural level we may make an operative distinction between the self-transparency of linguistic consciousness as rational and the obscurity of non-linguistic processes – generally emotional ones – as non-rational, neurological work has established the properly *evaluative* character of the pre-thematic emotion. This evaluation can itself be characterised as structured cognition or, to use Di Paulo and De Jaeger's phrase, as 'participatory sense-making' (Di Paulo and de Jaegher 2012). Here the definition of 'social cognition' found in the text by Kai Vogeley, Leonhard Schilbach and Albert Newen is important: 'We wish to define the concept of social cognition against the following background. The point of departure is a fundamental understanding of cognitive processes: a cognitive system is a system which in its reaction to environmental stimuli shows some degree of flexibility, a factor that is made possible by internal information processing' (Vogeley et al. 2014). Elsewhere we can read a description of the face-to-face encounter as an interaction which is 'complex, multi-layered, self-organizing', and which involves a whole series of mutual responses ranging from eye movement, facial expression and gesture to the synchrony of brain waves. This involves a subtle and pervasive 'alignment of behaviour' which includes 'synergies, co-ordination and phase attraction'. One person engages with another through neural coupling or imitation and through phase symmetry as the rhythms of breathing and heartbeat may align. In other words, not only do posture, gesture and speech become shaped to one another, but also the internal rhythms of brain and anatomy synchronize with one another. Again, the point here is that these mutual reflexes are 'self-organizing' and, as such, are 'outside our full control'. They have been described in the following terms: 'When we interact with another person, our brains and bodies are no longer isolated, but immersed in an environment with the other person, in which we become a coupled unit through a continuous moment-to-moment mutual adaptation of our own actions and the actions of the other' (Konvalinka and Roepstorff 2012). These adaptations actually occur in milliseconds and so are too fast for consciousness to be directly aware of them.

The nature of social cognition then as a form of continuing assessment of the other person, in the interests of establishing a bonded relationship involving judgments about the other and about the viability of the relationship with the other as potential social alliance, leaves us with the clear sense that what is being described here is something that is parallel to what we have described above as 'social or ethical reasoning'. Social or ethical reasoning is reasoning which takes place within a context of an other-person-centred encounter. It presupposes the complexity of the other as a living being who responds in kind to one's own communicative complexity. The unavoidability of a complex personal encounter with another human being is drawn out at the level of our pre-thematic 'self'. Moreover, this is a dimension of encounter which is characterised also as affective and empathetic (Schilbach et al. 2013). Here we cannot separate emotion or feeling from evaluation; each is integrated with the other.

Our question concerning the possible unity of the rational, linguistic self and the self that is pre-thematic and feeling, though also evaluating, leads us to ask a further question: Is it precisely in the managing of complexity as the site of reasoning that the possible unity of our elective (or free) linguistic consciousness and our ancient, socio-biological inheritance lies? Both of these layers, or aspects, of the self confront the complexity of the world. This occurs above all where it is made manifest in the human other. And about this human other we must either (a) arrive at clear evaluations at the pre-thematic, emotional level, or (b) as linguistic consciousness we must be able to reason effectively on their behalf because we have internalized their perspectives and interests, even though they may be different from our own. The difference between the two levels lies in the greater 'freedom' of our linguistic self who, in contrast with our inherited biology, can simply refuse to 'play along' with the pre-thematic processes of our social embodiment. Linguistic consciousness remains a 'trigger' or 'valve' which is both grounded in our pre-thematic self (or is at least in real continuity with it) while also possessing a reflexive power which allows mind to engage more dynamically and constructively with embodiment.

The final stage in posing our question about the potential unity of these 'two selves' is to ask: What are the conditions under which the 'higher', reflective self chooses to go with our pre-thematic, socio-biological self in a way that allows what we might call a certain 'convergence' between these two levels to come about? In other words, what drives the realization of that unity? We can even go further and ask whether that unity cannot also be described in terms of our human fullness, as something that comes about – or is accomplished – primarily within the face-to-face of immediate and dynamic encounter with the other. This turns our attention to something that is perhaps even more fundamental than the processes of 'participatory sense-making' discussed above. If what is coming into view in our final questioning concerns the realized unity of the human self as alive both in linguistic and pre-thematic ways, then can we also justifiably speak about how we are in the world as human beings? For linguistic consciousness to be in the body is surely also for us to be in the world: world and body are inseparable in this sense, since both are the – potential – object of mind's reflexivity. The source of the materiality of language, as that which grounds our reflexive consciousness, lies in our environment and is external to the human body (air as sound or shape as text). This is true even though the evolutionary passage into linguisticality is inevitably the internalisation of that external form within consciousness and within the human body, in parallel with the internalisation of external form, which characterizes technology and tool-use. We have to wonder whether the themes of human unity and the fullness of the human being do not already invoke a different and in fact specifically 'theological' register in light of its inherently cosmic dimensions?

3.3 A Theological Afterword

I conclude this paper then with a brief review of theological observations on the unity of the human being in specific terms regarding the combination of cognitive reason and affectivity (or feeling) as this manifests in medieval discussions of the beatific vision (which fulfils human life). I will also touch on the combination of knowledge and love, which according to theological precepts, is most characteristic of that ultimate human end.

In the medieval context, the unity of these two (reason and feeling) goes back most evidently to St Augustine's innovative reflections on the nature of faith as combining reason and personhood, specifically the will (Williams 2015). It is possible to read his discussion as initiating a distinctively Christian critique of the classical inheritance, which understated the role of will. What we see in Augustine can be read as an innovative response to the profound shift in understanding the human, which arises from Christian faith as reflection on, and response to, divine incarnation. This opens up new thinking about the human, and projects it along an axis of fullness and completeness. Since this is a divine incarnation, the human dimension, which is at once embodied, reasoning and intentional, is already taken up into a new, transformational horizon. Here the human self comes into view as being most fundamentally a project in time, of perfection, restoration and completion. Here the human is also radically opened up to new thinking and new imagining within the horizon of the theological reception of the incarnation of God in Jesus Christ, against a deeply paradoxical and dynamic framework of the Chalcedonian single *hypostasis* and dual *physis*.

The Augustinian synthesis of reason and will, or knowledge and love, appears again in a more direct form following Bishop Tempier's condemnation in 1277 of 219 propositions which represented rationalist Aristotelianism that was influential in Paris (Aertsen et al. 2001; de Libera 1991, 1998). We are generally better acquainted with how Thomas Aquinas succeeded in integrating the two domains before the condemnations, but in fact it was perhaps in a later generation, which included the Franciscan John Duns Scotus, that we find a more pointed attempt to take back ground lost to rationalism in the aftermath of the 1277 condemnations. Scotus specifically unites knowledge and love in his account of the beatific vision. This is of importance not only in terms of conceptions of the after-life but also, for Scotus, in terms of how we respond when we find ourselves in the presence of the real. God is the ultimate reality, whom we encounter ecstatically in heaven in the beatific vision. But following a Franciscan emphasis, Scotus understood there to be a continuity between our apprehension of God as the ultimate real in heaven and how we respond to his divine reality in the everydayness of our lives. For Scotus, the real comes to us in the moral, other-centred law which informs our decision-making in concrete situations of moral judgment. Moral judgments depend ‘upon the agent’s intellectual access to moral truth as it appears in the present situation as a form of learning in the particularity of our situational reality’ (Ingham and Dreyer 2004:193). This is not something that is simply given by a virtuous character, but is more akin to a way of being openly alive in the world as God’s world or reality. Scotus follows Augustine’s emphasis here on the attractive power of love to affect our cognitive unity with the good. At this point, he is adapting the standard position in the medieval conception of the Transcendentals that the beautiful is the *vis apprehensiva* or ‘haptic’ or ‘attractive power’ of the Transcendental of the Good (Aertsen 2012).

What we see in the medieval period therefore is the sense that reason alone cannot account for our apprehension of the real. In the terms we might use today, the view was that reason is neither sufficiently embodied nor contextual enough in itself to capture the real adequately but that other, intentional motivations of affective love, associated with the will, are required. Classically this did not replace reason, but rather combined it with what we would call values, and so also perhaps *humanized* it.

Discussion of the beatific vision was extended in the medieval period since the very nature of how human beings are in the world, concerning also the incarnation of God in human form, seemed to be at stake. It was a dynamic conversation. Where the issue of the unity of reason and love is in question, a leading modern commentator on this conversation, the Jesuit Pierre Rousselot, seems to capture its dynamic most succinctly where he says that reason and love co-exist in the medieval view in such a way that neither eclipses the other. Rather, in his phrase, ‘in faith these faculties “reciprocally cause each other; each brings the other into reality as condition of its own realisation”’ (Rousselot 1990).

4 Conclusion

‘Credition theory’ is a bold attempt to think through the role of emotion and cognition in the beliefs by which we live. In this paper we have focused upon the potential unity of emotion, affectivity, empathy and love with the movement of reason in its self-transparency. Following the insights of evolutionary biology and contemporary social neurology, this has led us to reflect upon the potential for human unity, and so also for our being more fully in the world. The cosmic dimensions of this reflection have in turn brought us back to religion and to the medieval discussion of the potential realization of the unity of our knowing and loving in the beatific vision which, for a thinker such as Scotus, represents our encounter, in heaven, with God as the ultimately real, in whose coming-to-be world we presently and dynamically live.

References

Aertsen JA (2012) Medieval philosophy as transcendental thought. Brill, Leiden, pp 161–176

Aertsen JA, Emery K, Speer A (eds) (2001) Nach der Verurteilung von 1277. Philosophie und Theologie an der Universität von Paris im letzten Viertel des 13. Jahrhunderts. Walter de Gruyter, Berlin/New York, pp 3–19

Angel HF (2013) Credition, the process of belief. In: Runehov A, Oviedo L (eds) Encyclopedia of sciences and religions. Springer, Dordrecht

Baars BJ (1997) In the theater of consciousness. Oxford University Press, New York

Cartmill EA, Beilock S, Goldin-Meadow S (2012) A word in the hand: action, gesture and representation in humans and non-human primates. Philos Trans R Soc 367(1585):129–143

Clark A (2011) Supersizing the mind. Embodiment, action and cognitive extension. Oxford University Press, New York

de Libera A (1991) Penser au Moyen Age. Seuil, Paris

de Libera A (1998) Philosophie et censure. Remarques sur la crise univer- sitaire parisienne de 1270–77. In: Aertsen JA, Speer A (eds) Was ist Philosophie im Mittelalter? de Gruyter, Berlin/New York, pp 71–90

de Saussure F (1986) Course in general linguistics, 3rd edn (Trans. Harris R). Open Court Publishing Company, Chicago

Di Paulo E, de Jaegher H (2012) The interactive brain hypothesis. Front Hum Neurosci 6:163

Ghazanfar AA, Takahashi DY, Mathur N, Tecumseh Fitch W (2012) Cineradiography of monkey lip-smacking reveals putative precursors of speech dynamics. Curr Biol 22:1176–1182

Hurford JR (2007) The origins of meaning. Language in the light of evolution. Oxford University Press, Oxford

Ingham M, Dreyer M (2004) The philosophical vision of Duns Scotus. CUA Press, Washington, DC, p 193

Janz PD (2009) The command of grace. A new theological apologetics. T&T Clark Continuum, London

Kant I (2006) Anthropology from a pragmatic point of view. Cambridge University Press, Cambridge

Konvalinka I, Roepstorff A (2012) The two-brain approach: how can mutually interacting brains teach us something about social interaction? Front Hum Neurosci 6:215

Lende DH, Downey G (2012) Neuroanthropology and the encultured brain. In idem (eds) The encultured brain. An introduction to neuroanthropology. The MIT Press, Cambridge, MA, pp 23–65

Noë A (2006) Action in perception. MIT Press

Nussbaum MC (2001) Upheavals of thought. Cambridge University Press, Cambridge, pp 19–88

Rousselot P (1990) The eyes of faith (Trans. Donceel J). Fordham University Press, New York, p 48

Schilbach L, Timmermans B, Reddy V, Costell A, Bente G, Schlicht T, Vogeley K (2013) Towards a second person neuroscience. Behav Brain Sci 36(4):393–414

Seitz RJ, Angel HF (2012) Processes of believing – a review and conceptual account. Rev Neurosci 23(3):303–309. doi:10.1515/revneuro-2012-0034

Solomon RC (1988) On emotions as judgments. Am Philos Q 25(2):183–191

Steele J, Ferrari PF, Fogassi L (2012) Theme issue “From action to language: comparative perspectives on primate tool use, gesture and the evolution of human language”. Philos Trans R Soc B 367(1585):4–9

Vogeley K, Schilbach L, Newen A (2014) Soziale Kognition. In: Hartung G, Herrgen M (eds) Interdisziplinäre anthropologie. Springer, Heidelberg, pp 13–39

Williams R (2014) The edge of words. God and the habits of language. Bloomsbury, London

Williams AN (2015) Mysterious reasons. In: Buygis E, Neuheiser D (eds) Desire, faith and the darkness of God. University of Notre Dame Press, Notre Dame (in press)

Recent Scientific Explanations of Religious Beliefs: A Systematic Account

Lluis Oviedo

Abstract The study of beliefs – both in a large sense and specifically religious – has had exponential development in the past number of years. The current research makes good use of cognitive and neuroscientific methods, allowing for a deeper insight into the structure of beliefs and believing as a complex process. Religious faith has received particular attention, giving rise to many studies. For clear access to its variety and value, a systematic review on the published material is presented in an Appendix, which includes – to date – 75 books and articles applying cognitive, evolutionary, and neurological approaches, and other new methods, in an attempt to better characterize religious experience and beliefs. As a result, a dynamic picture emerges and some development can be followed toward more complex and inclusive theories. A case is made for the utility that this research can offer for the study of broadly understood beliefs; the same can be stated regarding the application of research on general beliefs for a better knowledge on religious ones.

1 Introduction

Beliefs and believing are attracting great attention in recent years from several disciplinary settings. Part of the interest is due to the growing realization that human life and cognition depends on elements unique to humans such as ideas, representations, or future expectations, which cannot be entirely rationalized, but nevertheless are foundational to a normal existence. The study on a special kind of beliefs, 'religious beliefs', is possibly more mature and generated an extensive array of research, mostly applying cognitive and evolutionary methods. Several questions arise while browsing through this large research body concerning, for instance, the relationship between religious beliefs and other beliefs. Are the former just one kind inside a broad genre? A positive answer suggests the importance of understanding the dynamics of the general believing process in order to have better knowledge regarding religious ideas (Smith 2014). However, the answer could point in a different

L. Oviedo (✉)
Pontifical University Antonianum, Rome, Italy
e-mail: loviedo@antonianum.eu

H.-F. Angel et al. (eds.), *Processes of Believing: The Acquisition, Maintenance, and Change in Creditions*, New Approaches to the Scientific Study of Religion 1,
DOI 10.1007/978-3-319-50924-2_21

direction; in that case, we would have to start with the study of religions in order to better understand the general nature of beliefs, which would find their paradigmatic expression in the religious sub-set. In any case, a way to approach the issues arising from beliefs and believing is to follow the recent production in the field characterized as the 'new scientific study of religion' and to trace the main research lines and their conclusions, as a first step towards gaining knowledge about the general dynamics presiding over belief's formation and functions.

The scientific study of religion has produced a considerable amount of new contributions and models, applying diverse theoretical frameworks. The time is ripe to take stock of these new entries and to organize the different approaches in a systematic way. It can be expected that a complex panorama will develop and many questions will surface, allowing for a broader view and prompting a comparison between distinct proposals. This exercise should help to better address the pending questions, to draw some provisory conclusions and to trace hypothetical lines for future research. A 'systematic review' on the published material to the date appears as the best methodology for the proposed task. The proposed task makes sense in connection with the *Creditions* program, and its aim to better know the dynamics presiding over the formation, stability and changes in beliefs and believing. Indeed a wider knowledge about the many attempts to describe religious beliefs in naturalistic terms will shed light on the process bringing to beliefs formation.

The general label 'new scientific study of religion' can be understood in a broader sense. In the prompted survey, the term 'new' is applied to essays published in the last 16 years, i.e. after 1999. 'New' does not mean only recent, but a set of research programs resorting to original or innovative methods, and which could be listed in the order of: biological-evolutionary, cognitive, and neurological, and also approaches in new scientific anthropology and social psychology. In a broad understanding, the sample gathered under that label includes the so-called 'cognitive science of religion' (CSR), and assumes the many views that build on evolutionary criteria. But further on, it embraces all the attempts to explain religion in naturalist terms that respect the clauses of scientific or academic rigueur.

Summarizing the issue, it can be stated that the described approaches are new in the sense that they have not been previously applied during a long history of naturalistic accounts of religion. One reason is that these scientific methods have only recently been developed. They were lacking the kind of academic clout and recognition they enjoy nowadays. Furthermore, the new study of religion is scientific in the sense that it provides exclusively naturalistic views, which are devoid of supernatural or transcendent references when trying to explain what religion is about, its origins, evolution, and current dynamics.

The use of the term 'scientific' in the new series of theoretical explanations about religion is rather flexible, and has fuzzy contours. Despite the scarce presence of empirical or experimental evidence – an essential trait about what can be deemed as 'scientific' – all the proposed essays are clearly involved in a 'scientific program'. This point will be subjected to later scrutiny, since the epistemological status concerning current research is not easy to assess when standard scientific programs are taken into account. In any case, the new scientific study of religion is not being born in a void. Rather, it has been developed inside what can be described as 'matrix disciplines' like evolutionary biology, anthropology, and different orientations inside a more scientific psychology. The authors' academic affiliation could be revealing in that respect. In any case, the new approaches can be identified for their characteristic longing for 'scientificity', a quality perhaps less salient in the former developments that were grown inside more humanistic disciplines. Indeed, their hermeneutic character has frequently led to interference with ideological positions. This is one issue that needs greater clarification and discernment through the systematic review on the available material.

It is important to recognize that the new approaches collected here have, by and large, mainly contributed to expand the field of the scientific study of religion, introducing new elements or factors, and increasing the theoretical kit for an in-depth analysis of religious phenomena. However, not everything in this broad set can be assumed as convenient or will pass the test of scientific validity. In most cases, the contributions are rather theoretical, speculative and even conjectural, providing no empirical evidence. A deeper assessment of the available repertoire is badly needed as a condition to move forward in this scientific endeavor. Several essays have indeed, in the last few years, tried to undertake a necessary critical assessment regarding the standard forms that have been assumed in the new scientific study of religion (Laidlaw 2007; Day 2007; Barrett 2010; Visala 2011; Van Slyke 2011; Schüler 2012; Turk 2013; Watts and Turner 2014; Smith 2014). More work needs to be done in that direction as a condition for a healthy extension and renewal of the available models and research programs.

This chapter attempts a systematic review on the available published literature in the described research field as a first step in a critical evaluation. Its aim is to account for most of the existing proposals and to assess their specific contributions, their methods, and the levels of reported evidence. This exercise is necessary in the first stages of this young research field, mostly following an interdisciplinary approach, and needing to expand. The systematic review on published material will later lead to an assessment concerning the main consequences that can be deduced from these developments. In general, interesting issues are emerging, such as some extension regarding the factors involved in religious beliefs, like those symbolic and cultural; the need to apply more multi-level approaches, overcoming a very reductive original program; and then the disputed issue concerning the more or less specific nature of religious beliefs and the ways in which they provide meaning.

2 Results from a First Systematic Review

Following the standard method known as a 'systematic review', the present exercise has gathered and ordered selected studies published in the last 16 years that could be placed under the category of "scientific study of religion" and were aimed at 'explaining' the central aspects in the religious mind and behavior. To select this material, several databases have been explored: first, a personal archive of papers

Table 1 Number and proportion of publications on scientific study of religion, 1999–2015

Year	Number of essays	Proportion
1999	2	2,6
2001	3	3,9
2002	1	1,3
2003	1	1,3
2004	3	3,9
2006	8	11,0
2007	1	1,3
2008	5	6,6
2009	11	14,6
2010	7	9,3
2011	8	10,6
2012	5	6,6
2013	9	12,0
2014	10	13,3
2015	1	1,3
Total	75	100,0

and books dealing with scientific explanations about religion; additional research in international scientific databases has been endeavored to find new entries or to locate studies missed in the available personal collection.

The systematic review proposes a table that has been designed with five columns, which include: date of publication, complete quotation of the article or book, method applied in the research, content or description of the main points, and levels of evidence supporting the suggested thesis.

In this work, references for 75 authors were collected (see Table 2, the Appendix to this chapter). As a methodological choice, each author has been represented by one relevant study, even when many among the quoted scholars have published some books and several articles. In general, the quoted material was chosen to represent an author's better systematized position. It is now time to break down the analysis for each of the main columns in Table 2. For informational purposes, Table 1 indicates the proportionate temporal distribution of the published material.

2.1 About Theoretical Frames and Methods

Taking a descriptive approach, it is relatively easy to count the main disciplinary fields being applied in this endeavor. Of the 75 studies in Table 2, 45 make reference to a biological or evolutionary framework; these can be combined with 'evolutionary psychology' or anthropology, epidemiology, and even primatology and microbiology. The biological component is paramount in all these cases; i.e. the great majority of authors apply selectionist and adaptive perspectives to their analysis of religion. Also, the cognitive viewpoint is very prominent in the table; it appears in 37 of the registered contributions and is combined with varying disciplines in different versions: cognitive psychology (22), neurology (15) social cognition (2), and artificial intelligence (1). A point to remember is that the authors often take a pluralistic perspective combining more than one theoretical framework and therefore they do not assume exclusivist positions as could be expected in the first developments of the sub-discipline. The neurological approach, for instance, often combines with biological and other cognitive perspectives. There are some minor variations of interest that can be mentioned. Paleoanthropology appears in 6 instances; but in several more, the proposed reconstruction of the origins of religion draws on paleoanthropological scenarios or hypothetic reconstruction of human origins. The historical record often provides arguments to advance one's own hypothesis as well. In a similar way, 7 cases are clearly related to anthropological or ethnographic observations. There are some more particular approaches such as those applying game theory, resorting to thermodynamics, psychiatric enquiry and to developmental psychology.

As already mentioned, in many cases the methodological approaches to the new study of religion assume an explicit or latent 'multi-level' stance, combining different forms of observation and inference which include biology, cognition, emotions, symbols, and culture. Indeed a tension arises in the development of the new scientific study of religion between more multi-disciplinary studies and those that are more focused inside a unique paradigm, between less and more reductive perspectives. The impression is that in this endeavor, more authors try multi-level approaches to deal with the intricacies of religious experience, allowing them to overcome one-sided perspectives.

2.2 *About Results and Contents*

The contributions analyzed can be considered from a methodological point of view and from their content as theories or explanations about the functioning of the religious mind and behavior. The described record of applied methods already reveals the direction of the solutions given to the somewhat 'riddle' of religious origin and development. To be sure, if in most of the described works the biological or evolutionary stance is paramount, then more explanations in adaptive terms are to be expected. This is indeed the case for at least 35 of the studies listed in Table 2. The range of explanations about what renders religion adaptive in different environments, or at least in primitive ones, varies greatly. Examples include the following, with the number of relevant entries in Table 2 given in parentheses:

- Religion enhances pro-social behaviors or cooperation, often through a ritual system or behavior code based on costly signaling, or through supernatural punishment, or through ritual synchronization (18 entries).

- A similar function can be described as 'favoring moral commitment' (4 entries)
- Reproductive advantage and functional regulation of sexual activity (6 entries)
- Enhancement of cognitive abilities, like symbolization; expansion of mind; new forms of cognition or imagination (7 entries)
- Allaying anxieties or coping with contingency (7 entries)
- As a 'hazard precaution system' to avoid contagion (1 entry)

Obviously, in this case too, explanations are sometimes plural and combine two or even three factors that could be identified as adaptive with regards to religious beliefs and practices. It is important to note that in some cases the evolutionist's logic seems to be reversed, in the sense that religion's success does not depend on serving a particular interest but instead a universal one (Rolston 1999). In other cases, epigenetics could be an equally plausible explanation rather than traditional evolutionary gene-changing theory (Kellerman 2013). Furthermore, in several cases, much of the adaptive logic uses the still-controversial model of 'group selection', named such since the emphasis in these studies falls on the religion's prosocial performance and its contribution to group cohesion (Wilson and Sober 1994). In such cases, the advantage is experienced rather at group level. This clearly contradicts the more traditional view of individuals as the only unit of selection. The impression of this author in reviewing the available research and proposals is that the biological and evolutionary study of religion invites the expansion and modification of the existing theoretical frameworks to accommodate the 'new entry' of religion into existing models.

A different orientation is represented by the authors who are profound and more committed to a cognitive framework. About 22 of the studies discuss in explicit ways the so-called "cognitive science of religion"; however in at least 8 of these cases, their understanding of the cognitive pattern does not exclude an adaptive dimension to religion. Indeed, if the gathered entries list might help to settle the age-old discussion on how much of religion is adaptive or just a by-product of adaptive traits, the authors who hold the view that religion as a by-product are in the minority; furthermore, more recent contributions to the field are indefinitely committed to the adaptationist paradigm. Recent entries have increased and emphasized a kind of exaptation schema which states that religious origins are seen as a by-product of other cognitive functions, but in the course of time they become much more adaptive at different levels.

Interestingly, in 9 of the studies the authors utilized the cultural dimension in order to explain religious development and its current constitution. This socio-cultural dimension is somewhat connected to cognitive functions and appears necessary to better explain religious processes when a broader model of cognition is assumed. This is surely one trend very affirmed in the most recent contributions.

Then we find less frequent scientific methods applied to the study of religion, as for example: the thermodynamic view built on information theory (Dean 2014); the psychiatric perspective that observes hallucinations and delusions becoming functional for religious purposes (Rogers and Paloutzian 2006); or attachment theory, that looks at religion as a security provider before fear and uncertain situations (Kirkpatrick 2004).

An overview of the more than 70 research approaches that were identified and their proposals offers opportunities for further analysis. The first opportunity concerns the possibility of following some sort of development internal to this subdiscipline, from views stressing sheer biological factors, to views that enlarge or extend the range of what is involved in religion's origin and evolution. In a sense, what is at stake is a more reductive vs. a more inclusive perspective about fitness and the functionality of religious ideas and practices. Extending the range of variables involved means being able to include features like 'cognitive enhancement', 'symbolic ability', 'imagination', and a broad spectrum of cultural and social elements, which include 'enhancing group internal communication', 'motivating moral commitment', or 'enforcing social codes'. Obviously all these features could be subsumed inside a biological framework, but on the condition that such a frame is enlarged to include specific human traits that upgrade the biological dimension to make place to these emergent traits.

A second issue comes to mind when observing the panoramic view on this set of theories. In many cases, it would be possible to trace the roots of many proposed models and to elaborate a sort of 'genealogical tree'. As an example, many studies of cognitive ascendancy are inspired in the seminal work by Dan Sperber, (1985), or the proposed view about the modular mind by Jerry Fodor in 1983. The roots of many biologically-driven studies could be found in Wilson (1975) and other authors of what was called at the time 'sociobiology', and evolved into 'evolutionary psychology'. It would be interesting – again – to trace the developments of these origins toward more complex, elaborated and mature models and theories. Sometimes these more complex models and theories may need to depart from their original roots and become yet more complex and elaborate in order to be able to integrate different explanatory levels. This work on theoretical reconstruction could become very instructive and shed light on a scientific endeavor moving from some available paradigms towards more sophisticated representations after integrating more variables and theoretical frameworks.

2.3 About Evidence Levels

There is a broad agreement about the principle that a research program may be qualified as scientific when it provides enough evidence, especially through empirical observation or through experimental testing. In Table 2, the column describing 'levels of evidence' counts nine entries that are described as 'empirical', while five entries can be attributed as 'experimental' – at least in part. Four studies resorted to neuroimaging techniques in order to better support their proposals.

Perhaps the range of empirical proof might be extended considering that in many cases, authors build their theories on top of other forms of 'empirical observations', like: anthropological or ethnographic description, paleo-anthropological reconstruction, historical records and psychological description of human faculties. Nevertheless these theoretical approaches do not count towards the standard empirical observation or laboratory testing. However, such methods can be seen as a starting point in the study of religion. Then the analyzed theories present a 'hermeneutic challenge', in the sense that empirical observations are subjected to many interpretations, rendering them harder to redirect or to obtain a consensus.

Even considering the newness of this field, the scarcity of empirical and experimental studies projects some doubt on its scientific credits. Nevertheless, an alternative – more charitable – explanation could justify the label of 'scientificity'. Indeed, many among the reviewed studies clearly assume a character of theory-building, and in that exercise, they are involved in theoretical frameworks broadly accepted by the academic community. However, this is not always the case, especially when some of the original theories themselves are now being challenged by new data, or alternative theories with more heuristic power. This has happened with the connectionist theory of mind or the so called 'modular brain'; and with hypothesis like those associated with 'memes' and the 'selfish gene', which provided a basis for several theories on religion.

It can be conceded that in all the reported studies, the authors are looking for greater 'explanatory power' and 'parsimony' in their proposals. The first ideal is right but not easy to test; the second could become dysfunctional when trying to explain very complex phenomena requiring multi-level theories. In broad strokes, scientificity means not just being able to provide empirical evidence in support of one's own proposal, but also allowing the advanced view of the subject to be open to contrasting opinions, discussion and 'falsification' in a Popperian sense. This should be the case – or at least could be expected – in all the proposed theories aspiring to the status of 'scientific'.

3 Reviewing the State of Research: An Open Panorama

Placing together most of the current research on religious beliefs and behavior in a systematic way allows for a comparative analysis and the ability to draw conclusions about what is being done, especially the progress that might be observed, and the limits that still hinder this scientific endeavor. Taking stock on what has been published up until today will help to pay more attention to what is missed in the contemporary analysis on religion.

The extensive systematic review about existing research provides a descriptive catalog of the many relevant features in the religious mind, brain and behavior in terms of cognitive functions, neurological mechanisms and evolutionary processes. Combining these many contributions could lead towards the eventual integration of many elements into a more comprehensive, naturalistic explanatory framework, beyond the available philosophical and theological self-explanations.

Among the collected material, a significant subset provides analyses aimed at revealing the more or less adaptive traits in religion, or uncovering epiphenomenal, by-product, derivative characteristics about religion, whose functionality remains subject to discussion. Besides this, many quoted studies offer a competing list of factors or variables involved in religion's origins and formation, ontogenetic development, and social or historical evolution.

Trying to summarize the main achievements of the ongoing research, a list can be offered as a guide:

- The possibility to observe religion as a natural process in humans that reflects both mental schemas and forms of behavior that can be analyzed in cognitive and behavioral terms, revealing internal dynamics mostly shared with other human faculties.
- The observation of religion as a cognitive process that employs or re-employs specialized domains or schemas to deal with phenomena usually linked to supernatural agency, or beyond a more naturally available explanation.
- The distinction between two cognitive processes, the intuitive and the reflective, both influencing religious believing, and hence configuring a sort of 'dual schema' that needs to be accounted for a correct analysis of religious cognition.
- The exploration of distinctive bio-evolutionist processes that help to better know the adaptation of religious forms, pointing to features that increase survival or reproductive fitness.

A critical assessment of the state of research would help to orientate future decisions and to place the attention on what is still needed. Part of the critical discussion concerning the contemporary attempts to explain religion has been anticipated in the former paragraph, regarding issues that could help to verify the proposed theories. In a schematic way, the following lines denote the limits that have been observed in the course of the research to the present:

- Too many biases towards religious beliefs and believers; often, authors in this field dismiss the contents of professed faith and highlight the dysfunctional features that could be found in many religious expressions.
- Use or application of dated theories and frameworks; in many cases, authors were working with connectionist theories of mind, which have been mostly overcome by later developments; the same happens with views of evolution or natural selection that have been displaced by more complex models.
- Difficulties in accounting for the evolution of religious forms and ideas; it is evident that religions have evolved along the human history towards a plurality of versions still alive and with distinctive features; the difference between pre-axial and post-axial religions has been mostly neglected in many studies.
- The social and cultural aspects of religion have been, until quite recently, left out, even if they constitute central dimensions of religious mind and behavior, especially when the evolutionary perspective is assumed: genetic and cultural evolution are heavily entrenched.
- Aspects that appear as central to religion, like meaning, emotion and value, have been forgotten in most of its new scientific treatment; since religion can be recognized as a 'meaning system' such exclusion becomes suspect.

- An abuse of reductive models, going too far with the principle of parsimony, which has prevented a greater attention to the real complexity of many religious expressions or their actual presentation.
- Lack of empirical evidence in most cases, and especially troubles with experimental approaches. Then, some basic tenets of the standard model that defines that cognitive science of religion has not managed, so far, to provide the expected evidence, like regarding the 'minimal counterintuitive' status of religious ideas; the 'theory of mind hypothesis'; or, on the evolutionist side, the thesis that links religion to its capacity to enhance pro-social behavior.

The former list is not exhaustive and does not discredit every reported study; not every proposed research suffers in a similar way from the described flaws. Indeed, a distinction needs to be made between aiming to better clarify the ground and realizing the internal developments taking place in the last few years in this sub-discipline. This distinction should discriminate between a former wave of research, which possibly has its starting point in Pascal Boyer's seminal book *Religion Explained* (2001); and a second wave that emerges much later and finds expression in the programmatic papers collected in the section devoted to 'religion' in the collective book *Cultural Evolution* (Richerson and Christiansen 2013). A clear development can be described in the passage from Boyer's work to the new awareness expressed in a concluding chapter in that book, endorsed by 17 leading scholars in the field (Bulbulia et al. 2013).

The progress noted above can be characterized by a broadening of the original model towards the inclusion of formerly neglected variables and the application of a larger set of methods and perspectives, leading to a 'multi-level' approach. Such a move becomes especially apparent in the growing importance that 'culture' assumes as a central factor. Indeed, among the most recent entries in our list, some plead for a greater role played by cultural evolution in the configuration of religious beliefs (Norenzayan et al. 2015). Furthermore, the new wave has been much more prone to include dimensions like meaning and symbols in the scientific description of religious beliefs. Such a move could be quite surprising since such terms resonate more in humanistic than scientific settings. The fact is that the most recent scientific study of religion does not shy away from these almost neglected factors, even if a different language and approach is practiced when 'meaning' becomes a scientific term or is applied into that framework.

Supporting the described development, some leading authors in that field do not refrain from showing a clear paradigm change when their original proposals are compared with new ones. This might be the case observed in publications by Harvey Whitehouse (2013) and Ilkka Pyysiäinen (2014); both cases can be perceived as having a clear awareness concerning the excess of reductionism or one-sided methodologies in the first steps given in that sub-discipline. As a consequence, a plight for a more multi-level and plural approaches to the study of religion is justified.

Things are changing and it could be expected that – following that tendency – we might count on more elaborated, complex and rich models able to describe the religious mind and behavior in the future.

Taking a broader view, a striking feature arises from a more general perspective of the data in Table 2: there are a large number of new theories – perhaps too large – trying to explain religion in a scientific way. In principle, this perception should not be understood in a dismissive sense; indeed, many among the theories developed in the last several years could be seen as complementary, trying to explain or account for different aspects of a multifaceted experience. However, some suspicion is raised when so many different interpretations of the same phenomenon are noticed, with the emphases placed on several distinctive features in different studies. The project aimed at making a more unified theory that would be able to integrate the many aspects so far observed becomes less likely at the present time, despite voices claiming for the existence of a 'standard model' that could synthesize the main theories (Smith and Sankey 2012). What can be guessed is rather a 'change of paradigm' inside the field covering the scientific study of religion, one that renders still harder the unifying of the different streams of research, even if some fresh proposals try hard to achieve that goal. This is apparent in the quoted essay of Norenzayan, Shariff and their colleagues; nevertheless the discussion that this paper has invited – published and not-published – casts serious doubts about its viability and the suggested historical evidence for their model.

Several main approaches are competing with each other to offer the better explanation, and therefore, they become somewhat 'exclusive', rendering rival views less credible: accepting one often entails the negation of other, as has happened with the discussion between more adaptationist views vs. more epiphenomenalists. Such discussions may appear as less intense and even dated after new theories have been advanced. An example is the case of 'examptation', a term defining features originally related to some functions, but later re-used for new different ones. However, tensions still arise between other reported theories or emphases. As a result, the systematic review of available proposals should give rise to an exercise in ordering and clustering views that sometimes overlap or present similar aspects, or simply, are not incompatible between them. Possibly, competitiveness can be observed among theories in the science of religion 'market'. Eventually, 'one' theory will prevail when it can predict that which has not yet occurred and which cannot be predicted by common sense or by simple observation and deductive reasoning. Such predictions are far and few between in the literature. Additionally, the issue of "just so stories" need to be addressed and potentially regarded "hearsay," as many theoretical positions on religion are not testable empirically and could become less useful for the advancement in the scientific study of religion.

The question now is where are we going in the scientific/naturalist study of religion and religious beliefs? The balance sheet needs to account for the critical points that have been largely missed in the current state of research. First, we need a more ordinate schema on the factors involved in religious mind and behavior; that schema would help to place every factor in its appropriate or systematic arrangement into a greater complex whole. Second, we need to build theories connecting different viewpoints and paradigms, or providing some sort of 'consilience' and 'road map' between the several involved dimensions, as for instance: the cognitive and neurological with the biological, the social and the cultural, tracing the arrows that describe evolutionary directions. Third, we need to account for religion's evolution or the changes it has undergone along its extended history; to describe the rules that drive such developments through historical and social settings, from the most elementary forms until the secular or post-religious cultures. And fourth, an updating of current theories is required, that can take into account developments in their own scientific frameworks, as it happens with evolutionary studies, anthropological studies, cognitive psychology and neuroscience, which have undergone great progress and paradigmatic innovation in the last 20 years. What were assumed as broadly-accepted explanations no longer enjoy general recognition, and their updating claims for adaptations in the fields where they have found applications.

Expanding upon this last point, the case of human multi-level evolution, now broadly assumed, should be integrated as a basis and guide for the scientific study of religion (Jablonka and Lamb 2005). In that sense, what is still badly needed to assist in the progress of that scientific program, among other things, is an analysis and integration involving different hierarchical levels that try to explain religion as a multi-level, complex, phenomenon. Such a move would require the application of distinct paradigms such as physical or thermo-dynamic, biological or evolutionary, neurological and cognitive and social/cultural or symbolic. A further step would point to the achievement of an overarching theory able to encompass the dynamics involved in religion's evolution, which could account for different hierarchical selection levels: beliefs, behaviors, groups or social units, entire religions… taking into account the historical record and the ethnological data (Bellah 2011).

The last demand to integrate, or at least relate, the different aspects involved in religious dynamics that could be seen as an effort in meta-theory building. Possibly what is needed is at least some analysis on how biological and cognitive dimensions work together; or the cognitive and the social aspects that might be related and might collaborate to explain complex human and social phenomena. All this could yield a greater openness to receiving and integrating analysis from other disciplines traditionally related with the study of religion, which include theology, philosophy of religion, phenomenology, psychology, anthropology and sociology. Many insights from these more mature disciplines should not be ignored.

Examples of the possible directions that the scientific study of religion is going right now are recent proposals regarding genetic and cultural co-evolution. This point has been made by some pioneering authors (Richerson and Boyd 2006), and has been confirmed through biological evidence (Laland et al. 2010). In that sense, if religion is a substantial part of every culture, and culture is an essential component of human evolution, then we can somewhat reverse the logic that most biological accounts of religion have applied to the date: not only would biological pressures have conformed to religion, but vice versa, i.e. religious beliefs and behaviours would stamp their signature into evolutionary process. This means that religion's biological study could be followed in both directions of mutual determination, and scholars would need to identify the changes in religious patterns that have triggered changes in social structures, and the other way around. Such mechanisms could be located at different levels, from epigenetic to developmental and cultural.

The current scientific research just described can be further qualified through a practical test: its ability to engage in fruitful dialogue with humanistic and – particularly – theological studies concerning religion. If a new scientific approach to religious phenomena is unable to establish a meaningful dialog with those who study religious beliefs and behavior inside traditional frames of reference, then it will lose credibility and heuristic power.

4 Religious Beliefs and General Beliefs: The *Pars Pro Toto* Problem?

A pending question after reviewing the available literature on the new scientific study of religion is the relationship between specific religious beliefs and general beliefs; or between believing in a religious sense, and believing as a human attitude or broad cognitive disposition. Different orientations can be perceived and a latent discussion goes on to eventually cause understanding to emerge. Greatly summarizing the state of affairs, two basic tendencies may be described: The first considers religious beliefs as a rather specific and even *sui generis* or peculiar cognitive construction; and the second stresses the many common features and even overlapping of religious and general beliefs. In other words, religious faith would be just a sort of general belief which can be analyzed with the same means and tools applied to other beliefs. Indeed, the more or less similarity or integration would justify the application of the same or specific methods and heuristics regarding different beliefs. It is probable that things are more complex than that, and the issue cannot be reduced to an alternative between exclusive theories, but could be represented as a kind of spectrum comprising extreme and intermediate expressions.

The fact is that the last several years have registered greater attention paid to the study of beliefs, in the fields of philosophy, cognitive psychology and neurological studies (Spohn 2012). It is hard to state what preceded what, whether the interest on religious beliefs or the one on general beliefs. As an example, the recent book by Nilsson, *Understanding Beliefs* (2014), could be seen as a sign toward that growing interest. From this book many points can be recognized that clearly apply to religious beliefs: they are a form of 'declarative knowledge' with great versatility, whose level of certainty depends on many factors, like hints, relationships with other beliefs, habitual experiences, and other people's testimony… Their sources are our senses and the consequences derived from already held beliefs. Then, the author is convinced about the need to change or mature beliefs and to pay attention to the many biases that affect beliefs and which are often useful, but sometimes confusing and needing correction.

In my opinion, both branches of study should be complementary and need to mutually enrich each other in great measure. As far as I know, two programs have tried to develop a model to understand religious beliefs that is based on studying the structure and process of general believing. The first one is the so-called 'creditions program' promoted for several years by Hans-Ferdinand Angel and Rüdiger Seitz, a model extensively explained in the present volume; and the second is offered by Aaron Smith in his recent book *Thinking about Religion* (2014). In both cases, a functional schema is proposed to explain the many factors and the dynamics that nourish beliefs and allow for their formation, development, stabilization and eventual extinction. These two approaches present evidence from several sources about the cognitive and neuronal basis underlying such dynamics. Their axiomatic is similar, because both assume that religious beliefs are a specific case of general beliefs, and analyzing the general believing process would untie many closed or thorny issues concerning religious faith.

However, some doubts remain about the inclusive program here outlined. An example is the insistence from more authors to explain religion in terms of a 'meaning system' (Paloutzian and Park 2005; Park and McNamara 2006). Again, this point is easily traceable to the issue of beliefs; indeed, beliefs are connected with meaning-making in several ways. The risk that has been pointed out by critical voices (Wink 2015) is that such program could bring some confusion regarding the divisions between different beliefs and distinct sources of meaning or meaning-systems. The impression is that religious-specific ways to provide meaning could be too assimilated with other psychological ways to handle that seemingly important function, which is aimed at providing orientation in our complex environments. That discussion echoes former debates taking place during many years in other disciplinary settings, especially sociology, on 'religion' and 'spirituality', or on 'explicit' and 'latent' religious forms.

A further distinction discriminates between *religion* and *religiosity*. Even if the English language does not stress too much a contrast, other languages like German, point to a distinction between concrete religious forms and general dispositions that would be common to believers, a sort of shared basic traits that give rise to many developments or expressions. This difference could add further complexity to the study of beliefs and religion, or could help to better nuance the field. The term *religiosity* suggests a broad research program aimed at integrating the several aspects involved in this very human dimension (Angel 2013).

The current state of research does not allow us to settle the issue concerning how much 'exceptional' and how much assimilated are religious beliefs, related to other forms of believing. After all, the opening of this new approach is very promising and could allow for the future enlargement of the available scientific methods and the deepening of a more complete understanding about the dynamics of religious beliefs, and their greater or lesser particularity.

The many suggested approaches to the study of religious beliefs could still be enlarged with proposals trying to understand them as a sort of specialized language that mediates the communication regarding transcendence or ultimate values. Being that language is at the centre of human evolution and specificity, and being that religion and ritual behaviour are close to that specificity, it could be hypothesized that religious beliefs work as a set of codes that allow for a specific form of communication and socialization inside cultural settings, and contributing to cultural developments.

Appendix

Table 2 Seventy-five naturalistic explanations of religion: Theories and evidence

Year	Author and quotation	Theoretical frame, method	Content	Evidence
2011	Abelow, Benjamin, The Shaping of New Testament Narrative and Salvation Teachings by Painful Childhood Experience, *Archive for the Psychology of Religion* 33, 2011, 1–54	History of childhood, psychology of symbolic thought, psychology of trauma	Christianity – and other religions – are based on "mapping" of childhood experience onto a theologically imagined [or constructed] cosmos	Thematic parallels between childhood patterns and religious teachings
2006	Alper, Matthew, *The God Part of the Brain: A Scientific Interpretation of Human Spirituality and God,* Naperville,IL: Sourcebooks, 2006	Evolutionary psychology	Religion is hardwired in human brain, and its function is to cope with fear of death	Theoretical reconstruction, philosophical tradition
2010	Atran, Scott & Joseph Henrich (2010), The Evolution of Religion: How Cognitive By-Products, Adaptive Learning Heuristics, Ritual Displays, and Group Competition Generate Deep Commitments to Prosocial Religions. *Biological Theory*, 5 (1):18–30.	Evolutionary psychology, biology, cognitive studies	Religion enhances pro-social behavior, and has a cognitive base at inferring intentional agents. Rather a by-product	Historical reconstruction
2006	Bainbridge, William S., *God from the Machine: Artificial Intelligence Models of Religious Cognition*, Lanham, MD: Altamira, 2006.	Artificial intelligence, social cognition, systems modelling	Religion provides uncertain compensators and explanations favouring social aggregation	Computer simulations
2004	Barrett, Justin L., *Why Would Anyone Believe in God?* Lanham, MD: Altamira, 2004.	Cognitive psychology and anthropology	Religious beliefs are consequence of the natural structure of human brain, which biases some representations towards a supernatural format	Analysis of cognitive content; anthropological record; experimental

(continued)

Table 2 (continued)

Year	Author and quotation	Theoretical frame, method	Content	Evidence
2010	Barrett, Nathaniel F., Toward an Alternative Evolutionary Theory of Religion: Looking Past Computational Evolutionary Psychology to a Wider Field of Possibilities, *Journal of the American Academy of Religion*, 78–3, 2010: pp. 583–621.	Cognitive psychology, information theory, history and culture	Religion processes information embedded in cultural environment and not in isolated ways; faith as an interactive engagement with value	Criticism towards standard models of cognitive science of religion; broadening the model.
2011	Bellah, Robert, *Religion in Human Evolution: From the Palaeolithic to the Axial Age*, Cambridge, Ma., London: Harvard University. Press, 2011	Cultural history, paleoanthropology	Religion is awareness of an alternative reality, born from play and ritual, allowing for an expansion of mind and morality	Historical reconstruction, social history
2010	Bering Jesse, *The God Instinct: The Psychology of Souls, Destiny and the Meaning of Life*, London: N. Brealey, 2010	Evolutionary psychology, biology, cognitive studies	Agency attribution and theory of mind prompt religious beliefs that become adaptive enhancing reproductive advantage, and moral commitment through 'divine watching'	Psychological, neurological, historical
2008	Bloch, Maurice, Why religion is nothing special but is central, *Philosophical Transactions of the Royal Society*, doi:10.1098/rstb.2008.0007	Cognitive science, neurology, evolutionary biology, paleoanthropology, primatology	Religion helps to imagine other worlds, which are the foundation of the sociality of modern humans	Contrast with other species; paleontological and historical reconstruction
2009	Blume, Michael, The Reproductive Benefits of Religious Affiliation, in Voland and Schiefenhövel, *The Biological Evolution of Religious Mind and Behavior*, 117–126	Evolutionary biology, paleo-anthropology, genetics	Religion enhances cooperation and motivates successful reproductive behaviour beyond economic rationality	Paleo-anthropological reconstruction
2001	Boyer Pascal, *Religion Explained: The Evolutionary Origins of Religious Thought*, New York: Basic Books, 2001.	Cognitive psychology, epidemiology	Religion as by-products of cognitive functions, like theory of mind and agency attribution	Hypothetical reconstruction of mental processes

2014	Brazil, Inti A. and Miguel Farias, Why would anyone need to believe in Big Gods? *Behavioral and Brain Sciences*, 02 December 2014.	Cognitive and social psychology	The rise of Big Gods contributes to reduce uncertainty and to increase long-term predictability	Analysis of psychological needs and religious functions
2012	Bulbulia, Joseph, Religious costs as adaptations that signal altruistic intention, *Evolution and Cognition*, 10–1, 2004, 19–38	Social psychology; evolutionary psychology, game theory	Religious cognition as adaptation that enhances reproductive success by facilitating reciprocal altruism	Theoretical modeling
2014	Crespi, Bernard, Kyle Summers, Inclusive fitness theory for the evolution of religion, *Animal Behaviour* 92–2 (2014) 313–323.	Anthropology, evolutionary theory, psychology, neuroscience, genetics	The concept of God is represented by one's circle of kin and social salience, such that serving God and serving this circle become synonymous.	Hypothetical based
2014	Dean, Malcolm, (Forthcoming, St. George Publishing, Toronto, 2014; Working Paper #12http://vimeo.com/17463603)	Information macrodynamics, cognitive thermodynamics, complex systems theory	Religion is Physics, and religious systems are physical systems. Hierarchical Borromean interactions of Cognitive, Cultural, and Religious Systems. Sparse representations and dynamic Bayesian ontologies.	Observer-based Information Theory as a worldview. Cognitive Thermodynamics of object-creation by Cognitive, Cultural, and Religious Systems.
2013	Diamond, Mitchel, *Darwin's Apple: The Evolutionary Biology of Religion*, Terrapin and Hare Press, 2013	Evolutionary biology, cognitive psychology	Religion is biologically adaptive and genetically evolved through the co-evolution of religion, ritual, and advanced human cognition.	Ontogenetic reconstruction
2013	Doner, Jonathan, Self-Interest, Ultimate Meaning, and the Full Realization of Symbolic Consciousness (unpublished paper)	Phylogenetic reconstruction of human evolution	Mind, culture and religion are deeply entrenched: the emergence of spirituality/religion, or ultimate meaning, is a necessary condition for the emergence of culture.	Analysis of meaning systems in human mind and culture

(continued)

Table 2 (continued)

Year	Author and quotation	Theoretical frame, method	Content	Evidence
2011	Dulin, John, How emotion shapes religious cultures: A synthesis of cognitive theories of religion and emotion theory, *Culture Psychology*, 2011, 17–2, 223–240	Cognitive psychology, culture psychology	The transmission of common religious concepts is facilitated by the trajectory of the human emotional response and they are likely to be internalized, recalled, transmitted, and institutionalized.	Analysis of the heuristic dimension of emotions in social settings
2013	Dunbar, R. I. M., The Origin of Religion as a Small-Scale Phenomenon, in Steve Clarke, Russell Power, and Julian Savulescu, *Religion, Intolerance and Conflict: A Scientific and Conceptual Investigation*, Oxford, New York: Oxford University Press, 2013, 48–66.	Evolutionary biology, social psychology, primatology	Religion arose as a mechanism to facilitate social cohesion in (for primates) unusually large communities in order to ensure that these communities provided the ecological benefits they were intended to provide	Hypothetical reconstruction of human evolutionary scenarios
2011	Ellis, Thomas B., Disgusting Bodies, Disgusting Religion: The Biology of Tantra, *Journal of the American Academy of Religion*, 2011, 79–4, 879–927.	Biological evolutionary psychology	Tantra disgusting practices as a case of study for the maladptive forms of religion promoting disgust	Cultural anthropological observation and analysis of practices
2009	Epley, Nicholas, Benjamin A. Converse, Alexa Delbosc, George A. Monteleone, and John T. Cacioppo, Believers' estimates of God's beliefs are more egocentric than estimates of other people's beliefs, *PNAS* 106–51, 2009, 21,533–21,538.	Social psychology, questionnaire surveys and neuropsychology	People's own beliefs on important social and ethical issues were consistently correlated more strongly with estimates of God's beliefs than with estimates of other people's beliefs	Empirical and neuroimaging
2009	Feierman Jay R., How Some Major Components of Religion Could Have Evolved by Natural Selection?, in Voland and Schiefenhövel, *The Biological Evolution of Religious Mind and Behavior*, 51–66	Evolutionary biology, human ethology	Only structural design features of religion can evolve, like some forms of religious behaviour, becoming adaptive	Observation of shared features among religious behaviour

2014	Ferretti, Francesco, and Ines Adorneti, Biology, Culture and Coevolution: Religion and Language as Case Studies, *Journal of Cognition and Culture* 14 (4), 2014, 305–330.	Evolutionary study of culture	It is possible to interpret religion and language in terms of coevolution; religion and language are forms of biological adaptations	Reconstruction of human evolutionary processes
2009	Frey, Ulrich, Cognitive Foundations of Religiosity, in Voland and Schiefenhövel, *The Biological Evolution of Religious Mind and Behavior*, 229–241	Cognitive psychology, evolutionary biology	Religion explained by favourable mental structures or biases, cultural support and enhancing cooperation	Cognitive analysis, cultural observation
2010	Geertz, Armin W, Body and Culture. On what needs to be done in the cognitive science of religion, *Historia Religionum*, 2010–2, 21–38.	Social cognition, neurology	Religion is the result of an interaction between the functional organization of brain, the cultural world, and the development and flexibility of that brain	Observation and analysis of complex cognitive processes
2011	Gervais, Will, Aiyana K. Willard, Ara Norenzayan & Joseph M Henrich (2011). The cultural transmission of faith: Why innate intuitions are necessary, but insufficient, to explain religious belief. *Religion,* 41(3): 389–410.	Cognitive science, cultural evolution	Religion is based on cognitive biases and cultural support, providing motivation for commitment	Psychological and social research; cultural history; developmental empirical studies
2014	Girotto, Vittorio, Telmo Pievani, and Giorgio Vallortigara, Supernatural beliefs: Adaptations for social life or by-products of cognitive adaptations? *Behaviour* 151 (2014) 385–402	Evolutionary psychology and cognitive psychology	Supernatural thinking is a secondary effect of cognitive predispositions originally shaped for different adaptive reasons, but requires cultural scaffolding	Analysis of psychological predispositions that explain religious beliefs
2001	Guthrie, Stewart, Why Gods? A Cognitive Theory, in: Jensine Andressen, *Religion in Mind: Cognitive Perspectives on Religious Belief, Ritual and Experience*, Cambridge: Cambridge University Press, 2001, pp. 94–112	Cognitive psychology, evolutionary biology	Religion provides a view of the world alive and humanlike, a bias that is adaptive.	Anthropological observation, hypothetical reconstruction human evolution

(continued)

Table 2 (continued)

Year	Author and quotation	Theoretical frame, method	Content	Evidence
2009	Henrich, Joseph, The evolution of costly displays, cooperation and religion: credibility enhancing displays and their implications for cultural evolution, *Evolution and Human Behavior* 30 (2009) 244–260.	Cognitive psychology, evolutionary biology	Religion ensures association of costly acts, often in the form of rituals, with deeper commitments to group beneficial ideologies, and higher levels of cooperation within groups	Theoretical reconstruction of natural selection process
1999	Hinde, Robert A., *Why Gods Persist: A Scientific Approach to Religion*, London, New York: Routledge 1999	Cognitive psychology, evolutionary psychology	Religion is adaptive, helping survival of individuals and communities, and enhancing coherence and cognitive integration	Empirical observation, search for adaptive traits in religion
2011	Inzlicht, Michael, Alexa M. Tullett and Marie Good, The need to believe: A neuroscience account of religion as a motivated process, *Religion, Brain & Behavior* 2011, 1–3, 192–251	Neuropsychology and social neuroscience	Religious beliefs provide meaning and buffer the distress associated with disruptions to meaning, thus leading to decreases in distress.	Experimental, neuroimaging
2001	Irons, William. 2001. "Religion as a Hard-to-Fake Sign of Commitment" in *Evolution and the Capacity for Commitment*. R. M. Nesse (ed.), pp. 292–309. New York: Russell Sage Foundation.	Evolutionary psychology	Religion enhances prosocial behavior through a system of beliefs and practices that avoid free-riding	Reconstruction of social evolutionary scenarios
2006	Johnson, Dominic D.P. and Jesse Bering, (2006) Hand of God, Mind of Man: Punishment and Cognition in the Evolution of Cooperation, *Evolutionary Psychology* 4: 219–233.	Evolutionary Psychology, social psychology	Religion enhances pro-social behavior providing a cognitive system of supernatural agents watching and punishing	Speculative reconstruction of anthropological and social development
2014	Jong, Jonathan, Ernest Becker's Psychology of Religion Forty Years on: A View from Social Cognitive Psychology, *Zygon*, 49–4, 2014, 875–889.	Social cognitive psychology	Religion as terror management before death anxiety	Speculative building on experimental evidence about psychological needs.

2014	Kapogiannis, Dimitrios, Gopikrishna Deshpande, Frank Krueger, Matthew P. Thornburg, and Jordan Henry Grafman, Brain Networks Shaping Religious Belief, *Brain* Connectivity, 2014 Feb;4(1):70–9.	Neuropsychology, theory of Mind, cognitive psychology	Religious beliefs are founded both on propositional statements for doctrine, but also on episodic memory and imagery, using respective neural networks	Experimental, neuroimaging and analysis of directional connectivity.
2009	Kay, Aaron. C., Whitson, J.A., Gaucher, D., & Galinsky, A.D. (2009). Compensatory control: Achieving order through the mind, our institutions, and the heavens. *Current Directions in Psychological Science*, 18, 264_268.	Social and cognitive psychology, anthropology, institutional studies	Religion helps to protect the belief in a controlled, nonrandom world by imbuing people's social, physical, and metaphysical environments with order and structure when their sense of personal control is threatened	Analysis of the different processes to achieve compensatory control
2013	Kellerman, Henry, *The discovery of God: A psychoevolutionary perspective*, New York: Springer, 2013	Evolutionary biology, psychoanalysis, neurology	Religion as result of epigenetic processes from survival driven individuals in interplay with environmental pressures	Anthropological reconstruction, neurological hypothesis
2007	King Barbara J, *Evolving God: A Provocative View on the Origins of Religion*, New York, London: Doubleday, 2007	Evolutionary psychology, biology, comparative primatology	Religions are born from growing ties of social interaction moving up to conceiving interaction with supernatural agents.	Historical reconstruction
2004	Kirkpatrick, Lee A., *Attachment, Evolution, and the Psychology of Religion*, New York: The Guilford Press, 2004.	Evolutionary psychology, cognitive science, attachment theory	Religion is a by-product of attachment cognitive systems that provide safety before fear and a secure base.	Psychological observation of familiar attachment. Empirical correlation between forms of attachment and religious forms.
2009	Lahti, David, The Correlated History of Social Organization. Morality and Religion, in Voland and Schiefenhövel, *The Biological Evolution of Religious Mind and Behavior*, 67–88	Evolutionary biology, social history	Co-evolution of social forms, morality and religious expressions, driving to an ever more extended range of relationships until reaching a pattern of universality	Historical reconstruction, cultural anthropology

(continued)

Table 2 (continued)

Year	Author and quotation	Theoretical frame, method	Content	Evidence
2010	Lewis-Williams, David, *Conceiving God: The Cognitive Origin and Evolution of Religion*, London: Thames & Hudson, 2010	Cognitive and evolutionary psychology, neurology	Religion is the result of altered experiences, rightly interpreted and motivating behaviour and social cohesion	Historical record, compared religions, archaeological evidence.
2013	Martin, Luther H., The Ecology of Threat Detection and Precautionary Response From the Perspectives of Evolutionary Psychology, Cognitive Science and Historiography: The Case of the Roman Cults of Mithras, *Method and Theory in the Study of Religion*, 25, 4–5, 2013, 431–450.	Evolutionary psychology, biology, neurology	Religion allays anxiety and helps to cope with many threats	Historical and psychological observation
2012	Matthews, Luke J., The recognition signal hypothesis for the adaptive evolution of religion: A phylogenetic test with Christian denominations. *Human Nature.* Vol.23(2), Jun 2012, pp. 218–249.	Evolutionary psychology	Religions provide a system of signal recognition than enhances in-group cohesion	Empirical observation of Christian denominations
2011	McCauley, Robert N., *Why Religion is Natural and Science is Not*, Oxford, New York: Oxford University Press, 2011	Cognitive psychology	Religion is an intuitive set of beliefs based on agency attribution and theory of mind	Psychological observation
2013	McGuire, Michael, Believing: *The Neuroscience of Fantasies, Fears, and Conviction*, Prometheus 2013	Neuroscience, cognitive psychology, behavioural psychology	Beliefs are products of human neurological structure, interacting with environment; pleasurable and rewarding; do not influence behaviour, but are their consequence.	Neuroscientific observation; theoretical reconstruction of behavioural processes
2009	McNamara, Patrick, *The Neuroscience of Religious Experience,* New York: Cambridge University Press, 2009	Neuroscience, cognitive psychology	Religion helps to ‘decentering the self, and hence to ‘self-transformation’ from a passive to a more agent	Study of recurrent patterns in human history

2008	Newberg, Andrew B; Newberg, Stephanie K., Hardwired for God: A neuropsychological model for developmental spirituality, Authoritative Communities, 5, 2008, pp. 165–186	Neuropsychology	Basic mechanisms associated to religious experiences are correlated with essential brain functions, evolving together	Neurological observation, hypothetical reconstruction
2014	Norenzayan, Ara, Azim F. Shariff, et al. 2015. "The Cultural Evolution of Prosocial Religions". *Behavioral and Brain Sciences*, 02 December 2014. DOI: http://dx.doi.org/10.1017/S0140525X14001356;	Social psychology, evolutionary biology, cognitive science	Religious forms evolved to conceive more potent gods., motivating prosocial behaviors that gave rise to big and more integrated societies	Empirical, experimental, historical
2014	Panchin, Alexander Y., Alexander I Tuzhikov, Yuri V Panchin, Midichlorians – the biomeme hypothesis: is there a microbial component to religious rituals? *Biology Direct* 2014, 9:14	Microbial biology	Certain aspects of religious behavior could be influenced by microbial host control and that the transmission of some religious rituals could be regarded as the simultaneous transmission of both ideas (memes) and parasitic organisms.	Speculative derived from evidence on microbiotic influence on human behavior
2006	Park, Crystal L. P. McNamara, Religion, Meaning and the Brain, McNamara, Patrick (Ed.), *Where God and Science meet: How brain and evolutionary studies alter our understanding of religion, 3: The psychology of religious experience*. Westport, CT: Praeger, 2006, 67–89	Cognitive psychology, neuropsychology, evolutionary psychology	Religion as a means to build meaning – mostly through rituals – which is a human cognitive condition to process information	Psychological observation; hypothetical reconstruction
2013	Purzyck, Bengamin G., The minds of gods: A comparative study of supernatural agency, *Cognition* 129 (2013) 163–179	Cognitive psychology and anthropology	Religions attribute to their gods moralizing bias which influence social behavior	Anthropological field work and surveys
2004	Pyysiäinen, Ilkka, *Magic, Miracles, and Religion: A Scientist's Perspective*, Altamira Pr., Walnut Creek – Lanham – New York, 2004	Cognitive anthropology; evolutionary psychology	Religion as a complex set of counterintuitive beliefs linked to somatic markers and emotions	Psychological observation; philosophical analysis and hypothesis

(continued)

Table 2 (continued)

Year	Author and quotation	Theoretical frame, method	Content	Evidence
2006	Rogers, Steven A; Paloutzian, R. F., Schizophrenia, Neurology, and Religion: What Can Psychosis Teach Us about the Evolutionary Role of Religion? McNamara, Patrick (Ed.), *Where God and Science meet: How brain and evolutionary studies alter our understanding of religion, 3: The psychology of religious experience*. Westport, CT: Praeger, 2006, 161–165.	Evolutionary psychology, psychiatry, neurology	Religion as a result of hallucinations and delusions of schizophrenic origin, mediating access to the divine, but functional to cope with life contingencies of a group	Empirical: observation of schizophrenic symptoms, and hypothetical reconstruction; cross-cultural
2010	Rossano, Matt J., *Supernatural Selection: How Religion Evolved*, Oxford: Oxford University Press, 2010	Evolutionary biology, paleoanthropology	Religion enhances through ritual social cohesion and mutual support	Paleoanthropology; hypothetic reconstruction of human evolution
1999	Rolston, Holmes III, *Genes, Genesis, and God: Values and Their Origins in Natural and Human History*, Cambridge, New York: Cambridge University Press,1999.	Evolutionary psychology, biology, genetics	Religion evolves from functional local forms to universal ones, more fitting in the long run, challenging evolutionist rule	Historical, social or cultural
2009	Schiefenhövel Wulf, Explaining the Inexplicable: Traditional and Syncretistic Religiosity in Melanesia, in Voland and Schiefenhövel, *The Biological Evolution of Religious Mind and Behavior*, 143–164	Psychology, ethnography	Religion helps to allay anxieties by providing explanations for the unknown and the threatening aspects of their vulnerable life	Anthropological observation
2011	Schloss, Jeffrey P. and Michael J. Murray, Evolutionary accounts of belief in supernatural punishment: a critical review, *Religion, Brain & Behavior*1–1, 2011, 46–99	Evolutionary psychology, systematic-critical review	Reviews evidence about thesis of religion as forms of supernatural punishment that are adaptive for groups	Historical reconstruction; social observation
2012	Schüler Sebastian, *Religion, Kognition, Evolution: Eine religions-wissenschaftliche Auseinandersetzung mit der Cognitive Science of Religion*, Stuttgart: Kohlhammer, 2012	Evolutionary psychology, biology, cognitive studies	Religion as synchronizer of social groups through ritual activity	Historical, observation of behaviour

2012	Shenhav, Amitai, David G. Rand, and Joshua D. Greene, Divine Intuition: Cognitive Style Influences Belief in God, *Journal of Experimental Psychology: General*, 141(3):, 2012, 423–8.	Cognitive psychology; intuitive vs. reflective cognition	The extent to which one believes in God may be influenced by one's more general tendency to rely on intuition versus reflection	3 empirical and experimental studies
2008	Slone, Jason (2008): The Attraction of Religion: A Sexual Selectionist Account. In: Bulbulia J, Sosis R, Harris E, Genet R, Genet C, Wyman K (eds.): *The Evolution of Religion: Studies, Theories, & Critiques*. pp. 181–187. Santa Margarita, CA, Collins Foundation	Evolutionary psychology, biology	Religion enhances reproductive advantage, signaling individuals with more parenting availability	Hypothetical Paleolithic environment and some empirical evidence in USA context
2014	Smith, Aaron C.T. 2014. *Thinking About Religion: Extending the Cognitive Science of Religion*. Basingstoke UK, New York: Palgrave.	Cognitive psychology and evolutionary psychology	Religious beliefs are less 'special' and more as a version of the general tendency by humans to hold beliefs, required for orientation and social connection	Analysis of psychology of beliefs and its functionality
2003	Sosis, Richard and Candace Alcorta, Signaling, Solidarity, and the Sacred: The Evolution of Religious Behavior, *Evolutionary Anthropology* 12:264–274 (2003)	Evolutionary psychology, social psychology	Religion as a system of costly signalling mechanisms to enhance solidarity	Hypothetic reconstruction of ancient scenarios
2008	Steadman, Lyle B. and Craig Palmer, *The Supernatural and Natural Selection: The Evolution of Religion*, Boulder, Co, London, U.K.: Paradigm, 2008	Evolutionary biology, behavioural psychology, communication studies	Religion increases number of descendants: reproductive success and enhances family-like cooperation	Ethnographic descriptions of traditional kinship-based religions
2013	Talmont-Kaminski Konrad, *Religion as Magical Ideology: How the Supernatural Reflects Rationality*, Acumen 2013.	Evolutionary biology, cognitive science and culture	Religion adapts as a result of interaction between cognitive and cultural processes, prompting pro-social behavior and resistant cognition	Historical reconstruction, cognitive analysis

(continued)

Table 2 (continued)

Year	Author and quotation	Theoretical frame, method	Content	Evidence
2006	Thagard, Paul (2006). *Hot Thought: Mechanisms and Applications of Emotional Cognition*, Cambridge, Ma., London: MIT, pp. 237–250.	Multidisciplinary study of emotions and their interaction with cognitive processes.	Rel. not an adaptation, not related to evolutionary pressures; rel. Results from internal 'emotional coherence' satisfying some needs	Psychological analysis connected with evolutionary/ cognitive study of emotions
2010	Tiger, Lionel and Michael McGuire, *God's Brain*; New York: Prometheus Books, 2010.	Evolutionary biology, neurology	Religion is adaptive regulating sexual relationships, organizing hierarchies, and – specially – as a form of brainsoothing.	Historical, anthropological
2006	Tremlin, Todd, *Minds and Gods: The Cognitive Foundations of Religion*, Oxford, New York: Oxford University Press, 2006.	Cognitive psychology, evolutionary psychology	Religion is based on mental structures like theory of mind, and is prompted by forms of intuitive thinking	Psychological analysis
2012	Van Slyke, James A., *The Cognitive Science of Religion*, Farnham UK, Burlington VT: Ashgate, 2011	Multilevel analysis, including biological, emotional, symbolic, and cultural	Religion regulates sexual behavior; enhances the process of symbolic thinking	Historical, neurological
2009	Voland, Eckart, Evaluating the Evolutionary Status of Religiosity and Religiousness, in: Eckart Voland and W. Schiefenhövel (Eds.), *The Biological Evolution of Religious Mind and Behavior*, Springer 2009, 9–24.	Evolutionary biology, behavioural ecology	Most traits of religions are adaptive, like bonding, identity, morals, except rel. Cognition – a by-product; exaptation plays a role in this adaptive process	Analysis of religious behaviour
2009	Wade, Nicholas, *The Faith Instinct: How Religion evolved & Why it Endures*, New York: Penguin Press, 2009	Evolutionary psychology, cultural history, paleoanthropology	Religion is hardwired in humans because of its central survival role in early societies, as moral enforcer	Paleoanthropology record, historical reconstruction, social observation

2015	Watts, Joseph, Greenhill Simon J, Atkinson QD, Currie TE, Bulbulia J, Gray RD. Broad supernatural punishment but not moralizing high gods precede the evolution of political complexity in Austronesia. Proc. R. Soc. B 282: 20,142,556, 2015.	Evolutionary psychology, cultural history and anthropology	Broad supernatural punishment drives political complexity, whereas 'Moralizing High Gods' follow political complexity	Bayesian phylogenetic approach with a sample of 96 Austronesian cultures
2008	Whitehouse, Harvey, Cognitive Evolution and Religion; Cognition and Religious Evolution, in Joseph Bulbulia et al. *The Evolution of Religion: Studies, theories, and critiques*, Collins Foundation Press: Santa Margarita, CA, 2008, pp. 19–29.	Cognitive anthropology	Religion combines holding and turning functions – ratchet effect – in interaction with its environment	Anthropological observation and taxonomy
2013	Wiebe, Donald, Pseudo-Speciation of the Human Race: Religions As Hazard-Precaution Systems, *Method and Theory in the Study of Religion*, 25,3–4, 2013, 410–430.	Biology, epidemiology, group selection	Religion as 'hazard precaution system' enhancing immune boundaries between groups	Historical social
2002	Wilson, David Sloan, *Darwin's Cathedral: Evolution, Religion and the Nature of Society,* Chicago – London: Chicago University Press 2002	Evolutionary biology	Religion as a form of group selection, or multilevel selection, that favours better organized populations	Social anthropological observation
2006	Winkelman, Michael, Cross-Cultural Assessments of Shamanism as a Biogenetic Foundation for Religion, in McNamara, Patrick [Ed]. *Where God and Science meet: How brain and evolutionary studies alter our understanding of religion* (Vol 3): The psychology of religious experience. Westport, CT: Praeger 152–172	Ethnography, Biology, paleoanthropology	Shamanism as elementary religious form, helped to develop forms of thinking, healing, and group solidarity	Hypothetical reconstruction of Palaeolithic scenarios and ethnographic observation

References

Angel HF (2013) Religiosity. In: Runehov A, Oviedo L (eds) Encyclopedia of sciences and religions. Springer, Dordrecht, pp 2012–2014

Barrett NF (2010) Toward an alternative evolutionary theory of religion: looking past computational evolutionary psychology to a wider field of possibilities. J Am Acad Relig 78(3):583–621

Bellah R (2011) Religion in human evolution: from the palaeolithic to the axial age. Harvard University Press, Cambridge

Bulbulia J, Geertz AW et al (2013) The cultural evolution of religion. In: Richerson P, Morten H (eds) Christiansen, cultural evolution: society, technology, language, and religion. Harvard University Press, Cambridge, pp 381–403

Day M (2007) Let's be realistic: evolutionary complexity, epistemic probabilism, and the cognitive science of religion. Harv Theol Rev 100(1):47–64

Dean M (2014) Forthcoming, St. George Publishing, Toronto; Working paper #12. http://vimeo.com/17463603

Fodor J (1983) Modularity of mind: an essay on faculty psychology. MIT Press, Cambridge

Jablonka E, Lamb M (2005) Evolution in four dimensions: genetic, epigenetic, behavioral, and symbolic variation in the history of life. MIT Press, Cambridge

Kellerman H (2013) The discovery of God: a psychoevolutionary perspective. Springer, New York

Kirkpatrick LA (2004) Attachment, evolution, and the psychology of religion. The Guilford Press, New York

Laidlaw J (2007) A well-disposed social anthropologist problem with the cognitive science of religion. In: Whitehouse H, Laidlaw J (eds) Religion, anthropology, and cognitive science. Caroline Academic Press, Durham, pp 211–246

Laland KN, Odling-Smee J, Myles S (2010) How culture shaped the human genome: bringing genetics and the human sciences together. Nat Rev Genet 11(2):137–148

Nilsson NJ (2014) Understanding beliefs. MIT Press, Cambridge, MA

Norenzayan A, Shariff AF et al (2015) The cultural evolution of prosocial religions. Behav Brain Sci. Published online 2 Dec 2014. http://dx.doi.org/10.1017/S0140525X14001356

Paloutzian RF, Park CL (2005) Recent progress and core issues in the science of the psychology of religion and spirituality. In: Paloutzian RF, Park CL (eds) Handbook of the psychology of religion and spirituality. Guilford, New York, pp 3–22

Park CL, McNamara P (2006) Religion, meaning and the brain. In: McNamara P (ed) Where God and science meet: how brain and evolutionary studies alter our understanding of religion, 3. The psychology of religious experience. Prager, Westport, pp 67–89

Pyysiäinen I (2014) The cognitive science of religion. In: Watts F, Turner L (eds) Evolution, religion and cognitive science: critical and constructive essays. Oxford University Press, Oxford, pp 21–37

Richerson PJ, Boyd R (2006) Not by genes alone: how culture transformed human evolution. University of Chicago Press, Chicago

Richerson PJ, Christiansen MH (2013) Cultural evolution: society, technology, language, and religion. Harvard University Press, Cambridge/London

Rogers SA, Paloutzian RF (2006) Schizophrenia, neurology, and religion: what can psychosis teach us about the evolutionary role of religion? In: McNamara P (ed) Where God and science meet: how brain and evolutionary studies alter our understanding of religion, 3. The psychology of religious experience. Prager, Westport, pp 161–165

Rolston H (1999) Genes, genesis, and God: values and their origins in natural and human history. Cambridge University Press, Cambridge/New York

Schüler S (2012) Religion, Kognition, Evolution: Eine religionswissenschaftliche Auseinandersetzung mit der Cognitive Science of Religion. Kohlhammer, Stuttgart

Smith ACT (2014) Thinking about religion: extending the cognitive science of religion. Palgrave, Basingstoke/New York

Smith ACT, Sankey H (2012) Thinking about religion: examining progress in religious cognition. In: Dawes G, Maclaurin J (eds) A new science of religion. Taylor &Francis, London, pp 111–130
Sperber D (1985) Anthropology and psychology: towards an epidemiology of representations. Man [N.S.] 20:73–89
Spohn W (2012) The laws of belief: ranking theory and its philosophical applications. Oxford University Press, Oxford/New York
Turk M (2013) Being religious: cognitive and evolutionary theories in historical. Pickwick, Eugen
Van Slyke JA (2011) The cognitive science of religion. Ashgate, Farnham/Burlington
Visala A (2011) Naturalism, theism and the cognitive study of religion: religion explained? Ashgate, Farnham/Burlington
Watts F, Turner L (eds) (2014) Evolution, religion and cognitive science: critical and constructive essays. Oxford University Press, Oxford
Whitehouse H (2013) Proximate causation and development in religious evolution. In: Richerson PJ, Christiansen MH (eds) Cultural evolution: society, technology, language, and religion. Harvard University Press, Cambridge/London, pp 349–364
Wilson EO (1975) Sociobiology: the new synthesis. Harvard University Press, Cambridge
Wilson DS, Sober E (1994) Reintroducing group selection to the human behavioral sciences. Behav Brain Sci 17(4):585–654
Wink P (2015) Are religion and spirituality at the same order as other meaning systems? A case for partial exceptionalism. Relig Brain Behav 5(2):157–161

Soul and Body According to "De Fide Orthodoxa" of St. John Damascene

Dorin Oancea

Abstract The Christian and particularly the Orthodox understanding of belief sometimes might be seen as a matter of the soul and not a matter of the body. Based on such an understanding the binomial "creditions – neuronal processes" would not have any significance for an Orthodox anthropology. But such an understanding can be marked as reductionist regarding the broader conceptions that we can find in the positions of the Fathers. In this contribution, some aspects of the comprehensive anthropological understanding of humans and their relation to God will be presented as it is conceived in the famous synthesis of patristic thought, *De Fide Orthodoxa*, written by St. John Damascene (~ 650–before 755).

1 Theological Thinking and the Complexity of the Process of Believing

The question of how to relate faith and brain activity has led to interesting developments. Many of them are associated with the so-called "neurotheology" (Persinger 1987, d'Aquili and Newberg 1999; d'Aquili et al. 2001; Joseph 2002). But the neurotheological proposals do not provide an acceptable approach for bringing together religious experience with brain functions, as the proponents of this idea ignore the basic rules of hermeneutics. It might be possible to conceive the intention of "neurotheology" as an attempt to conceive a "neurobiology of religiosity" (Angel 2013b). Therefore, it is crucial not to confuse the question of the neural base of belief with any neurotheological concepts. On the contrary, one of the origins of the concept of credition was to explicitly avoid those theoretical traps that result from a lack of hermeneutics, which are elemental in the attempt to understanding religious experience as neurotheology (Angel 2006).

On the other hand, it cannot be ignored that religious experiences are part of the general possibilities of humans. In this there is an interest to better understand this

D. Oancea (✉)
Facultatea de Teologie Andrei Saguna, Lucian Blaga University of Sibiu, Sibiu, Romania
e-mail: oancead@yahoo.com; dorin.oancea@ulbsibiu.ro

H.-F. Angel et al. (eds.), *Processes of Believing: The Acquisition, Maintenance, and Change in Creditions*, New Approaches to the Scientific Study of Religion 1,
DOI 10.1007/978-3-319-50924-2_22

ability. It will be necessary to carefully separate different systematic approaches from one another and not to confuse incompatible terms and research interests.

One model that avoids the traps of neurotheology and even builds bridges between different approaches in science (esp. neuro-science), humanities, philosophy, and theology seems to be the model of creditions. Introduced a decade ago (Angel 2006), the "model of credition" (Angel 2013a) has meanwhile developed into a broader scientific context that includes different fields of science and humanities (Seitz and Angel 2012; Runehov and Angel 2013; Seitz and Angel 2014; Sugiura et al. 2015).

Regarding the concept of credition, three aspects seem to be of major interest for Christian anthropology and are fundamental at the same time:

- Creditions are not limited to solely religious belief, but include all other cognitive and emotional processes whose certitude comes from both repeatable observations of certain phenomena and subjective-emotional ways of understanding those phenomena. In this way, creditional processes may be interrelated with peoples' general worldviews. Similarly in mathematics, postulates do not need any demonstration in order to be approved. Creditions are basic assumptions, perfectly able to offer a coherent, present world view and to approximate a still unknown or uncertain future, but of course, only within this framework. Religious belief is only one part of a complex process through which persons understand the world. Because of this, the idea of credition may be more easily acceptable both for religious and non-religious people. More importantly, it suggests a systemic isomorphism between all forms of belief. This might be discussed as a question of anthropology, but it seems to me that this way of understanding is more suitable to understand acts of beliefs than any dichotomic concepts of belief. On the other hand, one should not ignore the significant differences between religious and non-religious experiences. Depending on the religious or non-religious orientation, deeper consequences might be expected for the subjective perception of the self and the world. It will be of major interest to define more clearly the subjective efficacy of different orientations if they follow most of the aspects of general biological rules of processing.
- In general, as in theological discussions, belief/faith in the sense of religious belief is often emphasized as content/contents of belief. This content orientation of belief tends to ignore its emotional dimension although the major obstacles in theological dialogues are of emotional origin. According to the "model of credition," creditions (including religious beliefs) and all processes related to them are not only specific to the cognitive dimension of man but also to his emotional life: "Credition is conceived as a psychological term in analogy to emotion and cognition that denotes the mental activity related to what we call 'he/she believes'" (Seitz and Angel 2012).
- The connection between creditions as processes of belief and neuronal processes allows an understanding of belief as embodied. This has a major implication for understanding religious cognition (see the contribution of Oviedo in this volume). Additionally, it helps to better formulate a central intention of Christian catechesis; it is not possible to pass over Christian Faith like an object. It has to

be undertaken by those who are interested in understanding the meaning of the Christian dogma. Contents of belief and dogmatic concepts are not "alive" without "embodiment" in individual humans, and consequently in Christian communities. This leads to the conclusion that in order to understand Christian belief and the "growing in Christ," one should keep in mind at least the bodily processes complementary to creditions.

One could argue that the Christian and particularly the Orthodox understanding of belief is a matter of the soul and not of the body. If one follows this argument, there is no observable benefit from any progress in studying the bodily life of humanity. At least, the understanding of the body seems to have little relevance for his/her communion with God. Therefore, the binomial "creditions – neuronal processes" would have no significance at all for an Orthodox anthropology, one and the same at all times.

To me this seems to be a reductionist outlook which is quite far from the much broader perspective of the Fathers. The openness of the Fathers, who have a comprehensive anthropological understanding of humans and their relation to God, can be verified by having a closer look into their anthropology.

It is not my intention to offer a more detailed presentation of the credition model, but to investigate the extent to which the above-mentioned basic ideas are consistent or not with the traditional Christian and Orthodox anthropology. In the case of an affirmative answer, they might be used to articulate an anthropological understanding of Christian belief. Methodologically, this might be seen as an attempt to describe the general structure of Christian Faith in a way that is appropriate from a scientific point of view and which is familiar to contemporary people. In this way, the concept of credition might be conceived as one possible explanation of Christian faith as a "normal" potentiality of humans. But this is not enough to clarify how the aspect of transcendence, which is impossible to express in terms of human language, can be formulated. It should be noted that the understanding of creditive processes theoretically refers to the concept of subconsciousness and that creditions are understood as being deeply rooted in subconscious processes. This allows us to explain Christian faith also as a "specific" potential of humans which finally transcends all attempts to explain it in terms of natural science.

Of course, there needs to be deeper theological and anthropological research to clarify more substantially the relationship between the concept of credition and traditional theological concepts regarding the role of belief for any understanding of Christian faith.

I intend to make nothing more than a first step to see how the compatibility of the concept of credition with the anthropological view of the Fathers might be verified. I refer to the famous synthesis of patristic thought, which is expressed in "*De Fide Orthodoxa*"[1] written by St. John Damascene (~ 650–before 755). This author

[1] *De Fide Orthodoxa* is divided in four books, each of them containing several chapters. All quotations are from the online edition of the revised version.

experienced the period of Islamic expansion and gives insight in the way of thinking in times of transition (Argárate 2013).

De Fide Orthodoxa is the third and most important book of the *Fountain of Wisdom*. It is divided into four books, each of them containing several chapters. From the very beginning, I want to avoid a misleading interpretation of this title: *fide* means here the entire Christian understanding of reality, with its two fundamental dimensions – God and His creation. St John makes it perfectly clear that each of these two dimensions is governed by specific rules, spiritual and mundane, and that humanity is expected to act in accordance with them, on the one hand without confusion, on the other without separation. This broad understanding is at the same time *Orthodox* and *Catholic* and this is the reason why the Damascene treatise has been highly regarded not only in the Eastern tradition but also in the Western one, here as the first important synthesis of the Christian world view before the *Summa Theologica* of St. Thomas AquinasThomas Aquinas. The subjective faith of an individual person is just a part of the ensemble, and I shall deal with it in the context of the three ideas already mentioned.

2 The Universal Character of Faith – Structures/Creditions

St. John Damascene deals with faith in Book IV, especially in chapters 9, 10 and 11. Important references can be found in Chapter 13 and 15.

To start with, I quote an important assertion St John makes on faith in Book IV, Chapter 11:

> … without faith it is impossible to be saved. For it is by faith that all things, both human and spiritual, are sustained. For without faith neither the farmer does cut his furrow nor does the merchant commit his life to the raging waves of the sea on a small piece of wood, nor are marriages contracted nor any other step in life taken. By faith we consider that all things were brought out of nothing into being by God's power. And we direct all things, both divine and human, by faith. Further, faith is assent free from all meddlesome inquisitiveness. (Book IV,11).

It is possible to identify several elements in this assertion, all of them important for our argument. I shall mention them one by one, but not in their original succession.

(a) With regard to creditions, the first would be the universal character of faith: "For it is by faith that all things, both human and spiritual, are sustained. For without faith neither does the farmer cut his furrow nor does the merchant commit his life to the raging waves of the sea on a small piece of wood, nor are marriages contracted nor any other step in life taken" (Book IV,11). On one hand, it is important to underline the unity of all forms of faith; we are not confronted with a particular religious way of understanding the world but with a general human reality – everyone exercises faith in one way or another, irrespective of his specific action.

On the other hand, of similar significance is the importance associated with faith. It is not only universal, but also of vital importance – all things are sustained by faith. In other words: no faith, no possibility of accomplishments in real life. One could say that faith receives an ontological significance in the dynamics of life. In Orthodox understanding, this would be an expression of the image-likeness dynamics as an essential communicatory feature of humanness, understood as a permanent movement from a given situation of the image towards the possible development of likeness. Humanity's choice to tread on this path always approximates the outcome according to a mental projection and to the hope that there will be a concordance between this projection and the outcome of this action. The farmer cuts the furrow according to a projection – covering the seeds with the earth from the furrow, he hopes to be able to harvest a crop several months later. His previous experience tells him that this is the way things happen. Cognitive processes on the basis of previous experiences, hope and action, these are constitutive elements of his faith. They are constitutive elements of any way of organizing life within the image-likeness dynamics, about which Christians are entitled to say that it is of an ontological character, because all humans were endowed with it from the very beginning.

Any faith-based project within mundane life can and must be verified according to certain rules specific to this mundane existence. Starting from early Greek beginnings, passing through the time of Aristotle and later developments, epistemology has established several criteria in this respect: inner coherence, concordance with reality, and the possibility of repeating an experiment. One could say that experience means to make use of these criteria without reflecting upon them. Therefore, under mundane circumstances, the assent to an action free from all meddlesome inquisitiveness is not possible, if I may paraphrase St John.

(b) The other project, the communion between God and humans, functions according to similar rules, but only up to a certain point, as far as humanity is concerned. This is so because no verification by means of repeatable experiments is possible in this case, as the reality of somebody's communion with God is fully visible for outsiders only during the eschaton (Pannenberg 1973). Nevertheless, its exterior signs can be perceived and correctly interpreted as communion with God or as faith in God, from one's perspective. At the same time for the faithful, the communion he/she experiences is as real as any mundane process; this is his/her way of understanding the world. Subjective experiences can be noticed[2] and shared, and they take on an objective character for those who participate in the process. Starting from these premises, *De Fide Orthodoxa* offers not only an almost all-encompassing image of man's communion with God, but also a behavioural pattern, with faith as the starting point and permanent support of the whole process: "… we direct all things, both divine and human, by faith" (Book IV,9).

[2] Mathew 5,16: "Let your light so shine before men, that they may see your good works, and glorify your which is in heaven."

As one can see, according to Damascene, the whole human life is based upon and directed by faith as an isomorphic process with as many particularities as the multitude of actions performed by a person. Faith is for him a universal reality "by that all things, both human and spiritual, are sustained" (Book IV,9). In my opinion, there is an impressive correspondence between the faith model of the Damascene Father and the credition model with regard to structures and processes of believing.

3 The Cognitive and Emotional Character of Faith

The second element of the credition model to be compared with the patristic outlook refers to the simultaneously cognitive and emotional aspect of faith. At first glance, one might think that faith, for St John of Damascus, is a cognitive reality without emotional components. In my opinion, both elements are present, probably in a way unfamiliar to modern understanding. In order to identify them, I shall start with an introduction to the cognitive dimension, keeping in mind that the emotional side is present too. The following reflections are based on different chapters of Book II.

3.1 The Cognitive Dimension of Faith

(a) When speaking about this cognitive faith, one should not forget that, according to the all-embracing model of *De Fide Orthodoxa*, the finality of a person's life is to be in communion with God. This is the Alpha and Omega of religious belief, and St. John knows that its accomplishment is possible because God endows him/her with essential virtues, necessary for working this out: "Bear in mind, too, that virtue is a gift from God implanted in our nature, and that He Himself is the source and cause of all good, and without His cooperation and help we cannot will or do any good thing. But we have it in our power either to abide in virtue and follow God, Who calls us into ways of virtue, or to stray from paths of virtue, which is to dwell in wickedness, and to follow the devil who summons but cannot compel us" (Book II,30). It is important to notice that humanity is never looked at as an object of analysis for itself but as a communicating person, in communion with God. He or she receives from his or her Creator uninterrupted impulses to do good things and can decide for or against them. This should not lead to the conclusion that God gives the original impulse, like a *primus movens*, and then retires, leaving the person all alone. After humanity's option in favour of virtue and against evil, He supports these endeavours: "… the choice of what is to be done is in our own hands: but the final issue depends, in the one case when our actions are good, on the cooperation of God, Who in His justice brings help according to His foreknowledge to such as choose the good with a right conscience" (Book II,29. Concerning Providence).

The option in favour of evil does not enjoy support from God, in this case man is "… liable to death and corruption, … to labour throughout a miserable life" (Book II,30).

(b) One can see the decisive significance of humanity's choice in St. John's argument. We name this basic concept in Christian anthropology *free will*, which makes the difference between humans and all of God's other creations, and makes understanding the Orthodox concept of *image-likeness dynamics* possible. St. John associates it both with the direct communion with God, who speaks to His creature and receives a corresponding dialogic answer, and to the indirect communion with Him – by means of the command God gives and one's decision for or against fulfilling it. The possibility of making a decision for or against a specific action is the link between reasoning and acting, according to the pattern: the situation – which demands an action decision, evaluation – the necessity and possibility to act or refrain from it, and the action or non-action itself. The necessary link between these three elements and free will is clearly stated by St. John: "Every one, then, who deliberates does so in the belief that the choice of what is to be done lies in his hands, that he may choose what seems best as the result of his deliberation, and having chosen may act upon it. And if this is so, free will must necessarily be very closely related to reason" (Book II,27).

The logic of the argument is perfectly clear up to now: a human's purpose in life is to be in communion with God; being endowed from the very beginning with free will, he or she achieves it by making choices in favour of and not against this essential exchange with his or her Creator; one can choose by means of deliberation and this is directly related to reason. Faith itself is the result of such an option, as one could see in Book IV, page 11: "… faith is assent …". Assent includes deliberation, making a certain decision in favour of a possibility or against it. This is the reason why the next step leads us to the anthropological foundation of reason and of knowledge as its result.

(c) St John Damascene offers a model of knowledge with several elements introduced in a precise, but inverted succession, if one considers the natural order of the events: "The faculties of knowledge are mind, thought, notion, perception/representation/presentation[3], sensation…" (Book II,22). In an abbreviated form, this model goes back to *De Anima* by Aristotle, as expected. Nevertheless, one can notice a difference of some importance, whereas in *De Anima,* representation is not an indispensable element of knowledge. However, it seems to be a necessary part of the process in *De Fide Orthodoxa*, as its second spiritual element after sensation. Further, it is interesting to note that these five elements

[3]The New Advent edition we use translates the Ancient Greek φαντασία with "presentation", ignoring other meanings like "apparition, impression, imagination, perception, representation". We think that in the context of its etymology - φαντάζω = "I make visible, I show at the eye or the mind" - a better translation might be "perception", but from Avicenna onward "representation" has been normally preferred, so that we shall use it too.

belong to an epistemic chain, so that sensation cannot be separated from mind, because it leads to notion, and the mind works with notions: "It is sensation that causes a passion, which is called presentation, to arise in the soul, and from presentation/representation comes notion. Thereafter thought, weighing the truth or falseness of the notion, determines what is true: and this explains the Greek word for thought, διάνοια, which is derived from διανοεῖν, meaning to think and discriminate" (Book II,22). The link between sensation and mind is interesting for the relationship between soul and body, but also for the emotional side of faith, which will be dealt with during the next step of our analysis.

Before doing so, we may conclude that as long as sensation, notion, thought, and deliberation belong to one and the same process, the cognitive dimension of faith is perfectly clear. And in addition, we may infer that faith as result of an assent belongs to the "reasoning mind".

3.2 The Emotional Dimension of Faith

At first glance, the association of faith and emotion cannot be easily sustained. Nevertheless, there are important elements which make it possible, provided one keeps in mind the large scope of the phenomena of emotions. Inner disposition to, liking and desire for, or the wish to do something – all these could be called emotions. They belong to the emotional side of humanity together with love and anger, fear, pain, anguish grief, the pleasure to do or experience something, and so on. I have mentioned only emotions present in St. John's argument. In order to identify the emotional side of faith I shall pick up only some of them.

(a) When speaking about cognitive faith, I said that the link between sensation and a reasoning mind is significant for the emotional faith. In order to see how this happens I go back to an already introduced quotation: "Thereafter thought, weighing the truth or falseness of the notion, determines what is true: and this explains the Greek word for thought, διάνοια, which is derived from διανοεῖν, meaning to think and discriminate" (Book II,22). Thought, the forerunner to the mind on the scale of knowledge, has the mission to deliberate and to decide upon falseness or truth, a "this is called judgment" if we use the same Damascene words. And this judgment, or deliberation or faith has an emotional side: "… this is called judgment (κρίσις). Thereafter, one becomes disposed to and forms a liking for that in favour of which deliberation gave judgment, and this is called inclination (γνώμη). … Then, again, after one has become so disposed, choice or selection (προαίρεσις and ἐπιλογή) comes into play. For choice consists of selecting one out of two possibilities in preference to the other" (Book II,22).

We have already seen that faith is the result of deliberation and a choice between two possibilities (to believe or not), in favor of one option. Major components of this process include disposition and liking, both of which belong to the emotional part of human makeup. Thus, a person can make a choice in favor of something, e.g., to act in faith, in a manner consistent with his or her inner disposition or liking for it.

(b) Desire belongs to the emotional part of human makeup, there is no doubt about it. But we may doubt whether having certain desires is legitimate. According to St. John, having desires is certainly permitted, because they activate a natural, and one may argue, a given faculty of human nature: "It should be understood that there is implanted in the soul by nature a faculty of desiring that which is in harmony with its nature, and of maintaining in close union all that belongs essentially to its nature: and this power is called will or θέλησις" (Book II,22). Desire is described not as a contemplative but as an active emotional characteristic of human nature – thus, no desire, no humanity. And if this is true and if faith is characteristic of human nature, then faith does not exist without desire. This should not lead to the conclusion that, according to the Damascene Father, faith has only an emotional side, because he underlines its rational character: "… there is seated in the soul of man a faculty of rational desire" (Book IV,22). "Rational desire" is the name for a reality that is at once cognitive and emotional. We could say instead "rational emotion," which brings us quite close to another reality called "credition".

St. John of Damascus mentions desire in the context of the Holy Eucharist and makes it clear that faith cannot be imagined without an emotional core: "… with all fear and a pure conscience and certain faith let us draw near … Let us draw near to it with an ardent desire, and with our hands held in the form of the cross let us receive the body of the Crucified One: and let us apply our eyes and lips and brows and partake of the divine coal, in order that the fire of the longing, that is in us, with the additional heat derived from the coal may utterly consume our sins and illumine our hearts, and that we may be inflamed and deified by the participation in the divine fire" (Book IV,13). There is a lot of emotion in these words, emotion of the faithful, directly connected to their faith. Key words like "certain faith", "ardent desire", "the fire of the longing", "inflamed" show beyond any doubt the intimate connection between faith and an emotion, desire, about which we have been told should be rational.

The Damascene Father goes very much along the same line when he urges all Christians to honour the apostles, the martyrs, the holy fathers, the ascetics, because of their "faith and love and hope and zeal and way of life, and endurance of sufferings and patience even to blood" (Book IX,15). On the one hand, they are praised for certain characteristics of their lives, about which one may say they are of emotional nature. All of them should be put together with cognitive faith, as together, they form a rational and emotional faith at the same time. This two-dimensional faith is not an ideal exception, but the rule for all the faithful, because we are urged again to "emulate" their faith and love.

It is obvious that in St. John Damascene's understanding, religious faith is both rational and emotional. Could we say the same about any kind of faith? Yes. I say this because the arguments provided for rational faith match inner-mundane processes too. Yes, because in daily life, people love, hope, show zeal, endurance of sufferings, and patience, which are all elements of that emotional dimension of existence which participates in religious belief. Given these similarities, we can conclude that, according to St. John, cognition and emotion are constitutive elements of all forms of faith, religious or non-religious. Another conclusion is directly related to my general theme: the simultaneously cognition- and emotion-coloured credition model is consistent with the faith model of the Fathers, as worked out by St. John Damascene.

4 The Soul – Body Complementarity

The existence of a soul complementary to a body has been a philosophical and theological theme for centuries at least, and nowadays it is being discussed in the context of the neurosciences. Theologians certainly would take it for granted, but some of them and many faithful could wonder whether faith and all spiritual processes have anything to do with the body at all, as long as spiritual matters are specific to the soul alone. We find a conclusive answer to these possible dilemmas in *De Fide Orthodoxa* and I shall refer to it quite briefly, not more than it is necessary to understand the neuroscientific efforts around the credition model.

With regard to the soul, St. John mentions – first of all, the general Christian conviction that it was created at the same time with the body: "… body and soul were formed at one and the same time, not first the one and then the other …" (Book II,12). Neither the successive nor simultaneous creation of soul and body are matters of interest now, but rather, the consequences of their simultaneity. The emphasis put upon them means that they are inter-conditioned and makes evident that humanness and personhood are possible only if they function together.

One should not forget that unity does not mean uncensored equality – the soul is the guiding force which makes "… use of an organized body …". Nevertheless, given the unity of the two, their inter-conditioning becomes evident by associating different parts of the brain with certain functions of the soul. I shall mention three pairs: "… the organ of imagination is the anterior ventricle of the brain" (Book II,17); " The organ of thought then is the mid-ventricle of the brain, and the vital spirit it contains" (Book II,19); "Now the organ of memory is the posterior ventricle of the brain, which the Greeks call the παρεγκεφαλίς, and the vital spirit it contains" (Book II,20). The way in which the soul and body work together is also examined in the context of sensation, as the Damascene Father is able to say something about the nerves as a connection between the organs of sense and the brain.

It is not my intention to go into any anatomical and physiological details, but rather, to make it clear that these connections between soul and body are so important to St. John that he feels it necessary to mention them[4] in their antinomic unity. The notion "antinomic" is important, as the two main components of man are contradictory, if one appreciates that the soul's being is simple, formless, and excludes the multiplicity of the material body. We shall not follow this idea much longer, although it belongs to the core of Christian and, actually, to any comprehensive understanding of the sacred. It is essential both for the complementary relation between the nature/ousia as the undefined, transpersonal being of God and His triadicity, as his defined, personal being, and the equally complementary relation between the same simple nature/ousia and the uncreated energies of His Grace by means of which he acts uninterruptedly upon any respect of complex creation. The first expression of this antinomic model was elaborated on by St. Basil the Great in the fourth century, and the second expression by St. Gregory Palamas in the fourteenth century, although both of them had been part of the genuine Orthodox life from the very beginning. Consequently, it is not surprising to see St. John Damascene making use of the same isomorphic model in the eighth century, more or less chronologically between the other two.

However, we can hardly appreciate his point of view as an innovation – St. Gregory of Nyssa had shown a similar way of thinking in *De Hominis Opificio*. In contrast, he offers a synthesis of his patristic predecessors, so that this unifying expression of their experience in Christian faith and life has become paradigmatic for Orthodox theology and for the Orthodox Church worldwide ever since. That is why the model of an antinomic unity between soul and body is, for contemporary Orthodox theologians, by no means obsolete, and draws attention to the necessity of a similar anthropological approach. Deepening the understanding of the way human brain works and is connected to the soul becomes imperative for the theologian who knows that everything he does is an answer to questions asked by the Holy Spirit uninterruptedly.

At the end of these reflections, I come to the conclusion that the credition model is consistent with the basics of patristic anthropology, as formulated by St. John Damascene. Its future development could also help theological reflection find more appropriate expressions of Christian faith and life in our time.

References

Ables S (2013) Did John of Damascus modify his sources in the Expositio fidei? In: Vinzent M (ed) STUDIA PATRISTICA. 16th international conferenceon patristic studies, Oxford 2011, vol LXVIII. Peeters, Leuven

Angel HF (2006) Religiosität als menschliches Potential. Ein anthropologisches Modell der Religiosität im neurowissenschaftlichen Horizont. In: Angel HF (et al) (eds) Religiosität. Kohlhammer, Stuttgart, p 62–89

[4] We know that St. John of Damascus was not a medical doctor, that he took these anatomical data from Nemesius of Emessa. (Ables 2013)

Angel HF (2013a) Credition, the process of belief. In: Azari NP, Runehov A, Olviedo L (eds) Encyclopedia of sciences and religions. Springer, Heidelberg/New York
Angel HF (2013b) Religiosity. In: Runehov A, Oviedo L (eds) Encyclopedia of sciences and religions, vol 4. Springer, Dordrecht/Heidelberg, pp 2012–2014
Argárate P (2013) Ἡ μέχρι τοῦ νῦν κρατοῦσα λαοπλανὴς θρησκεία τῶν Ἰσμαηλιτῶν. A study on De Haeresibus, 100. In: Kralides A, Gkoutzioukostas A (eds) Byzantium and the arab world encounter of civilizations. University of Thessaloniki, Thessaloniki, pp 45–70
D'Aquili E, Newberg A (1999) The mystical mind: probing the biology of religious experience. Fortress Press, Minneapolis
D'Aquili E et al (2001) Why God won't go away. Ballantine Books, New York
John of Damascus, An exposition of the Orthodox faith. In: Schaff P, Wace H (eds) Nicene and Post-Nicene fathers. Second Series, vol. 9. Christian Literature Publishing Co., Buffalo, 1989, Revised and edited for New Advent by Kevin Knight: http://www.newadvent.org/fathers/3304.htm
Joseph R (ed) (2002) NeuroTheology: brain, science, spirituality, religious experience. University Press California, San Jose
Pannenberg W (1973) Wissenschaftstheorie und Theologie. Suhrkamp, Frankfurt am Main
Persinger MA (1987) Neuropsychological bases of God beliefs. Praeger, New York
Runehov ALC, Angel HF (2013) The processes of believing: revisiting the problem of justifying beliefs. Stud Sci Theol 14:205–219
Seitz RJ, Angel HF (2012) Processes of believing – a review and conceptual account. Rev Neurosci 23(3):303–309. doi:10.1515/revneuro-2012-0034
Seitz RJ, Angel HF (2014) Psychology of religion and spirituality: meaning-making and processes of believing. Relig Brain Behav 5:22–30
Sugiura M, Seitz RJ, Angel HF (2015) Models and neural bases of the believing process. J Behav Brain Sci 5:12–23

Music as a Medium of Personal Motion and Belief: Some Phenomenological Reflections

Peter Ebenbauer

Five mysteries hold the key to the unseen:
the act of love, and the birth of a baby,
and the contemplation of great art,
and being in the presence of death or desaster,
and hearing the human voice lifted in song.

(Salman Rushdie 2000, 20)

Abstract Singing, dancing, and drumming are primordial phenomena of human culture. Throughout history, chanting and music have been important resources concerning the anchorage of beliefs, or 'creditions,' as well as existential perspectives of life. At the same time, they transcend common patterns and beliefs, and open a world beyond everyday life. Along with these insights, this contribution offers some ideas about how personal motions, beliefs and 'creditions' are generated and communicated by singing and music.

The process of believing seems to be structured in a way that shows a narrow interdependence of emotions and cognitions (cf. chapter Angel and Seitz in this book). From these neuroscientific insights one can conclude that the emotional side is of high relevance for the believing process. Any attempt to influence the emotionally shaped state of people is influential to the "modus" of how the believing process will take place. Thus, this presentation is based on the idea that the emotional aspect of music is an important means of affecting believing, one that shows impacts on the so called "modulator function".

P. Ebenbauer (✉)
Institute of Liturgiology, Christian Arts and Hymnology, Karl-Franzens University, Graz, Austria
e-mail: peter.ebenbauer@uni-graz.at

H.-F. Angel et al. (eds.), *Processes of Believing: The Acquisition, Maintenance, and Change in Creditions*, New Approaches to the Scientific Study of Religion 1,
DOI 10.1007/978-3-319-50924-2_23

1 At the Beginning – Where Does Music Come from?

We don't know exactly where music comes from and why our early ancestors started singing and playing instruments; however, they did, even in prehistoric times. For example, flutes made of wood or bones from animals were found in South-Germany (Schwäbisch Alb) dating back to the Paleolithic period. They are about 35,000–40,000 years old.

From the Old Stone Age onwards, man has been dancing and singing. Clapping hands and stamping feet mark the beginning of dance and of the performance of rhythmic patterns in groups. Wooden sticks or rods, rattles and drums support these rhythms; flutes, horns (from animals) and simple string instruments complete the prehistoric orchestra (Altenmüller and Kopiez 2013).

Such instruments were often venerated as sacred and only special persons like priests or shamans were allowed to play them in the context of special events or needs.

There is no doubt that singing, playing music, and performing rhythmic movements are intense ways of human communication which characterize even the earliest stages of human culture; be it for the purposes of communicating over long distances, hunting, military engagements, or certain biographical or social occasions connected with rituals, such as medical and healing rituals or the so-called "rites of passage" (Arnold v. Gennep/Victor Turner). Just think of pregnancy and birth, adolescence, marriage, or death and funeral. Singing, drumming, and dancing are primordial bridges of culture that have been with mankind from the earliest times until today (Finnegan 2012).

2 What Happens if Someone Is Singing, Playing Music or Listening to Music?

Music arises at the border between material and mental or spiritual reality. With very sensitive sensory receptors of our organism, we comprehend complex oscillations of the air. In the case of music, these are caused by instruments, for example our body with its organs to produce voice and songs, or the whole range of music instruments, or other sources of sound and rhythm. Material and body instruments on the one hand, and sensory receptors of our organs of perception and our neuronal systems on the other hand, are serving as the equipment of sending and receiving music. But three more components are necessary to enact and to experience music:

- the atmosphere, which enables and promotes audible oscillations, combined with the fact that every material thing is oscillating – up to the elementary particles of matter;
- the mental, psychological and emotional ability of resonance; and
- the phenomenon of the extraordinary temporality of musical experience.

Music requires the material nature of the world; at the same time, it requires the psychological, mental and emotional abilities of man, and it requires very complex patterns of time and rhythm, not just to fill them with sound, but to reach beyond our common patterns of experience.

There is another astonishing aspect connected with music:

If you intuitively sing a song or just a little melody, you are at the same time the creator, the actor, the interpreter, the instrument and the listener of your song or melody. The borders of subject and object are transcended and the common logic of production and reception does not work any longer.

In order to understand musical experience, it is necessary to go beyond the separations of creator, actor, interpreter and listener. This is true not only in relation to music, but also to theatre, opera and the performing arts as a whole. Music and arts are manifestations of the spirit floating into and floated by material concreteness. They point to areas of human expressiveness and receptiveness, which do not only touch man's rationality, desire and belief, but break them up, deepen and sometimes even shatter them.

If we speak about music, we must turn around and change the perspective: From the registration and description of objective facts on the one hand or pure individual emotions on the other hand, to the reflection of what happens through musical enactments, within a person as well as inter- and transpersonally, and also recognizing the idea or the genius of each composition.

3 Music and Brain, Music and Body

Recently, the relation between music, brain and body has become subject of intensive research. The focus was directed towards the complexity of multisensory processes (Engel et al. 2011), as well as to the question of how far one can understand the brain of a musician as a model of neuroplasticity (Münte et al. 2002). Multiple effects connected with performance and perception of music were shown to resemble the relation between repetition and memory effects for duration (Wiener and Thompson 2015) as well as the response of the auditory brain system at the detection limit (Lütkenhöner and Seither-Preisler 2008). These examples make it clear that listening to music is a highly complex activity that involves a wide range of neural subsets.

When we are listening to music, we convert the vibrations of the air reaching our ears in several steps. At first, we convert them into mechanical movements of the organic structure of the middle ear. Then we convert these beats into moving waves of the liquid within the internal ear, and afterwards these liquid motions are converted into neuronal pulses of energy within the central nervous system. At the end of these transformative motions, there stands the conscious experience of music and the cognition: "I hear music!" (Kapteina 2001)

It is very interesting to see that "differences between certain pieces of music [are not only recognized] in the upper, cortical regions [of the brain], but even earlier in deeper regions, where several systems of activation of musical motions are supposed" (Kapteina 2001:4–5). With these deeper regions, Kapteina addresses the limbic system or the formatio reticularis of the brain stem.

When someone listens to music, the neuronal pulses are initially converted within the brain stem. On this level, music has not yet reached our consciousness. This happens afterwards, when the stimuli reach the auditory centre and other areas within the frontal cortex of the brain.

Kapteina points out: "The most important finding of musico-psychological brain research during the last decade says: Before we become aware of music, before we convert music within the hemispheres of our cerebrum, before we can think about, judge, criticize, enjoy or reject what we are listening to, a totally diverse program has already happened unconsciously, based on the Limbic System. [...] Here we also find the neuronal connections that allow us the experience of emotions, and last but not least, this is where there is a direct connection to the areas of the long-term memory" (Kapteina 2001:5). In addition to this, we can observe hormonal reactions connected with this first area of converting neuronal musical pulses within the brain stem, for example endorphins (Dunbar et al. 2012), the so called happiness hormones, which are also produced when eating or playing sports or having sex or consuming drugs and so on.

Concerning the following considerations about the structures of 'creditions' and about music as a catalytic medium of exploring these structures, it is highly important to see that there is not just one region of musical experience within the brain. Music is activating several regions of the brain, both the brain stem and the cerebrum; both the right and the left hemisphere of the brain and obviously even Broca's area, one of the speech areas which influences both cognitions *and* emotions (Fadiga et al. 2009). "It might seem strange, but from a neuroscientist point of view it is evident that the most useless effort man has ever been able to fulfil – and doubtlessly this is spontaneous and unconcerned singing – shows the greatest benefit for the development of the brain (of children)" (see Hüther 2015). There are many explorations concerning the abilities of hearing, the physiological basics of musical experience and the neuronal abilities of the brain stem within the last 20 years. They all converge on the conclusion that music is one of the strongest stimulations of emotional and personal dynamics (Panksepp and Bernatzky 2002). Music is able to influence learning and education, mind and memory, health and social as well as spiritual abilities on a very high level.

4 Singing – Medicine Against Fear and Medium of Belief in Ritual Contexts

Now let us focus on one certain aspect of musical experience: It is evident throughout the history of singing in every culture that it is an effective way to reduce fear and to reach a strong inner feeling of self-efficacy and reassurance. To illustrate this,

I choose the phenomenon of lullaby-songs, and with this example we reach the field of 'creditions' in musical and ritual contexts. Mothers, fathers, grandmothers and other persons sing lullabies to babies and young children in order to get them to sleep and to manage the transition from the alertness of the day to the darkness embodying the uncertainty and danger of the night. Children ask questions that sometimes are not easy to answer: "Is the night dangerous? Who cares for me if everyone is sleeping? Will I wake up healthy tomorrow?", and so on. Lullabies give answers to these questions in the shape of sung beliefs, which are very effective on various bodily and mental levels, both consciously and unconsciously.

The elementary form of a lullaby reveals the wonder of music in a very clear dimension:

Music is able to touch a person in the very intimate zones of the heart or the soul beyond any fixed access. Music can move the body and spirit beyond order and arbitrariness. Music produces a secret agreement between singer and listener; an 'auditory picture' of another side of being, of another dimension of time; an 'auditive picture' which at an instant breaks through our finite life.

The belief or 'credition' experienced by a lullaby cannot be expressed in any other way. "The night is peaceful. The darkness cares for you. You will sleep in security and peace." – No one can guarantee that these propositions are true. But singing them in the way of a lullaby is convincing body, soul and spirit: "Yes, I believe it because as you are singing it for me; I cannot object."

Other examples concerning music as a medium of belief or 'credition' can be found within many traditions of religious worship. What is a liturgy without music and singing, for example in Jewish or Christian life? It would be very poor and miserable. One of the great Jewish scholars of the twentieth century, Abraham Joshua Heschel, has said: "Man is the cantor/singer of the universe […]. Singing means to feel and to confirm that the spirit is real and the glory and delightfulness (of God) is present within the world" (Heschel 1985:196). Within the context of worship, 'ritual singing' opens a special form of symbolic experience. It allows an entrance into the world of belief, which primarily is an auditive world. Singing and playing music allow for a deeper and more intense listening than any other modes of communication. Martin Luther, the great sixteenth century reformer, said:

"If they don't sing it, they don't believe it" (Harnoncourt 2009:21). And therefore, Luther emphasized congregational singing of chorals both within and outside the liturgy. Liturgical singing is able to transform reality, to go beyond everyday experience, to perform and to anticipate a hopeful life and future. This is valid not just within the Lutheran traditions, but within every liturgical tradition: The "sounding body of the word" – as it was called by Godehard Joppich (Behrendt 2012:377) is the main medium of liturgical communication. Worship lives and unfolds through the musically-sounding word which expresses belief, prayer, praise and testimony in a unique way.

Of course this is not only true with regard to religious belief or to peaceful and calm music, but also to ecstatic and chaotic music, which in the worst case can lead to violence and destruction. Music and singing are able to become means of transport of any kind of collective beliefs including political ideologies.[1]

5 Artificial Music – Transcending Consciousness and Imagining a Different World

But let us now turn to another question: What about artificial music and its transcending power? Artificial music brings us to areas of a different world, like a birdcall or a promise or a cry that disturbs and interrupts our everyday business. It probably encases us with a utopian possibility of life. Artificial music does so by moving and touching us in our bodily, psychological, emotional and mental dimensions, which are nearly immaterial, but do so with the highest effectiveness. It touches us in the totality of our personal being and motion.

This happens when we listen to music, and it happens even more intensely if we are singing or playing music.

There are lots of examples which show that playing music itself is seen not only as a process of 'production' or self-activity, but also as a process of perception; this dual-form process is connected with the experience that music streams from an inapprehensible source, through the body and the mind of the musician. Olivier Messiaen, one of the greatest musicians and composers of the twentieth century, once said:

"The more the notes are pushing and knocking at our inner ear and the more this colourful chaos moves and disturbs us, the more intensely we notice the contrast or the connection to another reality: so strong, that our closest, deepest, innermost 'Me' is transformed and affiliated with a higher truth, which we never could hope to reach for …" (Bubmann (1993:106) Let me just quote another testimony of the transcending power of artificial music. The pianist Lars Vogt expresses his experience of a certain passage of a sonata for piano from Ludwig van Beethoven with the following words: "This is the moment, which grants me the certainty (and not just the assumption), that there is a higher power than what we experience in this life. It is the moment of insight, of revelation. At this point you can't explain any more […] and after this tremendousness we very slowly get back to normality; the first flourish after minutes of pianissimo is like an embracement of the whole world and a thanks for a glimpse into eternity" (see Vogt 2001).

[1] As one important example, musical propaganda was an important factor in the Nazi-regime during the Second World War.

6 Music and 'Creditions'

Music is one of the strongest media of personal motion and belief. It can be as strong as death – a dictum which is usually dedicated to love (see the Biblical Song of Solomon 8:6, which says, "The passion of love bursting into flame is more powerful than death, stronger than the grave"). Loving or dying with a song on the lips is not just an exotic cultural custom, but the attestation of personal belief or existential conviction of life even in the moment of death.

Now we have arrived at the very point where we can consider some aspects of music and 'creditions', or more precisely, some aspects of how physiological and phenomenological research in music can contribute to important questions in order to explore the structure of 'creditions'.

Instructed by musical experience, I would say that 'credition' should be understood as a coherent cluster of affirmations including emotional, cognitive, volitional, bodily and sensitive-esthetical motions, including unconscious and conscious aspects.

Several regions of the brain (the brain stem, the left and the right hemisphere of the cortex, and so on) as well as other bodily processes are involved in the act of 'credition'. It is a complex act of personal motion, i.e., a personal act that exists and communicates between basic acts of emotional feeling, sensitive recognition, and spontaneous reflexes and reactions, as well as with personal acts of a higher level.

Without 'creditions' the higher abilities like argumentation, dialogue and discourse, cultural and artistic processes, creativity, science and technics, social skills and interpersonal interactions would not be possible. Such higher abilities are only possible within the fields of coherent personal affirmations, which constitute a stable network of communication; and – as I have already emphasised – they solely work under inclusion of emotional, volitional, bodily, cognitive and sensitive-aesthetic components.

In addition, all these higher activities are connected with and produce similar clusters of affirmations, i.e., new fields of 'creditions'. Culture, science, arts, ethics, and all manner of humanity's functions may proceed from relatively less to relatively greater complexity of 'creditions'. New aspects or fields of complex affirmations modify the landscapes of our mind, the horizon of spirit and rationality, of desire and human practice throughout history.

New stages of knowledge and science open new fields of 'creditions'. Both are not exclusive, but rather inclusive of each other. All attempts to exclude them alternately must fail. Liquid 'creditions' and liquid rationality are two sides of the same coin; that is, human evolution and civilisation including all dimensions of personality and social life.

Music constitutes an immediate expression of 'credition', a transpersonal and in many cases even a transcultural medium of motion and belief in the described way. Music and singing are catalytic media of 'creditions' *par excellence*. Interdisciplinary research in music and singing will detect more and important parameters that can help us to advance the theory of 'creditions'.

References

Altenmüller E, Kopiez R (2013) Starke Emotionen und Gänsehaut beim Musikhören: Evolutionäre und musikpsychologische Aspekte. In: 16. Multidisziplinäres Kolloquium der GEERS-Stiftung 2012 in Berlin; Zeitschrift für Audiologie/Audiological Acoustics, Sonderheft 1(19):51–58

Bubmann P (1993) Menschenfreundliche Musik. Politische, therapeutische und religiöse Aspekte des Musikerlebens. Chr. Kaiser, Gütersloh

Dunbar RIM et al (2012) Performance of music elevates pain threshold and positive affect: implications for the evolutionary function of music. Evol Psychol 10(4):688–702. www.epjournal.net

Engel AK, Senkowski D, Schneider TR (2011) Multisensory integration through neural coherence. In: Murray MM, Wallace MT (eds) The neural bases of multisensory processes. CRC Press, Abingdon

Fadiga L, Craighero L, D'Ausilioa A (2009) Broca's area in language, action, and music. The neurosciences and music III – disorders and plasticity. Ann N Y Acad Sci 1169:448–458

Finnegan R (2012) Oral literature in Africa, World oral literature series, vol 1. Open Book Publishers, Cambridge, pp 236–241

Harnoncourt P (2009) "... so sie's nicht singen, so gleuben sie's nicht" – Das gilt heute wie vor 50 und vor 500 Jahren! In: Prassl FK, Tarlinski P (eds) Bene Cantate ei. Festschrift 50 Jahre IAH, IAH-Bulletin 37. Selbstverl, Graz, pp 21–36

Heschel AJ (1985) Die ungesicherte Freiheit. Essays zur menschlichen Existenz. Neukirchener Verlag, Neukirchen-Vluyn

Hüther G (2015) http://www.gerald-huether.de/populaer/veroeffentlichungen-von-gerald-huether/texte/singen-gerald-huether/index.php. Accessed 8 July 2015

Inga B (2012) Gregorianischer Choral als "Klangleib des Wortes". Zum 80. Geburtstag von Godehard Joppich. In: Musica Sacra 132 (2012) Heft 6, p 377

Kapteina H (2001) Was geschieht, wenn wir Musik hören. Fragmente zur Psychologie des Hörens. http://www.musiktherapie.uni-siegen.de/kapteina/material/forschungsgebiete/neu_was_geschieht_wenn_¬wir_musik_hoeren.pdf. Accessed 21 Nov 2013

Lütkenhöner B, Seither-Preisler A (2008) Auditory brainstem response at the detection limit. J Assoc Res Otolaryngol 9(4):521–531. doi:10.1007/s10162-008-0131-1. Epub 2008 Aug 14. PMID: 18704580

Münte TF, Altenmüller E, Jäncke L (2002) The musicians's brain as a model of neuroplasticity. Nat Rev Neurosci 3(6):473–478. Review

Panksepp J, Bernatzky G (2002) Emotional sounds and the brain. The neuro-affective foundations of musical appreciation. Behav Process 60:133–155

Rushdie S (2000) The ground beneath her feet. London

Vogt L (2001) About Beethovens sonata for piano, op. 111. http://www.larsvogt.de/Uber_Musik.html. Accessed 15 Aug 2013

Wiener M, Thompson JC (2015) Repetition enhancement and memory effects for duration. NeuroImage 113:268–278

Part V
Social Sciences

Reconciliation After a Protracted Violent Conflict: Do Believing Processes Play a Role, and Which One? A Research Agenda

Joseph Marko

Abstract Twenty years after the conclusion of the Dayton Peace Agreement, the conflict between Bosnia and Herzegovina is still a prime example of the difficulties and challenges of reconstructing and reconciling deeply divided societies after protracted violent conflict, especially with ongoing ethnic mobilization of the population in the educational and political system. At the same time, there are ongoing theoretical battles between proponents and adversaries of the ethnic power-sharing system established by the Dayton constitution, as well as between methodologically individualist and neo-institutionalist approaches in the social sciences on how to understand and explain the phenomenon of "ethnicity." This chapter, therefore, tries to make use of credition theory in order to focus on the functions which "processes of believing" can play in the political mobilization of "ethnicity" and thereby to contribute to a better conceptualization for further research with regard to "ethnic" conflict and reconciliation.

1 Introduction: Problems of Re-construction and Reconciliation After Violent Conflict

As I have tried to demonstrate at some length elsewhere (Marko 2013a, b), all the efforts of state- and nation-building in Bosnia-Herzegovina (BiH) undertaken by various internal and external actors have led to nothing but a "defective democracy" and "failed state." Alhough political commentators and analysts do not disagree about this fact, they do have different opinions about whether BiH is therefore at the brink of collapse or, on the contrary, whether this state of affairs is a relatively stable political arrangement even for the long run. Based on conclusions of empirical studies of elections and the functioning of the party system as well as legal studies on jurisprudence, we can state that re-construction of the war-torn state and economy as well as reconciliation of society in BiH does not work on the basis of the

J. Marko (✉)
Institute of Public Law and Political Sciences, University of Graz, Graz, Austria
e-mail: josef.marko@uni-graz.at

H.-F. Angel et al. (eds.), *Processes of Believing: The Acquisition, Maintenance, and Change in Creditions*, New Approaches to the Scientific Study of Religion 1,
DOI 10.1007/978-3-319-50924-2_24

power-sharing system between the so-called "constituent peoples" of Bosniacs, Serbs, and Croats, established with the Dayton Peace Agreement in 1995. All efforts of reconciliation through international and national criminal jurisprudence – due to the genocide in Srebrenica and many war crimes committed during the war between 1992 and 1995 have failed to convince people on the ground that it is possible to live together in a common state, let alone to cooperate for a common future within the larger framework of EU integration.

Twenty years after the end of violent conflict, political mobilization along "ethnic" lines is still ongoing in the post-conflict phase. Thus, the question that must be posed is, "When does post-conflict all of a sudden turn into pre-conflict again?" To this very day, there is an institutionally segregated educational system with so-called "two schools under one roof", originally "invented" by the OSCE as tool for reconciliation. In addition, there are ethnically-biased school curricula. Moreover, the entire public as well as private media system is ethnically segregated, and additionally, there are no multi-ethnic NGO's operating in the entire territory of BiH. It can thus be no surprise that the assumptions made by Arend Lijphart, a political scientist that advocates power-sharing, about the functioning of a power-sharing system (namely, that power-sharing will lead first to inter-ethnic cooperation of elites which might then spill over to the mass level) does not work in BiH. Instead, what we can see in place is what I call a "negative" elite consensus of "divide and rule" the respective ethnic segments of society through "capture" of the respective state institutions which are ethnically predetermined by law as "possession" of one of the three constituent peoples. This ethnic predetermination and "state capture" by the leaders of mono-ethnic parties then leads to a vicious circle of legislative and executive "obstruction" of necessary reforms for EU membership which can, however, be rationally defended by the party leaders, forming in reality a predatory political cartel of power. This resulting cartel can then claim that they are "defending" the "vital national interests" of the respective ethnic group in order to get constantly re-elected, and thereby democratically legitimized, despite the fact that the standard of living of the population is deteriorating from legislative period to legislative period; at the same time, all media outlets report on wide-spread governmental corruption, through which these leaders get richer and richer.

In conclusion, Milorad Dodik, – "the" political leader in Republika Srpska since 2006 because it does not matter whether he holds the office of Prime Minister or President of the Republic – has announced referenda for secession from BiH almost on a monthly basis since 2011 and even denied that the genocide in Srebrenica constitutes "genocide" as this had been established by international courts. In addition, academics and leading experts in power-sharing and/or human rights protection have criticized the jurisprudence of the European Court of Human Rights (McCrudden and O'Leary 2013), having found that the corporate power-sharing mechanism constitutionally entrenched in BiH violates the right to stand as candidate in elections for every citizen irrespective of his ethnic affiliation as guaranteed by the European Convention on Human Rights.

However, the challenge posed by this state of affairs demonstrates that our social, political, and legal theories on the interplay between state- and nation-building on the one hand, and reconciliation after protracted violent conflict on the other, seem to create the infamous hen-and-egg problem: Does democracy require a functioning state which – in turn – needs a basis in a "collective identity" called "nation"? Is thus a "homogenous national identity" – which obviously does not "exist" in a deeply ethnically divided society – a prerequisite for both state-formation and democracy-building?

Hence, the interdependence of transitional justice (TJ), and state- and nation-building through reconstruction of institutions and reconciliation of ethnically conceived communities, is of particular interest for necessary reconceptualizations. That said, I follow a broader conception of TJ which is not confined to retributive justice, but has to embrace also all issues of restorative justice which, of course, do not necessarily exclude each other. Nevertheless, the "structural" problem of "security" and "stability" versus "justice" as – at least in the short-run – contradictory policy goals must not be underestimated (Leebaw 2008). At the same time, it is clear that in particular, all the goals and means of restorative justice in the "redefined" meaning of reconciliation[1] (Leebaw 2008; Skaar 2012) are intimately interwoven with the problems of what is called state- and nation-building in political science literature about transformation from authoritarian regimes to democratic systems. Such goals and means include healing the pain of victims not only through reparations but also truth-telling and public apologies, the integration of all affected parties into community-level confidence-building measures, instilling trust in the new legal and political system, and finally, through all these means, re-constructing social cohesion.

"Irreconcilable goals" (Leebaw 2008) are also a conceptual issue in this framework. Theoretically, the relationship between peace-building and state-building should be complementary (Call and Cousens 2007). State-building, after the cessation of hostilities, should support the consolidation of peace which is substantially more than the mere absence of violence, i.e. "positive" peace. Of course, state-building for democratic governance does not only require representative legislature and executive functions, but also the establishment of a well-functioning justice system that provides for security by peaceful conflict resolution. Additionally, an effective and equal public service delivery system is needed to provide welfare for all, irrespective of their group membership, so that the state and its institutions gain enough legitimacy again, combined with and based on a feeling of loyalty for the state or even "national" identity of its citizens. It goes without saying that such an "idealist" goal of state- *and* "nation"-building cannot be achieved overnight in a society deeply divided by war and protracted ethnic conflict.

Moreover, it follows from comparative research that state-building will not result in a "revolutionary" process to break away from the old regime to "find" a new political order, but only in a "cosmetic change and create weak, unstable, or even criminal state structures", if peace-making is a compromise with corrupt and

---

[1] This means, according to Leebaw, no longer a "short hand for compromises and bargains with the old regime" as necessary condition to stabilize newly democratizing governments, but "the aspiration for political community based on consent and shared norms" (Leebaw 2008: 98).

predatory elites (Samuels 2009:173). Hence, there are several dilemmas and paradoxes of state- and peace-building such as the short-term imperative to negotiate a ceasefire potentially through a tacit bargain with predatory elites, against the long-term need to build "depersonalised" democratic and effective state institutions, and international intervention in order to foster self-government (Paris and Sisk 2007).

But is it then the function of a newly adopted legal system as it was provided by the Dayton Peace Agreement to not only establish the normative framework for the process of decision-making in the exercise of state power, but also to provide legal rules and principles outlining how to overcome the consequences of the war through state- and nation-building? A "realist" political science approach informed by history will remind us that most constitutions are a political compromise that mirrors the balance of power at the time of drafting. A "positivistic" law approach will then warn that a "constitution" cannot do more than determine the rules of the game. Seen from this perspective, the text of preambles or the declaration of constitutional principles about how to "regain paradise" are mere constitutional rhetoric at best and thus superfluous; and they may also be harmful because they can create expectations that cannot be fulfilled and may therefore lead to disillusionment, fostering bitterness, or even exacerbate conflict.

In stark contrast, an "idealist" perspective of "constitution-building" in the broader sense of rebuilding institutions and creating an institutional culture of democratic governance has to develop new ideas about how to circumvent the paradoxes and dilemmas of state- and peace-building, and to bring about a change in expectations, claims, and behaviour not only of political elites, but also of society at large. Seen from this perspective, a constitution should also perform the function of integration of society and thereby, in the end, also the establishment of "the" state as a political entity. However, this raises even more intricate problems and dilemmas. Linz and Stepan, based on their comparative analysis of transformation processes in South America, Southern Europe and Post-Communist Europe, come to the conclusion that "without a state" – or at least the willingness to live together in a state – "no modern democracy is possible" (Linz and Stepan 1996:17). From this perspective, "constitution-building" in a deeply divided society seems to require state-building first. But, as Sarajlić convincingly argues in a book on the failures of internal as well as external state-building efforts in Bosnia-Herzegovina, "any talk about the state inevitably raises the issue of the nation upon which the state is formed" and "it is this tension that aids political players in rendering almost every political issue in the country as primarily an issue of identity rather than practical politics, economy or something else"[2] He then raises the provocative question for a deeply divided post-conflict society like Bosnia-Herzegovina: "Can there be a state without a nation … by any means of the word?" (Sarajlić 2011:11–13). Does this finally mean for deeply divided societies that, first, nation-building must come before state-building, and that second, there are no other choices for constitutional design than the civic "state-nation" or ethnic "nation-state" based on consociational

[2] I have labelled this phenomenon from my own participatory observations in BiH the "ethnic Midas effect." See Marko 2001:79.

institutional arrangements or, if this fails, the separation of the state along ethnic lines as this is claimed by the political elites in Republika Srpska and supported in parts of Western diplomatic circles?

Moreover, these conceptual and structural problems between state and nation have their analogy in the scholarly battles between "accomodationists" and "integrationists" for the "correct" form of consociationalism or power-sharing devices for post-conflict societies in the tradition of Arend Lijphart and Donald Horowitz (Choudhry 2008) as already indicated above. Accomodationists argue that institutional power-sharing on the basis of elite cooperation and co-existence of separated ethnic groups is all that can be achieved in deeply divided societies, whereas integrationists aim to transcend group antagonisms by mechanisms to cross-cut the ethnic division not only on elite level, but also through cooperation of societal groups around common political goals. They argue with convincing empirical evidence that instances of poorly-designed constitution-building and power-sharing that do not take into account the political context of severely divided societies might even firmly entrench ethnic division instead of triggering moderation and allowing for reconciliation, let alone transcending the divide. Moreover, as we can see from empirical evidence on power-sharing in BiH, there is also the normative and functional dilemma why outside intervention with the short-term goal to end violence shall create long-term "local ownership" through self-government. This creates the danger of a combination of dependency and resistance, provoking in the end renewed conflict, in particular if non-representative, corrupt or even criminal leaders are engaged in power-sharing who are, in reality, not committed to the implementation of the peace settlement, but see it as a "continuation of the war by other means." Hence, constitution-building, including its necessary constitutional amendments to adapt the original institutional mechanisms to the dynamic political context, is bound to fail, unless there is substantial domestic support for reform. In conclusion, "transitional constitutionalism" cannot only be enforced from the outside and from above, but needs "participatory and inclusive" constitution-building, in particular, if compromises with predatory elites had been necessary in the short-term to end the war.

All of these concerns have been addressed also in TJ literature. Both Paige Arthur and Will Kymlicka claim that TJ makes a difference from the classical Latin American cases when identity-based divisions of society come into play. Identity politics or, more specifically with regard to my case study of Bosnia-Herzegovina, ethno-confessional politics present different challenges for TJ efforts (Arthur 2011). Thus, TJ is not only a response to massive and systematic violations of human rights that aims to recognize victims and to prevent the recurrence of abuse, but has to work – after violent conflict and mass atrocities – in the context of "entrenched" identity-based divisions so that the theoretical distinctions between "primordialist", "instrumentalist", or "constructivist" views on ethnic identity formation no longer work in practice. A "neo-primordial", ethnic social reality (Marko 2009) cannot simply be transformed into "crosscutting and civic identities," as this has been suggested for South Africa, for instance, as goal of TJ in terms of broader societal transformation (Arthur 2011:6) and what is also the underlying rationale of

Horowitz's integrationist approach. Insofar, Arthur argues, TJ measures can contribute to the goal of reconciliation as a precondition for preventing ethnic conflict only if they actually address the key factors of ethnic conflict in operation (Arthur 2011).

In line with this argument, Kymlicka underlines the "instrumentalist" function of TJ, which is often described as its "nation-building" dimension. But he immediately highlights the conceptual difficulties when he argues that "…TJ can serve this nation-building function only if the national identity is indeed an inclusive one – if the members of different ethnic groups can see a place for themselves within this new national identity" and he warns: "If not, nation building can simply exacerbate the problem" (Kymlicka 2011:304), which has been the case with BiH. So what? Kymlicka thus argues for a "different sort of nation-building" which he calls "pluricultural" or "multination building", but the challenge for TJ with his conception of a "multinational federation" is not very different as he, I think rightly, argues: "The key challenge here … is to prevent TJ from being captured by, and subordinated to, the dynamics of ethnonational contestation" by "consensus and dialogue … on innovative forms of TJ that are endorsable by all parties despite their differing views of sovereignty." However, he sceptically continues: "… appealing to an ethos of consensus and of creative ambiguity over sovereignty as the basis for an effective TJ is putting the cart before the horse. … If a climate of trust and consensus across ethnonational lines had already existed in countries like Sudan, Iraq, Indonesia, Bosnia, or Sri Lanka, they would not have undergone years or decades of ethnonational civil war." In the end, he thus concludes: "All we can safely say at this point is that all the options require us to radically and creatively rethink current assumptions about how TJ relates to state legitimacy and nationhood" (Kymlicka:329–333).

In conclusion, we need much more basic research in terms of theoretical reflection and reconceptualization of collective identity formation and the social organization of groupings to be able to "creatively rethink" these problems of reconciliation. The book *Understanding Ethnic Violence* suggests that an "emotion-based approach to ethnic conflict", signifying, fear, hatred, and resentment as decisive causal factors in terms of "action tendencies" results in the individual preparing to change the environment. Fear, in this approach, prepares the individual to enact safety concerns with regard to "security dilemmas"; hatred prepares the individual to act on historical grievance; and resentment prepares the individual to address status/self-esteem discrepancies (Petersen 2002).

It goes without saying that all of these factors have played an important role in the processes of political mobilization of "ethnicity" leading to the dissolution of former Yugoslavia in 1991 and the following wars in the Balkans as I have tried to demonstrate elsewhere (Marko 2009). However, what is not clear until now is the interplay between these factors, in particular, why the "economic" interests of the Republics of Slovenia and Croatia became so easily re-interpreted and transformed into national "identity" politics of these Republics against the poor Southern republics and provinces, in particular Montenegro and Kosovo as part of Serbia, and why people were ready in the end to "believe" in a "security" problem triggering the "readiness" to use violence? Hence, how exactly does the interplay between cognition and emotion work in such a process? Obviously, two interdependent concepts require much more attention for empirical research: First, the concept of "ethnicity" and, second, to what extend people "believe" that their neighbors whom they are now ready to kill must be "seen" as the "enemy" because he/she seems to belong to another "ethnic," and therefore "dangerous," group. Is thus a "process of believing", theoretically already labelled as "credition" (Angel 2006, 2013; Seitz and Angel 2012), the "missing link" between the concepts of cognition and emotion so that they cannot be seen any longer as "independent" or even mutually exclusive elements in what is termed "rational" behaviour? Is not the "belief" in the "reality" of "ethnicity" and "ethnic belonging" the main obstacle in all efforts of state reconstruction and reconciliation, not only underlying legal and political theories of democratic power-sharing, but at the same time also guaranteeing the "stability" of the "hybrid regime" in BiH? Let us examine these issues.

2 Three Conceptulizations of "Ethnicity" and the Pitfalls of Political and Legal Theory

The first thing to consider is that social philosophy and political theory have not yet resolved the debate about whether we have to take the vantage points of Hobbes, Locke, or Kant to see how we could get from "civil" war within polities and "anarchy" between states to global governance and "eternal peace" and – at every critical juncture of history – how we can prevent a "return of history"? (Wendt 1999; Behr 2014) Or to phrase the same problem in another way: Can we dare to raise the question of how to turn a vicious cycle into a virtuous cycle without the immediate response of (neo-)"realists" in all academic disciplines that this is "utopian", i.e. wishful thinking at best but in "reality" something causing too often more harm than good for the particular "community," so that the old Roman saying *"si vis pacem, para bellum"* holds true until the very day?

Second, the so-called "Böckenförde dilemma"[3] - arguing that the liberal, secular state is based on (cultural) preconditions whose existence it cannot guarantee itself – (Böckenförde 1976) does haunt all social theories as long as the confusion of epistemology and ontology is not disentangled; we must not ask why "the" modern, secular state "is not able" to produce (any longer) the necessary trust and solidarity among citizens, let alone vis-à-vis "strangers." Phrasing the question in such a way, the "answer" offered by Böckenförde is already hidden in his "dilemma" in the form of a *petitio principii* based on the axiomatic premise of modernity, i.e. secularism: Hence, it must appear as if only "pre-political" homogenous language groups and/or religious "communities", in short "ethnic" groups, can produce trust and solidarity. Therefore, we must reformulate the Böckenförde dilemma in order to be able to "understand" its hidden ideological prescription: Why "shall" (!) trust and solidarity as allegedly necessary "feelings" for "cultural homogeneity", state

[3] "Der freiheitliche, säkulare Staat lebt von Voraussetzungen, die er nicht garantieren kann."

formation and "norm compliance" come only from "pre-existing" language groups or religious "communities" so that solidarity vis-à-vis strangers seems to be impossible?

The answer to this riddle must lay in the de-construction of the legacies of ancient Greek philosophy determining our ways of thinking about "Otherness" and "difference". The so-called Böckenförde dilemma is nothing but a "reification" of the triadic social relation of identity: equality – solidarity which is deeply embedded in Aristotle's political theory about the Athenian polity as a "closed system" in which equality and solidarity are seen as possible only between "equals", i.e. those enjoying the status of citizens and thereby excluding all others also living in the city-state, namely women, metics (foreign merchants), and slaves. With this thought "model" as vantage point, there would indeed be no way out of the "inescapable conflict between man and citizen" (Canovan 1996), i.e. (universal) human rights and citizens' rights granted only to members in a closed, i.e. "ethnic" polity. Thus, there could be no understanding of the "duality" of institutional "structures," not only in constraining actions but also (re-)creating *and* possibly transforming them so that the model of the modern democratic "nation-state," legally requiring and morally postulating equality and solidarity only among citizens, need not remain the "end of history" (F. Fukuyama). Ideally, such understanding would allow for the (re-)conceptualization of social ordering, including trust and solidarity among strangers, and transnational or cosmopolitan law-making beyond "existing" nations and states.

As I try to critically analyze in detail elsewhere (Marko 2017), the red thread running through all the variations of the ideologies of "classic", biological racism and the "differentialist" racism of right-wing extremist parties in Europe, of "ethnic" versus "civic"- liberal nationalism in the tradition of Hans Kohn, and of "individualistic" versus "communitarian" liberalism is a "meta-theory" of identitarianism (Malesević 1995). Within this "meta-theory," "identity" – be it the identity of "the" individual or "the" nation or "the" state – is conceived as pre-political "quality" or "essence" in strict separation from politics as process, so that all conceptualizations and theories of how to conceive, construct and create the "unity" of social, cultural or political "entities" remain trapped in either/or categorizations. Insofar the "deep" structure (Chomsky) of monistic *and* dualistic "models" of state, law and society "is" the same and remains trapped in the legacy of the bivalent structure of Aristotelian logics, the laws of identity, non-contradiction and the axiomatic conclusion of *tertium non datur*. Hence, basic divisions in social and legal theory follow from the dichotomic conceptions of monist/dualist versus pluralist theories.

However, as we know from human history, not every encounter between human beings can have started with a fight for survival as theorists like Carl Schmitt and Thomas Hobbes want us to believe with their definition of politics as friend-versus-foe antagonism in the "natural" state of affairs as *bellum omnia contra omnes*. Nor does every encounter – as we know from everyday practical experience – start as a love story. As a consequence, against all Hobbsian "realism" and methodologically individualist approaches in the social sciences, we must turn to an alternative which views the relationship between identity, equality, and solidarity from a constructivist and historic *as well as* sociological institutionalist perspective. This view no longer reifies trust and solidarity as if they were emotions in the form of specific psychological properties of individuals which they can "have" only in relation to their "family" members in the extended sense of fellow-citizens but never in relation to "strangers" which cause "fear", as anthropological "theories" want make us "believe" to be a universal "natural" phenomenon.[4]

This is now the place to ask for the added value which a new cognitive- and neuro-science-based theory of "credition" in terms of processes of "believing" might bring for understanding processes of "ethnification" of socio-cultural relations in pre-conflict phases and to "design" the framework conditions for successful "de-ethnification" as prerequisite for reconciliation in post-conflict phases.

In summarizing the elements of credition theory developed by Angel (2013), Seitz and Angel (2012), and Sugiura et al. (2015), we can state the following:

Believing is a self-organizing process composed of cognitive and emotional elements whereby new information from actions or the situation in the outside world is transformed into "perceptions" of objects or about persons due to the "attention" given to the respective phenomenon because of a "selection" among myriads of bits of information coming from the outside through the sensory system. This selection procedure is based on "personal relevance" on the basis of previously stored information, i.e. personal "memory", combined with a personal value matrix stemming from one's emotional states. In short, "believing" is thus an act of generating and maintaining a mental construct in terms of mental "representations" of self, other, and the environment as "real" or "true" forming a "cognitive space" or "disposition" in terms of readiness for action.

This framework concept of credition is based on four major functions:

- The enclosure function, which integrates different contents of information into a coherent set of knowledge thus conceived as "real" or "true";
- the converter function, which denotes the relationship between a specific belief and specific range of behavior (for instance: "danger"- "rescue");
- the modulator function, which highlights the influence of the individual state of cognitive and or emotional development as "space for action"; and
- the stabilizer function, which stabilizes beliefs into more long-lasting "values" and "attitudes" despite of changes in the environment.

Moreover, credition theory perceives that processes of believing take place at three analytically distinct levels which form a "nested" hierarchy:

- At the individual, physical level, "self-agency" is conceptualized as the association of motor action and its feedback sensation. In addition, the physical schema also considers the accommodation of one's own motor action and the perception of others' actions.

[4] I have critically analyzed this sort of anthropological "evidence" in Marko (1995:77–81) and demonstrated how "fear" as universal category can be and is misused to transform the "Other" into scapegoats for each and everything.

- At the interpersonal level, one's actions, which are directed towards other persons and the perception of others' response, are associated. This schema allows the conceptualization of social relationships between the self and others.
- At the collective level, the social-value schema associates one's behavior and the perception of the social evaluation by others responding to this behavior. This schema is concerned with the (social) self-concept, the context-specific self-value and social role.

How can we now make use of credition theory for a better understanding of the phenomenon of "ethnicity" in phases before and after violent (ethnic) conflict and the battles of interpretation in social, political, and legal theory over the "best" response to "ethnicity" or even how to "resolve" ethnic conflict?

The ideologies of ethno-nationalism and "primordial" social theories of "ethnicity" will tell us that "ethnicity" is based on the "common origin" of people in terms of "biological descent" called "kinship" or other forms of allegedly "natural" relationship as can be seen from Samuel Huntington's reasoning in his infamous book on the "Clash of Civilizations" when he argues: "In class and ideological conflicts the key question was 'Which side are you on?' and people could and did choose sides and change sides. In conflicts between civilizations, the question is: 'What are you?' That is a given that cannot be changed" (Huntington 1993:35–6). As a consequence, this form of "ethnic determinism" denies the possibility of changing your "ethnicity," so that "ethnic difference" can be "seen" as root-cause of conflict which would allow for peace-keeping, if that is possible at all, only through separation and segregation of territory or people in the forms of secession and/or "voluntary" population transfer before the outbreak or in the aftermath of violent conflict.

In striking contrast, more or less radical social constructivist theories will tell us that "ethnicity", for example, is nothing but the same wrong "belief" people held until very recently that red-haired women are, by definition, possessed with "witchcraft" with red hairs as "objective" marker of this capacity. In conclusion, they argue that we simply have to recognize that ethnicity as a "mental construct" is a false "belief" and to stop "believing" in such inaccurate "mental representations." As long as this is not achieved, the theory will tell us, "ethnic" entrepreneurs – be they political, economic, or cultural elites – will be able to (mis)use these beliefs as an instrument for satisfying their personal goals.

However, such a "constructivist-instrumental" approach in defining the "meaning" of the term and concept of "ethnicity" cannot answer two, interrelated questions: First, what causes people to "believe" in a concept against their own "interests" so that they – as we have argued above with regard to BiH as a form of "defective democracy" – reelect political leaders again and again who get richer and richer whereas, at the same time, they got poorer and poorer? Second, why does it not work to simply "de-construct" the concept of "ethnicity" in deeply divided societies by revealing the "belief" as "false consciousness," and start telling people that they simply have to stop perceiving each and everything in the outside world through an "ethnic lens," having been called the "ethnic" Midas-effect by me?

Hence, in contrast to all individualistic-liberal theories (based on the assumption of pre-given identities, and thus agencies of "persons" assembled like balls on a billboard for a game called "society") and communitarian theories (which assume that individual behavior is structurally "embedded" in the culture of an a priori given "community"), the axiomatic assumption of the neo-institutionalist approach presented here lies in a different "social fact". This social fact is that interaction and social relations, i.e. the formation of various kinds of "groupings", are always "embedded" in a "situative context," so that interactions in "situations" – not "individuals" with pre-given identities nor pre-given "communities" – are the basic units of analysis whereby "meaning-in-action" is created through speech acts over "norm contestation" (Searle 2010; Wiener 2014).

Following from the constructivist and interpretative turn in the social sciences, the starting point for any social analysis from this perspective must be the insight that *diversity* and *difference* are *not synonymous,* and thus, *not* identical terms. The various "diversities" among individual human beings with regard to sex, age, or "ethnicity" etc. are an only seemingly "obvious fact" according to which we "believe" to "observe" these diversities. Simultaneously, however, we suppress and thereby hide the fact that we could "discriminate" between individuals and myriads of their "elements" also in many other ways and not only with reference to any of those "imagined" *categories* (such as "ethnicity"). Accordingly, unlike the indeed "brute fact" of "diversity", "difference" can never "be" a "natural" property, but must be "constructed" from the perspective of a specific event or situation which forces us to make a "selection" among possible "pattern variables" on the basis of categorizations; this thereby enables us to give "meaning" to the situation through self-perception and the perception of "other," as this is also conceptualized by the elements of credition theory summarized above.

In line with credition theory, a neo-institutionalist approach must also – against all contestations between methodological individualism and holism in the social sciences (Moses and Knutsen 2012) – analytically distinguish between the *three* levels of subjective, inter-subjective, and collective intentionality and action (Searle 2010).

At the "subjective" and thus "intrinsic" level where actors and their intentions – which cannot be directly "observed" – do play a decisive role for interaction and the establishment of social relations, an actor's "understanding" of his or her position in a situation will thus not only depend on his or her mental and physical abilities, but also social capacities stemming from previous experiences and social learning processes, such as acquiring the capacity to use a "language." Thus, more or less habitualized *dispositions* in the form of internalized "social beliefs", stipulating rules and roles for living in groups, and the *perceptions* he or she already has, for instance in the form of prejudices.

Hence, the formation of personal and social "identity" must not be "perceived" as mutually excluding each other in the sense that "society" or other "institutionalized relations" such as family, "the" group etc. is – by definition – constraining the exercise of "free will", but personal and social identity formation are complementary. It is this "duality of structure and agency" (Giddens 1976) which allows us to recognize – i.e. to "imagine" and to "perceive" and not to "discover" (Searle 2010:105) – the interplay of the *reciprocal perception* and thus necessary "*recognition*" in the meaning of "acceptance" of self and other creating the notion of self as "I and me" (Mead 1967:196). Only this form of "mutual recognition" is providing the "sense" of "autonomy" and "distinctiveness" of identity *and/or* "belonging" (Massey and Abu-Baker 2010), as "disposition" for the possibility of communication since individual intentions together with perceptions about others' intentions are not sufficient for cooperation among people (Searle 2010), nor – I would like to add in our context of conflict prevention – to trigger violent behavior. Hence, following Petersen's approach with regard to fear, hatred and resentment as *necessary* factors for violent conflict (Petersen 2002), we must ask – in line with credition theory – where and how these alleged "emotional" factors come into play in addition to the cognitive elements?

Against the "primordialist" reification of emotions as "intrinsic properties of individuals", I would like to argue that the "emotional" components come into play already in the association of the subjective and intersubjective level through processes of *categorization* and *stereotyping* of self and other which necessarily include an evaluative, i.e. *normative*, assessment along the lines of "good/bad" for something. Hence, dispositions and perceptions are not simply modes of processing empirical information about an event as "situational context" through the sensory apparatus, but they necessarily also include normative assessments through a "selection" procedure producing "attention" to the phenomenon under observation.

This requires, first, that we have constructed or construct "categories" in our heads by "imagination" and "signification" which are part of what Searle calls the "human capacity for collective intentionality" and the possibility to impose "status functions" on others (Searle 2010:43; 59). Hence, what we "recognize" through observation with our biological sensory organs must already have a "name", be it an x-element in quantum physics having been sought after for decades and now "discovered" through a new experiment or be it imagined such as "ethnic difference".

Already the process of the construction of categories is thus both imaginative and normative in terms of "ordering" subjects/objects along the binary code of similarity/difference and good/bad for, i.e. functional/dysfunctional, when constructing a model of "entity"/"quality", i.e. a social "category" such as race, class, gender, or ethnicity. In social relationships, however, we frequently confuse good/bad for the performance of something with good/bad, such as an ethical or moral judgement about persons, groups, and the use of things, which becomes institutionally formalized into law and thereby transformed into the binary code legal/illegal.

Hence, against both Marxist as well as liberal assumptions, and in contrast to all ideologically inspired "naturalizations" of cultural diversity, we must be aware that we construct social, political and legal categories such as "race", "ethnicity", "gender", etc. through three analytically distinct though, in practice, simultaneous and thus inseparable steps:

- On the *epistemological* level, we have to make a choice based on the binary code of similarity/difference, which we combine with
- the *normative* level, where we have to make a choice based on the binary code of equality/inequality to give either similarity or difference valence so that

- we make, on the *empirical* level, a choice based on the binary code of inclusion/ exclusion.

Of course, the colour of my skin is an objective, "biological" factor. But, first and above all, it is a *normative* decision to give exactly that factor personal "relevance" for social and political behaviour based on an "evaluative appraisal" which creates "belief" as "cognitive faculty" and "desire" as "volitional faculty" formed by both "perceptional memory" and future-oriented "prior intentions" (Searle 2010:59, 41). Hence, already at this "abstract" epistemological level, we must recognize that the creation of perceptions requires not only "value-neutral" information processing, but also a normative "assessment" on the basis of the "value"-dichotomy equality/ inequality "of" and "for" and cannot be reduced to 'biological', 'anthropological' or 'psychological' predetermination of "individual" identities. Second, in defining a 'people' or 'nation' by so-called objective markers such as language or religious denomination, one again has to make a decision that a particular cultural marker out of a plurality of such markers *shall be* the 'common' characteristic to be found in a certain number of people, thereby constructing a 'category' and not a 'group' in the sociological sense. Hence, it is a normative decision and not an empirical fact that the characteristics that people have 'in common' constitute a particular people or nation in our "imagination" so that the alleged identity of 'common' characteristics is nothing else but the normative concept of equality with the demand to treat individuals with those ascribed 'common' characteristics equally.

However, ethnicity has no 'substantial' content or meaning, as I have demonstrated elsewhere through an analysis of all theories of nationalism and ethnicity (Marko 2017), but is "representing" the *dichotomisation* of group relations in line with credition theory into a "societal configuration" of an "us-versus-them" mindset as we will demonstrate below with the example of the process of dissolution of former Yugoslavia. In line with the enclosure and converter functions postulated by credition theory, 'ethnicity' is thus not an inherent, 'natural' trait or 'essential property' of people(s) or territories, but a *structural code* with the political *function* of *exclusion or inclusion*. And it is the political function of 'nationalism' as an ideology, be it ethnic or civic, to 'camouflage' these normative decisions in the social construction of political 'unity'. By pretending the existence of 'natural' characteristics, power relations are concealed, legitimised and, at the same time, immunised against critique.

Thus, very often, fear or hatred of others are also wrongly conceptualized, as when conceived as universal intrinsic, emotional properties of all human beings without recognizing that such an "essentializing" psychological approach overlooks that fear, hatred, and resentment are, first and above all, cognitive constructions. Thus, combined with *differentiated* emotional re-(!)actions called "affection" according to the converter function of credition theory, fear and/or hatred become part of the process of "believing" *specific* alleged "security dilemmas" or "status injustices" stemming from perceptions of *specific* situational patterns[5]. In conclusion, all of the ideas about the necessity of a pre-given or pre-political "community" or even more abstract "horizon of meaning" as (logically) necessary or even functionally required for "understanding", in itself then conceptualized as functional prerequisite of "feelings" of "mutual trust" and "solidarity", are nothing but an "essentialization" of functions or even "naturalization" of social relations when "trust" and "solidarity" are conceptualized as if they were only "emotions."

In conclusion, we can thus identify *three different 'meanings'* of the concept of ethnicity. So far, we have dealt with the dichotomic opposition of primordialist and constructivist theories:

- *Primordialist theories* and the *twin-ideologies* of *racism* and *ethno-nationalism* claim that ethnicity is a 'given' universal category insofar as the social world is divided into a plurality of ethnic communities based on 'common descent' and a 'homogenous culture' (language, religion, values and practices) which stand – by definition – in a position of latent conflict to each other.
- A *constructivist-instrumentalist* position understands ethnicity as the perceived expectation – i.e. generalised stereotype – that "diversity" in terms of fictitious, but imputed biological "descent" ("the" Jews) or "national"-geographic origin ("the" Italians, Turks, etc.) and thus "cultural differentiation" in terms of symbolic categorization and normative ordering of the social world can determine others' social behaviour. This can then lead to *"ethnic" boundary-making* by "ethnic" entrepreneurs through various political strategies. However, so the argument goes, a "non-ethnic", i.e. "civic" social world would be the "ideal" against any "essentialization" of *social* relations into *"cultures"*, let alone "ethnic groups", so that – in the end – "ethnicity" shall "wither away" like in Marx's and Engels' proposition for "the" state.

If we do not "believe" in any of the viewpoints above with regard to our research problem of how to assess the possibilities for reconciliation in deeply divided societies, we have then to conceptualize a third "perspective":

- A *constructivist-structuralist* position insists that there is also something like a *'neo-primordial'*[6] *deep ethnic division of societies* as this is the case in BiH, which is not "fictitious", but a mental representation of social reality constraining action at all levels and in all dimensions of what I have called the ethnic Midas effect above. In such a situation, individuals no longer have a "real choice" for action because of asymmetric power relations, which result in the socio-economic and ethnic stratification of societies, mutually reinforcing each other.

[5] Thus, the converter function also allows one to distinguish between "fear", "hatred" and "rage" as this is claimed in general by Petersen (2002), Prinz (2012), Ross (2014).

[6] I have to thank my colleague Benedikt Harzl for helping me to clarify this point through our debates on "ethnic" conflict.

Hence, as long as the ideologically constructed propositions of the so called Böckenförde dilemma discussed above and the opposition of equality and difference with the alleged predetermination for conflict and cooperation are not transformed into the *triadic structure* of identity: diversity and solidarity, *institutionalized* diversity management and governance will not be possible. Only when we no longer "believe" in the essentialized "nature" of social and political behavior do we approach – at least at the theoretical level – the possibility of looking for institutional arrangements of equality on the basis of diversity as the new "essential" task of constructive institution engineering for the purpose of multiple diversity governance.

These concepts of *institutionalization* and *structure* bring us now to the social and legal theory in line with the interplay of credition theory's second, intersubjective, and, third collective level and their "stabilizer" function, i.e. the processes of social integration and systemic integration.

Social integration is based on "enculturation" through the acquisition of knowledge and capacities, and varies according to "social distance" to a greater or lesser extent, created by "status positioning" through individual and social recognition in interpersonal contacts, in particular in the educational system, labor market, and through participation in institutional settings. This leads to "interperceptions", i.e. thinking of Me and other persons in a particular way from a "holistic" and therefore triangular perspective, which may lead to the development of distinctive (normative) standards and (behavioral) traditions (Massey and Abu-Baker 2010). In other words, socialization and internalization of such "social beliefs" lead to more or less cognitive and emotional "identification" with an "entity" the persons "believes" thus to "belong" to.

Social integration is thus dependent on the "openness" of dispositional attitudes of all actors involved in interaction. Hence, the decisive question is the *interdependence* of *identity* formation and the formation of different varieties of *groups* through symbolically institutionalized boundary-making (Wimmer 2013).

There are either "diffuse" or "clearly" demarcated symbolic and institutionalized boundaries following from identification with social beliefs. Hence, with "barricaded" or "corporate" identities, a person is classified as belonging only to a "fixed" category such as ethnicity and definitively distinguished thus from members of other groups. With a "bounded" identity, however, a person identifies with a group which partially defines self, but such an identity also allows for non-exclusive, complementary perceptions of self as belonging also to other categories or groups, in short, "multiple" identities.

Hence, contacts between persons "believing" to belong to different categories or groups do not automatically "re-personalize" and thereby "de-categorize" intersubjective relations and thus motivate peaceful cooperation, but contact between persons with "barricaded" identities in "diffuse" situations can also trigger aggression due to their, for instance, (social) beliefs in status inconsistencies, i.e. "resentment" in Petersen's terminology. The opportunity for reconciliation is thus improved only through contact when persons seen as belonging to other groups are evaluated as describable in multiple classifications, and not as members of essentialized categories. Conversely, the lack of contact may help polarize "us-vs.-them" images and emphasize in-group exclusiveness (Massey and Abu-Baker 2010), as we know from phenomena such as being an anti-Semite without ever meeting a Jew or fearing strangers without ever meeting a refugee.

In conclusion, we have to see that social integration and *systemic integration* in terms of social cohesion of a given society go hand-in-hand in what Searle signifies as "collective intentionality" and "assignment of status functions" through "declarations," thereby creating "human institutional ontology" (Searle 2010:59, 69). Through such speech acts, human beings are able to make themselves and others believe "in being" something that matters. This is the process by which institutions such as money or legal persons, for instance multinational corporations, are created *ex nihilo* and start to have a social reality of their own. Collective intentionality and the syntactical elements of language make it even possible to create an impossible, i.e. utopian, state of affairs.

From the perspective of ideal-types, the interplay of social and systemic integration through the assignment of status functions may lead to four different *"configurations" of society*, again "structured" around the basic normative value and principle of equality/inequality on the one hand, and the question of "boundedness" of groups on the other.

- Social and systemic integration are "successful" from a functional perspective – following Searle's observation that functional assessments lead us to use "normative vocabulary" – in the case of identity and group formation in terms of allowing for dual identities, excluding thereby the "closure" of group boundaries and thus fixed group "antagonisms." This then leads to the formation of *multicultural societies* based on the normative principle of *status equality* of *individuals* as well as *groupings* despite of *horizontal "cultural differentiation"* of society, so that cultural markers such as language or religion are not given social and political relevance with regard to access to education, the labor market, or political participation.
- However, as we could learn from socio-economic conflicts in European history from the development of capitalism not only as a mode of production, but also "structuration" of societies, if only a minority of persons with "barricaded", individualistic identities becomes economically and politically dominant with the vision of "social space" as a "market" where only competition to satisfy his/her own interests is the guiding principle, they bring about a *vertical hierarchy* in terms of *socio-economic stratification* and thus a *division* of society along these lines so that, for a historical example, Benjamin Disraeli could declare in the first half of the nineteenth century even before the publication of the Communist Manifesto for Great Britain that (only) "two nations", rich and poor, live in this country (Disraeli 1845).
- If *functional differentiation* through specialization is "re-interpreted" in cultural terms, this is the vantage point for a process of "ethnification" of society which can be observed through "ethnic *segmentation*", i.e. a *horizontal hierarchy* between groups because of their systemic, i.e. "structural" occupation of parts of

social subsystems. Hence, there may be "*separate, but equal*"[7] occupational sectors where only members of a grouping in the process of "closure" and thus process of "ethnification" get access; other empirical indicators for such a process are the separation of private and public educational facilities only for members of specific groups. Additionally, there may be the proposal to introduce different legal systems as an "exemption" from the monopoly in the exercise of "legitimate power" of the "modern" state, in this case a uniform legal system for the adjudication of conflicts within specific groups as this would be the case, for instance, with the introduction of a Sharia-court system in Western democracies in cases of family conflicts among Muslims. This form of society with an "ethnic segmentation" of social subsystems is what I call the "model" of a "*pluri-ethnic society*."

- Finally, the *mutually-reinforcing* socio-economic stratification and ethnic segmentation may lead to the socio-economic deprivation and cultural marginalization of entire groups of society, called "*ethclasses*" by Milton Gordon (1964), and thus to *deeply divided societies* as a consequence of the total failure of social and systemic integration. Examples for this case are Sinti and Roma all over Europe or so-called "first nations", i.e. Inuit and Indians, in Canada who suffer from multiple instances of "structural" discrimination.
- In stark contrast to this case, there are groups who were formerly conceived as national "minorities" in centralized nation-states who got, however, a strong political position in the process of transition into "pluri-national" states or federations over the last decades such as the Scots in Great Britain, Catalans in Spain, and the Flemish in Belgium, and who also belong to the richest regions in Europe but nonetheless *claim for secession* as a symbol for deep divisions.

So, how useful are these reconceptualizations of "ethnicity" in the process of social "identity" formation and the political mobilization of groupings with the help of credition theory to re-assess the possibilities of reconciliation in deeply divided societies such as BiH?

3 Conclusion

Credition theory can help us, first and foremost, to understand and explain the processes of "ethnic" mobilization of people (a singular term!) in both the pre-conflict and post-conflict phases. As the case of Bosnia and Herzegovina demonstrates, the process can become a vicious cycle in collective memory (Halbwachs 1967) as a stabilized "belief-system" *as if* "intergenerational vengeance" and not the former were the root cause of the renewed outbreak of violence in every new generation (Marko-Stöckl 2010:351). Thereby the "belief" in ethnicity as a root factor of intergroup violence is of central importance.

[7]This phrase is taken from the infamous decision of the US Supreme Court in Plessy v. Ferguson, 1896, adjudicating the claim for a "racially" segregated school system.

Hence, credition theory, with its focus on mental representations established as cognitive "certainties" without or even against the recognition of "objective truth,"[8] can help us to develop more specific research questions with regard to the seemingly "irrational" dichotomy of "knowledge versus acknowledgement" as a "kind of mental closure which makes people blind to facts … that has to be overcome, at the individual level as well as the societal level" (Marko-Stöckl 2010:8, 349, 351).

When we take the enclosure and converter function into account in political processes of ethnification of groups and society, we can (re-)interpret now the events which led to the dissolution of former Yugoslavia.

Already in the early 1980s, newspapers and other media in Slovenia and Croatia had started to interpret the economic gains made through exports of Slovene multinational companies and income generated by tourism along the Adriatic coast-line as "national" surplus, i.e. the "national property" of the Slovene and Croat "nations" which had to be given away to the "southern" republics of Yugoslavia (i.e. the Republics of Serbia, Montenegro and Macedonia) for the purpose of their economic "development." This was argued for on the basis of the mechanism of fiscal federalism imposed on them by the (in their opinion) communist, however, "in reality" Serb-dominated political system. These media discourses have to be seen thus as the vantage point in the processes of *categorization* and *de-personalization* in regards to the construction of "*ethnic*" *We-They* group *relationships* involved in the creation of a "pluri-ethnic" society described above. But, how "strong" are such processes of *stereotyping* based on "feelings" of justice and fairness with regard to economic redistribution? Do they already lead to a stabilized "belief" that the respective Other is "by nature" the "ethnic enemy" and thereby tip the balance for conflict versus cooperation?

Based on credition theory, we could thus hypothesize that self- and other stereotyping in terms of belonging to different "nations" does not yet automatically lead to a *stable*, "ethnic" re-configuration of society, and that because of this, parties in the process and external mediators could still prevent the "ethnification" of all social and cultural relations by giving political salience to other factors.

The next phase in the escalation of conflict can be "seen" from the perspective of credition theory when the media, but also religious and political leaders, started to interpret We-They group relationships in the mid- to late 1980s not only in terms of economic interests of federal entities, but to *denigrate* the "character" of the people in the "south" as "lazy", not interested in hard work etc. and thus to *stigmatize* them as an *inferior* class of peoples. Due to this, competing economic interests became coupled with "identity"-related evaluations in terms of negative coding of their social identities thereby creating an "ethnic social space" and thus dispositions for action. Hence, it became not only possible, but even much more easy through *enemy-stereotyping* between 1989 and 1991 to turn the already existing We-They group relationships into an *antagonistic structure of Us-versus-Them*, i.e. an ethnically and deeply divided society with mutually hostile attitudes of "closed" groups

[8]The best empirical example I can find to demonstrate this "fact" is the statement of an indictee before the ICTY: "You have your facts. We have our facts. You have a complete right to choose between the two versions", quoted after Marko-Stöckl (2010:348).

according to the typology elaborated above, and thus to create an alleged, but obviously "credible" security dilemma. This became obvious when political leaders in both Serbia and Croatia started to refer to the "collective memory" of – in actual fact, re-interpreted – past events of killing, ethnic cleansing and genocide during WWII and to "stigmatize" all Croats as *Ustaša* (fascists), all Serbs as *Četnici* having fought for the restoration of a Serb-dominated Kingdom of Yugoslavia, and all Muslims as religious fundamentalists who want to establish an Islamic state.

The same processes of ongoing *political* mobilization in ethnic terms can be observed also in the post-conflict phase. Twenty years after the conclusion of the Dayton Peace Agreement, primary and secondary students in Bosnia and Herzegovina, Kosovo, and Macedonia, and also students in universities, remain ethnically segregated. Additionally, even after this amount of time, religious leaders and the media have not stopped promoting ethnic propaganda.

We can now hypothesize that "ethnicity" under such a societal configuration of deep ethnic divide is not simply "false consciousness" which can and has simply to be "de-constructed" as such so that "enlightened" people will no longer give political salience in processes of (self-) "identification" to such a wrong "belief." The analogy that we no longer "believe" in the "existence" of witches as a sign of the development of "civilization" is simply wrong. Genocide against an "ethnic" group could be carried out in Europe even at the end of the twentieth century and women are still killed with the former allegation in other parts of the world. Hence, the central research question must be based on the need to analyse how "information" in communicative processes is "converted" into such a form of "certainty" in the pre-conflict phase that people are ready to even kill others? The same is true for the post-conflict phase: How is it possible to mobilize people along the same "ethnic" lines so that society remains deeply "ethnically" divided, and all efforts for reconciliation seem to fail on that account? These two scenarios bring us to two more specific research questions, noted below. This is not only because we need better theoretical clarification, but also for reasons of obvious practical importance for all efforts at reconciliation requiring "repersonalization" through contact and learning from intersubjective experience, such that "de-categorization" of neo-primordial ethnicity and a renewed "cross-categorization" allow persons to hold multiple identities through multiple classifications, and a "politics of pluralism" becomes possible. This – against the Hobbesian legacy – philosopher Hannah Arendt has already thought about when she prepared the shift from the identitarian to the "diversity paradigm," with her definition of politics as a permanent *task* to create unity out of diversity.[9]

But we will not be able to develop theories of reconciliation further by only making use of such theoretical reconceptualizations. For further progress, much more

[9] "Politik handelt von dem Zusammen- und Miteinander-Sein der Verschiedenen. ... Der Ruin der Politik nach beiden Seiten entsteht aus der Entwicklung politischer Körper aus der Familie. ... Insofern man in der Familie mehr sieht als die Teilnahme, das heißt die aktive Teilnahme, an der Pluralität, beginnt man, Gott zu spielen, nämlich so zu tun, als ob man naturaliter aus dem Prinzip der Verschiedenheit herauskommen könne" (Arendt 1993:9–10).

empirical testing is needed from the perspective of credition theory with its focus on processes of "believing" associating cognitive with emotional elements.

Hence, there are in particular two specific research questions which have to be empirically tested much more rigorously:

- First, what is the "specific" relationship between cognitive and emotional elements in the converter function? Is it true that "fear, hatred, and resentment" are the overwhelming "intrinsic" emotional properties which "ethnic" entrepreneurs can simply tap into? But why should people simply "believe" in the propaganda of ethnic entrepreneurs? In contrast to such an approach, the question can be raised about whether "fear, hatred, and resentment" are much more based on cognitive elements which stem from "collective memory" inculcated into individuals through processes of learning throughout socialization processes, so that these learning processes and thus cognitive elements have a much stronger influence on the creation of emotional "dispositions" which would be much more in line with the constructivist-structuralist theory of "ethnicity" elaborated above?
- Second, what is the relationship between "interest" and "identity"? Can these two analytical categories neatly be separated as different independent causal inferences? However, as our story on the process of dissolution of Yugoslavia above seems to indicate, there are again processes of "transformation" of "interests" into "identities" in play as "deep structure" so that identity formation cannot simply be divorced from interests. But is this also true the other way round? Can "identities" be transformed back into "interests", can "ethnic division" of society be "dissolved" and transformed into a "simple" multicultural society as Kymlicka (see above) seems to speculate?

References

Angel HF (2006) Religiosität als menschliches Potential. Ein anthropologisches Modell der Religiosität im neurowissenschaftlichen Horizont. In: Angel HF et al (eds) Religiosität. Anthropologische, theologische und sozialwissenschaftliche Klärungen. Kohlhammer, Stuttgart, pp 62–89

Angel HF (2013) Credition, the process of belief. In: Runehov A, Oviedo L (eds) Encyclopedia of sciences and religions. Springer, Dordrecht, pp 536–539

Arendt H (1993) Was ist Politik? In: Ludz U (ed) Aus dem Nachlaß. Piper, München, pp 9–10

Arthur P (2011) Introduction: identities in transition. In: Arthur P (ed) Identities in transition. Challenges for transitional justice in divided societies. Cambridge University Press, Cambridge, pp 1–9

Behr H (2014) Politics of difference. Epistemologies of peace. Routledge, London

Böckenförde EW (1976) Die Entstehung des Staates als Vorgang der Säkularisation. In: Böckenförde EW, Staat, Gesellschaft Freiheit. Studien zur Staatstheorie und zum Verfassungsrecht. Suhrkamp, Frankfurt/Main, pp 42–64

Call CT, Cousens EM (2007) Ending wars and building peace, Working paper series coping with crisis. International Peace Academy, New York

Canovan M (1996) Nationhood and political theory. Edward Elgar, Cheltenham, p 133

Choudhry S (2008) Bridging comparative politics and comparative constitutional law: constitutional design in divided societies. In: Choudhry S (ed) Constitutional design for divided societies. Integration or accommodation. Oxford University Press, Oxford, pp 3–40
Disraeli B (1845) Sybil, or the two nations. Oxford University Press, Oxford. 1998
Giddens A (1976) Central problems in social theory. MacMillan Press Ltd, London/Basingstoke
Gordon MM (1964) Assimilation in American life. The role of race, religion, and national origins. Oxford University Press New York, p 52
Halbwachs M (1967) Das kollektive Gedächtnis. Enke Verlag, Stuttgart
Huntington S (1993) The clash of civilizations. Foreign Aff 72(3):22–49
Kymlicka W (2011) Transitional justice, federalism, and the accomodation of minority nationalism. In: Arthur P (ed) Identities in transition. Challenges for transitional justice in divided societies. Cambridge University Press, Cambridge, pp 303–333
Leebaw BL (2008) The irreconcilable goals of transitional justice. Hum Rights Q 30:95–118
Linz JJ, Stepan A (1996) Problems of democratic transition and consolidation. Southern Europe, South America, and Post-Communist Europe. Johns Hopkins University Press, Baltimore/London, p 17
Malesević S (1995) Identity as ideology. Understanding ethnicity and nationalism. Palgrave, Basingstoke, p 4
Marko J (1995) Autonomie und Integration. Rechtsinstitute des Nationalitätenrechts im funktionalen Vergleich. Böhlau Verlag, Wien, pp 77–81
Marko J (2001) Friedenssicherung im 21. Jahrhundert: Bosnien und Herzegowina als europäische Herausforderung (Securing peace in the 21th century: Bosnia and Herzegovina as a European challenge). In: Ginther K et al (eds) Völker- und Europarecht. 25. Österreichischer Völkerrechtstag (International and European Law, 25th Austrian International Lawyers conference). Verlag Österreich, Wien, p 79
Marko J (2008) The law and politics of diversity management: a neo-institutional approach. Eur Yearb Minor Issues 6:251
Marko J (2009) Processes of ethnic mobilization in the former Yugoslav republics reconsidered. J South East Eur 2009:1–15
Marko J (2013a) Defective democracy in a failed state? Bridging constitutional design, politics and ethnic division in Bosnia-Herzegovina. In: Ghai Y, Woodman S (eds) Practising self-government: a comparative study of autonomous regions. Cambridge University Press, Cambridge, pp 281–314
Marko J (2013b) Ethnopolitics and constitutional reform in Bosnia-Herzegovina. In: Listhaug O, Ramet SP (eds) Bosnia-Herzegovina since Dayton: civic and uncivic values. Longo Editore, Ravenna, pp 49–80
Marko J (2017) Multiple diversity governance through law? Political theory, ideology and norm contestation in European context: an interdisciplinary approach (in press)
Marko-Stöckl E (2010) My Truth, Your Truth - Our Truth? The Role of History Teaching and Truth Commissions for Reconciliation. Eur Yearb Minor Issues 7:327-352
Massey RF, Abu-Baker K (2010) A systemic framework for forgiveness, reconciliation, and peace: interconnecting psychological and social processes. In: Kalayjian A, Paloutzian R (eds) Forgiveness and reconciliation. Psychological pathways to conflict transformation and peace building. Springer, New York, p 14
Mead GH (1967) Mind, Self, and Society, Charles W. Morris (ed) Chicago
McCrudden C, O'Leary B (2013) Courts and consociations. Human rights versus power-sharing. Oxford University Press, Oxford
Moses JW, Knutsen TL (2012) Ways of knowing. Competing methodologies in social and political research, 2nd edn. Palgrave, New York, pp 1–18
Paris R, Sisk TD (2007) Managing contradictions: the inherent dilemmas of postwar statebuilding. International Peace Academy, New York
Petersen RD (2002) Understanding ethnic violence. Fear, hatred, and resentment in twentieth-century Eastern Europe. Cambridge University Press, Cambridge

Prinz J (2012) Emotion. In: Frankish K, Ramsey WM (eds) The Cambridge handbook of cognitive science. Cambridge University Press, Cambridge, pp 193–211

Ross A (2014) Mixed emotions. Beyond fear & hatred in international conflict. University of Chicago Press, Chicago/London

Samuels K (2009) Postwar constitution building: opportunities and challenges. In: Paris R, Sisk T (eds) The dilemmas of statebuilding: confronting the contradictions of postwar peace operations. Routledge, London/New York, p 173

Sarajlić E (2011) Between state and nation: Bosnia and Herzegovina and the challenge of political analysis. In: Sarajlić E, Marko D (eds) State or nation? The challenges of political transition in Bosnia and Herzegovina. Centre for Interdisciplinary Postgraduate Studies, Sarajevo, pp 11, 13

Searle JR (2010) Making the social world. The structure of human civilization. Oxford University Press, Oxford, pp 69, 141

Seitz R, Angel HF (2012) Processes of believing – A review and conceptual account. Rev Neurosci:303–309

Skaar E (2012) Reconciliation in a transitional justice perspective. Transl Justice Rev 1:54–103

Sugiura M, Seitz R, Angel HF (2015) Models and neural bases of the believing process. J Behav Brain Sci 5:12–23

Wendt A (1999) Social theory of international politics. Cambridge University Press, Cambridge

Wiener A (2014) A theory of contestation. Springer, Heidelberg

Wimmer A (2013) Ethnic boundary making. Institutions, power, networks. Oxford University Press, Oxford

Understanding Young People's Worldview: A Practical Example of How to Work with the Model of Credition

Vasiliki Mitropoulou

Abstract Creditions are considered as cognitive processes, although all belief processes do not become conscious. The chapter aims to present some aspects of a small research project at the Aristotle University in Thessaloniki, Greece, which implements the theory of credition in examining young people studying theology, and to find out if their attitudes and beliefs were affected in accordance with the credition model.

1 The Problem with Beliefs

In everyday discussions of religious or non-religious content, we often hear the argument: *"That's a question of belief."* However, if our discussions about our problems and issues boil down to nothing more than what different people believe, then there is a high risk of becoming helpless. In complicated discussions, it may come to the point when we have to state: some believe this, others believe that, and there is no bridge between both positions.

But is this really the case? The concept of credition provides a tool that may help overcome the frontier of speechlessness and lack of answers. It can be helpful to see behind the acts of beliefs and to better understand the cognitive and emotional state of the participants. Thus, a person's belief is so strong that it can define decisions, form their attitudes and guide his/her actions. Regarding this kind of belief, a theory was formed, named with the new term "*credition*" aiming to state the "process of believing" (Angel 2011). The *theory of credition* suggests that the processes of believing are the result of attitudes, which act as a guide for our actions, influencing them and establishing new connections between old facts or ideas. (Davies 2007) This corresponds with basic anthropological considerations (Boyer 2003a). The concept of credition focuses on the process character, i.e., what happens when someone is doing what we call "he/she believes".

V. Mitropoulou (✉)
Aristotle University of Thessaloniki, Thessaloniki, Greece
e-mail: mitro@theo.auth.gr

H.-F. Angel et al. (eds.), *Processes of Believing: The Acquisition, Maintenance, and Change in Creditions*, New Approaches to the Scientific Study of Religion 1,
DOI 10.1007/978-3-319-50924-2_25

It was the *model of credition* [see chapter "Credition – From the Question of Belief to the Question of Believing (Angel)"] that prompted our research about how far we can come when applying the model within a defined set of communications. Our intention was to first conduct a small empirical research program to see whether the model of credition could help us to better understand the processes of believing. The target group was a small group of 4th-year (8th semester) students in the Department of Theology at Aristotle University in Thessaloniki, and the research method was qualitative, conducted with a personal, semi-structured interview.

2 Framework of the Credition Theory

The credition theory suggests that the believing process is based on four different functions: enclosure function, converter function, stabilizer function and modulator function (Angel 2013; Sugiura et al. 2015). I will briefly review these functions in the following paragraph.

The enclosure function is related to perception and is involved in modifying bab-configurations (ideas, values, ethical convictions). The converter function is related to action and activated when bab-configurations are transformed into action (in the space of action). Thus it reveals the relationship between a specific belief and the relevant behavior. The stabilizer function is responsible for maintaining the stability of the beliefs. Bab-configurations are constantly modified by new experiences that affect the actions. Therefore, the stabilization of bab-configurations is a precondition for the production of stable "spaces of action" (e.g. decision-making, planning, (re-)building of trust, etc). The modulator function shows the differences between individuals and/or situations, in which processes of believing may occur, given that credition is connected to body, memory, gender, cognitive and/or emotional development etc. Emotions influence the forming of a credition (e.g. stress, anxiety, anger, etc.) either consciously or unconsciously.

The analysis had its focus on the enclosure process of credition and was conducted in three main steps: definition of the clum, of the bab-configuration and mightiness.[1]

3 Intention of Research

Answering that one does or does not believe something nourishes the expectation that this belief is consequence of a stable bab-blob-configuration. Therefore, one might expect that a positive or negative response to the question, "Do you believe that…?" indicates a stable bab-blob-configuration. But that is obviously not the

[1] See chapter "Credition: From the Question of Belief to the Question of Believing", by Angel, for more introduction to these concepts.

case. The term "*bab*" was introduced to state or describe an item of knowledge that consists of the contents of beliefs (Angel 2013). Each "bab" could contain specific emotional value and describe an item. The same contents of a bab can exist with different values of "mightiness", expressing the varying personal relevance of the belief content. The collection of babs, or bab-configuration, comprises a new larger "bab" (the "*mega bab*"). Babs are organized as bab-configurations.

Because of this, one special point of observation was directed to the "ranking" of propositions and the mightiness of emotions. Interestingly, despite a remaining yes to the integration of a "clum", intrapersonal changes could be observed when the focus was directed to the (cognitive) relevance of a proposition and to the (emotional) mightiness of the same proposition.

- Attribution of cognitive relevance: The row of the propositions that pops up without a longer reflection was not stable. After some reflection the relevance of the different propositional arguments was rearranged.
- Sense of emotional mightiness: An astonishing observation was that the emotional mightiness, which was said to correspond to the proposition, produced again a different ranking.

Our intention was to better understand young people's worldview, which apparently is one of inner forces for shaping beliefs. We wanted to see whether it is possible to make the processes that are going on during the believing process more conscious and more transparent.

We followed the hypothesis that it is possible to more clearly express the cognitive and emotional components which underpin the different results of a believing process. Thus our research program provided a chance to check the adequateness of our hypothesis and to test whether the model of credition is understandable enough for everyday use.

There were some aspects that we introduced as important factors and we held them as indispensable when talking about believing.

One of these factors was the idea that there is a narrow link between propositional (content) aspects of beliefs and emotions, which are related to those propositions. This is why the participating students had to understand the concept of "babs" as well as the concept of "bab-blob-configurations". Further, they needed to understand why it is more adequate to the fluidity of the believing process when one uses the concept of "bab-blob-configuration" instead the concept of "mindsets," which creates the illusion of stability.

Since we needed examples close to reality, we started with the perception aspect of the believing process, which is expressed in the enclosure function. So some central aspects of the enclosure had been explained, especially the term "clum" and its meaning. In collaboration with Hans-Ferdinand Angel, we formulated a set of five *clums*, which were linked with an equal number of open questions.

The research mainly followed three steps.

- The participants should become aware that there are "contents" that we believe.
- The participants should understand that our "cognitive landscapes of contents" influence the decision about what we believe.

- The participants should understand that the propositional or content aspect is not sufficient to explain the deeper reasons for why we believe something.
- The participants should try to interrelate their own emotions (of course only those that they could talk about; the "blob" aspect of the enclosure process was explicitly excluded).
- The participants should check whether the aspect of mightiness of emotional loadings is helpful for their understanding of the believing process and the results of the process.

The questions were *open*, so that the subjects could have flexibility and freedom to answer them by fully stating their views. They were presented to the students during the interview procedure (Zafeiropoulos 2005). (As this was such a small research project, we decided not to discuss blobs but leave it for later). The open questions have the advantages of flexibility, and eliminating limitations to the way of answering. They allow the researcher to proceed more in-depth, provide the possibility to control the subject, encourage the collaboration/interaction between researcher-subject and produce unexpected answers. Among the disadvantages is the difficulty to compare the answers, which may lead to control loss. (Robson 2010).

The individual *interview* ensures that the subjects would not listen to the other's views, and thus there would not be any risk of getting the same answers. The difficulty inherent in this method was that we would not be able to compare the answers, because each student was influenced differently by their emotions as affected by their religious beliefs.

4 Procedure

We decided to proceed with a small group in the Department of Theology at Aristotle University in Thessaloniki. The research was initiated during a lecture in the course "*Teaching of Religious Education*" for 4th-year students. During the lecture, a discussion was started on whether one should believe certain content. After the lecture, their professor asked the students if they wanted to participate in an empirical research project to further investigate the thinking that led them to express their views. We invited those who were interested to participate in the research: 9 students stayed and we selected 5 of them. First, we set an appointment and tried to help them understand their own discussion process by clarifying their individual bab-configuration. Then we helped them understand that an individual operator transforms every individual bab–configuration into a certain space of action (which is preliminary for decision making). During the interview we discussed with them: (a) why they have come to their individual bab-configuration, (b) how to specify the mightiness of the babs, and (c) their emotions related to their babs configuration.

The research method we followed was the qualitative method, conducted with the personal interview because it fit better with the aim as well as with the theory of credition, and furthermore, it explained and analyzed the causes for the various phenomena under examination (Zafeiropoulos 2005). Qualitative research traces the causes of changes and describes and interprets the phenomena through the registration of the subjects' experiences. Given that the research took place in the Department of Theology in a university setting, and given the students' positive attitude towards the research and their willingness to provide answers, the research results reflected the real views of the participants and not formal or standardized answers. (Zafeiropoulos 2005). The interviews were conducted individually and were used as the main and unique approach (Robson 2010), which lately has been recognized to have an important place in the social sciences research (Zafeiropoulos 2005).

The personal interview is used more often because it is more flexible when carried out, its immediacy and intimacy is felt by the participants, and lastly, because of its low cost (Zafeiropoulos 2005). Interviews help to investigate the details about the subject matter of the research in more depth (Cajendra and Kanka 1999). However, it is a time-consuming procedure, because the views are registered and re-registered in order to write a structured text.(Zafeiropoulos 2005).

We used the semi-structured interview approach, because it contains pre-defined questions but the structure of a question can be modified and explanations can be added (Robson 2010). In a semi-structured interview, the questions are in a specific order, but the researcher can change their structures so that all subjects can understand them (Cajendra and Kanka 1999).

The interview is a flexible and adaptive way to learn things (Robson 2010). It is time-consuming, and the time that each interview takes can vary. In our research, the interview lasted up to half an hour (Robson 2010). Notes were kept during the interview and each question was written in a PowerPoint slide on a laptop. After each answer, a new slide showed the next question. Due to this design, the researcher can, after the examining the answers, investigate the emotions, the motivation, the experiences and the attitudes, something that cannot be achieved by any other technique (Cajendra and Kanka 1999).

The phases of the interview were: (a) Definition of the topic under investigation (questions construction), (b) guide for the conduct of the interview (list of topics which should be mentioned and arranged during the discussion), and (c) find the subjects (their number augments the time and the cost, registration of views, analysis and comments) (Zafeiropoulos 2005).

4.1 Sampling

The participants were selected according to the ease and availability of the subjects, in other words; these participants made up a voluntary convenience sample. (Zafeiropoulos 2005). The students' selection took place on the basis of their own choice. The 4th-year (8th-semester) students who attended the course entitled "Teaching of Religious Education" were asked if they wanted to participate in a research project on credition. The students who were interested in participating stayed in the classroom after the lecture and asked for more information. Explanations were provided and they were told that an interview would follow. After the explanations, those who were interested in participating remained in the classroom.

4.2 Working Process of Bab-Configuration and Enclosure Process

A bab-configuration and enclosure process are responsible for integrating a clum. The analysis of the enclosure process of credition was conducted in three main steps:

4.2.1 Definition of the Clum

The clum was fixed (e.g. theological studies makes the students better persons[2]). The instruction began in the following way: "*I believe….*". The aim was to very precisely work out the content of a clum, which was going to be included in an enclosure process, because the students were expected to provide different answers regarding the possible ways to integrate a clum into a bab-configuration. Thereafter, the students received the clum without any explanation and had to choose a position by answering YES or NO, i.e., if they thought the clum could be integrated or not. Then the researchers demonstrated for the student how the clum is dependent on the bab-configuration and asked them to think about it. The presentation of the clum was followed by the relevant question.

4.2.2 Bab-Configuration

The current given condition (clum) was defined first, followed by the accompanying question and then the contents of babs were written down (which are expected to define whether the clum was integrated or not). It was then pointed out which babs were available in the bab-configuration, followed by an analysis of the bab-configuration (by way of logical reasoning, i.e. the students had to state 5 phrases) and as well as an explanation of the babs. The number of babs at this stage we decided to be up to 5.

[2]A phrase repeated very often by the graduates of our Faculty.

4.2.3 Mightiness

The babs were sorted according to their mightiness, which resulted in the emergence of mega-babs. Following the 5 logical sentences (babs), the students organized the one according to how mighty they considered it to be. Obviously, the 5 babs were not deemed mighty to the same degree. The students organized the babs first in accordance to their content, and then to their mightiness. A mega-bab represents the strongest level of mightiness. There are also babs that are mighty to lesser degrees, called mini-babs. The degree of mightiness for each bab was scored on a 1–5 scale, with 1 representing a mega-bab, 5 representing the smallest mini-bab, and 2, 3, and 4 in between them.

4.3 Everyday Questions and Formulation of the Clums

The two first questions referred to the private sphere of the students.

Question No. 1 reflected a phrase that we heard very often by the graduate or last-semester students from the Department of Theology (these students were at the last semester of their studies and they would soon start looking for a job).

Question No. 2 referred to their graduation and reflected on the challenge of obtaining a Bachelor's degree.

Then *Question No. 3* followed was contextualized within the political sphere caused by the economic crisis in Greece and the blame that was cast on the politicians.

Finally, we posed a question (*No. 4*) in the sphere of religion, as the Church in Greece had taken a leading and very important role in social work aimed at helping the people suffering from the crisis.

The first task was to transform the colloquial question into a formulation which was able to serve as a clum. A clum is correctly formulated when a person can state "Yes" (which means: "I believe that this is right") or No" (which means: "I believe that this is not right").

The questions and clums were presented as follows:

No. 1

- Question: "Do you believe that your studies in the Department of Theology have changed you into a better person?"
- Clum: "The studies in the Faculty of Theology made me a better person."

No. 2

- Question: "Do you believe that your studies in the Department of Theology will help you find a job relevant to them?"
- Clum: "I will find a relevant job."

No. 3

- Question: "Do you believe that the politicians mean well when they vote for the economic measures, *and that they help to improve the present situation?"
- Clum: "The politicians mean well and wish to help improve the present situation."

No. 4

- Question: "Do you believe that the crisis has turned the people to religion for comfort?"
- Clum: "Religion offers comfort" (respectively: "People turn to religion for comfort").

Each student listened first to the clum. Then the student answered whether she/he accepted the clum or not by answering "Yes" or "No." Then he/she received the corresponding question and provided the babs related to it (up to five), first at random and afterwards in accordance to how mighty they were. This was important, because the results showed that on second thought, the string of babs changed for some of the students. In the end, they related each bab to their emotions.

5 The Results and Their Presentation

The presentation in this chapter of course cannot show the results of the research project in a more detailed way. It especially cannot give an adequate impression of the vivid discussions within the group.

Therefore, we decided to give only a very restricted insight into these discussions, and selected very few "results" which may give a first impression of how the model of credition might be used as tool of communication and solving conflict. The example is taken from the first research stage regarding the "sphere of privacy" and gives insight into the intra-babial changes of one participant (P 1):

The **question in a colloquial sense** was:

"Do you believe that your studies in the Department of Theology have changed you into a better person?"

Clum:

"The studies in the Faculty of Theology made me a better person."

The **question in the research setting** was:

"Can you integrate the clum into your bab-blob-configuration?"

The answer of P 1 was YES.

Participant 1 (P 1) could integrate the debated clum into the existing bab-blob-configuration. This means the participant believes that the studies in the Department of Theology have changed him/her into a better person. Contradicting the original hypothesis that a positive response indicates a stable bab-blob-configuration the bab-configuration of P 1 changed when the relevance of the proposition was reflected. The change is shown in the following figure.

Spontaneous ranking without reflection the relevance of the propositions (spontaneous proposition ranking: *s-PR*).

s-PR	Proposition
1	Was taught about moral values, freedom, justice, good/evil
2	Got answers to existential issues
3	Got in contact with many religions
4	Was informed on inter-religious issues
5	Learned methodology

Propositions ranked according *to a reflected relevance* (reflected Proposition Ranking: *r-PR*).

r-PR	Proposition
1	Was taught about moral values, freedom, justice, good/evil
2	Was informed on inter-religious issues
3	Got in contact with many religions
4	Learned methodology
5	Got answers to existential issues

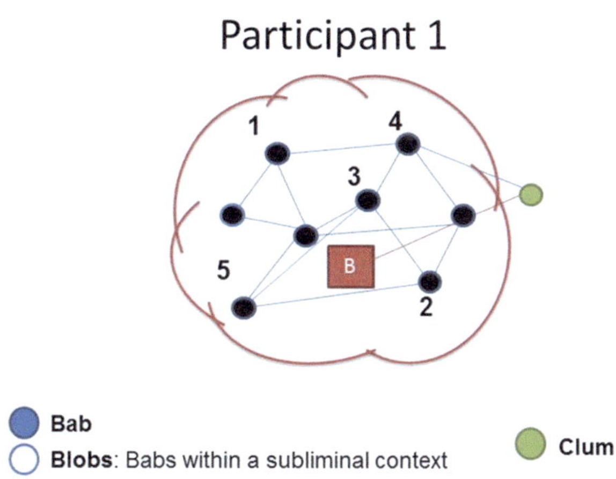

A key observation was that the introduction of *the emotional aspect* which was explained to correspond to the proposition produced again a different ranking (Emotional Aspect ranking: *EA-R*).

s-PR	Proposition	Emotion	EA-R
1	Taught moral values, freedom, justice, good/evil	Love, solidarity	1
2	Got answers to existential issues	Hope , anxiety	4
3	Knew many religions	Understanding, disappointment for the fierce behaviour of believers	3
4	Informed on inter-religious issues	Satisfaction	5
5	Learned methodology	Enthusiasm	2

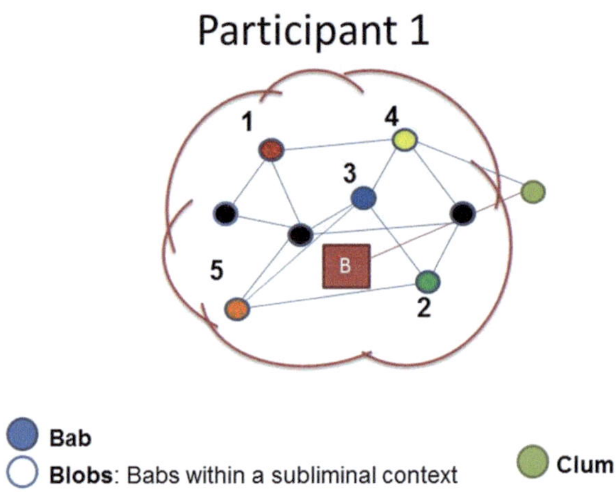

If we arrange the ranking according to *emotional mightiness,* which is connected with the different babs, we see again a different ranking (Emotional Mightiness-Ranking: *EM-R*):

s-PR	Proposition	Emotion	EM-R
1	Taught moral values, freedom, justice, good/evil	Love, solidarity	1
5	Learned methodology	Enthusiasm	2
3	Knew many religions	Understanding, disappointment for the fierce behaviour of believers	3
2	Got answers to existential issues	Hope , anxiety	4
4	Informed on inter-religious issues	Satisfaction	5

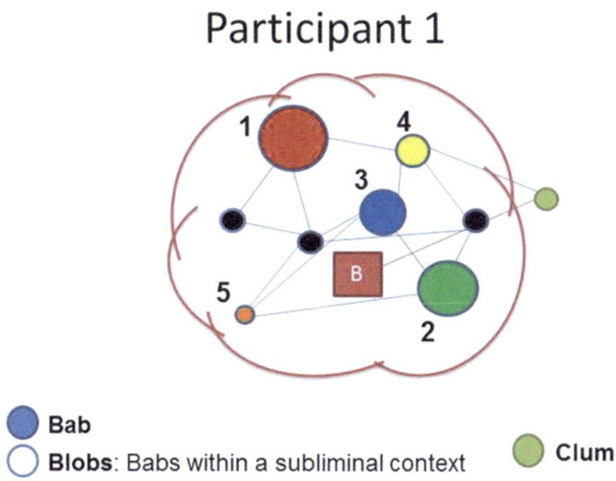

These results will make us much more careful regarding our own imputations which we attribute to others. Even if someone "believes" that "p" there might be extremely different bab-blob-configurations which "cause" this special belief.

6 Concluding Remarks

We tried to conduct our empirical research with participants from the 4th-year (8th-semester) students in the Department of Theology at Aristotle University in Thessaloniki. Our aim was to see the implementation of the theory of credition on young people studying Theology, and to investigate whether their attitudes and beliefs were affected in accordance with the credition model. The first results showed that when the emotions were taken in consideration, most of the time they influenced their initial bab configurations as well as the mega-bab, i.e. the most important bab, which was shown to be a different one than the one chosen before. The results were encouraging and prompted the continuation our research, and the first steps were taken to organize a comparative study together with the Karl-Franzens University of Graz.

References

Angel HF (2011) Can the concept of creditions be applicable to psychology of religion? Wege zum Menschen 63:4–26

Angel HF (2013) Credition, the process of belief. In: Azari NP, Runehov A, Olviedo L (eds) Encyclopedia of sciences and religions. Springer, Heidelberg/New York

Boyer P (2003a) Science, erudition and relevant connections. J Cogn Cult 3(4):344–358

Boyer P (2003b) Religious thought and behavior as by-products of brain function. Trends Cogn Sci 7(3):119–124

Cajendra V, Kanka M (1999) Educational research (trans: Griva E). Typothito-G. Athens, Dardanos

Davies O (2003) The sign redeemed: a study in Christian fundamental semiotics. Mod Theol 19(2):220–241

Robson C (2010) The research of the real world, 2nd edn (trans: Ntalakou V, Basilikou K). Athens, Gutenberg

Sugiura M, Seitz R, Angel HF (2015) Models and neural bases of the believing process. J Behav Brain Sci 5:12–23

Zafeiropoulos K (2005) How is a scientific research conducted? Critiki, Athens

Approaching Another Black Box: Credition in Economics

Richard Sturn

Abstract Credition processes are not a long–standing issue in economics, even though pertinent considerations never were completely absent from economic reasoning. But they were not historically a core part of the conceptual and analytical apparatus of the discipline of economics. In this chapter, I first give a brief overview of the ways in which related themes were more or less occasionally covered in the history of economic thought, including major figures such as Adam Smith and John Maynard Keynes. In order to place credition theory within the vast range of economic problems and approaches, I also will characterize the kinds of economic problems (and accompanying currents of quantitative economics) for which beliefs and creditions are not important. All this sets the stage for the discussion of game–theoretical frameworks in which issues of institutional economics and the economics of change can be analyzed. It is in the context of those frameworks that a more systematic account of the role of beliefs and creditions within economic processes becomes available.

1 Introduction and Overview

Some years ago, various aspects and episodes in the context of the financial crises reinvigorated discussions in economics about trust and trustworthiness. The perspective of bank runs and breakdowns of the interbank market in the presence of un-calculable uncertainties that were undermining the mutual relationship of trust supporting inter-bank lending not only highlighted the vulnerability of financial networks, but also dramatically illustrated a more theoretical issue: explanations of how the functions of basic institutions in capitalist market societies crucially hinge on assumptions about beliefs, and on beliefs about beliefs (higher order beliefs). To be sure: there is hardly any society that does not rely on beliefs. But it may be argued that the *complex and varying ways* in which capitalist market societies rely on beliefs—and in particular, the way in which the dynamics of credition

R. Sturn (✉)
Institute of Public Economics, Karl-Franzens University of Graz, Graz, Austria
e-mail: richard.sturn@uni-graz.at

H.-F. Angel et al. (eds.), *Processes of Believing: The Acquisition, Maintenance, and Change in Creditions*, New Approaches to the Scientific Study of Religion 1,
DOI 10.1007/978-3-319-50924-2_26

accompany socio–economic change including recurrent business cycles and crises is a specific characteristic of those societies. Hence, there are some *prima facie* reasons for thinking that it is unsatisfactory to treat *credition processes* as a black box. In a first approximation, credition processes are related to beliefs in the following way: credition processes are crystallizing in belief structures informing the choices of agents either in a specific situation, such as a bank run, or in recurring social interactions, which are the basis of socio–economic institutions.

Keeping in mind the pivotal role of credit markets for modern economies and recurrent episodes of financial instability, we may ask: Why is change and the dynamics of beliefs so important in modern societies? In traditional societies, social change was largely triggered by chance events or, at any rate, by forces that were external to the functioning of socio–economic mechanisms. This includes cases (such as the decline of civilizations like the Mayas) where the existing socio–economic mechanisms lacked the capacities to cope with emerging challenges and therefore underwent a crisis, eventually culminating in its breakdown. Moreover, change occurred in the context of military clashes between societies. Various levels of believing played a role, but the dynamics of beliefs were not so much related to endogenous (and more or less permanent) changes *within* the system than to much less frequent changes *of* system. Believing in such traditional societies can perhaps be described as equilibrium pattern of beliefs attuned to prevailing social practices, customs, internalized norms and power relations: crystallized beliefs, as it were. One of the protagonists of New Institutional Economics, Nobel laureate Oliver Williamson, summarizes all this under terms such as informal institutions/norms which embed or constrain formal institutions. He emphasizes that the informal embedding conditions of formal institutions change very slowly. He also stresses that a full analysis of economic institutions would have to consider an even more basic level, the working of the mechanisms of the mind. All this seems to entail a certain role of credition processes. Notice though that beliefs in that view belong to a slowly changing cluster of "informal" embedding conditions surrounding formal institutions and markets without constantly interacting with them; hence, those conditions can be taken as given as far as economic theories of market exchange and institutions are concerned.

The shortcomings of such approaches become visible when we are dealing with modern dynamic capitalism, as opposed to static exchange economies. The distinctive feature of capitalist market societies is restlessness, which does not need an external cause. It includes endogenous change, cumulative innovation, and associated updates of information. It even may include more comprehensive revision of knowledge beyond mere updating. Such a situation tends to be accompanied by a certain fluidity, a latent ambiguity and sometimes a reflected contingency of beliefs, few of which can be expected to gain the status of quasi–eternal truths. Hence it seems natural to view process–related aspects of the formation of beliefs as indispensable parts of a modern research program in economics. We have excellent reasons, it seems, to be interested in the circumstances and conditions under which beliefs are gaining ground, becoming stabilized, or facing abandonment.

Given the perspective which has been set up so far, it may come as a surprise that credition processes—or some closely corresponding concepts—are *not* a long–standing issue in economics. To be sure, pertinent considerations were never completely absent from economic reasoning. (How could they be?) But they were not a core part of the conceptual and analytical apparatus of the discipline of economics. In the remainder of this chapter, I will first give a brief overview of the way in which related themes were discussed by economists (Sect. 2). By contrast, in Sect. 3, I will characterize the kinds of economic problems in which the importance of beliefs and credition is hidden by a set of assumptions that specify an interesting border case of social interaction in great societies. Those interesting border cases were central to the development of economics as a mathematical and quantitative science in the twentieth century. While I certainly cannot do full justice to the merits and misses of this approach, this sets the stage for Sect. 4, where I discuss game–theoretical frameworks in which issues of institutional economics and the economics of change can be analyzed. In the context of those frameworks, a more systematic account can be given regarding the types of problems and the methodological perspectives of integrating beliefs and credition processes in economics.

2 Beliefs, Trust and Credition in the History of Economic Thought

As in most other fields of economics, Adam Smith provides at least a starting point and some essential insights into the problem. Regarding the theme of the present chapter, this is true on three levels at least. Here is the first of those insights, which is related to credit markets (the association between credit and credition is not merely coincidental) and the economics of regulation: In the context of the British banking crises of the early 1770s, Smith (1776) developed an acute understanding of belief–dependent contagion processes and called for "firewalls" (i.e. enforcement of suitable banking regulations) to prevent contagion. At a second level, a basic foundational level that on first sight seems to have little to do with the just-mentioned policy-oriented issue of credit market regulation, Smith was challenged by the problem of locating religious faith in the modern world. His concern was to develop an understanding of modernity which would provide conceptual resources to mitigate the imminent horrors of what he called a "fatherless world", ridden by distrust, uncertainty and fear. This was not easy for him, as he had fully grasped the power of the work of David Hume (a close friend of his), which had shown the scientific path to explaining social institutions and moral norms as part of "nature" by way of "experimental moral philosophy." The distinctive quality of Smith's own version of the Scottish Enlightenment is closely related to his perception of the ambivalences implied by Enlightenment programs of demystification. Smith's conclusion was that a rather specific form of regulation is needed in order to deal with those profound ambivalences and tensions of modernity; a form of regulation which he called "the system of natural liberty," indicating that this order must be neither static nor based on privilege, but rather based on a kind of reflective equilibrium sustainable in a society of free people overcoming the horrors of a fatherless world. For a third, intermediate level of economic theorizing, Jerry Evensky (2011) recently remarked that

> in Smith's real analysis we leave the realm of faith and the issue becomes trust. While engaged in the market we must ask ourselves: To what degree can we trust the integrity of the other individual(s) involved in a potential market exchange? To the degree that our trust diminishes, the transaction costs associated with protecting ourselves from the risk of immoral or unethical behaviors rise. Every market interaction involves a probabilistic calculus of the perceived risk so that the transaction costs can be assessed. This is a challenge in an intimate society. It is a daunting challenge in the global market system. In that larger economic system, one is unlikely to have direct information on the trustworthiness of the other parties involved, so in a laissez–faire environment, one must resort to proxies: risk assessments by others who, in turn, must themselves be assessed for risk. As the layers of this risk information filtering get thicker, the sources of the information move from almost transparent to almost opaque. In a complex economic system, we are often making risk assessments from behind something approaching an opaque 'veil of uncertainty' (250).

I will come back to this third level towards the end of the chapter and relate it to the second one in a specific way.

A second key figure not to be missed in a discussion on beliefs and expectations in economics is John Maynard Keynes, whose famous discussion of beliefs in the stock exchange touches upon many of the key issues, and highlights their pivotal role in times of accelerated change. I quote this passage at length, as it provides not only arguments and insights at more than one level in a condensed form, but also illustrates the difficulties of capturing such a kind of reasoning by means of formal economic models. It is no coincidence that Keynes's younger colleagues did not take up those aspects when they developed the basic models of Keynesian macroeconomics. Here is what he says:

> In abnormal times in particular, when the hypothesis of an indefinite continuance of the existing state of affairs is less plausible than usual even though there are no express grounds to anticipate a definite change, the market will be subject to waves of optimistic and pessimistic sentiment, which are unreasoning and yet in a sense legitimate where no solid basis exists for a reasonable calculation. But there is one feature in particular which deserves our attention. It might have been supposed that competition between expert professionals, possessing judgment and knowledge beyond that of the average private investor, would correct the vagaries of the ignorant individual left to himself. It happens, however, that the energies and skill of the professional investor and speculator are mainly occupied otherwise. For most of these persons are, in fact, largely concerned, not with making superior long–term forecasts of the probable yield of an investment over its whole life, but with foreseeing changes in the conventional basis of valuation a short time ahead of the general public. They are concerned, not with what an investment is really worth to a man who buys it 'for keeps', but with what the market will value it at, under the influence of mass psychology, three months or a year hence. Moreover, this behavior is not the outcome of a wrong–headed propensity. It is an inevitable result of an investment market organized along the lines described. For it is not sensible to pay 25 for an investment of which you believe the prospective yield to justify a value of 30, if you also believe that the market will value it at 20 three months hence. Thus the professional investor is forced to concern himself with the anticipation of impending changes, in the news or in the atmosphere, of the kind by which experience shows that the mass psychology of the market is most influenced. This is the inevitable result of investment markets organised with a view to so–called 'liquidity'. Of the

> maxims of orthodox finance none, surely, is more anti–social than the fetish of liquidity, the doctrine that it is a positive virtue on the part of investment institutions to concentrate their resources upon the holding of 'liquid' securities. It forgets that there is no such thing as liquidity of investment for the community as a whole. The social object of skilled investment should be to defeat the dark forces of time and ignorance which envelop our future. The actual, private object of the most skilled investment to–day is 'to beat the gun', as the Americans so well express it, to outwit the crowd, and to pass the bad, or depreciating, half–crown to the other fellow. … Professional investment may be likened to those newspaper competitions in which the competitors have to pick out the six prettiest faces from a hundred photographs, the prize being awarded to the competitor whose choice most nearly corresponds to the average preferences of the competitors as a whole; so that each competitor has to pick, not those faces which he himself finds prettiest, but those which he thinks likeliest to catch the fancy of the other competitors, all of whom are looking at the problem from the same point of view. It is not a case of choosing those which, to the best of one's judgment, are really the prettiest, nor even those which average opinion genuinely thinks the prettiest. We have reached the third degree where we devote our intelligences to anticipating what average opinion expects the average opinion to be. And there are some, I believe, who practice the fourth, fifth and higher degrees (Keynes 1936: 155–156).

Those insights were not developed in the format of a fully–fledged theory, but they also did not come out of the blue. In the introduction to his first great work (*Treatise on Probability* 1973), Keynes attempts to explain how a degree of belief could be rational and shared by all rational humans under similar circumstances, and thus not driven by psychological propensities or idiosyncrasies (cf. Keynes 1973, vol. 8, p. xxi). I will come back to this in the penultimate section.

More recently, some economists and rational–choice sociologists have attempted to integrate belief structures and processes in a more systematic way, not least in the context of issues such as "trust." Examples include Nooteboom (2005), Esser (2005), Gächter and Thöni (2005) and Held et al. (2005). I conclude this section with a quotation from Nobel prize winner Kenneth Arrow, perhaps the greatest living economist: "It strikes me that the essential point is the great importance of such a virtue as truthfulness in widely prevalent circumstances of economic life…. Virtually every commercial transaction has within itself an element of trust, certainly any transaction conducted over a period of time. It can be plausibly argued that much of the economic backwardness in the world can be explained by the lack of mutual confidence" (1972: 356–357). This statement is all the more remarkable as Arrow was one of the foremost contributors to a research program in economics where all this plays hardly a role, which will be outlined in the next section.

3 Pure Economics: Full Information "Without Credition"

Despite the insights and ideas discussed in the previous section, the most celebrated achievements of economic theory are related to the complex interdependences at the level of society. They were derived on the basis of theoretical models in which something like "credition" simply cannot play a systematic role. The most well–known class of theories includes the so–called Walrasian general competitive market equilibrium models, a strand of research to which Kenneth Arrow vastly contributed. Why are those models important? They stand out in the social sciences as a fairly fully-developed population–level approach capturing wide–spread interdependences (another population–level approach had been developed in the context of models of evolutionary competition in biology). But those interdependences are captured in a very specific way: the individual actor who maximizes his utility or her profit is confronted with a given vector of equilibrium prices; this equilibrium price vector captures all relevant aspects of what other actors are doing (demanding and offering goods etc.) in a world which is assumed to be finite. The market process is such that the envisaged kind of social interaction—market exchange—occurs if and only if this equilibrium price system obtains, i.e., a price vector equating supply and demand on all markets (so–called "market clearing"). Exchange out of equilibrium (at non-market clearing prices) is ruled out. Actors are not only rational but also fully informed about all relevant aspects of potential transactions. Contracts are enforced without costs; there is no cheating and shirking.

Pertinent achievements are related to the explanation of price–mediated interdependences and incentive mechanisms in which the element of strategic interaction (meaning that the outcome of my action depends on everybody else's actions) plays no big role. To be sure: analogous to situations of genuine strategic social interaction, the *game structure* in those Walrasian market games is guided by artificial rules and natural constraints. It also remains true that the outcome of my action depends on everybody else's actions. But everybody else's actions are summarized by the equilibrium price vector and allows me to maximize in the same way as Robinson Crusoe would: This price vector is a parameter for my choices analogous to the laws of nature—and the rest of society— and hence must be treated *as if it were "nature."* Put succinctly, very specific "rules of the game" (notably specifying a market process that does not allow out–of–equilibrium trading) are the key element in explaining some (unintended) aggregate outcome, while individual agency is represented in an extremely reduced form.

In this class of theories, we are generally not interested in developing a descriptively accurate account of human agency, as some very abstract conception of rationality does the job *on an as–if basis*. This works fairly well in certain environments, e.g. in private property market economies with perfect competition. The coordination function and the sometimes quite intricate interdependences of multi–market–systems can be explained while remaining largely agnostic about human agency.

But there are important problem settings for which this is not good enough. In a game–theoretic language, some of those problem settings are related to the existence of more than one equilibrium. (The most frequently used concept in that context is the Nash equilibrium, which is defined as a pattern of strategies such that nobody has a reason/an incentive to *unilaterally* change his or her strategy). With multiple equilibria, "equilibrium selection" becomes a problem—and beliefs become crucially important. A reasonable choice of strategies is not possible in the absence of reasonable conjectures (which can be ascribed to actors in a way consistent with the theory) regarding the question: On which of the many equilibria will the actors tend to coordinate their actions? Unfortunately (or fortunately for those who always had the suspicion that it is highly implausible to base all socio–

economic theory on abstract as–if rationality), it can be shown that conventional rationality assumptions do not help in determining the beliefs that agents would rationally develop in such situations. Beliefs with a wider, perhaps culturally informed background (or even more comprehensive mental models, e.g. what Nobel laureate Douglass North sometimes calls "ideologies"), may come into play at this stage. They may be thought of as closely associated with *rules/institutions operating as equilibrium selection devices in strategic interaction problems with many equilibria*. Moreover, in a long-term perspective, economic and institutional change is likely to be associated with some change regarding beliefs, preferences and even more comprehensive mental models. This in turn motivates further questions regarding the *plasticity* of beliefs, preferences and mental models. That is, when, why and how (incremental adjustment of beliefs or paradigm shift with regard to mental models?) are they subject to change? Analysis of credition processes may be expected to shed light on the properties of such processes of change and may complement existing approaches to explaining change.

In the remainder of this chapter (Sect. 4), I am going to highlight some answers to the following questions:

1. In which areas of economics are credition–related issues most important?
2. Which problems are appearing in conventional economic models attempting to approach those areas where there is some *prima facie* reason for the suspicion that credition may be important?
3. Which research strategies are pursued in order to address those problems and what might be the place of credition research in their context?

4 Credit Markets, Labor Exchange and the Economics of Institutional Change

In the 1970s, economists became increasingly aware of the fact that the dominant methodology discussed in the previous chapter may be misleading as far as some particularly important and complex markets are concerned: credit markets, insurance markets and labor markets. Notions such as incomplete contracts, moral hazard and adverse selection were introduced in that context. Moreover, the growing interest in the economics of norms and institutions (considered as an indispensable framework for market exchange) set the stage for an increasing importance of game theory (for a good overview and analytical introduction into those developments including behavioral economics see Bowles 2004).

In the economics of institutions, some typical assumptions of conventional Walrasian equilibrium theory are challenged almost from the beginning: for instance, in many contexts of institutional development, it is no longer plausible to assume given preferences and treat belief formation as a black box. Exogenous preferences imply ruling out the possibility that beliefs and preferences co–evolve with institutions, and in this sense, are an endogenous aspect of institutional development. Endogenous beliefs means (*inter alia*) that beliefs are to a certain extent shaped by institutions, whereas institutions in part can be understood as an "answer" to prevailing norms, which in turn may be shaped by beliefs. More generally, important classes of real–world problems are strategic interaction problems, where the above-mentioned research strategy of modeling rational individual behavior summarizing the actions of all other agents by a vector of prices (and thereby eliminating problems of strategic interaction) is not good enough. To cope with those challenges, new research strategies were developed, stressing or combining

1. Developments in game theory capturing strategic interaction and distribution problems;
2. frameworks where preference endogeneity is brought to the fore (e.g. adaptive preferences, second order preferences);
3. attempts to integrate economics and psychology (behavioral/experimental economics, neuronomics).

With regard to modeling individual behavior, three kinds of problems became most salient:

(a) Rationality assumptions may imply cognitive demands and calculative burdens which render rationality to be problematic as an as–if assumption in certain contexts. Alternatives include concepts of bounded rationality or integrating the role of routines or decision heuristics. Moreover, choice frames and biases are taken into account (for an overview see Esser 2005).
(b) An important group of experiments of strategic interaction problems suggest that individually and socially desirable outcomes under certain conditions may be supported by appropriate motivations or emotionally-anchored drivers of action (such as fairness, reciprocity, altruism, and inequality aversion). Variations of pertinent experimental designs under different cultural circumstances suggest that those motivations are likely to depend on the institutional–cultural environment, i.e. they may be "crowded out" in an environment where they can play no role or where the social structure is hostile to the kind of social learning which would lead to those motivations.
(c) Many real-world problems are best understood as strategic interaction situations with more than one equilibrium. In such situations, beliefs are essential, including in particular higher-order beliefs (beliefs about other's beliefs). And insofar as we are concerned with the processes of change out of equilibrium or the transition from one equilibrium to another equilibrium, the process of belief will be central.

In the first decades of experimental economics, there seems to have been a certain tendency to emphasize (or even isolate) one of the three above–mentioned aspects of (a), (b), and (c). For instance, the issue of cognitive/calculative demands and framing (a) is at the core of typical problems studied by experimental research dealing with choices under risk and uncertainty and by the literature on Libertarian Paternalism/Choice Architecture. Consider next the aspect of motivation (b). In the perspective of many designs in experimental economics, the classical public good game with its Prisoners' Dilemma–like structure (with one "bad" equilibrium where the benefits of cooperation are foregone) is a game where primarily the issue of motivation looms large, as people with selfish motivations are bound to end up as "rational fools" (to use a phrase coined by Amartya Sen). In the context of such games, the issue of beliefs only becomes salient if some aspects of the experimental design (such as repetition of the game and scope for reciprocity) make the people think that there might be a second ("good") equilibrium (c). Yet there is another game in which experimenters managed to almost isolate the issue of motivation (b): the Dictator game, where the outcome is unilaterally determined by the dictator, leaving little room for a role of second-order beliefs. For my choice as a dictator, it does not matter what I believe that the other believes that I believe …

By contrast, in many important real-world problems, *more than one* of the just–mentioned aspects plays a role. Think for instance of Keynes's beauty contest metaphor referring to the stock market, or imagine a bank run affecting a (healthy) bank with temporary liquidity problems in a situation of general financial turmoil. In a potential bank run situation, there is a good equilibrium (all individuals behave as they would do in normal times, basically leaving their money in their bank accounts) and a bad equilibrium (everybody tries to withdraw the money as quickly as possible, thereby turning a short–run liquidity problem into a solvency–problem). The details of such a model are of little interest here. Suppose, for instance, that if I am joining those queuing up at the bank counters, I will get my money with a 10% ex ante chance of success. Even if I knew that a better equilibrium were possible when all people were behaving "normally" (all keep 100% of their deposits), and even if I knew that my chance of getting my money is only 10%, it is individually rational for me to queue up, given that I believe that the others believe. Notice now that in principle, the logic of the two equilibria applies to any bank at any time. Hence, in order to understand a situation where, say, a good equilibrium breaks down and we move to a bad equilibrium, issues related to beliefs, choice frames and motivations must be taken into consideration.

One of the perspectives of future research designs is related to the fact that not seldom all three aspects (a) – (c) may play a role, and that they may interact in choice situations: e.g., motivations may interact with beliefs (cf. the "motivated beliefs" stressed by Jon Elster 2004: 3–4) or *cognitive/calculative stress may render motivations "narrower,"* as studied in some recent experiments (see Luchini and Teschl 2015).

Regarding all those problems, especially the mixed problems so important in the real world, credition *processes* may play an interesting role. For obtaining some initial ideas regarding the specific rationales for this role, it is useful to discuss the kind of problems that *mainly* hinge upon second-order beliefs. Those are situations with *more than one equilibrium* and naturally associated with "equilibrium selection" problems. In the case of the bank run example, one immediate question for me is: Are the other actors believing that the bank is sound? Which change of beliefs can I expect for the coming days? Etc. Along the lines suggested by such questions, considering credition processes as a dynamic environment of choice–relevant (higher order) beliefs supporting various outcomes is necessary for solving the problem.

This includes various types of situations, e.g. with

- good equilibria and bad equilibria (as in the example of the bank run)
- more than one good equilibrium (traffic rules: drive right or drive left)
- common interest (the same equilibrium is best for everybody, as in the bank run example)
- more or less divergent interests (different equilibria are best for different people, as stylized in a game called *Battle of the Sexes*)
- one equilibrium which yet may fail to be realized, as this is too demanding in terms of cognitive demands: playing the equilibrium strategy would require actors to engage in highly sophisticated reasoning in terms of what Keynes in the above-quoted passage called *forth, fifth or higher degree thinking*.

The various types of situations may be related to specific dynamics of interactions between motivations, framing effects, and beliefs, which cannot be discussed here. For the sake of illustrating the common structure of those problems, consider again the (relatively simple) bank run example—or any other example in which it is highly desirable for all individuals to coordinate their actions on the good equilibrium and not the bad equilibrium. The pivotal question here of course is: On which of the equilibria will actors coordinate their actions? It seems obvious that higher-order beliefs become crucially important in those situations. That is, belief not (only) *amounting to objective knowledge regarding the nature of the situation, but beliefs about beliefs*. As stressed in the above passages, conventional rationality assumptions do not help much in determining that beliefs agents would (rationally) develop in such situations. If I possess no evidence whatsoever for believing that other individuals will coordinate on the good rather than on the bad equilibrium and vice versa, I could assume a 0.5 probability. Given this, I can calculate that I had better do this or that. But such calculations do not lead very far. Hence, we are left with questions such as the following:

- Can we say something about the processes of belief formation?
- If yes, is this useful for answering the question: How do people develop shared beliefs?
- Which are the circumstances enhancing and obstructing shared beliefs?

The wording used in those questions is more or less congruent with some pertinent literature focusing institutional change. Using the noun "belief" seems to suggest that, as it were, single points (snap-shots) within belief processes are considered. This, of course, raises the question of how that can be properly conceptualized? Be that as it may, in seeking answers to those questions, it seems highly plausible to begin to study individual processes of belief, the way in which they may be influenced by social environments, and their dynamics so that they may be better understood. Analyzing a credition as a bundle of processes of belief is a promising research strategy from that point of view. This may shed light on the role of the formation of social networks with strong and weak links, rituals, and power-preserving structures in socio–economic situations.

An initial illustration of such ideas is again found in Adam Smith's (1776, V.i.g.iii) account of the role of religious education in a largely anonymous commercial society with no traditional social bonds, ranks and norms that could function as orientation. In the language of game theory, Smith's story can be summarized as follows: proper embedding of agents in religious credition is associated with the development of "character," which is not merely an individual process, but a process relevant for social coordination; it helps to support a no–cheat equilibrium.

5 Conclusion

Processes of belief are likely to be important with regard to certain levels and problems of economic analysis. This includes markets such as the financial market and the labor market where the assumption of full and symmetric information has long been recognized as problematic. It also includes economic phenomena in which change plays a major role. As a first way of approaching those problems, beliefs may be thought of as closely associated with rules/institutions operating as equilibrium-selection devices in strategic interaction problems with multiple equilibria. In a long-term perspective, economic and institutional change is likely to be associated with some change regarding more comprehensive mental models. Those changes could be thought of as specific phases within processes of creditions. For instance, discussions referring to the issue of *plasticity* in institutional economics may be taken as a foreshadowing of the integration of more process–related views and concepts. Analysis of credition processes may be expected to shed light on the properties of such dynamics of change in an open–ended universe, which is perhaps the most important and most difficult agenda for the social sciences.

References

Arrow KJ (1972) Gifts and exchanges. Philos Public Aff 1(4):343–362

Bowles S (2004) Microeconomics. Princeton University Press, Princeton

Elster J (2004) Cost and constraints in the economy of the mind. In: Brocas I, Carrillo JD (eds) The psychology of economic decisions. Oxford University Press, Oxford, pp 3–14

Esser H (2005) Rationalität und Bindung. Das Modell der Frame–Selektion und die Erklärung des normativen Handelns. In: Held M, Kubon-Gilke G, Sturn R (eds) Reputation und Vertrauen. Normative und institutionelle Grundfragen der Ökonomik, Jahrbuch, vol 4. Metropolis, Marburg, pp 85–111

Evensky J (2011) Adam Smith's essentials on trust, faith, and free markets. J Hist Econ Thought 33(2):249–257

Gächter S, Thöni C (2005) Vertrauen und Reputation: Beiträge der experimentellen Ökonomik. In: Held M, Kubon-Gilke G, Sturn R (eds) Reputation und Vertrauen. Normative und institutionelle Grundfragen der Ökonomik, Jahrbuch, vol 4. Metropolis, Marburg, pp 257–281

Held M, Kubon-Gilke G, Sturn R (2005) Ökonomik des Vertrauens – Stellenwert von Vertrauen in der Ökonomik. In: Held M, Kubon-Gilke G, Sturn R (eds) Reputation und Vertrauen. Normative und institutionelle Grundfragen der Ökonomik, Jahrbuch, vol 4. Metropolis, Marburg, pp 7–33
Keynes JM (1936) The general theory of employment, interest and money. Macmillan, London
Keynes JM (1973) The collected writings, vol 8. Treatise on probability. Cambridge University Press, Cambridge
Luchini S, Teschl M (2015) Effort and redistribution: is more than value judgement involved? Jahrbuch für normative und institutionelle Grundfragen der Ökonomik 14:165–184
Nootebom B (2005) Forms, sources and limits of trust. In: Held M, Kubon-Gilke G, Sturn R (eds) Reputation und Vertrauen. Normative und institutionelle Grundfragen der Ökonomik, Jahrbuch, vol 4. Metropolis, Marburg, pp 35–58
Smith A (1776) An inquiry into the nature and causes of the wealth of nations. Strahan, London

Credition in Business – Innovations with Crowdbusiness

Reinhard Willfort and Conny Weber

Abstract It is obvious that all kind of businesses need innovations, as the lifetime of new products or services is steadily becoming shorter and increased competition forces companies to surprise their customers with new products or services more frequently. Innovation management aims to systematically implement innovation in organizations. More specifically, innovation management focuses on how to derive profitable products and services from creative outputs within an organization. The underlying decision-making processes which lead to successful innovations are significantly influenced by *beliefs*. Most businesses, ranging from start-ups to established organizations, believe that they are making rational decisions. However, the decisions made within an innovation management processes are often based on a subjective assessment of different indicators including *gut feelings* and *beliefs*. Using digital technology allows for the assessment of the beliefs of many people, and the so-called "wisdom of the crowds" supports decision-making in innovation management. This chapter takes a closer look at how to increase transparency and democratization of beliefs that influence decision-making processes within the field of innovation management by systematically taking into account the concept of *credition*.

1 Rational Decision Making vs. Disruptive Innovations

In business theory, there are different theories of decision-making. Most of them are based on the concept of rationality. Rational decision-making consists of systematically selecting from among possible choices that are based on explicit reasons and facts. In a rational decision-making process, different analytical tools and models allow one to review relevant facts and derive possible outcomes, and finally the best option leads to a decision. And what about business practice? For Simon (1947, 1997), decision-makers cannot have complete knowledge about and be able to anticipate all of the possible alternatives to, as well as the consequences of, a

R. Willfort (✉) • C. Weber
ISN – Innovation Service Network GmbH, Graz, Austria
e-mail: reinhard.willfort@innovation.at; conny.weber@innovation.at

H.-F. Angel et al. (eds.), *Processes of Believing: The Acquisition, Maintenance, and Change in Creditions*, New Approaches to the Scientific Study of Religion 1,
DOI 10.1007/978-3-319-50924-2_27

decision. As these consequences exist only in the future, imagination and experience are required, and values can be only imperfectly applied. Rationality is bounded. A decision cannot be made by finding the optimal solution to a problem; rather, it is made by a satisfying choice. Thus, managers make individual decisions using different methods that lead to different conclusions not based on a rational choice, but influenced by individual personality, management style, and experience (Keen and Morton 1978).

Especially in the field of innovation, the real and disruptive innovations cannot rely on figures and facts analyzed by a rational homo oeconomicus, simply because there are not any figures and facts about unknown markets, unknown customers, and their behaviors. Real innovations rely simply on strong *beliefs*, *emotions*, and *gut feelings* (Willfort et al 2007a). These are also results of current research, e.g. in the field of trust, which show that decisions are strongly influenced by emotions and cognitions (Angel and Willfort 2013).

The most prominent and well-known example in the context of disruptive innovation is in Henry Ford's quote regarding faster horses. In fact, in 1894, the London *Times* estimated that by 1950, every street in the city would be buried ninefeet deep in horse manure. In light of this predicted issue, researchers tried, e.g., at the 1898 International Urban Planning Conference summit in New York, to find a solution for the faster-growing cities and the problems associated with horse transportation: thousands of tons of manure produced each day, locations around the city where the horses could be tethered, finding adequately-sized stables, and growing food for more than hundred thousand horses (e.g. Johnson 2015). Ford solved this dilemma by making the automobile available to the common person, instead of focusing on ways to remove horse manure. He came up with a solution that no one had ever thought about before, and it solved multiple issues stemming from one problem.

2 The Role of Emotions and Creditions – The Credition Theory in a Nutshell

Whether an organization can establish an innovative and creative environment or not cannot be influenced by a rational analysis. But as we have learned, the results of theses analyses will always contain challenging questions and cannot guarantee if the organization will manage to develop a new and profitable innovative product or service. Additionally, establishing and restructuring new processes in an organization involves fear, tremendous joy and desperation, which may also influence the results. In the end, organizations can only initiate or establish a sustainable and value-creating innovation management process if all members strongly believe in its success and meaningfulness.

"Believing" in the success of innovations requires a more in depth observation of the processes of believing. Recently, this new research field has developed under the term "credition" (Angel 2013) and covers research on the processes of beliefs. An

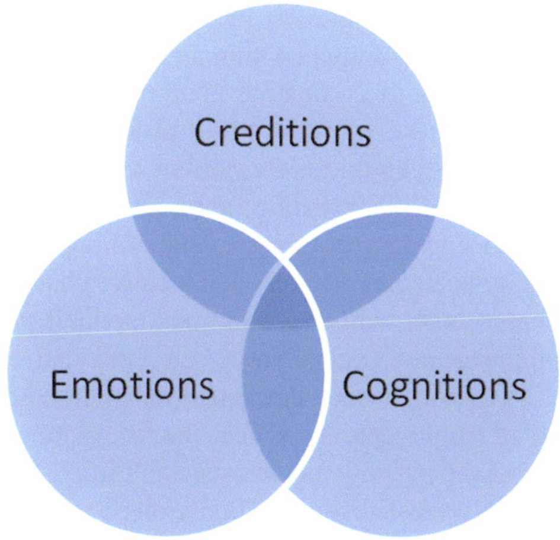

Fig. 1 Creditions as interdependent interaction with emotions and cognitions (Angel and Willfort 2013)

important aspect is that these beliefs are not only coined as "religious" but rather, they are seen as having the potential to deal with emotions and cognitions. Topics cover a broad range such as the structure of creditions, i.e. the role of cognition, emotion and appraisal; neuroscientific observations, i.e. how emotions influence credition processes, or the impact of beliefs, e.g. the phenomenon of the self-fulfilling prophecy described by Merton (1948) which describes a prediction that causes itself to become true, due to positive feedback between belief and behavior.

The term "credition" is a neologism, which is conceived in analogy to emotion and cognition and denotes the process of believing as it appears in religious and in non-religious contexts (Angel 2006). Processes of belief shape our lives to a great extent, and the sciences have just started their research on creditions.

To date, it is not quite clear yet how to qualify creditions, but there is a common agreement among academics that they are interrelated with emotions and cognitions (Fig. 1), and that they can influence our inner stability.

In the context of creditions, recent neuroscience research has shown that human behavior is influenced by different regions of the brain, depending on whether the respective person is concerned with the emotion-based search for short-term goals or a reflected development of more rationality inherent to long-term goals. In the end, the decision-making process is a consequence of subjective evaluation processes, which are closely related with beliefs.

3 Applying Credition Theory in Innovation Management

The need for innovation is obvious, as the lifetime of new products is steadily getting shorter, and increased competition forces companies to surprise customers with new services or products more often. Innovation management aims to systematically implement innovation in organisations (Schumpeter 1911). More specifically, innovation management focuses on how to derive profitable products and services from creative outputs within an organisation (Cooper 1987).

The idea of combining neurophysiologic perspectives with innovation, as it is based on research of Willfort et al. (2007b), is obvious in order to enrich these results with cognitions, emotions and creditions. The strongly-required innovation capabilities of companies are mainly determined by the willingness of its staff to embrace and enact change. And coming up with successful innovations requires a strong balancing act between creative chaos and systematic-methodical innovation management, while at the same time taking into account the psychological aspects of change and change processes (Fink et al. 2007).

A thorough consideration of innovation processes can reduce the fears and barriers of employees, and reduce the risk of failure of innovation projects. From a motivational perspective, it is especially important to highlight the short-term results of an innovation process. This strongly supports the acceptance and motivation of decision-makers to support the innovation process both in terms of resources and commitment for innovations. The underlying decision-making processes for innovation processes are highly complex, strongly interrelated and thus always contain a portion of *beliefs*.

4 A Tool Supporting the Communication of Creditions in Innovation Management Processes

The research field of credition is still in its beginnings, and many aspects are unclear and require further scientific discussion. Nevertheless, there exist early ways for grasping the influence of creditions in decision-making processes.

Angel and Willfort (2013) assume that it is possible to determine creditive values in processes and to quantify their importance. This allows one to determine the influence of creditions based on a so-called credition index, and to include this assessment in planning and decision-making processes.

The ISN (Innovation Service Network; www.innovation.at) has started to develop together with the Credition Research Network a *credition-tool* (www.credition.at) aiming at visualizing beliefs in decision-making processes. This tool allows for the analysis of the emotional and cognitive bases which underlie decision-making processes, and help to visualize the influence of beliefs. This tool represents more a gamified approach rather than an exact calculation for visualizing the credition-index of decision-making processes and aims to inspire further discussions (Fig. 2).

We believe that this tool provides insights into and transparency about innovation-oriented decisions and supports communication about the underlying processes. Innovation decisions are always decisions covering complex tasks with a high risk of failure. Dealing with innovations always means questioning existing practices in order to achieve new and better conditions. The credition theory supports both the explanation and the creation of such complex decisions.

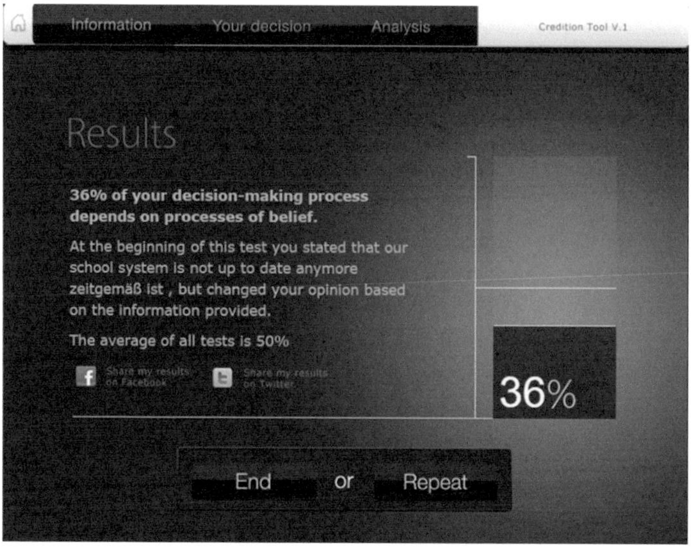

Fig. 2 Screenshot of the credition tool indicating the credition index of a decision

5 A New Perspective – Innovation, Credition and the Crowd

In the last few years, influenced by the possibilities of modern web technologies, several things have changed in business. A new and disruptive component has enriched traditional factors of production and thus innovation – *the crowd*. Crowd-based business models are springing up as we speak. Nowadays, the crowd decides whether a company, a product, a service, or a business model is successful or not. This phenomenon has initiated disruptive changes in traditional marketing concepts.

Thus, innovation management has significantly changed, especially towards approaches for supporting the innovation process and gathering ideas from outside the organization. Recently, these approaches have become increasingly computer-based while enabling access to large user communities. This phenomenon is summarised under the term "open innovation" (Chesbrough 2003) and goes one step further by including external resources, i.e. shareholders, end-users or communities in the innovation process. According to Chesbrough (2003) open innovation "is a paradigm that assumes that firms can and should use external ideas as well as internal ideas, and internal and external paths to market, as the firms look to advance their technology"(24).

Even more precise is the term "crowdsourcing," which was coined in 2006 by Jeff Howe, and describes an organisation leveraging the power of crowds for generating and assessing new ideas as well as for developing and marketing new products and services (Howe 2006).

A special form of crowdsourcing is crowdfunding. The idea of crowdfunding is to collect many small amounts from members of a community in order to support and realise a certain project, thereby providing a new dimension of venture capital financing (De Buysere et al. 2012). Similar to crowdsourcing, all shareholders interested in a project idea can support the realisation of the project with their funds. Recognition of the funders ranges from a “thank you” to a prize or other rewards. In a nutshell, crowdfunding is when *co-thinking* micro-investors provide small amounts for big ideas. Combined with the intelligent use of *crowd-technologies*, crowdfunding shapes new ways of decision-making and innovations. The difference between crowdsourcing and traditional ways of financing such as credits or individual investors is mainly that a larger group of people who *believe* in the success of the idea decides to realise a project with their funds.

That means in terms of the credition model, a larger group shares a common “mega-bab.” “Bab” is a novel term which was introduced in the framework of credition “to denote a knowledge item that consists of the contents of beliefs. Each ‘bab’ can carry specific emotional value and describes an item at any levels of complexity. The term “bab” is a meta-theoretically conceived neologism inspired by the hierarchical organization of the Babushka doll. Similarly to such a doll of different “sizes”, the same contents of a “bab” can exist with different values of “mightiness”, expressing the different personal relevance of the belief content” (Sugiura et al. 2015, 14).

Major babs are titled as “mega-babs” (cf. Angel in this volume). Mega-babs are highly relevant for one of the central functions of believing processes, namely the enclosure function, which influences decision-making. It is due to the enclosure function this “bab” may be enclosed into the bab-configuration of the agent (Angel 2013). Therefore, a commonly shared mega-bab of “co-thinkers” is supporting group coherence and common strategy-finding.

Superficially considered, enhancing business with the crowd can be seen as a more effective and efficient way to perform certain business functions. From a strategic advisory point of view, crowdbusiness can be considered as a systematic approach for business model innovation by including the creditions, cognitions and emotions of many people in the decision-making processes through crowd-based technologies. Crowdbusiness fosters the evolution of a new ecosystem for innovations by combining open innovation approaches with the latest crowd technologies and democratizing processes of belief.

6 A Framework for Crowdbusiness

Including the “wisdom of the crowd” (Surowiecki 2005) in innovation management processes supports credition-based innovation processes. Following Willfort and Weber (2015), the secret of success lies in the combination of professional

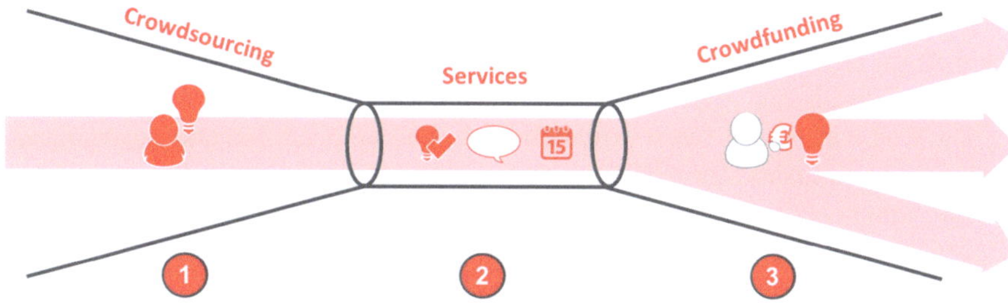

Fig. 3 The Crowdbusiness framework (Willfort and Weber 2015)

innovation services and crowd-based mechanisms supported by social media. The crowdbusiness framework describes a holistic approach for crowd-based innovation management covering all phases of the innovation process and has been developed by the ISN and implemented in several pioneering projects in Austria.

The threefold approach (Fig. 3) covers all phases of the innovation management process, i.e. the creation, the selection, the realization and financing of project ideas through democratizing the beliefs of the crowd.

1. Through crowdsourcing, credition aspects can improve and support the collaborative creation of innovative ideas. Further, engaging with a creative community provides valuable insights, creates connections, and thus provides value for the innovation success. The aim of the crowdsourcing phase is to generate ideas, to receive feedback and to further develop ideas by taking advantage of credition-based decision-making of many people. Thus, innovations can evolve within a network consisting of *co-thinkers*, creatives, entrepreneurs and organizations, who collaboratively submit ideas, evaluate the ideas and shape them into a final concept for a new product, service or start-up. All kinds of organizations can collect feedback and reduce the innovation risk at a very early stage and at the same time leverage the chance for a successful innovation.
2. Innovation services aim to support the presentation and realization of a promising project idea by providing the know-how of experienced innovation experts, investors and multipliers. This second phase provides complementary support for the presentation, realization and communication of a project idea.
3. Finally, crowdfunding services provide valuable means for funding a project by raising money from a community. Crowdfunding services provide information and support on potential financing and (further) funding opportunities and professionally influence factors associated with success and failure among crowdfunded projects. These factors are very diversified and may depend not only on the project quality, but also on e.g., the communication in social networks, geographical aspects, the duration, domain or the funding goal etc.

The crowdbusiness framework provides digital market places in which to combine crowdsourcing and crowdfunding principles.

In principle there are not any constraints with regards to company size or market segment for crowdbusiness. Several crowdsourcing and crowdfunding success stories demonstrate that especially established industries can achieve very good feedback on concepts or reach extremely high funding goals and take advantage of the crowd participation for further marketing and distribution activities.

The main benefits that the crowdbusiness framework might deliver are:

- Gathering new ideas (crowdsourcing) and financial support (crowdfunding) from the crowd, i.e. people who believe in the project idea
- The interaction with the crowd and their individual creditions validates ideas for products, services or business models in an early stage
- Crowdbusiness is a powerful tool for market analysis, because it allows testing whether there is a demand for an innovation or not
- Crowdsourcing and crowdfunding are perfect marketing instruments as they promotes an idea to early adopters
- Crowdbusiness allows lowering the innovation risk, as the community of "believers" and co-thinkers, e.g. investors or other shareholders, can provide direct feedback and share their experiences and know-how with the entrepreneur
- Crowdsourcing and crowdfunding initiatives are emotionally and personally motivated, which increases the guarantee of success

7 Conclusion – Credition in Crowdbusiness

Most businesses, ranging from start-ups to established organizations, believe that they are making rational decisions. However, the decisions made within an innovation management process are often based on a subjective assessment of different indicators including *gut feelings* and *beliefs*. Using digital technology allows a person or company to assess the beliefs of many people, and the so-called "wisdom of the crowds" supports decision-making in innovation management.

Crowdbusiness constitutes a new paradigm in innovation management by democratizing the processes of belief of many individuals through web-based crowd technologies. The combination of the credition and crowdbusiness approach can provide much added value for decision-making processes in all types of organisations.

Probably the most important and interesting aspect regarding credition-based innovations through crowdbusiness, is the "community of belief" behind the idea, consisting of the *co-thinkers* of a project, who are emotionally and personally motivated and deal in trust relationships.

References

Angel HF (2006) Religiosität als menschliches Potential. Ein anthropologisches Modell der Religiosität im neurowissenschaftlichen Horizont. In: Angel HF et al (eds) Religiosität. Kohlhammer, Stuttgart, pp 62–89

Angel HF (2013) Credition, the process of belief. In: Azari NP, Runehov A, Olviedo L (eds) Encyclopedia of sciences and religions. Springer, Heidelberg/New York

Angel HF, Willfort R (2013) Die Systematik hinter "Bauchentscheidungen". In: Lutz B (ed) Wissen im Dialog, Krems, pp 21–28. http://www.donau-uni.ac.at/imperia/md/images/department/wissenkommunikation/news/wima-2012-sammelband.pdf. Accessed 1 Aug 2015

Chesbrough HW (2003) Open innovation. The new imperative for creating and profiting from technology. Harvard Business School Press, Boston

Cooper RG (1987) New products: what separates the winners from losers. J Prod Innov Manag 4(3):169–184

De Buysere K, Gajda O, Kleverlaan R, Marom D (2012) A framework for European crowdfunding. http://www.crowdfundingframework.eu. Accessed 1 July 2014

Fink A, Benedek M, Neubauer A (2007) Möglichkeiten zur Steigerung der kreativen Produktivität aus Sicht der Psychologie und der Neurowissenschaften. In: Willfort R, Tochermann K, Neubauer A (eds) Creativity@Work für Wissensarbeit. Aachen, pp 27–38

Howe J (2006) The rise of crowdsourcing. http://archive.wired.com/wired/archive/14.06/crowds.html. Accessed 1 July 2014

Johnson B (2015) Great horse manure crisis of 1894. http://www.historic-uk.com/HistoryUK/HistoryofBritain/Great-Horse-Manure-Crisis-of-1894/

Keen PGW, Scott-Morton MS (1978) Decision support systems: an organizational perspective. Addison-Wesley, Reading

Merton RK (1948) The self-fulfilling prophecy. Antioch Rev 8:193–210

Schumpeter JA (1911) The theory of economic development: an inquiry into profits, capital, credit, interest and the business cycle. Harvard University Press, Cambridge Mass

Simon HA (1947) Administrative behavior [1997]: a study of decision-making processes in administrative organizations, 4th edn. Free Press, New York

Sugiura M, Seitz RF, Angel HF (2015) Models and neural bases of the believing process. J Behav Brain Sci 5(1):12–23. doi:10.4236/jbbs.2015.51002

Surowiecki J (2005) The wisdom of crowds. Anchor Books

Willfort R, Weber C (2015) The crowdpower 2.0 concept- An integrated approach to innovation that goes beyond crowdfunding. In: Brüntje D, Gajda O (eds) Crowdfunding in Europe. State of the Art in Theory and Practice. Springer, Cham

Willfort R, Tochtermann K, Neubauer A (2007a) Creativity@Work für Wissensarbeit. Kreative Höchstleistungen am Wissensarbeitsplatz auf Basis neuester Erkenntnisse der Gehirnforschung. Shaker Verlag, Aachen

Willfort R, Köck AM, Hartlieb M (2007b) Neurovation. Die Idee der Verbindung von Neurophysiologie und Innovation. In: Willfort R, Tochermann K, Neubauer A (eds) Creativity@Work für Wissensarbeit. Shaker, Aachen, pp 53–56

Part VI
Natural and Computer Sciences

Creditions and Modern Computer Science

Horst Bischof

Abstract This short chapter describes the relationship between computer science and creditions, and shows that any subfield of computer science that deals with data needs to make assumptions, and that these assumptions (we call them priors) are nothing else than beliefs or creditions. Two simple examples from computer vision and machine learning demonstrate the effect of priors. Finally, Bayesian inference is introduced as a principle method to handle priors in a rigorous manner.

1 Introduction

Computer science, like mathematics, is an exact science that is based on strict rules (axioms) where there seems to be no place for beliefs. This is true if one looks just at the formal nature of computer science. But since computer science is more than just formalisms, it is also about the application of formal methods to real world data. Therefore, we have to deal with the aspect of data interpretation.

The goal of this chapter is to discuss some inherent relationships between computer science and creditions. At first glance, this might seem quite far-fetched, and one is inclined to say that they are two completely separate things. But I will argue that parts of computer science (especially those that deal with the interpretation of data, e.g. computer vision, speech processing, machine learning etc.) are inherently confronted with belief systems. I will illustrate this using one example from computer vision (Szeliski 2010) and one example from machine learning (Mitchell 1997). But the same line of argumentation is true for other sub-fields of computer science as well. The argument is that in order to make "sense" of complex data, we need prior knowledge, and it is exactly this prior knowledge that encodes our beliefs. The essence of the problem lies in the fact that many complex problems are ill-posed i.e. Hadamard (1902) said that a problem is well-posed when:

1. A solution exists
2. The solution is unique
3. The solution's behaviour changes continuously with the initial conditions.

H. Bischof (✉)
Institute for Computer Graphics and Vision, Graz University of Technology, Graz, Austria
e-mail: bischof@icg.tugraz.at

H.-F. Angel et al. (eds.), *Processes of Believing: The Acquisition, Maintenance, and Change in Creditions*, New Approaches to the Scientific Study of Religion 1,
DOI 10.1007/978-3-319-50924-2_28

If one of these conditions is violated, then we say that the problem is ill-posed. In fact, in the examples we consider, we are very often confronted with a violation of the second condition, i.e., the available data allows for multiple solutions. In order to select one of those solutions, we have to introduce additional constraints or prior knowledge. And it is exactly this additional knowledge that we can interpret as a credition process. If we do not introduce additional constraints, there is no solution to the problem. In this sense, the process of creditions is inherent to the problem.

The rest of the chapter is organized as follows. I will first present a few examples from computer vision and machine learning that illustrate ill-posed problems and how they can be solved using additional information. Then I will present Bayes inference as a principle mechanism to illustrate how prior knowledge can be incorporated to an inference problem.

2 Examples

Let us first look at computer vision. The goal of computer vision is to build machines that are able to see and interpret their environment. All of us can tell a story about an arbitrary image that is presented; this is the ultimate goal of computer vision. To achieve this goal, we need to recognize all objects in an image, recognize the context they are in, recognize actions etc. All these are non-trivial tasks. Even for humans, this is sometimes not easy; just think about all the optical illusions (see for example Fig. 1 the Müller-Leyer illusion).

2.1 Image Denoising

Let us consider a basic image processing problem and let us illustrate the usage of priors. In image denoising, one is given an image $I_n(x, y)$ that is contaminated with an unknown noise $n(x, y)$, i.e., $I_n(x, y) = I(x, y) + n(x, y)$. The task is now, just given I_n[1] to infer I without any other knowledge. This is a classical ill-posed problem

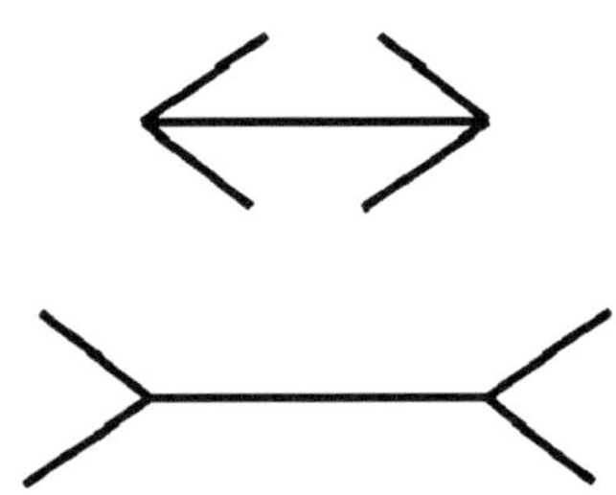

Fig. 1 The classical Müller-Leyer illusions. Despite having the same length the *upper line* appears to be shorter compared to the *lower* one

[1] To simplify the notation we skip the two-dimensional indices when there is no danger of confusion.

because there infinite many possibilities (i.e., the noise is a random process) regarding how the original images I might look like. A classic way of solving this problem is to set up an optimization problem with the following form:

$$\min_{I} \|I - I_n\|$$

i.e. we look for an image I that is close to the given image I_n. Of course, this does not work because in this case the optimal solution is $I = I_n$ so we need to impose additional constraints, e.g., we might assume a certain type of noise, or we might assume properties of the original image I. For example, we can assume that the image I is smooth (i.e., nearby pixels have almost the same colour), or we might assume that I is smooth and has sharp edges etc. This results then in the following optimization problem

$$\min_{I} = \lambda R(I) + \|I - I_n\|$$

where we have introduced an additional term $R(I)$ (called regularization) which expresses our prior assumptions we have about the image, and the scalar λ controls the influence of the prior. Typical priors are of the form:

$$R(I) = |\nabla I|^{\alpha}$$

where ∇I is the image gradient and depending on α, we get different solutions. With $\alpha = 2$ we favour smooth images, with $\alpha = 1$ (called total variation) we favour sharp edges.

See Fig. 2 for an example of such a denoising model. One can clearly see how our prior assumptions influence the solution. In this case, the total variation prior is closer to what we expect from natural images.

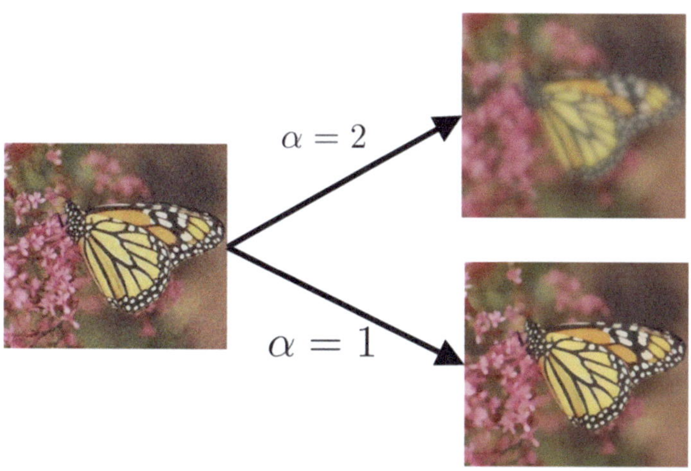

Fig. 2 Image denoising example with quadratic ($\alpha = 2$) and total variation ($\alpha = 1$) regularization

Though this example might look simple, it carries over to many computer vision problems. Depending on how we set up the energy functional, we can solve a variety of computer vision problems such as 3D reconstruction, segmentation or even recognition. In all these cases the prior influences the solution heavily (see also Zach et al. 2007a, b, Pock et al. 2009).

2.2 *Supervised Learning*

Another example that has lots of potential applications is supervised learning. The set-up is as follows: we are given a set of training examples $X = \{(x_i, y_i) | 1 \leq i \leq n, x_i \in \mathrm{IR}^m, y_i \in \mathrm{IR}\}$ and based on these, we want to infer an unknown function $f(x)$ that "explains" the training data. Figure 3 illustrates the situation in 2D.

The applications are numerous and range from all recognition tasks (speech, images etc.) to decision support systems and pattern classification tasks.

In Fig. 3 we see two possible functions that "explain" the data. Therefore, this problem is again a classical ill-posed problem, and we need to select a solution based on prior knowledge. For example, when we assume that the data is noisy and we prefer a "simple" function, we will select the solution on the right, whereas when we know that the data is noise-free we might select the solution at the bottom of Fig. 3. Again, the data alone cannot tell us which solution is the correct one. In fact, there is a huge amount on theory in machine learning that is concerned with priors and how to choose different solutions. In general, the theory tells us that usually simple functions are to be preferred, because it is more likely that those functions will deliver correct answers for unseen data (and this is the only reason why we want to learn such functions).

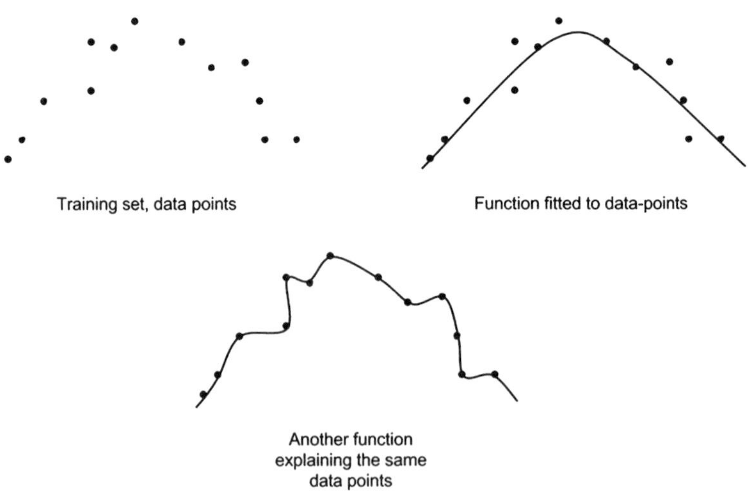

Fig. 3 Illustration of supervised machine learning for a 2D function

This example illustrates how our assumptions about the data influence the solutions we obtain. And no matter what we do, we always have to make assumptions, otherwise the problem is not solvable. This carries over to more complex and realistic problems.

3 Bayes Formula

The two examples from the previous section illustrate how prior knowledge influences solutions and makes proper solutions feasible. The question one might ask is if there is a principled way of how we can formulate our prior knowledge (beliefs) and how to use it to derive solutions to problems similar to the ones illustrated above. In fact, there is a very principled way of handling this, in the form of Bayesian statistics (Stone 2013), or more exactly, Bayesian inference. Bayesian inference is a method that uses the Bayes' theorem to update the probability for a hypothesis as more evidence is acquired. Bayesian inference has found application in a wide range of different fields of science, even philosophy. In the philosophy of decision theory, Bayesian inference is closely related to subjective probability, often called "Bayesian probability." The Bayesian probability provides a rational method for updating beliefs. In order to make things simple (and for the sake of the argument), we describe here only a simple case. This allows us to avoid excessive use of mathematics.

Bayesian inference derives the posterior probability of a hypothesis H as a consequence of the prior probability of the hypothesis ($P(H)$) (this is our belief we have) and a "likelihood function" that depends on the observed data (D). The posterior probability of the hypothesis given the data ($P(H|D)$) is computed according to Bayes' theorem:

$$P(H|D) = \frac{P(D|H)P(H)}{P(D)}$$

The term $P(H|D)$ measures the compatibility of the data with our assumptions and usually involves some modelling and assumptions about the noise. For example, in the curve-fitting example above, this measures the deviation of the data points from the curve. A typical assumption is that the noise of the data point is distributed normally.[2] $P(D)$ is sometimes termed the marginal likelihood. This factor depends just on the data and is the same for all possible hypotheses H. If we would like to compare different hypotheses, such as H_1 and H_2 we do not need to consider this factor (which sometime is complicated to compute). We could ask

$$P(H_1|D) = P(D|H_1)P(H_1) > P(H_2|D) = P(D|H_2)P(H_2)$$

[2] This was the assumption to obtain the simple solution in Fig. 3.

and select H_1 if this is true, and H_2 otherwise.

Using the Bayes formula, one can express the beliefs one has in a principled manner and one does not need to rely on ad-hoc models. There are numerous theorems that prove that this is a very fundamental way of handling inference.

Despite its elegance, it should also be noted that very often, the methods derived from Bayesian inference involve heavy computations. First of all, the involved probabilities P need to be known or estimated. Usually complex models cannot be processed in closed form by a Bayesian analysis, therefore complex simulations based on Monte-Carlo methods need to be performed

4 Summary

This short chapter has demonstrated that prior knowledge or belief is of eminent importance in computer science. This is true, in particular for those cases that deal with data. In order to deal with data in a proper manner, one needs models, and these models express our prior belief. A principled way of dealing with these priors is rooted in Bayesian statistics, which where originally invented by a monk (Thomas Bayes 1701–1761), but was never published by him, which nicely closes the circle to credition.

References

Hadamard J (1902) Sur les problmes aux drives partielles et leur signification physique. J Princeton Univ Bull 4952

Mitchell TM (1997) Machine learning, 1st edn. McGraw-Hill, New York

Pock T, Cremers D, Bischof H, Chambolle A (2009) An algorithm for minimizing the mumford-shah functional. In: 12th international conference on computer vision, pp 1133–1140

Stone JV (2013) Bayes rule: a tutorial introduction to Bayesian analysis. Sebtel Press

Szeliski R (2010) Computer vision: algorithms and applications, 1st edn. Springer, New York

Zach C, Pock T, Bischof H (2007a) A duality based approach for realtime tv-l 1 optical flow. In: Pattern recognition. Springer, Berlin/Heidelberg, pp 214–223

Zach C, Pock T, Bischof H (2007b) A globally optimal algorithm for robust tv-l 1 range image integration. In: 11th international conference on computer vision, pp 1–8

Public and Personal Causations of Creditions

Javier Leach

Abstract In this chapter, I classify the causes of the processes of believing (creditions) into two types: the causes of public processes, and the causes of personal processes. Public creditons are so characterized because they mean the same for everyone. Personal creditions are so characterized because they can have different meanings for different people. Each causal type of a credition corresponds to a kind of language. We use a language that tends to be formal and objective to express the causes of public creditions and we use a symbolic language to express the causes of the processes of personal creditions.

1 Introduction

Science studies the causes why things happen. With the use of mathematics as language of modern science, a unification of the causes occurs. Science does not understand the Aristotelian division between efficient and final cause. We say that the fact A is due to the fact B when we can prove that there is a relationship between the occurrence of A and the appearance of B. In this chapter, I shall distinguish between two types of causes: public causes and personal causes, and in particular, I will discuss the relationship between these two types of causes in processes of believing (creditions).

I will start with an example from Physics: In the field of physics, we talk about causes that are public; for example, we say that the force we put on a body causes an acceleration of that body because we can establish a relationship between the two. In this case, we put the two events in connection with the mathematical formula:

$$F = m \times a$$

In the case of the relationship between force and acceleration, I will say that the force *(F)* is a public cause of the acceleration *(a)*. I say that this physical cause is

This is a posthumous publication. The author died on 3rd August 2016; if anyone has any interest relative to his publication contact, at *University Complutense de Madrid*, I. M. Gómez-Chacón email address: igomezchacon@mat.ucm.es.

J. Leach (Deceased)
Facultad de Informática, Universidad Complutense, Madrid, Spain

H.-F. Angel et al. (eds.), *Processes of Believing: The Acquisition, Maintenance, and Change in Creditions*, New Approaches to the Scientific Study of Religion 1,
DOI 10.1007/978-3-319-50924-2_29

public or independent of the subject who observes, because I trust everyone to believe that the mathematical relationship between the two events ($F=m\times a$) is always fulfilled, under any circumstances, and for any person who observes.

However, there are cases in which not all subjects believe the same causal relationships. Depending on personal and community circumstances of different subjects, it may happen that a subject (S1) thinks there is some relationship between the occurrence of the fact A and fact B's appearance, while another subject (S2) does not think there is such a relationship. In such cases, we say that the cause is personal because the subject person is free to believe or not believe in the cause.

I propose a second example of a Personal Cause from the philosophy of mathematics. Some philosophers of mathematics believe in Platonism, according to which among the reasons why we know the mathematical abstract objects (A) is the fact that these objects exist independently of our thinking (B). Other philosophers of mathematics do not believe in Platonism, but instead believe that the cause for which we know the mathematical abstract objects (A) is because they are a mental construct, i.e., these other philosophers believe that mathematical objects exist independently of our thinking (not B).

The first example about force and acceleration is intended to illustrate a public cause and the second example about Platonism is intended to illustrate a personal and community cause. The first example is taken from physics and is based on the belief in the existence of a public and objective relationship between the force exerted on a body and the acceleration; we believe that everyone can understand in just the same way the relationship between force and acceleration. In the second example taken from philosophy, it is the personal belief that divides philosophers of mathematics into two distinct groups, those who believe in Platonism and those who do not believe in Platonism.

In both examples, there are processes of believing (creditions). In the first case, it is a process of public belief, based on physical facts. We believe that everybody can understand it in the same way, and in the other case, it is a personal process of believing, based on personal motivations and reasons that the subject can accept or reject freely and divides philosophers of mathematics into two distinct groups.

In this chapter, I will study these two kinds of belief processes (creditions) and I will point to the causes differentiating them: the public and the personal causes, which primarily differ by the language we use to express these causes. First, I will describe these two kinds of causes of belief processes. Then I will discuss the relationships between both kinds of belief processes.

As we will see, the public causes of creditions tend to be expressed by *formal languages* (Leach 2010). Formal languages are precise languages that can be understood and executed by a machine. These languages were first used in the context of mathematics, and now are used in the context of computer science. They are public languages because they intend to have always the same meaning for everyone.

Public causal explanations of creditions intend to be objective because they intend to have the same meaning for everyone, and therefore, they intend to have a semantic meaning that can be objectively studied, independent of any particular subject. The mathematical-empirical study of the public causes of creditions is analytical, and their causal action is explained by analyzing various aspects or parts of the causal systems of such creditions.

The incompleteness and undecidability theorems of mathematics show that there are internal constraints of formal languages to express the public causes as mathematical relations in a deductive causal system. Moreover, quantum theory shows the limitations to determining the causes of the public empirical evidence.

The personal causes of creditions are not public, that is, they do not have the same meaning for everyone. They depend largely on each person and his or her community context. The causes of these creditions are expressed by means of *languages* and systems that I call *symbolic*.

Nevertheless, as we will see, this second kind of personal causes of creditions logically includes the first one of the public causes, because the personal causes need to be consistent with the public causes. On the other hand, personal causes of creditions provide answers to questions that cannot be answered by public causes (Leach 2014a).

Although the semantics of the *symbolic languages* and systems include the semantics of formal languages and systems, the former have broader semantics than the latter. Symbolical languages and systems have a wider range of semantic meaning, because their semantic meaning is explicitly and directly affected by the internal motions of confidence, hope, and love, rooted in the liberty of the believer of such system.

The meaning of symbolic personal statements affects the personal identity of the speaker and his/her relationship with the world around him/her. Therefore, the meaning of personal statements is not necessarily the same for different individuals and communities. The same sentence can have different meanings to different people. For example, the statement *God is the Creator of the Universe* has a personal meaning for many people shaping the way they relate to the world, while for others, it means nothing. Personal creditions can be theistic, atheistic or agnostic. In any of these three cases, personal causes of creditions are related to the believer's personal language.

2 Public Causes of Creditions and Formal Languages

The use of formal languages can give an explanation of what reality is based on public beliefs, regardless of other personal beliefs, which scientists assume freely.

To describe reality based on public beliefs, mathematics has refined certain languages that I call formal languages over several centuries. These are characterized by transmitting a semantic meaning which is fixed and public. These languages are therefore autonomous from the personal beliefs of the subject using these formal languages. Formal languages are contrasted with other languages whose semantic meaning depends on the free personal consciousness of the subject that uses them; I will call these personal languages.

An example of a computer formal language is the language Pascal, and a Pascal statement may be, for example, the statement: 'write (hello)' which commands the program to type the word hello. Any programming language, like C ++ or Fortran, are also examples of formal languages. An example of formal language used in mathematics is the decimal representation. We use it to write the numbers we call natural: 0, 1, 2, 3, …. Another example of a formal statement can be any logical formula of any formal logic. For example, the formula $(A \vee \neg A)$, which expresses the logical principle of the excluded middle, states that given a statement A, A is true and thus we write A, or A is false and thus we write $\neg A$. The disjunction between A and $\neg A$ that we express in English with the disjunctive conjunction 'or' is formalized with the sign $\vee$.

I consider the use of formal languages as a cause of the belief in the public value (equal for all) of some beliefs. By having formal languages as a public value, beliefs caused by relationships expressed in a formal language can be applied technologically. The technology is based on the belief that it is possible to interact with reality from a public perspective, which is independent from the cultural context in which this interaction takes place. That is, formal languages and the technology that they describe have the same meaning and the same applications anywhere on earth, in China, in Europe or in America. Thanks to their universal validity and the precise and objective formulation of their results, formal languages and technology are based on the belief that they are able to predict the behavior of the objects they study and that prediction makes it possible to apply technologically the results of science.

The use of formal languages is currently helping to create a global culture based on a public technological belief that transcends particular beliefs. Technologies tend to be the same and serve as a link connecting to very different cultural contexts. For example, information technology is the same in all countries of the world, unless you have political restrictions.

I understand that the belief in the knowledge of the reality by technology is public because it aims to have always the same meaning for everyone, regardless of the personal beliefs characteristic of a particular culture. The belief in the knowledge of science and technology intends to be independent of the social and religious context to which each one belongs. Belief in the value of a public description of reality, and the value of scientific and technical knowledge based on that description, are public beliefs with an autonomous meaning that seeks to transcend all other personal beliefs.

For being a public knowledge, the belief in the value of science and technology is a result of human activity that, in principle at least, is a universal one because, by itself, that activity does not fall under the control of personal and community options for any human group but only under the control of the laws of nature as such.

Mathematical Platonism is an example of inter-connection between public and personal beliefs. The quality that mathematics and computer are public knowledge based on public beliefs has been made so repeatedly throughout history, that many mathematicians attribute to mathematical objects a real existence independent of the language and mathematical activity that produces them. Platonism is a philosophical personal belief that gives real and independent existence to formal mathematical objects, and reduces the activity of the mathematician to discover pre-existing mathematical objects.

While one statement made in a personal language can have different meanings for different individuals, formal languages are characterized contrarily by their ability to have a semantic meaning that is independent of the subject who uses it. This is because it can be built using rules that mechanically produce the meanings of well-formulated statements of each particular formal language. We can say that formal languages are artificial languages whose syntax and semantics depend solely on mechanical rules that govern their construction.

Formal languages have developed historically in the context of mathematics and logic; but formal languages are currently experiencing a great development due to their mechanical structure, which allows them to be used by computer technology.

An example of a personal language statement is the statement 'God exists.' This statement is true for a believer and is false for a non-believing subject. Another example of personal language is the statement 'I trust you,' that can be true when John states it in reference to his personal confidence in Mary, but can be false when Mary states it in reference to her personal confidence in John. The truth or falsity of these personal statements lies in the personal conscience of Mary and John.

Both formal and personal languages have grown and developed within broader languages we call natural languages as in, for example, English, Spanish or Chinese.

Natural languages also are called mother tongues because they are given to us in a social context, a family, a community of belonging.

3 Personal Creditions and Formal Languages

The ability of formal languages to transmit public and universal beliefs has inherent limits. By the intrinsic limits of formal languages, they are open to expressing personal beliefs.

Expressing the intrinsic limits of formal languages, meta-mathematics has served as a bridge between the physical beliefs and personal beliefs. We begin by showing what meta-mathematics is, its reason for being, and its historical significance.

By formal languages having an objective syntactic structure, which is fixed and public, and also an objective semantic meaning, which also is fixed and public, formal languages can become objects of mathematical study. We call meta-mathematics the mathematical study of the properties of formal languages. The mathematician Hilbert heavily contributed to the field meta-mathematics being able to propose a demonstration of the properties of formal languages by using meta-mathematical methods. Among the properties that Hilbert proposed to prove this is the property of the completeness of mathematical systems. A mathematical system is complete when all true statements can be deduced from a consistent and finite set of axioms (Hilbert 1928).

In 1931, Kurt Gödel proved, using meta-mathematical methods, the incompleteness theorem of arithmetic that says that it is impossible to deduce all true formulas of arithmetic from a finite set of axioms and be consistent. This proposal showed that Hilbert's quest was intrinsically impossible (Gödel 1931).

The crisis of meta-mathematics emphasizes the processes of personal belief. Not all mathematicians believe the truth of their statements in the same way. Among mathematicians, there is a plurality of criteria defining the real existence of a formal mathematical object. As early as Hilbert, there was a diversity of approaches to affirm the existence of mathematical objects. Hilbert's proposal aimed at finding a criterion that was accepted by all mathematicians, but that proposal was not successful. Some mathematicians only admitted to the existence of those formal objects whose existence could be proved mechanically in an effective way, while many other mathematicians also admitted to the existence of any formal object whose existence cannot be proven to be contradictory (Troelstra 1991).

A particular case within mathematical pluralism is a concept called the mathematical infinite. Some mathematicians support the current existence of sets with infinite elements, such as the set N = {1, 2, 3, …} of all natural numbers. Other mathematicians only support the current existence of finite sets that can have as many items as you want, without ever reaching an infinite number of elements, such as any finite subset n = {1,…, n} formed by the first n elements of the set N. Mathematical objects with an infinite number of elements currently do not exist for the latter mathematicians, as they only support as existing as formal objects those objects whose existence can be effectively demonstrated mechanically. However, for the classical mathematicians, the existence of mathematical objects with an actually infinite number of elements can be proved by *reductio ad absurdum.*

A concrete example is the demonstration of the existence of the infinite set of decimals from the root of 2. Indeed, if the root of 2 only had a finite number of decimal places, it could then be written as a ratio of two integers *a* and *b,* which would be in contradiction with the fact that the integers *a* and *b* have a unique prime factorization (Fig. 1).

$$\sqrt{2} = \frac{a}{b} \quad \Rightarrow \quad 2b^2 = a^2$$

Fig. 1 Decomposing a and b into its prime factors, 2 appears an odd number of times on the *left side* of the equation $2b^2 = a^2$ and an even number of times on the right side of this equation, which is a contradiction with the fact that every integer has a unique prime factorization

Another example is computable functions. What are actually executable by a computer, following the instructions of a program, are called computable functions. Some mathematicians only admit to the existence of computable functions, i.e., they only support those functions as actually existing if a computer program can execute them, at least theoretically. However, classical mathematicians support the existence of non-computable functions, which can be thought but not be executed by a computer program.

The Church-Turing (Church 1936; Turing 1936–1937) hypothesis, currently accepted as valid by mathematicians and computer scientists, states that any computable function is executable by a Turing machine and vice versa. Therefore, the Church-Turing hypothesis admits that a function that is mechanically executable by a Turing machine contains two equivalent concepts.

But not all functions that can be described by a formal language are executable mechanically. A famous case is the halting problem. This problem involves finding a function that, given any program and any input the function, effectively determines whether or not the program stops. That is, the halting problem seeks to find a meta-computable function separating programs that stop from those that do not stop. Alan Turing proved that there is not a computable function that solves the halting problem.

3.1 Procedural Pluralism

We have seen that among mathematicians, there is a plurality of views on the existence of formal mathematical objects. The formal meta-mathematical results are the same for everyone but their meaning is interpreted differently by different mathematicians. Throughout the twentieth century, different interpretations of the meaning of the meta-mathematical results, especially the negative results such as Gödel's incompleteness theorem, have led to different interpretations of what is meant by 'real' existence of a 'formal' system. We can say that there is currently no uniform opinion among mathematicians about what it means that a 'formal' system has a 'real' existence.

The plurality of criteria necessary to define what is meant by a formal object and to decide the existence of that formal object leads to the need to make a personal choice.

3.2 Formal Pluralism

The need to make a personal choice does not imply opting exclusively for any of the possible definitions of what it means that a mathematical object has real existence. Within the variety of formal languages, we can choose among a number of different definitions of what it means to really exist. Moreover, to admit a plurality of options as possible is currently the most common position among mathematicians. In some cases, it is more useful to consider constructivism as an option. In other cases, it is more useful a choice for a classical view of mathematics. Any mathematician can opt for one or the other as he or she finds that it is technologically more useful.

But in any case, it is inevitable that a personal choice has to be made, either for pluralism, which leads us to accept one definition or another depending on the circumstances, or for a precise definition of the meaning and existence of formal objects.

3.3 Consistent Systems

We can say that now in principle, any formal system is technologically valid provided that it helps us to handle situations in which we need to control a given problem technologically. We can even say that contradictory or inconsistent systems are valid. The reality is often contradictory and can be represented by an inconsistent formal system. The problem of the inconsistent systems, i.e. systems including contradictions, is that they can be deductively uncontrollable because they can lead to an explosion of the deduction tree. In the inconsistent systems, the explosion of the deduction tree is formed by the traditional logical principle 'ex falso quodlibet', that is, from a falsehood, we can deduce anything.

To avoid this explosion, it is necessary to limit the use of the classical rules of deduction. There are different types of logical systems, so-called para-consistent systems, that support contradictions but prevent the explosion of a deduction tree. They control the deduction rules that can be used as currently defined.

4 Interaction Between Public and Personal Creditions

4.1 Open Road to Personal Beliefs

The aim of this chapter is not only to distinguish between two types of languages and two types of causes, but also to interrelate them. Public causes are transmitted by formal languages, and personal causes are expressed in symbolic languages.

Formal languages are suitable, due to their syntactic and semantic accuracy, for describing physical and technological beliefs, while symbolic languages, due to their semantic richness, also communicate other beliefs that I call personal beliefs, as opposed to public beliefs, which can be expressed by formal languages.

The halting problem is an example of the functions that we can formally define but we cannot give them a computable solution. Alan Turing was aware of this situation, and in his works during the years 1937–1938, extended the definition of Turing machines by adding to them the ability to incorporate a mathematical instrument called 'oracle' which was able to make decisions that could not be made by a Turing machine. Turing says about the oracles:

> *We shall not go any further into the nature of this oracle apart from saying that it cannot be a machine* (Turing 1939).

Thus, Turing states that any formal language allowing us to define the oracles allows us to describe certain formal functions that are not computable.

We have seen that the incompleteness and undecidability theorems show that we cannot reduce the significance of formal languages to the meaning of a finite set of axioms and inference rules applying to these axioms. These theorems show that it is not enough to build a unique and formally 'closed' mechanical system in order to obtain mathematical theorems. These theorems show that intuition and creativity are also necessary for obtaining mathematical theorems. After the effort of the foundations of mathematics throughout the twentieth century, the meaning of formal languages remains 'open' and allows a plurality of different personal and community semantic criteria.

According to the incompleteness and undecidability theorems, we cannot explain everything by formal languages deductively that we can grasp intuitively. We can talk consistently about sets of mathematical elements whose existence we cannot deduce.

4.2 *Ineffable Semantics*

We cannot deductively control all the processes of believing that we can formally express because their semantic meaning cannot be formally described within a single deductive system. Their semantic meaning is so complex that there is not a deductive system that can describe it.

Formal languages do not allow deductively expressed scientific theories governing the behavior of nature and ensuring the validity of technological intervention. Thus, we can say that mathematics is 'deductively apophatic', in a way similar to negative theology, also called apophatic, i.e., because the experience of the divine cannot be described with words. In both cases, what can be intuited with mathematical or theological perception cannot be described by a language.

Personal and formal semantics are the result of two asymmetrical ways of believing in the same reality: Formal semantics cause a public and universal belief that is able to create technology. On the contrary, personal meaning is based on personal trust; trust in the person and the community. These two semantics are not symmetrical because while formal semantics can dispense with the personal meaning and remain isolated in itself, personal semantics cannot deny the formal truth of its own sentences because it is public and is equal for all (Leach 2014b).

The current search for knowledge is characterized by a great paradox produced by the enormous potential of formal and computer knowledge along with the limitations of that knowledge. This paradoxical situation causes a deep search of personal knowledge based on personal beliefs in today's culture, along with a technological development based on formal knowledge.

5 Personal Motions and Public Emotions

In this last part of this chapter, I will compare public emotions to personal motions. I call personal motions "free and emotional movements" that are the cause of our personal beliefs, and I call public emotions "unfree emotional movements" that can be described in a formal language and can, therefore, be imitated by a humanoid robot. Public emotions are causing public beliefs while personal motions are due to personal beliefs.

5.1 Belief in Motions and Symbolic Personal Language

Belief in personal freedom is, in itself, a free act. Belief in personal freedom is to believe in the existence of personal inner movements that are not public and which I shall call motions. Personal motions are personal internal movements including the experience of freedom. Not everyone believes in the existence of the experience of personal freedom. There are some people who believe in personal freedom as an experience that constitutes them as human beings and there are others who do not believe in the existence of the inner experience of personal freedom.

The experience of freedom is a personal belief that is not public, and therefore we cannot explain it by public formal causes (Leach 2012). The awareness of the power of liberty is personal and can only be communicated in a symbolic language through which we express confidence in what our partner says he or she has experienced.

5.2 The Emotions and the Public Formal Beliefs and Language

The existence of humanoid robots that capture and imitate human emotions shows that certain emotions are public and can be described in a formal public language that even robots understand. There are also public emotions that may be expressed by their effects in a formal language and can be imitated by a humanoid robot. I call such emotions human sensations expressed in a formal language. The formal languages with which robots and humans communicate restrict the ability of humanoid robots to capture human emotions and react mechanically according to these captured emotions.

6 Conclusion and Future Work

I began this chapter by saying that the causes of facts are expressed as relationships in a language that talks about these facts. In the introduction, I have raised the consideration of two types of languages to study the causes of creditions: the formal languages that are public and the symbolic languages that are personal.

Next, I showed that one reason for introducing these two types of languages is in the way in which modern science uses mathematical language. Modern science has tried, since the sixteenth century, to express the causes of events in a mathematical language. Since then, has been an increasing ability of science to express different relationships between facts in formal languages. That has produced unification in the study of the scientific causes due to the attempt to explain all of them in a formal mathematical language.

This unification of the types of causes has led to a deep divide between the study of the causes by the sciences and the study of the causality by philosophical traditions. For much of the philosophical traditions, it is important to consider the distinction between efficient causes and final causality. The philosophical traditions have often continued to distinguish between the causes of the facts and the motives for these causes that cause action The philosophy of mathematics has difficulty in making this distinction and seeks to explain all the facts by a unique type of causality. Consequently, many scientists renounce the existence of a purpose.

But science has only partially achieved this philosophical attempt to express all the causes as mathematical relationships with mathematical clarity. The first task of this philosophical attempt in the field of mathematics has been the effort to define what a mathematical language is. The works of Frege, Cantor, Brower, Hilbert, Gödel, Turing and Church, among others, have made significant advances in the foundations of mathematics but have not achieved their aim of obtaining a single foundation of mathematics. Pluralism has been imposed on the foundations of mathematics.

Pluralism in the foundations of mathematics opens the door to pluralism in the treatment of scientific causes. This chapter is a contribution to the scientific treatment of the causes of creditions, without falling into the unscientific separation between efficient causes and final causes. In this chapter, I introduced public and personal causation of creditions. Hereby, I attmtped to define and inter-relate both causalities, public and personal, thus looking to explain scientifically also the causality that cannot be expressed in mere formal languages.

This chapter opens some new perspectives for future work in the connection of the causation of creditions to the philosophy of language. It leaves us with several open questions in this area: How have the formal computer languages influenced the language of science? How do we currently understand, and will we understand in the near future, the role of mathematical intuition and creativity? And specially, how will we understand in the near future the use of formal languages and mathematical intuition and creativity in order to scientifically explain the causation of creditions?

References

Church A (1936) An unsolvable problem of elementary number theory. Am J Math 58:345–363

Gödel K (1931) Über formal unentscheidbare Sätze der Principia Mathematica und verwandter Systeme I. Monatshefte für Mathematik Physik 38:173–198

Hilbert D (1928) Die Grundlagen der Mathematik. Abhandlungen aus dem Mathematischen Seminar der Hamburgischen Universität 6:65–85

Leach J (2010) Mathematics and religion: our languages of sign and symbol. Templeton Press, West Conshohocken

Leach J (2012) Taking options and decisions. Revista portuguesa de filosofía 68(1–2):87–104

Leach J (2014a) Matemática e metafísica. *Civiltà Cattolica* Quaderno N°3931

Leach J (2014b) The languages of artificial intelligence, the languages of metaphysics, and the languages of faith. Scientia et Fides 2(1):81–98

Troelstra AS (1991) A history of constructivism in the 20th century. University of Amsterdam, ITLI Prepublication Series ML-91-05. https://www.illc.uva.nl/Research/Publications/Reports/ML-1991-05.text.pdf

Turing AM (1936–1937) On computable numbers, with an application to entscheidungs problem. Proc Lond Math Soc 2(42):230–265

Turing AM (1939) Systems of logic based on ordinals. Ph.D. thesis, 1938. Princeton

Wave-Particle Duality and Quantity-Quality Complementarity in Natural and Human Sciences: Implications for Credition Research

Sungchul Ji

Abstract As predicted by the American chemist, logician, and philosopher Charles Sander Peirce (1839–1914), there appears to be a set of simple concepts that applies to every subject. The Golden Ratio and the Fibonacci series that appear in systems ranging from atoms to DNA, human anatomy, architecture, arts, and the cosmos are well-known examples. During the past 6 years, two additional principles have been recognized and characterized that apply to many organized processes, (i) the Planckian distribution equation (PDE) and (ii) the irreducible triadic relation (ITR) first articulated by Peirce and found to be related to the concept of the category in mathematics. PDE and ITR, being universal principles, may apply to the process of believing in the form of the 'emotion-cognition-credition' (ECC) triad which may be irreducible in characterizing and understanding any human goal-directed actions including believing.

1 Introduction

According to the American chemist, logician, and philosopher Charles Sanders Peirce (1839–1914), there are three irreducible aspects to all phenomena in the Universe, which he called Firstness, Secondness and Thirdness (see Table 1). During the past 6 years, two additional principles have been recognized and characterized that apply to many organized processes in both biotic (e.g., cells, brains, societies) and abiotic systems (e.g., atoms, chemical reactions, the cosmos): (i) The Planckian distribution equation (PDE) that was derived in 2008 from the blackbody radiation equation of M. Planck (1858–1947) by replacing its universal constants and temperature with three free parameters, A, B and C, and (ii) the irreducible triadic relation (ITR) first articulated by Peirce and found to be related to the concept of the category in mathematics. PDE and ITR, being universal principles, may apply to the process of believing in the form of the 'emotion-cognition-credition' (ECC)

S. Ji (✉)
Department of Pharmacology and Toxicology, Rutgers University, Piscataway, NJ, USA
e-mail: sji@rci.rutgers.edu

H.-F. Angel et al. (eds.), *Processes of Believing: The Acquisition, Maintenance, and Change in Creditions*, New Approaches to the Scientific Study of Religion 1,
DOI 10.1007/978-3-319-50924-2_30

Table 1 Peirce's categories (technical name: the cenopythagorean categories)[a]

Name	Typical characterization	As universe of experience	As quantity	Technical definition	Valence, "adicity"
Firstness	Quality of feeling.	Ideas, chance, possibility.	Vagueness, "some".	Reference to a ground (a ground is a pure abstraction of a quality)	Essentially monadic (the quale, in the sense of the *such*,[11] which has the quality).
Secondness	Reaction, resistance, (dyadic) relation.	Brute facts, actuality.	Singularity, discreteness, "this".	Reference to a correlate (by its relate).	Essentially dyadic (the relate and the correlate).
Thirdness	Representation, mediation.	Habits, laws, necessity.	Generality, continuity, "all".	Reference to an interpretant.	Essentially triadic (sign, object, interpretant).

[a]Reproduced from https://en.wikipedia.org/wiki/Categories_(Peirce)#cite_note-13

triad which may be irreducible in characterizing and understanding any human goal-directed actions including believing.

The empirical evidences supporting the universality of PDE and ITR have been reviewed and possible common mechanisms underlying the universality of PDE have been discussed. PDE and ITR may be related to the mathematical functors, the former *quantitative* and the latter *qualitative.* The relation between these two functors, in turn, is suggested to be the *principle of complementarity* advocated by Niels Bohr (1928).

Since credition (Angel 2013, 2014, 2015), or the process of believing, is one of the most characteristic phenomena of *Homo sapiens*, it seems reasonable to assume that the Peircean categories apply to credition. One way to apply the Peircean categories to credition is suggested by the triadic models of the world proposed by Plato, Popper, and Penrose as discussed by Burgin (2010:58–60) which can be summarized by Burgin's triadic model of the world (Fig. 1).

Grossmann, as cited in Burgin (2010: 69) defines structure thus: "A structure is (a representation of) a complex entity that consists of parts in relations to each other." In this sense, credition as described in (Angel 2013, 2014, 2015) has a structure consisting of parts called "babs" and "blobs" in interaction with one another (Sect. 2.5.5). Thus, I postulate that the phenomenon of credition possesses three irreducible aspects – (1) physical, (2) mental, and (3) structural. One of the key objectives of this contribution is to present a very broad outline of what these three aspects of credition might be. Toward this end, two concepts will be discussed that have been found to apply universally to numerous fields of inquiries ranging from atomic physics, to molecular biology, to cell biology, to brain neuorophysiology, to psychology, to economics, and to cosmology, and these concepts are ITR (Irreducible

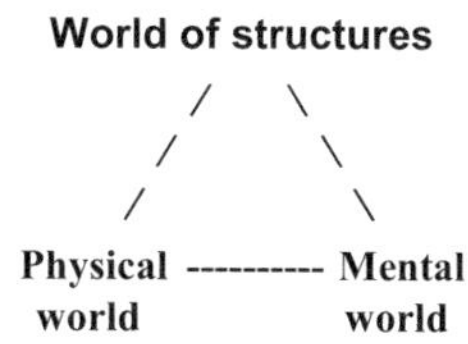

Fig. 1 The Existential Triad of the world (Reproduced from Burgin 2010: 60)

Triadic Relation of Peirce; see Sect. 2.6.1) and PDE (Planckian Distribution Equation).

In the following quote, Peirce predicted that there exists a set of simple concepts that apply to every subject: "The undertaking which this volume inaugurates is to make a philosophy like that of Aristotle, that is to say, to outline a theory so comprehensive that, for a long time to come, the entire work of human reason, in philosophy of every school and kind, in mathematics, in psychology, in physical science, in history, in sociology, and in whatever other department there may be, shall appear as the filling up of its details. The first step toward this is to find simple concepts applicable to every subject" (Hartshorne and Weiss 1931: vii).

During the past several years, we have found that two principles apply to many organized systems and processes, including (i) atomic emission of photons, (ii) protein folding, (iii) single-molecule enzyme catalysis, (iv) mRNA metabolism in cells, (v) brain functions such as consciousness, decision-making, and speaking, and (vi) the polarization of the cosmic microwave background (CMB) radiation (Ji 2015a, b). These principles are the Planckian distribution equation (PDE) that was derived from the blackbody radiation formula discovered by Max Planck in 1900 (Ji 2012e) and the Irreducible Triadic Relation (ITR) that was first articulated by Peirce and is synonymous with the concept of 'category' in mathematics (Spivak 2013; Brown and Porter 2006).

This chapter begins with a brief review of the basic concepts in thermodynamic and semiotics (i.e., the study of signs) that are deemed essential to understanding PDE and ITR and the empirical evidence for their universality.

Since the process of believing, called credition (Angel 2013; Seitz and Angel 2012; Sugiura et al. 2015), can only occur as the result of the dynamic interactions among a large number of physicochemical and neural processes that occur inside the brain under the influence of its physical and social environment, it seems logical to consider credition as an example of self-organizing process referred to as "dissipative structures" by Prigogine (1977) and "dissipations" by Ji (2012a). Since PDE and ITR have been found to apply to many organized systems and processes, both living (e.g., enzyme catalysis, cell metabolism) and non-living (e.g., the flame of a candle, Belousov-Zhabotinsky reaction), it is reasonable to anticipate that these principles will apply to credition as well, which will facilitate our understanding of these important brain functions that underlie most, if not all, human activities both personal and social.

2 Basic Terms, Laws, and Principles

2.1 Equilibrium vs. Dissipative Structures

Prigogine (1977, 1980) distinguished two types of structures in the Universe – (i) equilibrium structures that do not consume any energy to exist (e.g., nucleotide sequences in DNA or RNA, rocks, sheet music) and (ii) dissipative structures that absolutely require free energy dissipation for their existence (e.g., the flame of a candle, action potentials, EEG, audio music). *Free energy* is different from *energy* in that it is a function of both energy (obeying the First Law of thermodynamics) and entropy (obeying the Second Law of thermodynamics), and all living processes (including the *process of believing*) are driven by decreases in free energy and not by any changes in energy alone (Callen 1985; Lauffer 1983). Dissipative and equilibrium structures are also called "dissipatons" and "equilibrons" for convenience (Ji 2012). Since the process of believing requires dissipation of free energy (in order not to violate the laws of thermodynamics), it naturally belongs to the family of dissipatons.

2.2 Information

Just as 'energy' can be defined as the ability of a system *to do work*, so 'information' can be defined as the ability to *control work*. Information has three aspects – (i) amount, (ii) meaning, and (iii) value (Volkenstein 2009). The Shannon formula for quantifying information deals only with the first aspect while ignoring the other two (Shannon and Weaver 1949). In contrast, the concept of information used in biology is concerned with all of the three aspects of information. This probably accounts for the fact that the information provided by the Shannon theory is little known among biologists, since they find no critical use of it in their experimental research. But the qualitative use of the concept of information is essential in all aspects of biological research, since it is well-accepted that *information is required to control* physicochemical processes in all levels of biological organizations.

2.3 Energy

Although energy is defined as the ability for a system to do work (Callen 1985; Lauffer 1983), not all forms of energy can perform work. For example, thermal energy can perform work if and only if a device is available to harness its tendency to flow from a hot spot to a cold one.

2.4 *Entropy*

Entropy (S) is defined as the heat (Q) absorbed reversibly (or very slowly) by a material body divided by the temperature T at which the heat absorption takes place; i.e., $\Delta S = \Delta Q/T$, where ΔX is the change in quantity X in a system undergoing a change from the initial state, X_i, to the final state, X_f, i.e., $\Delta X = X_f - X_i$. The Second Law of thermodynamics dictates that ΔS accompanying any spontaneous process in an isolated system (e.g., the Universe itself) must be negative (Kodepudi and Prigogine 1998).

2.5 *Gnergy*

2.5.1 Definition

The term, gnergy, was coined by combining two Greek stems, "gn-" (from *gnosis* meaning knowledge or information) and "-ergy" (from *ergon* meaning work or energy) to indicate the ability of a system to perform "controlled work" or "to organize" (Ji 1991). Discrete units of gnergy were termed "gnergons". The relation between gnergy and gnergons is that the former is a *type* and the latter its *tokens*. Examples of gnergons include concentration gradients (e.g., action potentials), mechanical stress gradients in biopolymers called *conformons* (Ji 1974, 1979, 2000, 2012d) that are postulated to be necessary and sufficient to drive all goal-directed molecular motions, and sound waves carrying a message. More generally, it was postulated that *gnergy is necessary and sufficient to drive all goal-directed self-organizing molecular processes in both living and non-living systems* (Ji 1991: 1, 1995, 2004: 8, 2012a: 27).

2.5.2 Experimental Evidence

Probably the most direct evidence for the existence of gnergons (in the form of conformons) is provided by the circular DNA duplexes in prokaryotes (i.e., single-celled organisms without nuclear membranes) (Benham 1992, 1996). The circular DNA duplex can exist in two structural states – supercoiled and relaxed. There are enzymes in prokaryotes called DNA gyrases and topoisomerases that can cut the circular DNA and rotate the cut end around the long axis of the circular DNA using the free energy of ATP to introduce the so-called supercoils into the DNA molecule, thereby storing mechanical energy therein. This stored mechanical (also called conformational) energy is essential for DNA function, i.e, transferring its genetic information to mRNA. Relaxed circular DNA molecule loses this function. Benham (1992, 1996) has demonstrated that the conformationally-strained regions of the supercoiled DNA (called SIDD, Stressed-Induced Duplex Destabilization) are not randomly distributed along the circular molecule, but rather located in specific regions before and after genic regions (i.e., DNA segments containing genes). Thus, it is clear that the sequence-specific conformational strains (i.e., SIDDs) found in supercoiled circular DNA in the 1990s are synonymous with conformons first postulated to exist in biopolymers (Ji 1974, 2000).

Another piece of evidence for the role of gnergy (i.e., the combination of information and energy) is provided by the single-molecule experiments on myosin molecular motions and the kinetics of ATP hydrolysis accompanying the myosin motion (Ishii and Yanagida 2007). As described in detail in Ji (2012), Ishhi and Yanagida succeeded in demonstrating that, in order for the myosin molecule to move along the actin filament, the myosin molecule must be mechanically (i.e., conformationally) *energized* through the ATP hydrolysis it catalyzes. That is, the chemical energy of ATP hydrolysis must be transformed into the mechanical energy of the myosin head (i.e., *conformons*) before it can execute molecular motions along the thin filament (Ji 2012).

A third piece of evidence supporting the role of gnergy in living processes is the well-known fact that most cell functions require both ATP as a source of free energy, and DNA as a source of genetic information.

2.5.3 The Gnergy Principle of Organization (GPO)

In Ji (1991), it was postulated that all organizations in the universe, both biotic and abiotic, are driven by the combination of energy (ergon) and information (gnon), i.e., by gnergy. This postulate will be referred to as the Gnergy Principle of Organization (GPO).

Just as energy is associated with force and force carriers (e.g., photons), so it is assumed that gnergy is associated with its own force and force carriers, referred to as conformons in enzymes (Ji 2000), cytons in the cell (Ji 1991), 'cerebrons' in the brain, and 'societons' in human societies. It should be pointed out that I needed to coin the new terms, 'cerebrons' and 'societons' in Ji (2014a).

Organizations are found in atoms, enzymes, living cells, human bodies, societies, and the universe. All organizations that result from selecting components or component processes from random sets of components or processes made available by thermal motions (also called Brownian motions, or Wiener processes) generate data that fit the Planckian distribution (Ji 2015a, b). The degree of the non-random organizations resulting from Brownian motions 'rectified' (i.e., made non-random or asymmetric) by free energy dissipation can be quantified in terms of the *Planckian information*, I_P, defined as the binary logarithm of the ratio between the Riemann sum (or the area under the curve) of the Planckian distribution over that of the associated Gaussian-like distribution, in the units of bits.

2.5.4 Gnergy, Practopoiesis, and ITR (Irreducibole Triadic Relation)

The theory of mind recently proposed by Nikolic (2015) is based on the concept of 'practopoiesis' – a neologism combining Ancient Greek words 'praktis' meaning 'action', 'activity', or 'practice' and 'poiesis' meaning 'to make.' Nikolic explains the meaning of 'practopoiesis' as follows:

> "The term practopoiesis refers to 'creation of actions', emphasizing the fact that physiological mechanisms at any level of adaptive organization operate through actions – and requires mechanisms to be put in place capable of executing those actions" (41).

Practopoiesis thus defined is a 'creative action' or 'goal-directed action' and not a random one, and hence requires dissipating free energy under the guidance of control information: i.e., practopoiesis is driven by gnergy. Also 'practopoiesis' of Nikolic can be represented as an ITR (Irreducible Triadic Relation defined in see Sect. 2.6.1) as shown in Fig. 2, just as the Peircean sign can be so represented (Fig. 3).

Anapoiesis, defined as "reconstructing knowledge" (Nikolic 2015), i.e., Step g in Fig. 2, bridges two time domains: the relatively slow process of forming neural networks and the very fast neural firing activities that constitute behavior. I have considered a similar problem in Ji (2012c) and came to the conclusion, based on the Generalized Franck-Condon Principle imported from quantum mechanics, that such kinetically disparate processes can be coupled if and only if the slow process precedes the fast one.

Anapoiesis of Nikolic (2015) reminds us of the principle of rule-governed creativity (PRGC) in linguistics (Hockett 1960; Ji 1997). PRGC captures the property

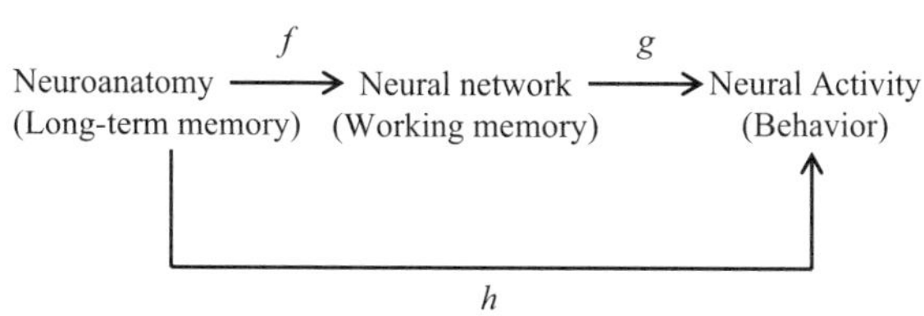

Fig. 2 A diagrammatic representation of practopoiesis of Nikolic (2015). f = memory recall; g = anapoiesis (i.e., reconstruction); h = genetic constraint, genetic information flow

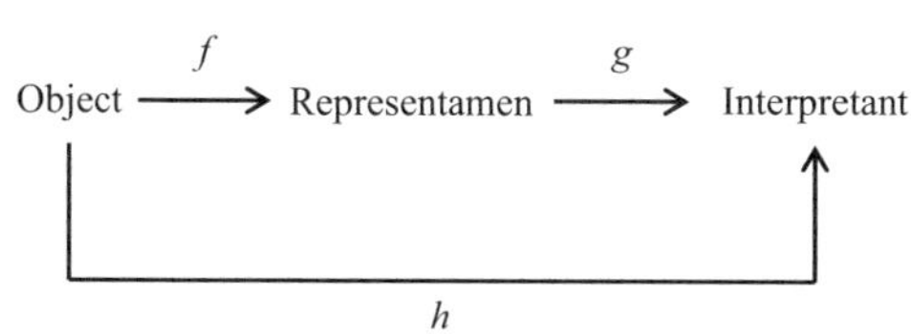

Fig. 3 Semiosis (also called the Peircean sign) as a commutative triangle and a member of the ur-category. f = sign production; g = sign interpretation; h = information flow, or grounding, or meaning of the sign

of a language that enables native speakers to construct an indefinitely large number of sentences out of a finite number of elements and to understand them even when they are encountered for the first time. According to the cell language theory, PRGC operates in living systems ranging from DNA (d) to RNA ®, proteins (p), metabolic network (m), cells ©, organs (o) and whole animals (a), leading to the coining of the terms d-, r-, p-, m-, c-, o- and a-creatons, where creatons are defined as the physicochemical systems capable of instantiating PRGC (Ji 1997, 2001).

If we define the physicochemical systems that implement practopoiesis as 'practopoiesis-executing agent' or 'practopoietons' for brevity, anapoiesis can be regarded as an essential component process performed by practopoietons. *Practopoietons* would then be 'isomorphic' with *creatons* as defined in the cell language theory (Ji 1997).

2.5.5 Gnergy and the Concept of Babs in the Credition Theory

To fix a theoretical base for a process oriented model of credition there was given the need to introduce the term "bab" in order

> to express that the same proposition can differ in its emotional relevance or meaning in analogy to the well-known Russian toy "babuschka". Similarly to a babuschka that accommodates a couple of figures of the same shape but of different sizes the same abstract proposition can occur with different emotional loadings ("Babuschka-Effect" or "bab") (Seitz and Angel 2014: 27).

In consequence of recent neuroscientific findings (cf. Chap. 2 in this book) the introduction of the term "bab" provided an innovative possibility to express the interdependence of emotion and cognition:

> As far as the term "bab" is accepted to represent an indispensable cognitive-emotional interconnection, a new dimension of conceiving the character of babs can be opened. When we have accepted the concept of an emotional tinge of a proposition represented by the term "bab", then we have to realize that the same type of emotion can be different with respect to its intensity. Thus, obviously, there is a need to express the different intensity of emotional loadings of a bab. Propositionally identical babs can differ by the "weight" or "mightiness" of their emotional loadings. To express this dynamic we proposed to introduce the terms "mega-babs" or "mini-babs" to identify the mightiness of an emotion (Angel 2015: 219)

The ITR (see Sect. 2.6.1) that is depicted in the diagrams in Figs. 2 and 3 and the ur-category in Fig. 7 are synonymous, since they can be represented using the same scheme (Fig. 7). Both ITR and the ur-category are recursive in the sense that they can be manifested within a system repeatedly, reminiscent of Babushka dolls. In other words, the diagram in Fig. 7 called the ur-category can be viewed as the largest Babushka doll in the universe that encloses all the other smaller Babushka dolls, or 'babs' of Angel (2016). I postulate that these smaller babs divide into three types, each belonging to one of the three worlds (see Fig. 1) proposed by Plato, Popper, and Penrose as dicussed by Burgin (2010: 58–60) (Physical world (denoted as 1), Mental world (2), and World of structures (3)), which may thus be named as Bab (1), Bab (2) and Bab (3) (see Table 2) (Fig. 4).

Table 2 The 6 elements of 'babology' or 'babushkology,' neologisms defined as the study of babs and blobs of Angel (2016)

	World		
Energy	Physical (1)	Structures (2)	Mental (3)
Dissipative structure	Bab (1)	Bab (2)	Bab (3)
Equilibrium structure	Blob (1)	Blob (2)	Blob (3)

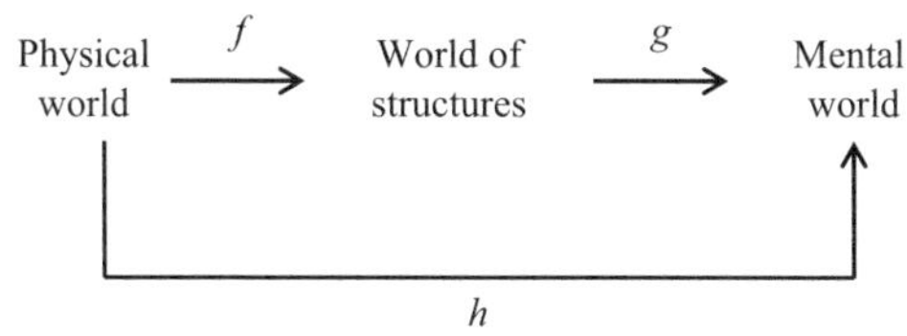

Fig. 4 The Existential Triad of Burgin (2010) as a Peircean (or irreducible) triad. f = natural science; g = human science; h = information flow to give rise to the innate knowledge of the human mid (?). I suggest that -h (the reverse of h) can be related to belief or the process of believing (called 'credition' in (Angel 2013, 2014, 2016).

Since babs are organized objects, they must require energy and information, i.e., gnergy, for their genesis and maintenance. Until now, only the informational aspect of babs (i.e., their shapes and sizes) have been considered, but we can also attribute energetic properties to babs as well (e.g., stability, rates of change, homeostasis, free energy costs, bab-bab interaction energies, etc.). For example, babs may be polarized with excess negative charges on the bottom and excess positive charges on the top in some babs and the other way around in some other babs, thus imparting different energy levels to different combinations of babs (or 'bab configurations' (Angel 2016)). Another example of the energetic aspect of babs would be the energy requirement for bab configurations, i.e., some bab configurations may be at equilibrium and stable while others are far from equilibrium, thus requiring free energy dissipation for their maintenance. We can identify the former as examples of Prigogine's equilibrium structures and the latter as the examples of his dissipative structures. Hence we can distinguish between two kinds of babs based on their energetics: (i) equilibrium babs (or e-babs) and (ii) dissipative babs (or d-babs). Combining these informational and energetic aspects of babs, we can infer that there would be a total of $3 \times 2 = 6$ types of babs as listed in Table 2. There is some theoretical and neurophysiological evidence for assuming that what is here called 'e-babs' may be closely related to the concept of 'blobs' proposed by Angel (2016) as the unconscious counterparts of babs, which explains why the new term 'blob' appears in the bottom of Table 2.

The neologisms 'babology' and 'babushkology' introduced here for the first time, with further refinement, may prove to be a convenient visual scheme to represent ITR in action in integrating (i) the triadic world models of Plato and others and (ii) the energetic aspects of living processes (e.g., stability, homeostasis, growth, etc.) including the process of believing. This integration may implicate the information-energy complementarity as the principle of organization (Ji 1991, 2012b).

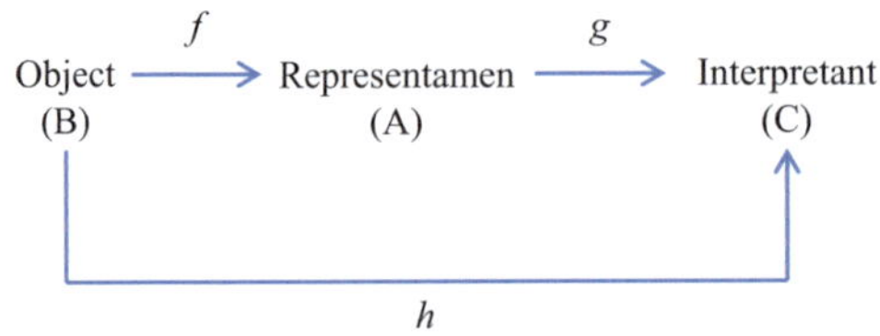

Fig. 5 A diagrammatic representation of the Peircean sign. This diagram is a re-drawing of Fig. 3 with new labels A, B and C that appear in Definitions (2.4) and (2.5). f = sign production; g = sign interpretation; and h = information flow, or grounding. The *arrows* f, g and h are called "structure-preserving mappings" in category theory (Spivak 2013). Mappings, f, g and h, are said to satisfy the commutativity condition, i.e., f followed by g leads to the same result as h, written as $f \times g = h$

2.6 Peircean Semiotics

2.6.1 The Peircean Sign and the Irreducible Triadic Relation (ITR)

In a letter written in 1902 to the Carnegie Institution, Peirce defined a sign as:

- "Anything that stands to someone for something other than itself."
- "Anything which determines something else (its interpretant) to refer to an object to which itself refers (its object) in the same way, the interpretant becoming in turn a sign, and so on an infinitum."
- "I define a sign as something, A, which brings something, C, its interpretant, into the same sort of correspondence with something, B, its object, as that in which itself stands to C."

The Peircean sign defined above can be diagrammatically represented as shown in Fig. 5.

The "structure" in "structure-preserving mappings" in Fig. 5 does not mean visual structures but rather "mathematical structure" of the kind discussed by Burgin (2010: 70–71), i.e., "…(a representation of) a complex entity that consists of parts in relation to each other".

The content of Fig. 5 can be expressed in words thus:

"B determines (or constrains) A which in turn determines C in such a way that C is indirectly determined by B."

Figure 5 is almost identical to another definition of a sign given by Peirce, if the following identities are recognized:

f = Þ
h = μ
g = missing in Peirce's definition

A = Representamen
B = Object
C = Interpretant

Peirecan definition of signs, reproduced from the online work of Robert Marty, "76 Definitions on The sign by C.S. Peirce":

A "sign" is anything, A, which,

1. in addition to other characters of its own,
2. stands in a dyadic relation Þ, to a purely active correlate, B,
3. and is also in a triadic relation to B for a purely passive correlate, C, this triadic relation being such as to determine C to be in a dyadic relation, μ, to B, the relation μ corresponding in a recognized way to the relation Þ.

Peirce discovered that the relation among object, representamen, and interpretant cannot be reduced to any combinations of two or less of the 3 nodes of the network. This idea of Peirce is often referred to as the "irreducible triadic relation (ITR)", which is also involved in the definition of a category in mathematics. (Hausman 1997: 13)

2.6.2 Possible Molecular Mechanisms Underlying Peirce's Hypostatic Abstraction

In his book, *Natural Propositions* (2014), Stjernfeld writes:

> ..., Peirce adds the idea that it is the very capacity of hypostatizing an abstract relation, representing it as if it were a thing, which is the key to self-control: 'The process consists, psychologically, in catching one of the transient elements of thought upon the wing and converting it into one of the resting places of the mind'.... (195).

When I read this paragraph, I scribbled on the margin of the page as follows: "hypostatizing = transforming dissipative structures to equilibrium structures." In other words, this states that the molecular mechanisms underlying the psychological process of hypostatizing (e.g., converting the predicate, "is sweet", to the noun, "sweetness") may be akin to transforming *dissipative structures* (e.g., neural firing patterns underlying the experience of the sweet taste; DS) to *equilibrium structures* (e.g., the structural changes in some neural network in the brain; ES) in non-equilibrium thermodynamics pioneered by Prigogine and his colleagues (1968, 1977, 1980) and others.

According to Prigogine (1991), the DS to ES conversion provides the general molecular mechanism for "encapsulating time into matter," which idea may be symbolically represented as follows (Fig. 6).

For convenience, I will refer to this idea as the *Prigoginian mechanism of encoding time into matter* (PMETM). All of the abiotic structure formations in the universe, beginning with the Big Bang, may be said to involve PMETM.

Fig. 6

$$\text{DS} \longrightarrow \text{ES} = \text{Time} \longrightarrow \text{Matter}$$

However, to account for the structure formation in biotic systems, ranging from unicellular organisms to multicellular ones such as the brain, the reverse process is required, i.e., the ES to DS transformation, e.g., genotype to phenotype, or gene expression (Fig. 7).

Although molecular mechanisms underlying the DS-to-ES transformation are relatively straightforward, as Prigogine's simplified example given in Prigogine (1991) clearly shows, the reverse mechanism, i.e., the ES-to-DS transformation, is not well understood, except for the fact that it requires an input of free energy to drive the process. One possible mechanism to effectuate the ES-to-DS transformation is to utilize *conformons*, the mechanical strains resident in biopolymers (DNA, RNA, proteins) that store free energy and genetic information necessary and sufficient to drive all goal-directed molecular processes in the living cell (Ji 1974, 2000, 2012a).

The content of Fig. 8 may be referred to as the "conformon mechanism of molecular functions" (CMMF), first proposed in (Ji 1974) (errata corrected in (Ji 1979)).

It is here suggested that the processes demonstrated in Figs. 6 and 8 constitute the components of a mathematical category (or an ITR) as shown in Fig. 9, which in turn may be viewed as a bridge (or a functor) connecting semiosis (including hypostatizing) and natural sciences:

Some mathematicians may object to my liberal use of the term "mathematical category" in connection with the diagram in Fig. 9 But my understanding of "mathematical category" (MC) as defined in Spivak (2013) and Brown and Porter (2006) indicates that MC embodies ITR (Irreducible Triadic Relation) as does the Peircean sign and hence it is justified to view Fig. 9 representing a MC.

Fig. 7 ES ⟶ DS = Information ⟶ Matter

Fig. 8 ES ⟶ DS ⇒ Molecular Functions

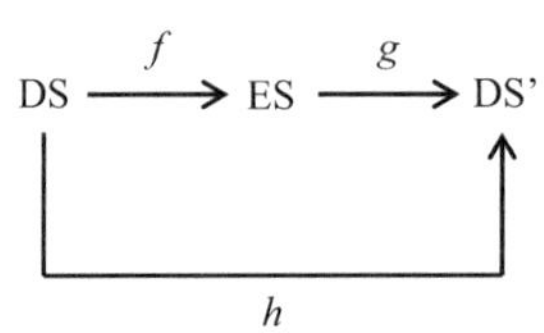

Fig. 9 A postulated universal molecular mechanism underlying semiosis (UMMS) that satisfies the thermodynamic and enzymological requirements. *DS* dissipative structure of Prigogine (1977), *ES* equilibrium structure, *DS'* a partial replica of DS. f = information production or encoding based on PMETM (Prigogine 1991); g = information utilization or decoding based on CMMF (Ji 2000); h = information flow, representation, self-replication, inheritance.

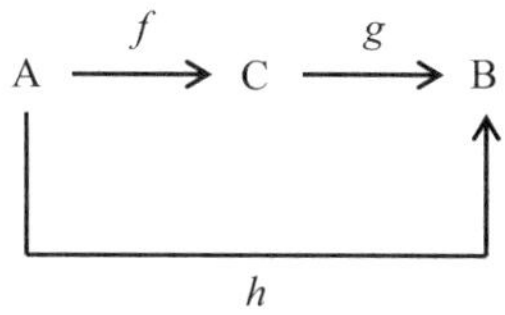

Fig. 10 The ur-category. A diagrammatic representation of the ur-category, i.e., the category to which all categories belong. The commutativity condition of the category theory is satisfied (which is denoted as f × g = h), if the operation f followed by operation g leads to the same result as operation h (Spivak 2013; Brown and Porter 2006).

2.7 *Category Theory*

2.7.1 What Is a Category?

*The category theory is a mathematical theory of comparison, as succinctly stated by Brown and Porter (*2006*):*

> Comparison and analogy are fundamental aspects of knowledge acquisition. We argue that one of the reasons for the usefulness and importance of Category Theory is that it gives an abstract mathematical setting for analogy and comparison, allowing an analysis of the process of abstracting and relating new concepts. This setting is one of the most important routes for the application of Mathematics to scientific problems (p.1).

> We view a category as giving a fairly general abstract context for comparison. The objects of study are the objects of the category. Two objects, A and B, can be compared if the set **C**(A,B) is non-empty and various arrows A ---> B are 'ways of comparing them'. The composition corresponds to: If we can compare A with B and B with C, we should be able to compare A with C (p.5)

2.7.2 The ur-Cateogry and Its Diagrammatic Representation

The ur-category ('ur' meaning 'earliest' or 'original' in German) is defined as the primal category to which all other categories belong. Figure 10 indicates that the ur-category embodies ITR (Irreducible Triadic Relation) of Peirce discussed in Sect. 2.6.1.

The 3-node diagram in Fig. 10 satisfying the commutativity condition, is also called a "commutative triangle" in category theory. The ur-category embodies the Irreducible Triadic Relation (ITR) that is intrinsic to the definition of the sign given by Peirce (see Fig. 5 and Sect. 2.6.1). Hence, it seems justified to regard Peirce as the originator of ITR. So, the terms, *mathematical category, commutative triangle, Peircean sign*, and *ITR* are synonymous.

2.7.3 What Is a Functor?

Spivak (2013) defines a 'functor' as different branches of mathematics (or *human knowledge; my addition)* can be formalized into categories. These categories can then be connected together by functors. And the sense in which these functors provide powerful communication of ideas is that facts and theorems (*regularities*) proven in one category (*discipline*) can be transferred through a connecting functor to yield proofs of analogous theorems in another category. A functor is like a conductor of mathematical truth (cf pp. 93–158).

In this chapter, I will be assuming that the mathematical concept of "functor" can be generalized to include *qualitative* connections between two objects, processes, or domains of human knowledge, in agreement with the concept of "functor" described by Brown and Porter (2006) and Spivak (2013).

2.8 *Complementarity vs. Supplementarity*

The term "complementary" first appears in William James' book, *Principles of Psychology* (1890), in the context of the idea that human consciousness consists of two parts:

> …in certain persons, at least, the total possible consciousness may be split into parts which coexist but mutually ignore each other, and share the objects of knowledge between them. More remarkable still, they are *complementary…* (p. 204).

There is a great similarity between the concept of complementarity that James introduced to psychology in 1890 and that Bohr introduced to physics about four decades later. Bohr discussed his philosophy of *complementarity* publicly for the first time at a meeting held in Como, Italy, in 1927 and published the first paper on complementarity in 1928 (Bohr 1928, Camillieri 2007; Plotnitsky 2006). In 1958, Bohr summarized the concepts of *supplementarity* and *complementarity* as follows:

> … Within the scope of classical physics, all characteristic properties of a given object can in principle be ascertained by a single experimental arrangement, although in practice various arrangements are often convenient for the study of different aspects of the phenomenon. In fact, data obtained in such a way simply supplement each other and *can be combined* into a consistent picture of the behavior of the object under investigation. In quantum mechanics, however, evidence about atomic objects obtained by different experimental arrangements exhibits a novel kind of *complementary relationship*. Indeed, it must be recognized that such evidence which appears contradictory when combination into a single picture is attempted, exhausts all conceivable knowledge about the object. Far from restricting our efforts to put questions to nature in the form of experiments, the notion of *complementarity* simply characterizes the answers we can receive by such inquiry, whenever *the interaction between the measuring instruments and the objects forms an integral part of the phenomenon. …* (p. 4)

The *supplementary* and *complementary* relations defined above can be conveniently represented as triadic relations among three entities labeled A, B, and C. *Supplementarity* refers to the relation in which the sum of a pair equals the third:

$$\text{Supplementarity}: \ C = A + B$$

As an example of supplementarity, Einstein's equation in special relativity, $E = mc^2$, may be cited. Energy (A) and matter (B) may be viewed as extreme manifestations of their source C that can be quantitatively combined or added to completely characterize C. In contrast to supplementarity, *complementarity* is non-additive: i.e., A and B cannot be combined to obtain C. Rather, C can be said to become A or B, depending on measuring instruments employed: i.e., C = A or C = B, depending on measurement. We can represent this complementary relation symbolically as shown in the following equation:

$$\text{Complementarity}: C = A^{\wedge}B$$

where the symbol ^ denotes a "complementary relation". The principles of *complementarity* and *supplementarity* defined above may operate not only in physics but also in biology and beyond as first suggested by Bohr (1933) and noted by others (Pais 1991; Plotnitsky 2006; Camillieri 2007).

3 Conclusion

One significant outcome of the Emotion-Cognition-Credition (ECC) triad is that it is implicated in all human actions and decision-making. Thus, it is underlying all human behaviors both common and uncommon, such as self-immolations and suicide bombings. The concept of the emotion-cognition-credition triad makes it interesting for discussions related to the Peircian postulate that there are three irreducible aspects to all phenomena in the universe, which he called Firstness, Secondness and Thirdness. And it might be discussed where and under which conditions the Planckian Distribution Equitation may open new perspectives for credition research. In general, it is suggested that the concept of credition might be an interesting topic for scholars dedicated to the study of the Peircian concept of the irreducible triadic relation observed throughout the universe.

References

Angel HF (2013) Credition, the process of belief. In: Runehov A et al (eds) Encyclopedia of sciences and religions. Springer, Dordrecht, pp 536–539

Angel HF (2014) Introduction. The conference on the structure of Credition – valuation, association and decision making, University of Graz, Graz, 26–29 November 2014

Angel HF (2015) No believing without emotion. The overlapping of emotion and cognition in the model of credition. In: Studies in science and theology, vol 15, pp 215–222
Benham CJ (1992) Sites of predicted stress-induced DNA duplex destabilization occur preferentially at regulatory sites. Proc Nat Acad Sci USA 90:2999–3003
Benham CJ (1996) Duplex destabilization in supercoiled DNA is predicted to occur at specific transcriptional regulatory regions. J Mol Biol 255:425–434
Bohr N (1928) The quantum postulate and the recent developments of atomic theory. Nature 121:580–590
Bohr N (1933) Light and life. Nature 133:421–423 (Part 1) and 457–459 (Part 2)
Bohr N (1958) Quantum physics and philosophy – causality and complementarity. In: Klibansky R (ed) Philosophy in the mid-century. La Nouva Editrice, Florence
Brown R, Porter T (2006) Category theory: an abstract setting for analogy and comparison. http://citeseerx.ist.psu.edu/viewdoc/download?doi=10.1.1.65.2083&rep=rep1&type=pdf.\
Burgin M (2010) Theory of information: fundamentality, diversity and unification. World Scientific, Hackensack
Callen HB (1985) Thermodynamics: an introduction to the physical theories of equilibrium thermostatics and irreversible thermo dynamics. Wiley, New York, pp 90–101
Camillieri K (2007) Bohr, Heisenberg and the divergent views of complementarity. Stud Hist Philos Mod Phys 38:514–528
Hartshorne C, Weiss P (1931) Collected papers of Charles Sanders Peirce, vol 1. Harvard University Press, Boston, p vii
Hausman CR (1997) Charles S. Peirce's evolutionary philosophy. Cambridge University Press, Cambridge
Hockett CF (1960) The origin of speech. Sci Am 203(3):89–96
Ishii Y, Yanagida T (2007) How single molecule detection measures the dynamics of life. HFSP J 1(1):15–19
James W (1890) The principles of psychology, vol 1. Dover Publications, New York, p 206
Ji S (1974) A general theory of ATP synthesis and utilization. Ann N Y Acad Sci 227:211–226
Ji S (1979) The principles of ligand-protein interactions and their application to the mechanism of oxidative phosphorylation. In: Yagi K (ed) Structure and function of biomembranes. Japan Scientific Societies Press, Tokyo, pp 25–37
Ji S (1991) Biocybernetics: a machine theory of biology. In: Ji S (ed) Molecular theories of cell life and death. Rutgers University Press, New Brunswick, pp 1–237
Ji S (1995) Complementarism: a biology-based philosophical framework to integrate western science and eastern Tao. In: Psychotherapy east and west: integration of psychotherapies. Korean Academy of Psychotherapists, pp 178–23; Sungbuk-dong, Songbuk-ku, Seoul, pp 136–020; Korea, pp 517–548. http://www.conformon.net
Ji S (1997) Isomorphism between cell and human languages: molecular biological, bioinformatics and linguistic implications. BioSystems 44:17–39
Ji S (2000) Free energy and information contents of conformons in proteins and DNA. BioSystems 54:107–130
Ji S (2001) Isomorphism between cell and human languages: micro- and macrosemiotics. In: Simpkins JD (ed) Semiotics 2000: "Sebeok's Century". Legas, Ottawa, pp 357–374
Ji S (2004) Semiotics of life: a unified theory of molecular machines, cells, the mind, Peircean signs, and the universe based on the principle of information-energy complementarity. In: Reports, Research Group on Mathematical Iinguistics, XVII Tarragona Seminar on Formal Syntax and Semantics, Rovira i Virgili University, Tarragona, 23–27 April 2003. http://www.conformon.net
Ji S (2012a) Principles of self-organization and dissipative structures. In: Molecular theory of the living cell: concepts, molecular mechanisms, and biomedical applications. Springer, New York, pp 69–78. http://www.conformon.net
Ji S (2012b) Complementarity. In: Molecular theory of the living cell: concepts, molecular mechanisms, and biomedical applications. Springer, New York, pp 24–50

Ji S (2012c) The kinetics of ligand-protein interactions: the"Pre-fit" mechanism based on the generalized Franck-Condon principle. In: Molecular theory of the living cell: concepts, molecular mechanisms, and biomedical applications. Springer, New York, pp 209–214. PDF at http://www.conformon.net under Publications>Book Chapters
Ji S (2012d) The Conformon. In: Molecular theory of the living cell: concepts, molecular mechanisms, and biomedical applications. Springer, New York, pp 231–253. PDF at http://www.conformon.net under Publications > Book Chapters
Ji S (2012e) Isomorphism between blackbody radiation and enzymic catalysis. In: Molecular theory of the living cell: concepts, molecular mechanisms, and biomedical applications. Springer, New York, pp 343–368. PDF at http://www.conformon.net under Publications > Book Chapters
Ji S (2014) Gaussian and Planckian distributions in brain processes underlying decision making and mind-body coordination. Lecture notes presented at the Conference on "The Structure of Credition – Valuation, Association and Decision Making", 24–29 November 2014. University of Graz, Graz
Ji S (2015a) Planckian distributions in molecular machines, living cells, and brains: the wave-particle duality in biomedical sciences. In: Proceedings of the international conference on biology and bioedical engineering, Vienna, 15–17 March 2015, pp 115–137
Ji S (2015b) Planckian information (IP): a new measure of order in atoms, enzymes, cells, brains, human societies, and the cosmos. In: Amoroso R, Rowlands P, Kauffman L (eds) Unified field mechanics: natural science beyond the Veil of Spacetime. World Scientific, Hackensack (to appear)
Kondepudi D, Prigogine I (1998) Modern thermodynamics: from heat engines to dissipative structures. Wiley, Chichester
Lauffer MA (1983) The significance of entropy-driven processes in biological systems. Comm Mol Cell Biophys 2(2):99–109
Marty R (2011) 76 definitions of the sign by C. S. Peirce. http://www.cspeirce.com/rsources/76defs/76defs.htm
Nikolic D (2015) Practopoiesis: or how life fosters a mind. J theoret Biol 373:40–61
Pais A (1991) Niels Bohrs' times. In: Physics, philosophy, and polity. Clarendon Press, Oxford, pp 438–447
Peirce CS (20xx) http://en.wikipedia.org/wiki/Charles_Sanders_Peirce
Plotnitsky A (2006) Reading Bohr: physics and philosophy. Springer, New York
Prigogine I (1977) Dissipative structures and biological order. Adv Biol Med Phys 16:99–113
Prigogine I (1980) From being to becoming: time and complexity in physical sciences. Freeman and Company, San Francisco, pp 19–26
Prigogine I (1991) Schrödinger and the riddle of life. In: Ji S (ed) Molecular theories of cell life and death. Rutgers University Press, New Brunswick, pp 239–242
Prigogine I, Lefever R (1968) Symmetry-breaking instabilities in dissipative systems. II. J Chem Phys 48:1695–1700
Seitz RJ, Angel HF (2012) Processes of believing –a review and conceptual account. Rev Neurosci 23(3):303–309
Seitz RJ, Angel H-F (2014) Psychology of religion and spirituality: meaning making and processes of believing. Relig Brain Behav:22–30. doi:10.1080/2153599X.2014.891249
Shannon CE, Weaver W (1949) The mathematical theory of communication. University of Illinois Press, Urbana
Spivak DI (2013) Category theory for the sciences. The MIT Press, Cambridge. http://category-theory.mitpress.mit.edu/
Stjernfelt F (2014) Natural propositions: the actuality of Peirce's doctrine of dicisigns. Docent Press, Boston
Sugiura M, Seitz RJ, Angel HF (2015) Models and neural bases of the believing process. J Behav Brain Sci 5:12–23
Volkenstein MV (2009) Entropy and information. Birkhäuser, Basel

Interoception and Gut Feelings: Unconscious Body Signals' Impact on Brain Function, Behavior and Belief Processes

Peter Holzer

Abstract The term "gut feelings" is widely used in everyday language and has a number of connotations ranging from intuition, instinctive feeling, making decisions without rational underpinnings, to serendipity. While in a psychosomatic context the gastrointestinal tract has long been known to respond to emotions and stress, exactly how the gut itself could be a source of feelings/emotions has remained elusive. Neurobiological research in the past two decades has revealed that there is a continuous flow of information from the digestive tract and other internal organs to the brain. A large part of this information does not reach the level of consciousness, but is important for the autonomic control of body functions. In addition, brain imaging techniques have revealed that part of the subconscious information that flows from internal organs is also fed into the corticolimbic system where it is very likely to influence thinking, emotions, and mood. This process is embodied in the term "interoception," and it is emerging that - via the process of interoception - signals from the gut and other internal organs exert an influence on our "feelings" (emotion, cognition, and mood), and that a disturbance in this interoception has an impact on neuropsychiatric diseases. In this relationship, interoception is also very likely to have an impact on the neurobiological basis of belief processes.

1 Introduction

The term "gut feelings" is frequently used in everyday language and has a number of connotations such as intuition (instinctive feeling), decisions made without rational underpinnings, decisions made on the basis of reasons (emotions, memories) that cannot easily be verbalized, decisions made quickly (e.g., fight or flight), to serendipity. "Gut feelings" imply a particular connection between the gastrointestinal tract and the brain, the neurobiological underpinnings of which are gradually

---

P. Holzer (✉)
Institute of Experimental and Clinical Pharmacology, Medical University of Graz, Graz, Austria
e-mail: peter.holzer@medunigraz.at

H.-F. Angel et al. (eds.), *Processes of Believing: The Acquisition, Maintenance, and Change in Creditions*, New Approaches to the Scientific Study of Religion 1,
DOI 10.1007/978-3-319-50924-2_31

emerging to be understood. Nevertheless, a relationship between the gut and brain has long been recognized, as is evident from old translations of the Hebrew and Greek texts of the Bible such as the King James Bible of 1611. In these quotations, it is not only the bowel that is affected by emotions ('my bowels are troubled'), but it also appears as if the bowel symbolizes emotional movement and expression ('my bowels were moved for him').

These expressions attest to an experience that mankind must have acquired far back in its evolution and refer to a relationship that has been delineated by neurogastroenterologic research only recently. While psychosomatic medicine has long contested that the gastrointestinal tract can, in some instances quite disturbingly, respond to emotions and stress, it has gone largely unnoticed that signals from the gut, as well as from other internal organs, have a noticeable impact on emotions, affective, and potentially cognitive, processes. Neurobiological research on the interdependencies of the gut and brain has revealed that there is a continuous flow of information from the digestive tract and other internal organs to the brain (Mayer 2011; Holzer and Farzi 2014). A large part of this information does not reach the level of consciousness, but is important for the autonomic control of body functions. The 'gut-brain axis' represents a fairly well-studied component of the interoceptive circuits that carry information from internal organs to specific areas in the brain where they influence various aspects of brain activity, emotional-affective processing, and behavior (Mayer 2011). Increasing evidence also indicates that a disturbed gut-brain axis may contribute to a variety of neuropsychiatric disorders ranging from anorexia, autism spectrum disorders, multiple sclerosis to anxiety disorders, depression, and dementia.

In this chapter, I will attempt to link gut feelings to the increasing knowledge of gut-brain interactions, trying to integrate this knowledge into the concept of interoception, and consider their potential involvement in belief processes.

2 The Gut-Brain Axis

The terms "gut-brain axis" and "brain-gut axis" refer to the bidirectional exchange of information between the gut and the brain (Fig. 1).

On the one hand, the central, parasympathetic, sympathetic, and enteric nervous systems, as well as neuroendocrine factors (derived from the adrenal medulla and cortex) participate in the autonomic regulation of digestion (motor activity, secretory and absorptive processes, and excretion). On the other hand, there is ongoing communication from the gut to the brain, in which multiple pathways are also involved, as will be discussed below (Mayer 2011; Holzer and Farzi 2014). Normally, most information that is transmitted from the digestive system to the central nervous system does not reach the level of consciousness. However, visceral information is continuously transmitted to subcortical regions of the brain, including the limbic system and the autonomic and neuroendocrine centers in the hypothalamus and brainstem (Craig 2002; Mayer 2011). Under pathological conditions,

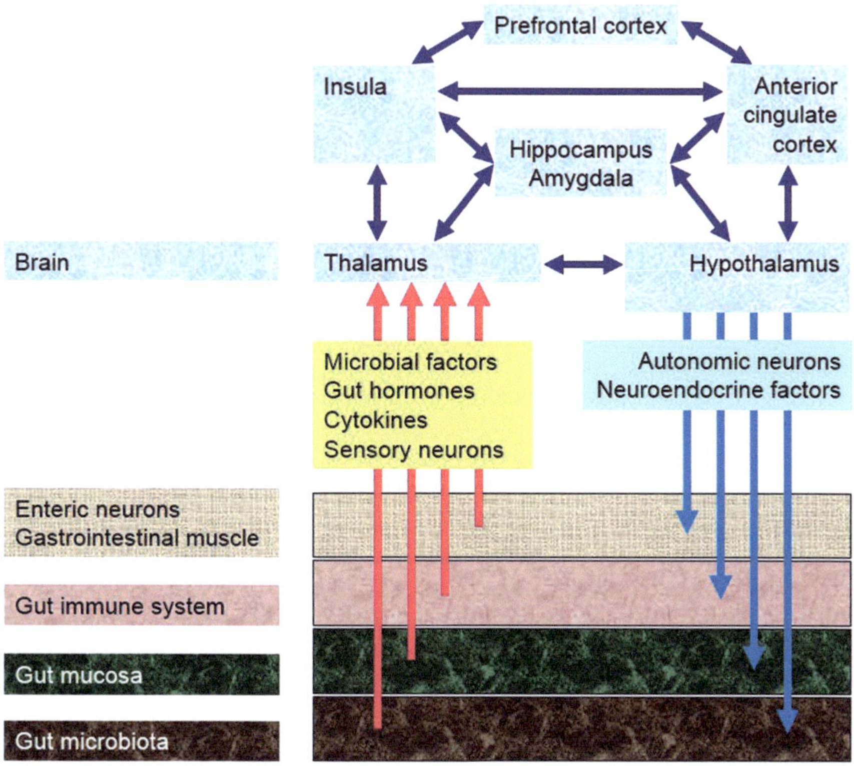

Fig. 1 Schematic illustration of the bidirectional exchange of information between the gut and the brain and the interoceptive processing of this information in the brain

the input from the gut can reach the cortex, giving rise to the sensation of nausea, discomfort, or pain. This afferent part of the gut-brain-gut axis has recently been the focus of investigation why gastrointestinal disease is associated with pain and a number of psychiatric disturbances, including anxiety, neuroticism, and depression (Mayer and Tillisch 2011). It has also contributed to advances in the understanding of interoception, i.e., how signals from internal organs impact on well-being/sickness and the state of mind.

The "gut-brain axis" uses several major information carriers for the communication between the gut and the brain (Fig. 1): metabolites generated by the microbiota in the lumen of the gut, immune messages carried by cytokines, endocrine messages carried by gut hormones, and neural messages carried by vagal and spinal afferent neurons. In addition, the enteric nervous system, which lies in the wall of the gut and can coordinate digestion independently of the brain, has the capacity to interact with afferent neurons (Perez-Burgos et al. 2014) and, via this route, to send signals to the brain. Each of these communication systems is abundantly present in the gastrointestinal tract, which for this reason has been designated as a major neurological (Holzer et al. 2001), immune (Wittig and Zeitz 2003) and endocrine (Ahlman and Nilsson 2001; Murphy and Bloom 2006) organ. Specifically, the gastrointestinal tract is supplied by a dense network of neurons of intrinsic and extrinsic origin (intrinsic enteric neurons and extrinsic afferent neurons as well as autonomic neurons). In addition, enteroendocrine cells in the gastrointestinal mucosa produce more than 20 hormones ("gut hormones") that play a role in the regulation of digestion, metabolism, appetite, energy homeostasis, and mood. The extensive gastrointestinal immune system is important in defending the body against foreign antigens and pathogens that enter with the food and in maintaining homeostasis with the extensive microbial community living in the intestine. The gut microbiota and the gastrointestinal immune system interact with each other via the gastrointestinal mucosa, and this interaction has important functional implications within and outside the gastrointestinal tract.

In the past decade, the gut microbiota has in fact turned out to be a major factor in the gut-brain axis (Collins et al. 2012; Cryan and Dinan 2012; Holzer and Farzi 2014; Mayer et al. 2015) because this enormous microbial community in the intestinal lumen (estimated to consist of 10^{14} cells) produces a huge number of signaling molecules. On the one hand, these microbial signaling molecules can enter the circulation and in this way themselves transmit information to the brain and other distant organs. On the other hand, the microbial signaling molecules can interact with the other information carriers of the gut-brain axis, i.e., they can activate afferent neurons, causing the release of gut hormones or stimulate immune cells. This is the case, for instance, with lipopolysaccharide and peptidoglycan components, which act on the innate immune system to generate and release cytokines and at the same time can directly signal to the brain to alter cerebral activity and elicit a sickness response (Farzi et al. 2015). Current research on the physiological and pathophysiological roles of the symbiotic microbiota in the gut suggests that the microbial signals have an important impact on mental health. Many neuropsychiatric disorders including autism spectrum disorders, multiple sclerosis, Parkinson's disease, chronic fatigue syndrome, depression, and dementia either are associated with a disturbance of the gastrointestinal microbial community ('dysbiosis') and/or can be ameliorated by interventions that normalize the composition and/or activity of the gut microbiota (Holzer 2015).

As is obvious from these findings, the multiple communication pathways constituting the gut-brain axis do not operate in isolation, but are closely interrelated with each other. For instance, cytokines and gut hormones can act on afferent neurons in the vagus nerve, and in this way send messages to the brain (Holzer 2008). The afferent vagus nerve also plays a particular role in transmitting the beneficial impact of a physiological gut microbiota on brain activity and mental well-being (Collins et al. 2012; Cryan and Dinan 2012). The communication between the gut and brain is not unidirectional, however, as the brain sends feedback messages to the gut. This bidirectional gut-brain communication not only ensures the proper maintenance of gastrointestinal function, but is also likely to have multiple effects on affect, motivation and higher cognitive functions, including intuitive decision-making (Mayer 2011), a process embodied in the term "gut feeling". Understanding the operation of the gut-brain axis in health and disease is thus relevant to several medical disciplines, ranging from gastroenterology to neurology and psychiatry, and has important implications beyond. The question is how signals from various internal organs influence mental processes. This issue touches on some fundamental aspects of brain research: how does the brain use and process the information it continuously receives from the outside world and from inside the body? How much do these inputs influence emotional, and in particular, cognitive processes? Can humans think, argue, discuss, assess, judge, contemplate and believe independently of such influences?

3 Interoception

The term interoception used here refers to the integrated sense of the physiological condition of the body (Craig 2002) and the representation of the internal state in the brain (Craig 2009). Interoception includes a wide range of conscious sensations such as pain, nausea, gastrointestinal discomfort, gastrointestinal tension, hunger, and thirst, as well as signaling processes that go virtually unnoticed although they impact on brain activity. There is good reason to assume that there is a continuous stream of interoceptive signals from the gut and other internal organs to the brain, although only a small fraction of this information is consciously perceived, triggering a conscious behavioral response such as ingestion and defecation (Mayer 2011). Emerging evidence suggests that various forms of subliminal interoceptive inputs from the gut may influence memory formation, emotional arousal, and affective behavior (Berntson et al. 2003; Mayer 2011).

Neuroanatomical and neurophysiological investigations hold that there are two neural pathways from the periphery (via spinal and vagal afferent neurons) to a thalamocortical relay that feeds into the primary interoceptive cortex (Fig. 1). It has not yet been fully delineated how microbial, hormonal, and immune signals from the gastrointestinal tract contribute to interoception, but it is very likely that they also participate in this process as is evident for the sensations of hunger and thirst and the pleasure of tasty food. In elaborating on the concept of interoception, Craig (2002) proposed that the interoceptive inputs lead the primary interoceptive cortex, located in the insula, to create an image of the homeostatic state of the body and contribute to self-awareness. The image generated in the insula is modulated by inputs from affective, cognitive, and reward-related brain circuits (Craig 2002, 2009). This image, as well as parallel signal processing in the anterior cingulate cortex, gives rise to a homeostatic emotion, made up of a feeling dimension represented in the anterior insula and a motivation dimension represented in the anterior cingulate cortex (Craig 2002, 2009; Paulus and Stein 2010; Mayer 2011). Importantly, interoceptive images cannot only be generated by signals from the gut and other internal organs but also by the recall of interoceptive memories (Mayer 2011).

Gut-related interoception includes the hedonic effects of signals related, for instance, to food intake, and the aversive effects of gastrointestinal inflammation or irritation by luminal toxins and pathogens (Mayer 2011). The ingestion of food that is beneficial to the organism is associated with a feeling of pleasure, whereas the ingestion of potentially harmful foods elicits negative emotions such as nausea (Mayer 2011). However, activation of the anterior insula and anterior cingulate cortex also occurs in the absence of interoceptive signals from the gut when subjects experience disgust or view images of others experiencing disgust (Wicker et al. 2003). This finding has been taken as an argument that interoception-like processes take place in the absence of interoceptive input, presumably through the recall of interoceptive memories (Mayer 2011). The mechanisms and pathways underlying the formation of interoceptive memories of gut-related signals await to be fully delineated, although it is known that the anterior insula, orbitofrontal cortex, amygdala, and hippocampus are involved (Mayer 2011). The recall of such memories without conscious awareness may bias behavioral responses, and such behavioral biases may be a reflection of an internal value map based on "gut feelings" (Mayer 2011).

Given the multiplicity of gut-brain signaling systems (Fig. 1), gut-brain interactions may make a significant contribution to emotional and motivational self-awareness in the absence of any conscious sensations. In this context, the popular reference to decisions based on gut feelings may have an actual neurobiological basis in unconscious signals from the gut or the recall of interoceptive memories that influence the state of mind (Mayer 2011). This contention is backed by neuroimaging studies that implicate sub-regions of the anterior insula in intuitive decision-making (Mayer 2011). Intuitive decision-making can be defined as the rapid assessment of the probability of a favorable or unfavorable outcome of a planned behavior in a situation of uncertain outcomes, which is dependent on previous experiences, rather than on processes of inductive or deductive reasoning (Preuschoff et al. 2008; Singer et al. 2009).

Disturbances in the process of interoception are increasingly implicated in neuropsychiatric disorders, such as anxiety and depression (Paulus and Stein 2006, 2010; Furman et al. 2013; Harshaw 2015). Neuroimaging studies attest to alterations in the function of the insula, the major hub of interoceptive awareness, and GABAergic deficits in this region (Binkofski et al. 1998; Wiebking et al. 2014). Paulus and Stein (2006) have proposed that, in anxiety disorders, there may be a mismatch of actual interoceptive input reaching the anterior insula with a falsely predicted interoceptive state (from interoceptive memory and/or influences from prefrontal and limbic regions). This mismatch results in the engagement of the anterior cingulate cortex, and thus leads to emotional arousal, increased activity of the autonomic nervous system, sensory facilitation, and a conscious feeling of anxiety and worry (Paulus and Stein 2006; Mayer 2011).

4 Interoception, Gut Feelings and Belief Processes

The contention that unconscious interoception can impact both emotional awareness and motivation provides a neurobiological explanation for gut feelings and intuitive decision-making. Although direct evidence for this relationship is scarce, intuitive decision-making has been linked to the insula, a key region involved in interoceptive processing (Craig 2009; Mayer 2011). In discussing the potential role of disordered interoception in anxiety and depression, Paulus and Stein (2010) argue that dysfunctional belief processes make an important contribution to these neuropsychiatric disorders. This contention is deduced from the finding that the experience of the individual with respect to self, others, and the future is altered in anxiety and depression, and that this alteration of self-awareness is governed by interoceptive changes and misleading belief processes (Paulus and Stein 2010). Specifically, the insula as the interoceptive center of the brain is critically involved in evaluating the potential impact of internal as well as external stimuli on the body. A mismatch between the actual interoceptive input and a disturbed interoceptive memory may give rise to false predictions and belief processes (Paulus and Stein 2006; Mayer 2011). Paulus and Stein (2010) define beliefs as propositional mental constructs that affirm or deny the truth of a state of affairs and are closely linked to basic judgment processes. Beliefs are frequently used to build mental models of the state of the world and are therefore important constructs to guide decision-making (Paulus and Stein 2010). Although the relationship between gut feelings, interoception, and belief processes requires experimental proof, the current knowledge of gut-brain communication (Fig. 1) provides a valid framework on which to base these research efforts. The study of interoception has already revealed that several cerebral functions, including creditive processes, are under the influence of unconscious inputs to the brain, a relationship that should not be underestimated.

References

Ahlman H, Nilsson O (2001) The gut as the largest endocrine organ in the body. Ann Oncol 12(2):63–68

Berntson GG, Sarter M, Cacioppo JT (2003) Ascending visceral regulation of cortical affective information processing. Eur J Neurosci 18:2103–2109. doi:10.1046/j.1460-9568.2003.02967.x

Binkofski F, Schnitzler A, Enck P, Frieling T, Posse S, Seitz RJ, Freund HJ (1998) Somatic and limbic cortex activation in esophageal distention: a functional magnetic resonance imaging study. Ann Neurol 44:811–815

Collins SM, Surette M, Bercik P (2012) The interplay between the intestinal microbiota and the brain. Nat Rev Microbiol 10:735–742. doi:10.1038/nrmicro2876

Craig AD (2002) How do you feel? Interoception: the sense of the physiological condition of the body. Nat Rev Neurosci 3:655–666. doi:10.1038/nrn894

Craig AD (2009) How do you feel – now? The anterior insula and human awareness. Nat Rev Neurosci 10:59–70. doi:10.1038/nrn2555

Cryan JF, Dinan TG (2012) Mind-altering microorganisms: the impact of the gut microbiota on brain and behaviour. Nat Rev Neurosci 13:701–712. doi:10.1038/nrn3346

Farzi A, Reichmann F, Meinitzer A, Mayerhofer R, Jain P, Hassan AM, Fröhlich EE, Wagner K, Painsipp E, Rinner B, Holzer P (2015) Synergistic effects of NOD1 or NOD2 and TLR4 activation on mouse sickness behavior in relation to immune and brain activity markers. Brain Behav Immun 44:106–120. doi:10.1016/j.bbi.2014.08.011

Furman DJ, Waugh CE, Bhattacharjee K, Thompson RJ, Gotlib IH (2013) Interoceptive awareness, positive affect, and decision making in major depressive disorder. J Affect Disord 151:780–785. doi:10.1016/j.jad.2013.06.044

Harshaw C (2015) Interoceptive dysfunction: toward an integrated framework for understanding somatic and affective disturbance in depression. Psychol Bull 141:311–363. doi:10.1037/a0038101

Holzer P (2008) The role of the vagus nerve in afferent signaling and homeostasis during visceral inflammation. In: Jancsó G (ed) Neurogenic inflammation in health and disease, Neuroimmune biology, vol 8. Elsevier, Amsterdam, pp 321–338

Holzer P (2015) Das Gehirn unter dem Einfluss des Darmmikrobioms. Neurologisch 01/2015:45–49

Holzer P, Farzi A (2014) Neuropeptides and the microbiota-gut-brain axis. Adv Exp Med Biol 817:195–219. doi:10.1007/978-1-4939-0897-4_9

Holzer P, Schicho R, Holzer-Petsche U, Lippe IT (2001) The gut as a neurological organ. Wien Klin Wochenschr 113:647–660

Mayer EA (2011) Gut feelings: the emerging biology of gut–brain communication. Nat Rev Neurosci 12:453–466. doi:10.1038/nrn3071

Mayer EA, Tillisch K (2011) The brain-gut axis in abdominal pain syndromes. Annu Rev Med 62:381–396. doi:10.1146/annurev-med-012309-103958

Mayer EA, Tillisch K, Gupta A (2015) Gut/brain axis and the microbiota. J Clin Invest 125:926–038. doi:10.1172/JCI76304

Murphy KG, Bloom SR (2006) Gut hormones and the regulation of energy homeostasis. Nature 444:854–859. doi:10.1038/nature05484

Paulus MP, Stein MB (2006) An insular view of anxiety. Biol Psychiatry 60:383–387. doi:10.1016/j.biopsych.2006.03.042

Paulus MP, Stein MB (2010) Interoception in anxiety and depression. Brain Struct Funct 214:451–463. doi:10.1007/s00429-010-0258-9

Perez-Burgos A, Mao YK, Bienenstock J, Kunze WA (2014) The gut-brain axis rewired: adding a functional vagal nicotinic “sensory synapse”. FASEB J 28:3064–3074. doi:10.1096/fj.13-245282

Preuschoff K, Quartz SR, Bossaerts P (2008) Human insula activation reflects risk prediction errors as well as risk. J Neurosci 28:2745–2752. doi:10.1523/JNEUROSCI.4286-07.2008

Singer T, Critchley HD, Preuschoff K (2009) A common role of insula in feelings, empathy and uncertainty. Trends Cogn Sci 13:334–340. doi:10.1016/j.tics.2009.05.001

Wicker B, Keysers C, Plailly J, Royet JP, Gallese V, Rizzolatti G (2003) Both of us disgusted in My insula: the common neural basis of seeing and feeling disgust. Neuron 40:655–664. doi:http://dx.doi.org/10.1016/S0896-6273(03)00679-2

Wiebking C, Duncan NW, Tiret B, Hayes DJ, Marjańska M, Doyon J, Bajbouj M, Northoff G (2014) GABA in the insula – a predictor of the neural response to interoceptive awareness. NeuroImage 86:10–18. doi:10.1016/j.neuroimage.2013.04.042

Wittig BM, Zeitz M (2003) The gut as an organ of immunology. Int J Color Dis 18:181–187. doi:10.1007/s00384-002-0444-1

Decision-Making and Credition Under a Microbial Perspective

Gabriele Berg and Maria Sensen

Abstract The human body is home to a highly diverse microbial community. Next-generation sequencing-based technologies have drastically revolutionized our knowledge of the human microbiome; now we see them together as a tight association called meta-organism or holo-biont. We have learned from the analysis of the human microbiome that it is involved in many more processes and diseases than recently thought, including heart diseases, cancer, autism, obesity, and others. Less is known about how the microbiome affects brain function and our behavior. There is evidence that the brain and the gut are well connected. Here we present and discuss examples that our microbiome is vital in inter-kingdom communication and interplay. This overview of the state-of-the-art findings in current literature shows that the analysis of the human microbiome data has brought about a paradigm shift in our understanding of its role in diseases and decision-making. In contrast, credition - processes of belief – and microbiome shifts need further research. Taken together, we would like to postulate that our microbiome has to be considered as an essential partner in decision-making and credition processes, and propose the need for a tighter connection between microbiome research, neurosciences, and psychology.

1 The Healthy Microbiome

1.1 Basic Insights into the Human Microbiome

We are never alone, because during natural birth, we get a microbiome from our mother as a first gift upon our entry into the world, which provides us with the ability to develop our individual microbiome, which aids in protecting us against diseases (Blaser 2014). We are recognized as meta-organisms or holo-bionts because we contain ten times more microbial cells than human cells (Blaser et al. 2013). At least 40,000 bacterial strains (1800 genera and thousands of different species) in

G. Berg (✉) • M. Sensen
Institute of Environmental Biotechnology, Graz University of Technology, Graz, Austria
e-mail: gabriele.berg@tugraz.at; maria.sensen@tugraz.at

H.-F. Angel et al. (eds.), *Processes of Believing: The Acquisition, Maintenance, and Change in Creditions*, New Approaches to the Scientific Study of Religion 1,
DOI 10.1007/978-3-319-50924-2_32

abundances up to 10^{11} per gram, which collectively harbor at least 9.9 million non-human genes, colonize our body (Stilling et al. 2014). Surprisingly, these 100 trillion non-human-associated cells make up 1–2 kg in an adult body; comparable to the weight of the adult human brain (approximately 1.5 kg) (Forsythe and Kunze 2013).

There are many similarities between host-associated microbiome functions and ecology (Mendes and Raijmakers 2015). For example, the microbiome structure varies during life cycle, and the rhythm of their host and microbes is connected (Thaiss et al. 2014). Eukaryotic organisms co-evolve with their microorganism during their whole existence, and still today, the latter shape their evolution. Most host-associated microbiomes represent the interplay of *Bacteria*, *Archaea* as well as eukaryotic microorganisms. All of these microbial phyla contain viruses, which together form the virome, and contribute to co-evolutionary processes. A high taxonomic diversity was visible in the published metagenomes; *Bacteria* are often the most abundant micro-organisms in host-associated microbiomes and act as a key player (keystone species). *Archaea*, formerly considered to be inhabitants of extreme environments, were also found to be host-associated, e.g. in the human gut, on human skin, as well as in the endosphere of plants (Probst et al. 2013; Berg et al. 2015). Less is known about the functional interplay between individual different microbial kingdoms (Berg 2015). Bacteria-fungi networking was shown to be very important; however the function of *Archaea* in relation to eukaryotic hosts is not yet understood (Berg 2015).

To define a healthy microbiome is very difficult. The highly individual microbiome explained by both cohort effects and individual host genotype is only one of the factors (Benson et al. 2010). Another one is the immense loss of human-associated microbial diversity, which was shown in comparison to African and Amazon tribes (Schnorr 2015). Both functional and structural diversity within a microbiome seems to be important. The dilution effect theory that posits that diverse ecological communities limit disease spread via several mechanisms was recently strongly supported by Civitello et al. (2015). Although structural diversity was identified as paramount to the prevention and avoidance of pathogen invasion/outbreaks (van Elsas et al. 2012), we also learned that the individual component is important for the microbiome structure and, finally, the functional diversity is often crucial (Carrara et al. 2015). The beneficial potential of the microbiome is not yet fully understood, but now we realize that the extent of interplay and communication is much higher than ever thought. Developing predictable strategies to control the microbiomes are a future challenge (Berg et al. 2013; Berg 2015).

1.2 Our Eating and Sexual Behavior Is Influenced by the Gut Microbiome

First, the birth-giving mother's microbiome colonizes the lining of a newborn baby's gut; however the breast milk microbiome seems to play even more of an influential role for the lifetime development of the gastrointestinal ecosystem (Daft et al. 2015). After this early period of life, diet has the capability to change the microbiome rapidly and reproducibly, but also unsustainably; once a special diet is over, the microbial diversity can return to the pre-diet level within few days (David et al. 2014). The brain-gut axis (hypothalamic–pituitary–adrenal [HPA] axis) is a bidirectional communication system between the central nervous system and the gastrointestinal tract. Via this axis, bacteria send molecular information to influence what "we" want to eat, and it is sometimes difficult for us to change this behavior as studies with obese patients showed (Alcock et al. 2014).

The decision regarding which partner we select is very important for healthy children with a strong immune system, which is one of our most complex organs, and heavily educated by the composition of our microbiome. Moreover, the neuroendocrine system determines our personal smell partially via bacterial volatiles. People with different smells are much more interested in each other than those with similar smell, which helps to maintain and develop the strong immune system for further generations with the highest possible diversity rates and combinatorial variations. In general, the microbiome has a crucial role in social development (Desbonet et al. 2014).

2 The Unbalanced Microbiome

2.1 Depression and the Role of the Microbiome

Depression is believed to be the result of both chronic stress and stressful life events, or the imbalance of the neurotransmitters in the brain. Depressed persons are under stress when they have to make even small decisions. Depression treatments are based on this belief. Major depressive disorder (MDD) is the third most prevalent and costly disease worldwide, and it is projected to become number one by 2030 (WHO, GBD report, 2004). Antidepressants were the third most common prescription drug taken by Americans of all ages in 2005–2008, and the most frequently used by persons aged 18–44 years. From the periods of 1988–1994 and 2005–2008, the rate of antidepressant use in the United States among all ages increased nearly 400% (Pratt et al. 2011).

Interestingly, recent animal experiments have shown that in gene expression patterns triggered either by stress or in depressed animals, out of the approximately 1500 affected genes, there were only five genes shared between endogenous depressive behavior and chronic stress-related molecular mechanisms. Although chronic stress may trigger depressive behavior, it cannot be detected on a molecular expression level in the hippocampus/amygdala. Also, the animal model of depression could not identify alterations on the levels of genes controlling neurotransmitter functions. The biochemical events that ultimately result in depression actually may start in the development and functioning of neurons (Andrus et al. 2012). The gut microbiota played a critical role in the production of neurotransmitters, e.g. norepinephrine and dopamine in the gut of mices (Asano et al. 2012). In addition, **Candida** spp., **Streptococcus** spp., **Escherichia** spp. and **Enterococcus** spp., have been shown to directly produce serotonin (Cryan and Dinnan 2012). Further research is going to reveal whether the decreased level of properly functioning neurotransmitters is due to a dysbiosis of the gut where their production is abnormal or whether depression is more a consequence of a malfunctioning neuron system.

2.2 Social Anxiety Disorders and the Role of the Microbiome

When people are embarrassed or feel uncomfortable in public, their behavior is often linked to low serotonin availability. Interestingly, recent research results show that fermented foods and drinks are able to help curb that disorder (Hilimire et al. 2015). Dysbiotic gut flora often contain excessive amount of yeasts and their toxic metabolites, which can pass through the blood-brain barrier and alter neurological functioning, causing "brain fog"-related behavioral problems and learning difficulties. Excessive dysbiotic bacterial byproducts can interfere with neurotransmitters and cause chronic fatigue, while the beneficial bacteria helps with vitamin absorption and preventing infections (Hilimire et al. 2015). Fermented foods are a good source of both vitamins and vitamin-producing beneficial bacteria, such as *Lactobacilli* sp. as well (LeBlanc et al. 2011). In addition, *L. plantarum* was shown to exert its benefit by acting genetically upstream of the TOR (target of rapamycin)-dependent host nutrient sensing system controlling hormonal growth signaling (Storelli et al. 2011). Another experiment shows that anxiety-like behavior can be normalized by probiotic *Bifidobacterium longum* NCC3001 (Bercik et al. 2011). It has been shown that four weeks of dietary intake of fermented milk product with probiotics can modulate brain activities in healthy individuals. The experimental group in this study had increased activity in the areas of the prefrontal cortex associated with cognition, in contrast to the control group, which showed greater connectivity of the periaqueductal grey to emotion- and sensation-related regions (Tillisch et al. 2013).

A new microbiome study indicates how parasites are capable of provoking behavioral changes. *Toxoplasma gondii,* a well-known protozoan parasite in immunocompromised patients, can travel from the stomach to the brain. It was well known that a *Toxoplasma* infection can be detrimental during pregnancy for the developing baby's brain, however, in experimentally-infected rats, it triggered behavioral changes, evidenced, for example, in the lack of recognition of cats (or their odor) as dangerous (Blanchard et al. 2015).

2.3 Chronic Diseases and the Role of the Microbiome

During the last decade, a so-called personalized medicine system started to be developed based on the sequenced human genome. In chronic diseases, the identification of genetic abnormalities made a huge impact on understanding the underlying processes; however, it did not reveal the cause or origin of the chronic diseases. By gaining deeper insight into the microbiota component, great additional progress has been achieved; however, we are still far from understanding our complex microbiome-driven ecosystem. Furthermore, the environmental triggers should be identified too. Each chronic disease has a set of mental symptoms, sometimes it is mental fatigue or anxiety, but it can reach very severe levels like in Alzheimer's, as evidenced as a total loss of memory in some cases.

Inflammatory bowel diseases (IBD), like Crohn's disease (CD) and ulcerative colitis are chronic diseases, in which insomnia and depression are very common symptoms among the patients. Initially, research concentrated on the identification of the genetic alterations. So far 163 genes have been identified as necessary, but not sufficient, factors. Even though it is a very impressive contribution, these necessary genes alone are not enough to manifest the symptoms (Sartor 2014). By now, it is evident that the symptoms of inflammatory bowel disease (IBS) come from a series of strong immune responses to a shifted intestinal microbiome. The shift is visible already at phylum level: enrichment in *Firmicutes* and decrease of *Bacterioides* are consistent findings. In the lumen of the intestine, the level of the oxygen increases due to an increased inflammation of the mucosal layer and oxidative stress is well-reflected in the aerotolerant shift of the bacterial composition (Kennedy et al. 2014). The disease severity and location are microbiota-dependent (Schaubeck et al. 2015). Since the microbiome varies even for the same person based on diet, age, stress factors, and sampling location, it is very challenging to establish a dysbiotic pattern characteristic of different subtypes of IBS. Recent methods provide an assessment of the "dysbiotic index" based on the evaluation of a rectal mucosal-associated microbiome. Although antibiotics are the first line of treatment of IBS, analyzing patient data proves that application of antibiotics amplifies the microbial dysbiosis (Gevers et al. 2014). Dietary factors play a crucial role in the development of IBS, but other environmental triggers still remain debated. In animal experiments in the presence of soy protein, similar atrophy of the microvilli of the small intestine together with dysbiotic changes in the feces can be detected, as it is characteristic in some IBS types (Lim et al. 2015).

The faster the food travels through the gastrointestinal track, the less chance the pathogens have to successfully colonize the surface of the gut. This is a self-defense mechanism of our body. In contrast, the passage is much slower in germ-free mice compared to normal gut microbiome-baring animals. Early studies indicate that environmental stress factors, like deprivation of food and water, even bedding change in mice, can result in a dramatic decrease of the *Lactobacilli* in the small intestine, stomach, and the colon, while aerobic coliforms and enterococci can increase (Tannock and Savage 1974).

A harmoniously-functioning microbiome is capable of supplying the host with sufficient energy and micronutrients, among them the epigenetic role of short-chain fatty acids has been studied for decades (Hullar and Fu 2014). They possess particular importance in gut-brain axis signaling (Evans et al. 2013). The microbiota itself may be viewed as an epigenetic entity (Dinnan et al. 2010), which plays its crucial role, both in health and disease, via its specialized metabolites (Sharon et al. 2014).

3 Decision-Making and Credition Under Microbiome Influence

The brain-gut axis is modulated by the microbiome and it has been shown that the gut microbiota can be a key regulator of mood, cognition, pain, and obesity, as well as our decisions (Burokas et al. 2015). The central and the enteric nervous system are interconnected via the vagus nerve, which extends from the brainstem through the lung and heart to the abdomen. Beside the electric signals, it transports neurotransmitters and participates in controlling the heart and breathing rate, appetite, and many more elements affecting our conscious and unconscious decisions. Our overview of the state-of-the-art outcomes in current literature shows that the analysis of human microbiome data has brought about a paradigm shift in our understanding of its role in diseases and decision-making. The impact of the microbiome was shown under healthy and diseased conditions and is always connected with balanced/unbalanced microbiome structure and functions.

Research on the relationship between processes of believing and the microbiome has yet been published. However, we expect that practices like meditation, prayer and fasting, which are involved in processes of belief, have a strong link to the microbiome. Nutritional modulation of the microbiome by reduced food intake (avoiding malnutrition) was shown, and long-term, including inter-generational, effects of diet have been identified (Fontana and Partridge 2015). It has been experimentally supported that meditation significantly elevates the whole blood serotonin level while improving negative mood (Yu et al. 2011), and even has a potential for age-defying effects on the brain (Luders et al. 2015). Traditionally, all religions and atheistic views support both the spiritual and the physical (microbiome) "cleaning" in connection with credition.

Understanding microbiota-brain interactions is a promising area of research, which may contribute new insights into individual variations in cognition, personality, mood, sleep, and decision-making processes, which we historically recognized as intuition or "gut feeling. Credition - processes of belief – and microbiome shifts need further research. The microbiome has to be considered as an essential partner in our behavior. Finally, microbiome research should be integrated in concepts for healthy diets and also in mental disorder treatments, and needs a tighter connection to be made to neurosciences and psychology.

References

Alcock JM, Maley CC, Akipis CA (2014) Is eating behavior manipulated by the gastrointestinal microbiota? Evolutionary pressures and potential mechanisms. Bioassays 36:940–949

Andrus BM, Blizinsky K, Vedell PT et al (2012) Gene expression patterns in the hippocampus and amygdala of endogenous depression and chronic stress modells. Mol Psychiatry 17:49–61

Asano Y, Hiramoto T, Nishino R et al (2012) Critical role of gut microbiota in the production of biologically active, free catecholamines in the gut lumen of mice. Am J Physiol Gastrointest Liver Physiol 303:1288–1295

Benson AK, Kelly SA, Legge R et al (2010) Individuality in gut microbiota composition is a complex polygenic trait shaped by multiple environmental and host genetic factors. Proc Natl Acad Sci U S A 107:18933–18938
Bercik P, Park AJ, Sinclair D et al (2011) The anxiolytic effect of *Bifidobacterium longum* NCC3001 involves vagal pathways for gut–brain communication. Neurogastroenterol Motil 23(12):1132–1139
Berg G (2015) Beyond borders: investigating microbiome interactivity and diversity for advanced biocontrol technologies. Microb Biotechnol 8:5–7
Berg G, Zachow C, Müller H et al (2013) Next-generation bio-products sowing the seeds of success for sustainable agriculture. Agronomy 3:648–656
Berg G, Grube M, Schloter M, Smalla K (2015) The plant microbiome and its importance for plant and human health. Front Microbiol, e-book 5:189
Blanchard N, Dunay IR, Schutler D (2015) Persistence of *Toxoplasma gondii* in the central nervous system: a fine-tuned balance between the parasite, the brain and the immune system. Parasite Immunol 37:150–158
Blaser MJ (2014) Missing microbes. Oneworld Publications, London
Blaser MJ, Bork P, Fraser C et al (2013) The microbiome explored: recent insights and future challenges. Nat Rev Microbiol 11:213–217
Burokas A, Moloney RD, Dinan TG, Cryan JF (2015) Microbiota regulation of the Mammalian gut-brain axis. Adv Appl Microbiol 91:1–62
Carrara F, Giometto A, Seymour M et al (2015) Experimental evidence for strong stabilizing forces at high functional diversity of aquatic microbial communities. Ecology 96:1340–1350
Civitello DJ, Cohen J, Fatima H, Halstead NT, Liriano J, McMahon TA, Ortega CN, Sauer EL, Sehgal T, Young S, Rohr JR (2015) Biodiversity inhibits parasites: Broad evidence for the dilution effect. Proc Natl Acad Sci U S A A112:8667–8671
Cryan JF, Dinan TG (2012) Mind-altering microorganisms: the impact of the gut microbiota on brain and behaviour. Nature 13:701–712
Daft GJ, Ptacek T, Kumar R et al (2015) Cross-fostering immediately after birth immediately induces a permanent microbiota shift that is shaped by the nursing mother. Microbiome. doi:10.1186/s40168-015-0080-y
David LA, Maurice CF, Carmody RN et al (2014) Diet rapidly and reproducibly alters the human gut microbiome. Nature 505:559–563
Desbonnet L, Clarke G, Shanahan F, Dinan TG, Cryan JF (2014) Microbiota is essential for social development in the mouse. Mol Psychiatry 19:146–148
Dinan TG, Cryan J, Shanahan F, Keeling PW, Quigley EM (2010) IBS: an epigenetic perspective. Nat Rev Gastroenterol Hepatol 7:465–471
Evans JM, Morris LS, Marchesi JR (2013) The gut microbiome: the role of a virtual organ in the endocrinology of the host. J Endocrinol 218:R37–R47
Fontana L, Partridge L (2015) Promoting health and longevity through diet: from model organisms to humans. Cell 161:106–118
Forsythe P, Kunze WA (2013) Voices from within: gut microbes and the CNS. Cell Mol Life Sci 70:55–69
Gevers D, Kugathasan S, Denson LA (2014) The treatment-naive microbiome in New-Onset
Hilimire MR, DeVylder JE, Forestell CA (2015) Fermented foods, neuroticism, and social anxiety: an interaction model. Psychiatry Res 228:203–208
Hullar MAJ, Fu BC (2014) Diet, the gut microbiome, and epigenetics. Cancer J 20:170–175
Kennedy PJ, Cryan JF, Dinan TG et al (2014) Irritable bowel syndrome: a microbiome-gu-brain-axis disorder? World J Gastroenterol 20:14105–14125
LeBlanc JG, Lain JE, del Valle MJ et al (2011) B-Group vitamin production by lactic acid bacteria – current knowledge and potential applications. J Appl Microbiol 111:1297–1309
Lim J, Kim S, Choi J, Chen X et al (2015) Changes in microbiome profiles and nutrient absorption in intestine by soy protein. FASEB J 29:914–915

Luders E, Cherbuin N, Kurth F (2015) Forever Young(er): potential age-defying effects of long-term meditation on gray matter atrophy. Front Psychol 5:1551

Mendes R, Raaijmakers JM (2015) Cross-kingdom similarities in microbiome functions. ISME J [Epub ahead of print]. doi:10.1038/ismej.2015.7

Pratt LA, Brody DJ, Gu Q (2011) Antidepressant use in persons aged 12 and over: United States, 2005–2008. NCHS Data Brief 76:2011

Probst AJ, Auerbach AK, Moissl-Eichinger C (2013) Archaea on human skin. PLoS One 8:e65388

Sartor RB (2014) The intestinal microbiota in inflammatory bowel diseases. In: Lewis JD, Ruemmele FM, Wu GD (eds) Nutrition, gut microbiota and immunity: therapeutic targets for IBD. Nestlé Nutr Inst Workshop Ser. Nestec Ltd. Vevey/S. Karger AG Basel 79:29–39

Schaubeck M, Clavel T, Calasan J et al (2015) Dysbiotic gut microbiota causes transmissible Crohn's disease-like ileitis independent of failure in antimicrobial defense. Gut:1–13. doi:10.1136/gutjnl-2015-309333

Schnorr LS (2015) The diverse microbiome of the hunter-gatherer. Nature 518:14–15

Sharon G, Garg N, Debelius J et al (2014) Specialized metabolites from the microbiome in health and disease. Cell Metab 20:719–730

Stilling RM, Dinan TG, Cryan JF (2014) Microbial genes, brain and behavior: epigenetic regulation of the gut-brain axis. Genes Brain Behav 13:69–86

Storelli G, Defaye A, Erkosar B et al (2011) *Lactobacillus plantarum* promotes *Drosophila* systemic growth by modulating hormonal signals through TOR-dependent nutrient sensing. Cell Metab 14:403–414

Tannock GW, Savage DC (1974) Influences of dietary and environmental stress on microbial populations in the murine gastrointestinal tract. Infect Immun 9:591–598

Thaiss CA, Zeevi D, Levy M et al (2014) Transkingdom control of microbiota diurnal oscillations promotes metabolic homeostasis. Cell 159:514–529

Tillisch K, Labus J, Kilpatrick L et al (2013) Consumption of fermented milk product with probiotic modulates brain activity. Gastroenterology 144:1394–1401

Van Elsas JD, Chiurazzi M, Mallon CA et al (2012) Microbial diversity determines the invasion of soil by a bacterial pathogen. Proc Natl Acad Sci U S A 109:1159–1164

Yu X, Fumoto M, Nakatani Y et al (2011) Activation of the anterior prefrontal cortex and serotonergic system is associated with improvements in mood and EEG changes induced by Zen meditation practice in novices. Int J Psychophysiol 80:103–111

Part VII
Conclusion

Structuring Credition

Hans-Ferdinand Angel, Lluis Oviedo, Raymond F. Paloutzian, Anne L.C. Runehov, and Rüdiger J. Seitz

Abstract The chapter provides some synthesis to the contributions to this volume on the "process of believing", called "credition". In contrast to much of the traditional literature, which treats "belief" or "faith" as if it is a static phenomenon (i.e., talking about it as a noun), it summarizes the scientific and communicative transformation that is going on with the change from "belief" to the "process of believing". The contributions provide three different ways to illustrate the consequences of this transformation. We call them bridging (i.e., to clarify its implications for the concept of "belief" in a static sense), translation or modification (i.e., to discuss context-related changes in religious beliefs and religious cognition), and transfer (i.e., to illuminate the conceptual implications of credition from one scientific discipline to another, including psychological, general biological, molecular, genetic, and neurophysiological approaches). The chapter also provides another way to structure the variety of contributions. The Credition Research Project has elaborated a "model of the believing process" (model of credition) and a "conceptual framework of the believing process". Some chapters contribute more to the conceptual understanding of the believing process and aim to enrich its theoretical foundations. Other chapters explicitly take a more applied approach in exploring

H.-F. Angel (✉)
Institute of Catechetics and Religious Education, Karl-Franzens University of Graz, Graz, Austria
e-mail: ferdinand.angel@uni-graz.at

L. Oviedo
Pontifical University Antonianum, Rome, Italy
e-mail: loviedo@antonianum.eu

R.F. Paloutzian
Department of Psychology, Westmont College, Santa Barbara, CA, USA
e-mail: paloutz@westmont.edu

A.L.C. Runehov
Department of Theology, University of Uppsala, Uppsala, Sweden
e-mail: annerunehov@gmail.com

R.J. Seitz
Department of Neurology, Centre for Neurology and Neuropsychiatry, LVR-Klinikum Düsseldorf, Heinrich-Heine-University Düsseldorf, Düsseldorf, Germany
e-mail: seitz@neurologie.uni-duesseldorf.de

H.-F. Angel et al. (eds.), *Processes of Believing: The Acquisition, Maintenance, and Change in Creditions*, New Approaches to the Scientific Study of Religion 1,
DOI 10.1007/978-3-319-50924-2_33

how creditions might be relevant for social sciences and economic fields. For example, creditions are discussed in context of politics as related to understanding societies trying to undergo a transition from war to peace.

The propensity of humans to believe has interested philosophers since antiquity. One of the most common definitions is that, "beliefs, according to the tradition in philosophy, are states of mind that have the property of being about things" (Churchland and Churchland 2013, 1). Thus, beliefs are mental states that may be about things that seem predominantly associated with religions and spiritualities. However, people have beliefs about all sorts of things, many for unexplained or non-conscious reasons, not only objects or events called "religious" (Pechey and Halligan 2012). This occasional lack of explanation for believing something invokes the topic of epistemology and the issue of how knowing and believing are or ought to be related to each other.

Accordingly, this book does not focus on beliefs in terms of content or states, and especially is not about beliefs in a religious sense. On the contrary, the overarching topic of this book concerns what is going on inside a person's mind while he or she is believing. This refers to the process of believing, coined "credition" in this book. Semantically, believing connotes a person's assumption that something is probably true or that one can fully trust in something or someone. In common speech believing signifies the probabilistic perspective of an individual. This probabilistic perspective constitutes the degree or strength, but not necessarily the accuracy, of a belief. It is a general concept and should not automatically be associated with religions. Nevertheless, we think that many processes of believing occur in the contexts of religion(s), in both modern knowledge-based societies as well as so-called primitive societies. Overall, this book introduces a novel approach to interdisciplinary discourse for how to address the concept of believing as a process.

1 Transformation of How We Talk: From Belief to the Process of Believing

There is a fundamental difference between beliefs and the process of believing. A belief is the result of an ongoing mental process. The traditional discussions of "belief" in epistemology, theory of mind, religious cognition, and neuroscience is mainly noun-oriented. That is, the focus of most literature on "belief" or "faith" treats it as if it is a static thing. Even if process aspects of believing are on the table, linguistically the use of nouns remains predominant as illustrated in expressions like "formation of belief", "belief change", or even "mechanics of belief". Such wording gives the impression that beliefs are (at least implicitly) regarded as states.

Although we acknowledge that the fluidity inherent in the processes of believing can come to be perceived as a stable state, research has almost totally neglected the process of believing. But restricting "belief" to only noun-like functions is not sufficient to explain how believing operates in human lives. Therefore, in order to account for the mental processes related to believing, the concept of "credition" was conceived in analogy to the concepts of cognition and emotion. As such, the concept of credition serves as a bridge between various interrelated and interdependent processes such as cognition, emotion, belief formation, and evaluation. From a neuroscience point of view credition is best conceived of as a physiological mental operation in the same sense as for any non-pathological believing (Angel and Seitz 2016).

Because this book focuses on the "fluidity of beliefs", one of the challenges is how to define the process of believing when an accepted definition of belief as state does not exist. To this end we posit the question, "What is taking place in those moments when the believing process is going on?" To account for such operations "while someone is believing" (Angel, *Credition: From the Question of Belief to the Question of Believing*) a model was presented framing identifiable components of this mental process (Angel 2013). Specifically, it touches all discussions on "states" of belief. Beyond that opening chapter, the book focuses on the transformation of traditional static concepts of beliefs into the new fluid perspective of the process of believing.

2 Consequences of the Transformation

Addressing the question of what a "process of believing" is, we are confronted with the need to transform how we talk about belief in a way that touches all relevant scientific fields. For example, various traditional debates in fields such as epistemology, philosophy of mind, and neuroscience are implicated because research in these fields may bear upon our understanding between, e.g., believing and knowing. Therefore, in this book the transformation from a noun-based discussion of "beliefs" to a verb-related understanding of "while believing" is both explicit and implicit. Because all chapters aim at contributing to this transformation, most of the chapters address more than one of the below topics.

1. In order to analyze the process of believing in its behavioral, scientific, and epistemic complexity, we need to bring together concepts from research fields that may seem unrelated. Many scholarly fields have not shown much interest in interdisciplinary collaboration until recently. Because of this, some contributions to this book are intended to clarify the implications for the concept of "belief" in a static sense (i.e., as a noun) that have to be taken into account as we engage in any transformational work through which we change from talking about "belief" to talking about the process of believing.

From a neuroscientific perspective, this is the approach of the chapters by Cristorori and Grafman (*Neural Underpinnings of the Human Belief System*) and Conners and Halligan (*Belief and Belief Formation: Insights from Delusions*). From a philosophical point of view Visala and Angel (*The Theory of Credition and Philosophical Accounts of Belief: Looking for Common Ground*) hightlight the need of bridgebuilding and provide some perspectives how this task could be undertaken. This approach is evident also in the chapters of Kraals (*Hume on the Origins of Religious Belief*) and Weber (*A Process Pragmatist Heuristics of Believing*). Many additional chapters on epistemology, philosophy of mind and language, general philosophy, and cognitive science can be envisioned that would reflect the relevant aspects of this transformation.

2. Recent debates in epistemology, philosophy, and cognitive science give us insights into a wide field of expertise that reflects on the notion of beliefs in their noun-related sense. Thus we have much expertise about their content, apparent static nature, presumed roots, the kinds of propositions that comprise them, and what people who purport to believe them claim they do. How do these factors bear upon our need to make the change from research on beliefs to research on the process of believing (credition)? First, the emphasis on credition results in modifications in the questions asked about believing. Such modifications are illustrated in context of religious beliefs and religious cognition. They are highlighted in the chapters by Oancea on the history of religious thinking (*Soul and Body According to "De Fide Orthodoxa" of St. John Damascene*), Oviedo on religious cognition (*Recent Scientific Explanations of Religious Beliefs: A Systematic Account*), and Davies on theologically based anthropology (*Cognition, Emotion, and the Ethics of Authenticity*). The effects of neuroscientific and psychological approaches are reflected in the chapters by Seitz (*Beliefs and Believing as Possible Targets for Neuroscientific Research*) and Paloutzian and Mukai (*Believing, Remembering, and Imagining: The Roots and Fruits of Meanings Made and Remade*).
3. A further consequence of examining the process of believing instead of static beliefs is that the canon of relevant scientific disciplines that can converge on interdisciplinary research on credition seems exceptionally large. Even if there is no comprehensive definition of the believing process, it is obvious that it takes place in humans. This allows new approaches from fields that did not previously examine this fundamental human process. Thus, there also will be new opportunities to integrate psychological, biological, molecular, genetic, or neurophysiological approaches. This means that an integration of knowledge from diverse disciplines is relevant to understanding the believing process because the process can be analysed at different levels of analysis, e.g., in individuals, groups, and society (Sugiura et al. 2015). New questions of scientific interest will arise that could not be explored with "belief" understood as a noun or a point of stasis. However, when we conceive of belief in its fluid or process mode, it is possible to bridge different hitherto seemingly unrelated fields.

Some chapters in this book reflect this enlargement and argument for synthesis of disciplinary approaches and topics. The chapters by Aguilar-Ditzen (*Neurobiological Factors underlying Attachment and Trust in the Believing Process*), Berg and Sensen (*Decision-Making and Credition Under a Microbial Perspective*), and Meißner (*Believing in the Effectiveness of Treatment: From Placebo to Credition and Back*) highlight this approach.

3 Conceptual or Functional Explanation of the Believing Process

Most contributions to this volume enrich the understanding of the concept of a believing process, although they do so from different scientific disciplines. The various approaches can be seen as attempts at functional explanations of what is going on "while someone is believing". The contributions highlight different aspects of the process, all of which are relevant to understanding the credition concept and their relations to it. They endeavor to explain different putative connections between different levels (Sugiura et al. 2015).

For example, from the perspective of cognitive neuroscience, the meaning making process is central to the process of believing as meanings are constructed from incomplete bits and pieces of information (Seitz and Angel 2014). The resulting belief is represented by mental codes that are thought to be generated from the signals from the external physical world, allowing for generation and selection of appropriate action. The process may occur non-consciously and effect brain function, behavior, and belief processes, as well as the so-called "gut feeling" that humans commonly report (Holzer, *Interoception and Gut Feelings: Unconscious Body Signals' Impact on Brain Function, Behavior, and Belief Processes*). The mental operations are processed in extensive cortico-subcortical neural networks. Believing, therefore, occurs in a complex social-interactional framework under the influence of the neuroendocrine system.

Furthermore, the processes underlying believing on the individual, interpersonal, and societal levels (creditions) determine public and personal language. On the societal level moral, legal, political, and religious beliefs are important determinants guiding human behavior. Thus, illustrated as it pertains to the notion of contextual factors such a medical or mental patient's expectations, emotions, and beliefs, the argument can be extended to the role of beliefs in the will or power to live. Illustrated another way, the topic of emotion integrates the aspects of emotion regulation and emotionally relevant influences such as, for example, in music and dance. Conversely, pathological and dysfunctional religious or spiritual beliefs, as manifest in delusions, may be effective modulators of neuropsychiatric diseases.

There may also be some key concepts – labeled as "bridging", "translation", and "transfer" – that shed special light on our efforts to help transform the study of beliefs to the science of the process of believing. Although such terminology is somewhat schematic and may overlap in various chapters, the distinction among them may help us understand what the chapters contribute to the concept of credition.

3.1 Bridging

Some chapters aim at bridging different traditional fields of research with the concept of the believing process. This is the case with the chapters by Auletta (*Connections between Scripts Embedding Motor Schemes and Decision-making*), Buccino and Colagè (*New Concepts on the Motor System: Implications for Emotions and Credition*), Colagè and Gobbi (*Creditions and Self-Identity: Embodiment between Actions and [Life] Decisions*), Holzer (*Interoception and Gut Feelings: Unconscious Body Signals' Impact on Brain Function, Behavior, and Belief Processes*), Suguira (*The Power to Live with Disasters: Adaptive Believing Processes of the Self and the World*), and Northoff (*Brain and Self – A Neurophilosophical Account*).

3.2 Translation

Another approach is to take the concept of credition as given, and then see whether some of its terms and ideas can be translated into other concepts or theoretical approaches, or how they might be used in connection with other concepts and thereby be influential for the credition research project. This approach is evident in the chapter by Maaßen (*The Structure of Credition in Whitehead's Metaphysics of Experience*), who connects the concept of credition to various metaphysical aspects of Whitehead's philosophy.

3.3 Transfer

Some chapters intend to transfer (or transport) the concept or credition to be used in other areas of research, such as psychiatric disorders (Unterrainer, *Functional and Dysfunctional Religious/Spiritual Beliefs in Psychotic Disorders*) or music (Ebenbauer, *Music as a Medium of Personal Motion and Belief: Some Phenomenological Reflections*).

4 Process of Believing: Theory and Model

The Credition Research Project has elaborated a concept of the believing process. However, talking about the process of believing requires that we have two perspectives at different levels of complexity in mind, each of which needs to be further developed. They are (a) the model of the believing process and (b) a theory of the believing process. Progress toward developing more mature ideas about the model and theory is included in this book and summarized below.

4.1 *Model of the Believing Process*

We stress that it is not the same whether one is interested in providing an understanding of the believing process or in developing a functional model that makes "visible" how putative processes are involved in it. Sometimes an almost perfect concept cannot be transformed into an adequate model. Nevertheless, the process of believing (credition) has been modeled from a psychological perspective in a heuristic manner (Angel 2013), which was then set into an interdisciplinary context by applying a neuroscientific framework (Angel and Seitz 2016). To understand the developmental path that lead to this "model of credition", it is necessary to be aware of the conceptual work on which the model is based. The model of the believing process and its implications serve as the through-line for the composition of the volume – the idea that we hope helps to connect its different parts from beginning to end.

4.2 *Theory of the Believing Process*

So far, no theory in a strict sense has been elaborated. For such a theory to be useful, it has to have sufficient substance to address the question, "What is the process involved in the phenomenon of concern?" This question invokes the issue of where to find basic information about what a process is. Directions to such information are presented in the chapters that seek to relate the concept of credition to the framework of information theory (Bischof, *Creditions and Modern Computer Science*), logic and language (Leach, *Public and Personal Causations of Creditions*), and statistical aspects as discussed within Wave-Particle Duality and Quantity-Quality Complementarity (*Ji, Wave-Particle Duality and Quantity-Quality Complementarity in Natural and Human Sciences: Implications for Credition Research*).

5 Application of the Model

Whereas the above mentioned chapters aim at enriching the theoretical foundations of the concept and model of credition, there are other chapters that take a more applied path in exploring how creditions might be relevant for social sciences and economic fields. For example, creditions are discussed in context of politics as related to understanding societies trying to undergo a transition from war to peace (Marko, *Reconciliation after a Protracted Violent Conflict: Do Believing Processes Play a Role, and Which One? A Research Agenda*). One chapter presents a potential field of application that may be relevant to building economic theory (Sturn, *Approaching Another Black Box: Credition in Economics*). Another contribution stresses the opportunity to innovatively implement the model of credition in business, illustrated especially in context of crowd funding (Willfort & Weber, *Credition in Business – Innovations with Crowdbusiness*). Initial results of an application of the model of credition for practical educational work are presented in by Mitropoulou (*Understanding Young People's Worldview: A Practical Example of How to Work with the Model of Credition*). The possibility of using the model of credition as a retrospective interpretation tool to understand personal and scientific development is presented by Runehov (*Credition and Justification*), which retraces the scientific development of Albert Einstein in terms of the credition model.

6 Future Perspectives

The information about credition provides the basic concepts on which the model can be built and used for further innovative theorizing and research by scholars from specialties and domains that have not yet been involved in research on believing.

Because we structured the book according to traditional scientific fields -- Psychology and Neuroscience, Philosophy, Theology, Religious Studies, Anthropology, Social Sciences, Natural and Computer Sciences – we highlight that the transformational aspects of the model of credition can apply to the concerns, ideas, theoretical frameworks, and beliefs that comprise all these scientific fields. We are, therefore, convinced that developing and applying the concept and the model of credition will give opportunities to many young researchers in many fields – even those who never thought of sharing a belief.

References

Angel HF (2013) Credition. In: Runehov A, Oviedo L (eds) Encyclopedia of Sciences and Religion, vol 1. Springer, Dordrecht, pp 536–539. http://www.springerreference.com/docs/html/chapterdbid/357430.html

Angel HF, Seitz RJ (2016) Processes of believing as fundamental brain function: the concept of credition. In: Khalili S (ed) SFU Research Bulletin, Special Issue: Science and/or religion: a 21st century debate. SFU Res Bull 3:1–20. doi:10.15135/2016.4.1.1-20

Churchland PS, Churchland PM (2013) What are beliefs? In: Krueger F, Grafman J (eds) The neural basis of human belief systems. Psychology Press, Hove, pp 300–329

Pechey R, Halligan P (2012) Using co-occurrence to evaluate belief coherence in a large non clinical sample. PLoS One 7:e48446. doi:10.1371/journal.pone.0048446

Seitz RJ, Angel HF (2014) Psychology of religion and spirituality: meaning-making and processes of believing. Relig Brain Behav 5:139–147. doi:10.1080/2153599X.2014.891249

Sugiura M, Seitz RJ, Angel HF (2015) Models and neural bases of the believing process. J Behav Brain Sci 5:12–23

Author Index

A
Aguilar-Raab, C., 10, 29
Angel, H-F., 8, 10, 11, 17–22, 25–27, 30, 41, 70, 72, 73, 77, 78, 85, 89, 106, 125, 133, 134, 139, 140, 149, 168, 187, 190, 201, 214, 220, 222, 248–250, 258–260, 263, 277, 302, 319, 320, 331, 363–365, 388–390, 392, 418, 419, 424, 425, 455, 456
Anselm of Canterbury, 188
Arendt, H., 359
Aristotle, 183, 184, 264, 265, 268, 271, 323, 325, 348, 364, 366, 373, 419
Arthur, P., 345, 346
Audi, R., 186, 189, 192
Augustine, 19, 188, 285, 286
Auletta, G., 10, 29, 51, 53, 55–57, 59, 65, 71, 256, 257, 458

B
Barlev, M., 41
Berg, G., 14, 28, 444, 457
Bergson, H., 22, 272
Bischof, H., 14, 24, 71, 399–404, 459
Böckenförde, E-W., 347, 348, 355
Boyer, P., 70, 78, 120, 298, 304, 363
Brodmann Korbinian, 75, 98, 252, 257, 258
Buccino, G., 11, 24, 98, 101, 103, 105, 458

C
Cabeza, R., 47
Cantor, Georg F.L.P., 415
Cardeña, E., 41
Chomsky, N., 58, 348
Churchland, P., 18, 232
Clemens of Alexandria, 188
Cobb, John B., 220
Colagè, Ivan, 11, 12, 24, 250, 256, 257, 458
Connors, M.H., 11, 20, 23, 73, 153–155, 157, 160
Cristofori, I., 11, 20, 76, 118

D
Damasio, A., 25, 104, 234, 257
Daniels, P., 47
Debiec, J., 47
Descartes, R., 188, 196, 227, 231, 271
Ditzen, B., 10, 29, 84, 87, 457
Dodik, M., 342
Duns, S. J., 188, 277, 285

E
Ebenbauer, P., 13, 26, 458
Einstein, A., 196–199, 201–203, 205, 431, 460
Erikson, E.H., 169

F
Festinger, L., 30, 139
Fodor, J., 18, 65, 295
Folkman, S., 41, 169
Ford, H., 388

H.-F. Angel et al. (eds.), *Processes of Believing: The Acquisition, Maintenance, and Change in Creditions*, New Approaches to the Scientific Study of Religion 1,
DOI 10.1007/978-3-319-50924-2

Frege, G., 415
Friedlander, E., 40
Fukuyama, F., 348

G
Gallese, V., 98, 99, 104, 250
Gallagher, H.L., 233
German, T., 17, 18, 25, 172, 173, 188, 215, 231, 302, 429
Gettier, E., 22, 185
Giddens, A., 351
Gobbi, N., 12, 24, 29, 260, 458
Gödel, K., 410, 411, 415
Goldman, A., 12, 185, 187, 204–206
Goldstein, E.B., 40, 42, 43
Gorgias, 183
Greyson, B., 41

H
Halligan, P.W., 11, 20, 23, 70, 73, 76, 153, 154, 156, 157, 161, 456
Hebb, D., 32
Heraclitus, 22
Heywood, B., 40
Hilbert, D., 409, 410, 415
Hobbes, T., 211, 271, 347, 348
Holzer, P., 14, 28, 72, 436–438, 457, 458
Horowitz, D., 345, 346
Howe, J., 391
Hume, D., 12, 23, 188, 209–215, 231, 377, 456
Huntington, S., 350
Hurd, R., 212, 213

J
James, W., 155, 168, 264, 267–272, 314, 430, 436
Jeannerod, M., 53, 61–64, 66, 71, 250–255
Ji, S., 14, 24, 417–425, 427–431, 459
John of Damascus, 188, 324, 327, 329
John, Apostle, 187

K
Kahneman, D., 73, 158, 159
Kant, I., 188, 278–280, 347
Kaptchuk, T. J., 40, 130
Kelley, J.M., 40, 158
Kerenyi, K., 268
Keynes, J.M., 378, 379, 383, 384
Kinsella, M., 41
Kirkpatrick, L.A., 45, 169, 294, 309
Kluender, K.R., 40
Kohut, H., 169
Kokkotou, E., 40
Kraal, A., 12, 23
Kraus, E., 220
Krippner, S., 41
Kymlicka, W., 345, 346, 360

L
Lazarus, R., 26
Leach, J., 14, 29, 406, 407, 413, 414, 459
LeDoux, J.E., 47
Levi, Dennis M., 40
Libet, B., 62, 255
Lijphart, A., 342, 345
Lindeman, M., 40
Luther, M., 188, 310, 335
Lynn, S.J., 41

M
Maaßen, H., 12, 22, 218, 220, 458
Makkonen, T., 40
Marko, J., 13, 33, 349, 357, 358, 459
Mead, G.H., 352
Meissner, K., 73, 78, 128, 131, 132
Metzinger, T., 231–233, 235
Mitropoulou, V., 13, 33, 460
Mukai, K. J., 9, 10, 29, 78, 456
Murken, S., 40, 43

N
Nader, K., 47
Nash, J.F., 40, 380
Nilsson, Nils J., 8, 301
Northoff, G., 12, 29, 73, 230, 236, 243, 458
Nyberg, L., 47

O
Oancea, D., 13, 33, 456
Otto, R., 264, 267
Oviedo, L., 9, 13, 21, 320, 456

P
Paloutzian, R.F., 9, 10, 21, 29, 40, 41, 43, 44, 70, 78, 172, 294, 302, 312, 456
Pannenberg, W., 323
Park, C.L., 21, 41–44, 47, 70, 78, 302, 311

Parmenides, 22, 266
Paul, Apostle, 187
Planck, M., 417, 419
Plato, 183, 184, 218, 263–266, 269–271, 418, 424, 425
Poincaré, H., 205
Prigogina, I., 419–421, 425, 427, 428
Pyysiäinen, I., 298, 311

R
Riekki, T., 40
Rizzolatti, G., 57, 98, 99, 250
Rizzuto, A.M., 169
Robson, C., 366, 367
Rößler-Namini, S., 40, 43
Runehov, A., 8, 12, 22, 23, 25, 30, 187, 192, 201, 214, 320, 460

S
Sanchez, M.N., 40
Schachter, S., 26, 222
Schleiermacher, F., 264, 267
Schmitt, C., 348
Scotus, J.D., 188, 277, 285, 286
Searle, J., 62, 253, 352, 356
Seitz, R. J., 9, 10, 18, 20, 21, 25–27, 29, 33, 41, 58, 65, 72–74, 77, 78, 85, 89, 105, 106, 125, 133, 134, 139, 140, 150, 168, 190, 214, 222, 249, 250, 258, 259, 277, 302, 320, 331, 419, 424, 456
Sensen, M., 14, 457
Simplikios, 22
Smith, Aaron, 289, 291, 302
Smith, Adam, , 378, 377, 385
Sperber, D., 157, 295
St. Augustin. *See Augustine*
St. John. *See John, Apostle*
St. John Damascene. *See John of Damascus*
St. Paul. *See Paul, Apostle*
St. Thomas. *See Thomas Aquinas*
Strawson, P.F., 218
Streib, H., 43
Sturn, R., 13, 33, 459
Sugiura, M., 11, 20, 27, 29, 30, 73, 106, 133, 140–142, 148–150, 228, 248–250, 258, 320, 364, 392, 419

T
Taves, A., 47
Theaitetos, 183, 184
Thomas Aquinas, 188, 285
Troelstra, A.S., 410
Turing, A., 411–413, 415

U
Unterrainer, H-F., 11, 32, 168, 169, 171–175, 458

V
Visala, A., 11, 17, 19, 191, 291, 456
Voltaire, 188

W
Weber, C., 13, 392, 393
Weber, M., 12, 33, 183, 266, 267, 269, 456, 459
Whitehead, Alfred, North, 12, 201, 217, 218
Whitehouse, H., 298, 315
Wiener, A., 333, 422
Willfort, R., 13, 33, 388–390, 392, 393, 459
Wilson, D.S., 294
Wilson, E.O., 295
Winnicott, D., 169
Wolfe, J.M., 42

Z
Zahavi, D., 233, 235
Zajonc, R., 26, 222

Subject Index

A

Action, 9, 24, 26, 29, 32, 52, 70–75, 89, 97, 112, 140, 186, 197, 202, 214, 220, 230, 247, 268, 280, 322, 346, 363, 380, 400, 407, 457
- action-perception-value triad, 78, 140, 144, 250
- "action tendencies" and ethnic conflict, 346–355
- beliefs and actions, 250–259
- goal-directed actions, 417–418
- mirror neuron system and action, 99–105
- motor neurons and, 54–59, 98
- ritual actions, 77
- theory of mind and, 59
- three levels of action, 61–63

Activation, 75, 77, 83, 87, 101–105, 115, 118, 120, 130, 131, 134, 150, 214, 238, 241, 252, 256
Adaptation, 89, 283, 294, 297, 299, 300, 305, 307, 314
Adrenocorticotropic hormone (ACTH), 86
Aggression, 18, 30, 87, 114, 169, 175, 355
Altruism, 58, 65, 86, 116, 130, 141–145, 148, 282, 305, 382
Amygdala, 26, 86, 104, 113, 118, 213, 214, 440, 445
Anapoiesis, 423
Anselm of Canterbury, 188
Anterior cingulate cortex, 131, 134, 439, 440
Anthropology, 10, 12, 18, 19, 21, 25, 26, 140, 209, 277, 278, 290–292, 295, 300, 303–309, 311–315, 320, 321, 325, 329, 349, 353, 363, 456, 460
Anticipation, 72, 77, 78, 126, 254, 297, 335, 378–379, 387, 419
Antidiuretic hormone (ADH). *See* Vasopressin (VP)
Anxiety, 40, 45, 83, 87, 127, 130, 131, 156, 158, 168, 173, 175, 211, 294, 308, 310, 312, 364, 372, 436, 437, 440, 446, 447
Archaea, 444
Arginine vasopression (AVP). *See* Vasopression (VP)
Aristotle, 183, 184, 264, 265, 268, 271, 323, 325, 348, 364, 366, 373, 419
Arousal, 32, 87, 155, 439, 440
Association task, 117
Atheist, atheism, 21, 40, 407, 448
Attachment, 83–92, 169, 294, 309
Attitude, 18, 21, 22, 29, 32, 39, 43, 44, 75, 77, 78, 91, 117, 126, 141, 142, 144, 145, 147, 161, 174, 184–186, 189, 197, 200, 202, 244, 249, 250, 259, 260, 301, 349, 355, 358, 367, 373
Attribution, 21, 27, 31, 45, 48, 64, 72, 77–78, 113, 115, 147, 156, 158, 222, 235, 237, 244, 249, 252, 253, 295, 304, 310, 311, 365, 373, 409, 425

B

Bab, 26–28, 249
Bab-blob-configuration, 30–32, 249, 364, 365, 370, 373
Bacterial volatiles, 445
Bacterioides, 447

H.-F. Angel et al. (eds.), *Processes of Believing: The Acquisition, Maintenance, and Change in Creditions*, New Approaches to the Scientific Study of Religion 1,
DOI 10.1007/978-3-319-50924-2

Balance, 25, 43, 170, 265, 271, 299, 344, 358, 390, 448
Bayesian inference, 57, 403–404
Behaviour, 18, 22, 26, 70, 74, 76, 78, 104–106, 155, 160, 169, 171, 174, 176, 213, 249, 253, 254, 256, 257, 259, 282, 283, 300, 302, 304–307, 310, 312–314, 323, 344, 347, 353, 354, 372, 399
Behavioral science, 455
Belief, 3–14, 17–33, 40, 65, 69–78, 84, 106, 111–121, 125, 139, 153–161, 167–176, 183–192, 196, 209–215, 219, 244, 248, 263, 277, 289–315, 331–337, 363, 375, 388, 399, 406, 425, 435–441, 454
  "belief-as-noun" problem, 18–19
  characteristics, 278
  dispositional beliefs, 186
  distinction between belief and faith, 197–198
  distinction between belief and religion, 301
  internal-schema framework
    hierarchical levels, 141
  legal beliefs
    associated neural structures, 116
    relationship with hormones, 116
  moral beliefs
    aspects, 112
    associated neural structures, 112–114
  political beliefs
    associated neural structures, 117–119
  processes of believing (*see* Belief processes)
  relationship with knowledge, 184–186
  relationship with microbiome, 448
  relationship with religion
    contemporary thought, 189
    early Christianity, 187–188
    enlightenment thought, 188
    medieval thought, 188
  religious beliefs
    associated neural structures, 119–120
    causes of belief (according to Hume), 211
    characteristics, 119
    neurophysiological substrates, 213–215
    purpose, 169, 176
    role of anxiety/fear, 211–213
  social beliefs, 111–112
Belief evaluation, 20, 155, 159–161, 249, 258
Belief formation, 11, 12, 14, 20, 71–73, 106, 107, 153–161, 249, 381, 384, 455, 456
  five-stage model
    acceptance stage, 160
    consequences stage, 160–161
    precursor stage, 157–158
    proto-belief evaluation stage, 159–160
    search for meaning stage, 158–159
  mental/psychological processes, 200
  natural processes, 200
  neural substrates, 249–250
  occurrent beliefs, 186
  processes of change, 200
  project processes, 200
  psychological roots
    imagination, 47–48
    implementation, 46
    intuition, 44–46
    learning, 43–44
    memory, 46–47
    perception, 42–43
  structural processes, 200
Belief processes, 14, 21, 134, 168, 169, 176, 190, 384, 406, 435–441, 457, 458
Belief systems, 8, 9, 11, 21, 22, 47, 77, 78, 85, 91, 112, 114–121, 132, 168, 399
Believing, 3–14, 17–33, 39–48, 65, 69–78, 83–92, 106, 115, 125–134, 139–151, 154, 184, 196, 213, 217, 248, 263–272, 277, 289, 319, 331, 341–360, 364, 376, 388, 405, 417, 448, 454
Biases, 73, 156, 158, 159, 161, 210, 297, 301, 303, 307, 311, 342, 382, 440
Big Five, 168
"Big Four" model of religious dimensions, 85
Biology, 279, 282, 284, 291–293, 303–315, 319, 418, 420, 431
Bio-psycho-social (BPS) model, 168
Body, 13, 14, 24, 62, 72, 87, 92, 98, 104, 128, 131, 202, 227, 229, 231–233, 249, 266, 279–281, 319, 332–336, 435, 444, 447
Bonding, 85, 87–89, 169, 223, 282, 283, 314, 385
Brain, 10, 19–23, 42–43, 51, 70, 86–87, 89–91, 99–107, 112, 125, 169, 190, 201, 214, 222, 227, 247, 278, 296, 319, 333, 389, 417, 435, 444, 457
  brain areas and functions, 70–78, 112–120, 256–258
  and existential meaning making, 77
  and mirror neuron system, 99, 101, 102
  organic brain syndrome, 171
  probabilistic representations, 71

recent resources on brain and believing, 303–315
and self, 227–245
and symbolic systems, 55
Brain function, 10, 14, 26, 30, 70, 77, 190, 222, 311, 319, 419, 435–441, 457, 458
Brain-gut axis, 445
Brainstem, 86, 436, 448
Business theory: Decision-making theories, 387–388

C

Capgras, 155, 157
Category theory, 429
ur-category, 429
Causations, 29, 405–415, 459
Causes, 12, 20, 30, 41, 45, 104, 116, 144, 148, 154, 159, 176, 186, 187, 204, 210–215, 224, 230, 252, 253, 255, 257, 270, 286, 301, 324, 326, 349, 350, 357, 366, 373, 376, 389, 405–408, 412–415, 446
personal, 406–407, 409–412
public, 405–409, 412, 414
Central nervous system
F5 neurons
canonical neurons, 98
mirror neurons
definition, 98
function, 98–102
location in the brain, 99
mechanism for emotions, 103–105
mirror neuron system (MNS) function, 99–102
shared circuits, 105
sub-classes, 100, 102
motor cognition
associated neural areas, 257–258
conscious control, 252–256
implications, 252
internal forward model, 251
motor system
anatomical divisions, 98
Childhood, 21, 78, 89, 191, 198, 303
Christ, 19, 188, 285, 321
Church-turing hypothesis, 411
the halting problem, 411–413
Classical conditioning, 127, 128
Codes
basic aspects, 53
need for, 53
Co-evolution, 300, 305, 309, 444
Cognition, 7, 18, 21, 25–27, 39, 52, 59, 64–66, 70, 84–88, 104–107, 116, 125, 154, 172, 187, 201, 222, 239, 248–251, 277, 289, 320, 331, 333, 346, 388–389, 417, 446, 454
appraisal of social interactions, 73
decision-making
neural substrates, 75
role of probabilistic mental representations, 74–75
mental representation formation, 73–75
motor cognition, 64–66
social cognition
simulation theory approach, 105
theory of mind, 47, 102–103
table of references, 303–315
Cognitive dissonance theory, 30
Cognitive neuropsychiatry, 154
Cognitive psychology, 233, 293, 300, 301, 303–308, 310, 311, 313, 314
Cognitive science, 6, 18, 21, 141, 161, 187, 190, 290, 294, 298, 304, 307, 309–314, 456
Complementarity, 430–431
Comprehension, 13, 27, 72, 91, 149, 168, 173, 197, 202, 249, 259, 296, 321, 329, 376, 381, 385, 419, 456
Computer science, 399–404, 406, 459, 460
definition, 399
Computer vision, 399, 400, 402
image denoising, 400–402
supervised learning, 402–403
Conflict
Böckenförde dilemma, 347–348
ethno-nationalism, theoretical perspectives, 350–357
post-conflict societies
power-sharing, perspectives, 345
state-building, purpose, 343–344
Consciousness, 12, 44, 62, 133, 219, 223, 228, 229, 231–233, 235, 236, 239, 252–259, 266, 279–284, 305, 334, 336, 359, 407, 419, 430, 435–436
Consilience, 299
Constitution-building, 344, 345
Converter function, 31–32, 106, 133, 140, 143–144, 146, 149, 150, 201, 248, 249, 258, 349, 353, 358, 360, 364
Coping, 11, 91, 169, 176, 294
future planning, 75–78
role of religion, 76–78
Corticolimbic system, 437

Corticotropin-releasing hormones (CRF), 86
Cortisol, 86
Credition, 8, 17, 41, 51, 70, 85, 106, 125, 140, 168, 190, 196, 213, 219, 228, 247, 263, 277, 290, 319, 334, 347, 363, 375, 388, 399, 407, 419, 448, 454
  applications to Orthodoxy, 322–324
  applied research, 364–373
  bab-blob configuration, 30
  bab, characteristics, 27–29
    definition, 26–27
    dissipative babs (d-babs), 425
    equilibrium babs (e-babs), 425
    relationship to irreducible triadic relation (ITR), 424–425
  blob, 28
  challenges, 28–29
  characteristics, 320–321
  cognitive elements, 324
  converter function, 31–32
    connection to factors of power to live, 143–145, 149
  emotional elements, 324, 326–328
  enclosure function, 30–31
    connection to factors of power to live, 142–143
  modulator function, 32
    connection to factors of power to live, 146–148
  necessity, 20–21, 23–24
  purpose, 25–26, 190
  relationship with business, 388–389, 392–393
  relationship with conflict, 350–351
  relationship with emotion and cognition, 26
  relationship with gut-brain axis, 440–441
  relationship with music, 337
  relationship with socio-economics, 375–379, 383–385
  stabilizer function, 32
    connection to factors of power to live, 145–146
Credition research project, 10, 12, 217, 458
Crohn's disease (CD), 447
Crowdbusiness, 13, 387–394
Crowdfunding, 392–394
Crowdsourcing, 391, 393, 394
Culture, 6, 23, 57, 58, 60, 84, 114, 116, 118, 170, 173, 222, 272, 282, 298, 300, 304–307, 332, 337, 351, 354, 408, 414
Cytokines, 437, 438

D
Dayton Peace, 13, 342, 344, 359
Death, 6, 41, 45, 76, 114–115, 170, 173, 200, 211, 303, 308, 325, 332, 337
Decision, 4, 7, 10, 12–14, 18, 31, 54–59, 74–76, 112, 115, 143, 219, 243, 281, 394, 413
De-ethnification, 349
Default network, 257, 258
Delusion, 4, 18, 70, 154, 170, 294, 456
  cognitive explanations, 154–156
  persecutory delusions, 156
  prediction error, 156
  theory of mind in delusions, 156
  two-factor theory, 155
Desire, 62, 74, 76, 116, 144, 145, 203, 210, 212, 252, 326, 327, 333, 337, 353
Dionysian Mysteries, 265
Disaster, 11, 139–151, 458
Disbelief, 8, 18
Dissapatons. *See* Structures, dissipative structures (DS)
Dorsolateral prefrontal cortex (dlPFC), 75, 116–119, 131, 132, 134, 249, 252, 258
Dorsomedial prefrontal cortex (dmPFC), 118, 236, 237, 239
Dual cognitive model, 24
Dysbiosis, 438, 446, 447

E
Economics, 7, 10, 13, 33, 168, 202, 203, 205, 304, 346, 350, 354, 356, 358, 369, 375–385, 418, 431, 459, 460
  Walrasian general competitive market equilibrium markets, 379, 381
    problems, 380–383
Eleusis, 268
Embodiment, 12, 24, 247–260, 280, 284, 321, 458
Emotion, 8, 21, 47, 51, 71, 85, 100, 113, 125, 140, 154, 171, 188, 201, 210, 219, 229, 249, 265, 278, 293, 320, 332, 346, 364
  emotional regulation, 120, 141
  emotion characteristics, 278
  neurophysiological substrates, 26, 106, 107, 117, 120, 258, 446
  two-factor theory of emotion, 26, 222
Emotion-cognition-credition (ECC) triad, 417–418

Empathy, 58, 60, 66, 75, 90, 116, 126, 129, 133, 144, 235, 249, 282, 284, 286
Empirical evidence, 72, 154, 176, 215, 245, 255, 291, 296, 298, 313, 345, 407, 418, 419
Enclosure function, 24, 30–31, 106, 107, 140, 142, 146, 150, 248, 249, 258, 349, 364, 365, 392
Endogenous depressive behavior, 445
Energy, 420
Enlightenment, 29, 188, 210, 377
Enteric nervous system, 436, 448
Entropy, 421
Epigenetic role, 447
Epiphenomenal, 296, 299
Epistemic theory, 204–206
Epistemology, 196–205
  justification, 196, 204
    epistemic, 204
    non-epistemic, 204–205
Equilibrons. *See* Structures, equilibrium structures (ES)
Equilibrium, 376, 378–383, 420, 425, 427, 428
Etiquette, 141, 142, 147–148
European Enlightenment, Influence on Biblical narrative, 210
Event-feature-emotion complex (EFEC) framework, 114
Event-related potentials (ERPs), 117
Evolution, 9, 41, 54, 72, 86, 112, 169, 198, 222, 269, 279, 289, 337, 343, 380, 392, 436, 444
Evolutionary roots of meaning making and believing, 42–48
Evolutionary study of religion, 294
Examptation, 299
Expectation, 9, 11, 78, 84, 125, 127–129, 131–134, 211, 258, 289, 344, 354, 364, 378, 457
Explanatory power, 296

F

Face expression, 71, 75, 105
Faith, 12, 17, 57, 78, 168, 186, 248, 263, 285, 319, 377, 454
  characteristics, 199–200
Fear, 6, 12, 23, 28, 45, 72, 76, 104, 130, 161, 170, 211–215, 294, 303, 309, 310, 326, 327, 334–336, 346, 349, 352, 353, 356, 360, 377, 388, 390
Fides qua, 19
Fides quae, 19
Firmicutes, 447
Fluidity, 9, 22, 24, 27, 190, 365, 376, 455
fMRI. *See* Functional magnetic resonance imaging (fMRI)
Forgiveness, 18, 172
Formal languages
  decimal representation, 408
  meta-mathematics, 409–410
  role in personal causes, 409–411
  role in public causes, 408–409
Forward model, 251, 253, 255
Framing, 5, 13, 29, 62, 218, 224, 225, 249, 253, 295, 303, 382, 384, 455
Free-energy principle, 30
Functor, 430
Function, 17, 20, 24, 30–33, 43, 44, 46, 51, 70, 84, 99, 113, 140, 153, 167, 189, 196, 212, 222, 230, 233, 240, 242, 248, 258, 294, 319, 331, 341, 364, 392, 402, 411, 419, 436, 444, 455
  brain function in believing, 70–78, 242–244, 248–249
  four credition functions, 30–33, 349
  four credition functions assigned to Kosovo conflict, 353–360
  four credition functions related to three levels of internal schema, 142
  function of mirror neurons in believing, 99–107
  functions of scripts and motor schemes, 51–64
Functional and dysfunctional beliefs in delusions and psychosis, 170–171
Functional magnetic resonance imaging (fMRI), 100, 102, 104, 105, 114, 117, 118, 230, 236, 242
Future, 7, 23, 46–47, 56, 74, 91, 112, 140, 157, 172, 189, 200, 211, 225, 256, 289, 320, 335, 379, 388, 415, 441, 460
  attitudes, beliefs, and future conduct, 256–260
  beliefs and coping with the future, 75
  evolutionary roots of sense of future, 46–47

G

Gamma, 72, 76, 228, 239, 242
Game–theoretical frameworks, 377
Generation Sequencing, 443, 445, 448
Gnôsis, 12, 263–266, 270

Gnosticism, 266
Goal, 43, 44, 47, 59–65, 72, 74, 77, 99, 100, 103, 144, 154, 203, 252–254, 257, 299, 343, 345, 350, 389, 393, 394, 399, 400, 418, 421, 423, 428
God, 13, 19, 40, 70, 85, 111, 169, 197, 271, 285, 321, 335, 407
Gorgias, 183
Gnergy
  definition, 421
  evidence of, 421–422
  Gnergy Principle of Organization, (GPO), 422
Gnosis
  characteristics, 264–266
  role in Grecian Mystery religions, 265
  role in Grecian Orphic mysteries, 265
Gut-brain, 436–441, 447
Gut-brain axis, 436–438
Gut feeling, 14, 72, 388, 394, 435–441, 448, 457
Gut hormones, 438
Gut microbiota, 438, 445, 448

H
Hallucinations, 170–171
Hebbian principle, 32
Holo-biont, 443
Hope, 14, 43, 45, 46, 75, 130, 172, 176, 186, 189, 200, 211, 225, 271, 323, 327, 335, 336, 372, 407, 459
Hormone, 86, 87, 90, 116, 130, 334, 437, 438
Human philosophy: Views on religious beliefs, 210–215
Hypothalamic–Pituitary–Adrenal (HPA) Axis, 86, 445
Hypothesis, 57, 78, 104, 129, 150, 155, 159, 267, 293, 296, 298, 309–311, 365, 370, 378, 403, 411

I
Identity formation, 345, 346, 351, 355, 369
Illusion, 18, 21–22, 72, 171, 231, 344, 365, 400
Imagination, 47, 120, 211, 294, 295, 328, 352, 353, 388
Imagining, 10, 39–48, 154, 285, 336, 456
Imitation, 60, 104, 268
Infancy, 21, 131
Inflammatory bowel diseases (IBD), 447
Information, 10, 20, 40, 54, 70, 99, 117, 126, 144, 156, 218, 231, 279, 349, 367, 393, 408, 420, 436, 445, 457
Innovation, 13, 21, 285, 290, 300, 329, 346, 376, 387–394, 424, 459
  management, 389–390
  open innovation, 391
Innovation Service Network (ISN), 390
Institutional economics, 377, 385
Insula, 104, 105, 115, 120, 131, 439, 440
Intelligence, 57, 58, 60, 75, 149, 280, 293, 303, 379
Intention, 25, 46, 58, 90, 98, 113, 156, 199, 228, 252, 272, 285, 303, 319, 351, 364
Intentionality, 63, 228, 351, 352, 356
Internal schema, 140–147, 149, 150
Interoception, 14, 115, 147, 435–441, 457, 458
  definition, 439
  physiological processes, 439–440
Intuition, 23, 45–46, 73, 192, 196, 199, 200, 202, 223, 265–267, 307, 313, 413, 415, 435, 448
  in meaning making and believing, 44
Intuitive, 20, 24, 73, 74, 77, 252, 268, 297, 298, 310, 311, 313, 314, 333, 413, 438, 440
Irreducible aspects, 417–418
Irreducible triadic relation (ITR), 417–418, 426–427

J
Judgment, cognitive processes in, 279

K
Knowledge
  conditions, 184–185
  Jamesian process pragmatism
    knowledge-about, 26
    knowledge of acquaintance, 267
    reality, 269

L
Language, 14, 18, 45, 58, 69, 120, 184, 197, 225, 234, 271, 278, 298, 321, 347, 380, 405, 424, 435, 456
  function and development, 279–281
Lateral prefrontal cortex, 26, 75, 131

Leadership, 141, 143–145, 148, 149
Learning, 9, 14, 22, 26, 43–44, 56, 58, 87, 91, 127–129, 132, 214, 286, 303, 334, 351, 359, 360, 382, 399, 400, 402–403, 446
Linguistics
  cell language theory, 424
  principle of rule-governed creativity (PRGC), 423–424
Long-term memory, 334
Lullaby, 335

M
Machine learning, 14, 399, 400, 402
Magical thinking/ideation, 173
  in schizotypy, 174
Markov blanket, 54, 55
  representational (model-building), 55
Mathematics, 14, 58, 71, 222, 320, 377, 399, 405, 417
Meaning, 4, 17, 41, 53, 73, 85, 99, 146, 168, 187, 219, 266, 291, 343, 365, 406, 420, 457
Meaning making, 10, 29, 42–48, 77, 78, 91, 457
Meaning system, 9, 42–48, 297, 302, 305
Medial frontal cortex (MFC), 73, 75, 77, 78, 105–107, 134, 214, 249, 258
Mega-bab, 27, 28, 369, 392
Memes, 296, 311
Memory, 26, 46–47, 54, 56, 73–75, 202, 230, 249, 280, 309, 328, 333, 349, 364, 423, 439, 447
  collective memory of war in Ksovo, 359–360
  and meaning, 158–160
Mentalizing, 11, 105, 106, 116
Metagenomes, 444
Meta-mathematical, 409, 411
Meta-organism, 443
Microbiome, 14, 443–448
  early development, 444–445
  ecology, 443–444
  gut-brain axis
    definition, 436
    physiological processes, 436–439
  impact on mental health, 445–447
  impact on physical health, 438, 446–447
Mini-bab, 27, 28, 369, 424
Mirror neuron, 57, 59, 98–104, 129, 133, 144, 250
Mirror system, 105, 106, 250
Model, 10, 22, 24, 51, 72, 84, 105, 114, 126, 133, 141, 156, 168, 188, 210, 217, 249, 290, 320, 333, 348, 364, 378, 387, 401, 418, 441, 445, 455
  "Big Four" model of religious dimensions, 85
  bio-psycho-socio-spiritual model of health and disease, 168
  credition model, 22–34
  enlightenment period and the medieval model, 188
  internal forward model, 249–253
  models of brain function, 69–78
  the nature and variations of models, 51–65
  neurocognitive models, 149
  placebo effects and the predictive coding model, 133
  self-models, 231–232
Modulator function, 32–33, 46, 106, 140, 146–147, 150, 206, 248, 249, 331, 349, 364
Mood, 14, 71, 74, 159, 438
Moral dilemmas, 113
Morality, 113, 304, 309
Motion, 13, 22, 26, 31, 101, 223, 331–337, 407, 414, 421, 422, 458
Motor programs, 63, 64, 75
Motor schema, 141
Motor systems
  levels, 61–62
  scenes, 63–64
  scripts, elements of, 63–64
Music, 13, 26, 265, 331–337, 420, 457, 458
  components of experience, 332–333
  history of instruments, 332
  physiological perception, of, 333–334
  purpose, 334–336

N
Narratives, 77, 78, 158, 210, 253, 254, 256, 257, 259, 280, 303
Nation, 210, 341–344, 346, 348, 353, 356–358
Naturalist, 13, 210, 290, 296, 299, 303–315
Near death experience (NDE), 41
Neural synchronizing processes, 32
Neuroendocrinological mechanisms, 90
Neuroimaging, 9, 10, 12, 26, 29, 75, 77, 112, 113, 117, 131, 134, 141, 213, 214, 295, 306, 308, 309, 440
Neurosis, 6, 18
Neurology, 25, 69, 83, 200, 222, 227, 280, 283, 286, 290, 293, 296, 299–301, 304, 307, 309–312, 314, 437, 439, 446
Neuron, 24, 57, 59, 98–104, 129, 133, 144, 231–232, 250, 437–439, 445, 446

Neurophysiology, 9, 10, 29, 72, 91, 98, 100, 103, 213–215, 390, 425, 439, 456
Neuroplasticity, 89, 333
Neuropsychiatric disorders, 11, 14, 78, 171, 436, 438, 440, 457
Neuroscience, 9–12, 19, 20, 26, 69, 84–86, 90, 114, 120, 140, 149, 187, 190, 213, 215, 222, 228–231, 233, 236, 240, 242, 247, 250, 256, 259, 278, 300, 305, 308, 310, 328, 389, 448, 454, 455, 457, 460
Nucleus accumbens (NAcc), 87

O
Orbitofrontal cortex, 26, 131, 134, 440
Ontological principle, 218–219
Oxidative stress, 447
Oxytocin (OT), 10, 86–90, 116, 130, 132
  function, 86–87, 89–90
  production, 86

P
Pain, 32, 40, 75, 104, 127–132, 212, 229, 235, 303, 326, 343, 437, 439, 448
Paleoanthropology, 293, 304, 312, 314, 315
Pantheism, 271
Peircean sign, 426–427
Perception, 9, 10, 20, 24, 26, 29, 30, 33, 42, 44, 58, 63, 70–73, 78, 85–87, 100, 106, 111, 116, 140, 144, 146, 147, 149, 150, 160, 161, 169, 171, 172, 185, 231, 242, 248–250, 252, 258, 269, 280, 299, 320, 325, 332, 336, 349–353, 355, 360, 364, 365, 377, 413
  perception-action-value triad, 26, 33, 73, 78, 144, 249
  substrate of meaning making, 42, 44
Personal value, perception of, 72
Personal motions, 414
Personality, 11, 85, 89, 116, 130, 141, 142, 144, 145, 168, 173–175, 268, 337, 388, 448
  Eysenck's model of personality factors, 174–175
    relationship with spirituality and schizophrenia, 174–175
  personality disorders, 174
Personalized medicine, 446
Perspective, 4, 8–14, 20–33, 63, 69, 71, 73, 77, 85, 89, 91, 100, 140, 141, 146, 169, 176, 189, 214, 229, 231, 235, 239, 248–250, 256, 257, 277, 278, 282, 293–295, 297, 299, 307, 309–311, 333, 344, 348, 351, 354–356, 358, 360, 375, 377, 381–383, 385, 390–392, 408, 415, 443–448, 454, 455, 457–460
  change from "belief" to "believing", 4, 8–14, 20–33
  as cognitive mechanisms, 189
  embodied perspective, 248, 256
  existential, 331–333
  first-person/third-person perspectives, 91, 229, 235–236, 239
    second person perspective, 235–236
  perspectives on state-building following war, 347–357
  probabilistic default first person perspective, 69–73
  psychodynamic and clinical perspectives on religious/spiritual beliefs, 169, 176
  subjective perspective-taking, 214
  visual perspective and mirror neurons, 100
Philosophy of mathematics, 406, 415
Philosophy of mind, 184, 186, 190, 192, 455
Pistis, 12, 187, 263, 264, 266, 267, 270
  characteristics, 264
  religion in classic Greece, 265
  role in Grecian Orphic mysteries, 265
Placebo, 11, 18, 30, 40, 73, 78, 116, 125–134, 457
Placebo effect
  associated personality traits, 130
  definition, 126
  expectations, 127–128
  involvement of emotions, 130
  learning processes
    conscious learning processes, 129
    unconscious learning processes, 128–129
  neurobiological mechanisms, 131–132
  predictive coding, 132–133
Planckian distribution equation (PDE), 417–418
Plato, 183, 184, 218, 263–266, 269–271, 418, 424, 425
Pluralism, 359, 410–412, 415
Postero-medial cortices (PMC), 257, 258
Power-sharing, 342, 345, 347
Power to live, 11, 139–151, 457, 458
  definition, 141
  factors
    active well-being, 147
    altruism, 144
    emotion regulation, 143
    etiquette, 147–148

leadership, 144–145
problem-solving, 142–143
self-transcendence, 146
stubbornness, 145–146
Practopoiesis, 423
Pragmatism, 250, 267–272
Precuneus, 77, 105, 237, 239, 249, 252, 257, 258
Prediction, 9, 26, 31, 33, 74, 116, 120, 132, 149, 156, 160, 251, 253, 258, 299, 305, 388, 408, 419, 440, 444
Prediction error, 132, 156
Predictive coding, 132
Prefrontal cortex (PFC), 11, 75, 98, 103, 105, 106, 120, 131, 150, 446
Primary interoceptive cortex, 439
Prior, 14, 62, 63, 73, 75, 126, 132, 149, 233, 243, 253, 254, 256, 265, 279, 353, 399–403
Probabilistic, 21, 31, 33, 70, 72–74, 77, 378, 454
Problem solving, 143, 150
Process, 5–14, 19–24, 28, 40, 42–44, 53, 70–78, 83, 88, 98, 102, 105, 114, 125–126, 128, 132, 139, 154, 157, 168, 185, 190, 196, 198, 200, 213, 217, 229, 248, 263, 278, 289, 319, 331, 333, 341, 352, 363–366, 376, 387, 405, 417, 435, 443, 454
Processes of believing, 7–10, 12–14, 22, 23, 29, 30, 40, 41, 43, 48, 78, 88–90, 146, 150, 187, 188, 191, 196, 197, 201, 202, 205, 206, 214, 215, 278, 324, 349, 363, 388, 405, 406, 413, 448, 454, 455
Proposition, 27–29, 31, 69, 70, 184–186, 189, 191, 197, 201, 217–225, 250, 270, 285, 309, 335, 354, 365, 366, 370–372, 424, 427, 441, 456
Pro-social behavior, 86, 293, 298, 303, 308, 313
Psychiatry, 169, 170, 173, 176, 293, 294, 312, 437, 439, 458
Psychological well-being, 172
Psychology, 4, 6, 8–11, 19–21, 24–26, 40, 43, 46, 48, 70, 84, 89, 113–116, 119, 125, 127–132, 143, 146, 154, 168, 170, 172, 184, 185, 187, 192, 222, 228, 230, 233, 236, 240–242, 244, 291–293, 295, 300, 301, 303–315, 320, 332, 334, 336, 349, 353, 378, 382, 390, 418, 427, 430, 448, 456, 459, 460
credition and emotion, 26
folk-psychology, 6–7, 19
placebo research, 125
psychological roots of meaning making and believing, 39–49
psychology, neuroscience, and self, 228–241, 244
psychology of delusions, 154
psychology of meaning making, 4
psychology of psychotic disorders, 167
psychology of religion, 21, 70, 119
Psychopathology, 154
Psychosis, 170–171, 176, 267, 312
Psychotic disorder, 11, 32, 167–176, 458
Public emotions, 414

Q

Quattrocento, 271

R

Rationality, 184, 187, 188, 202–204, 213, 219, 223, 304, 313, 333, 337, 380, 382, 384, 387, 389
characteristics, 203
deontological rationality, 203
means-end rationality, 203
Reality, 20, 24, 47, 57, 92, 112, 128, 139, 159, 161, 170, 186, 198, 201, 217, 219–224, 231, 233, 266, 269, 271, 285, 286, 304, 322, 323, 327, 332, 335, 336, 342, 345, 347, 354, 356, 358, 365, 407, 408, 412, 413
facing the reality of disasters, 139
imagining, step-by-step goals, and reality, 47
merging internal and external reality, 24, 57
placebos and reality, 128
Plato on knowing, believing, and reality, 266
reality and delusions, 153, 170
Whitehead process and reality, 217
Reality testing, 159
Reasoning, social/ethical, 282–285
Reassurance, 334
Receptor, 86, 90, 332
Reconciliation, 13, 341–360, 459
Religion, 4–9, 17–18, 21, 42, 65, 70, 78, 85, 112, 168, 170, 176, 187, 189, 198, 209, 222–225, 248, 263, 290, 354, 369, 448, 454
communities, purpose of, 89, 169
dimensions, 85–86
experience, explanations of, 20–21, 78
religious/spiritual well-being, dimensions, 172–173

Religiosity, 18, 19, 24, 26, 76, 168, 172–174, 263, 267, 269, 270, 302, 307, 312, 314, 319
Religious, 4, 5, 7, 9, 11–13, 17–21, 23–26, 33, 40, 43, 47, 70, 78, 84–91, 111, 119–120, 134, 140, 167–176, 187–191, 198–200, 202–205, 209–215, 220–225, 248, 249, 259, 264, 266–269, 271, 278, 282, 290–300, 302–315, 319, 320, 322, 324, 327, 335, 347, 353, 358, 363, 366, 367, 371, 372, 377, 385, 389, 408, 454, 456–458, 460
  belief (*see* Belief)
  characteristics, 119
  conversion, 40, 43
  community/group, 89, 169, 264–265, 270, 271, 282, 347–348, 353
  coping, 91, 169, 176
  dimensions, 11, 85
  education, 366–373, 385
  experience, 4, 9, 10, 20, 21, 23, 24, 141, 176, 198, 214, 215, 222–225, 267–270, 293, 319, 320
  faith (*see* Faith)
  fanatic, 6
  intuition, 223
  meaning/meaning making, 77, 169, 302
  movements, 175
  narratives, 259
  neurophysiological substrates, 120
  purpose, 169, 176
  religiousness, 19
  ritual/practices (*see* Ritual)
  studies, 4, 8, 12, 271
  well-being, 172
  world, 6
  Worldview, 3, 6, 212
Religious/spiritual well-being, dimensions, 172–173
Representation, 23, 33, 62–64, 69–75, 77, 98, 100–106, 114, 119, 121, 131, 140–147, 150, 153, 173, 191, 227–237, 248–250, 254–258, 280, 303, 325, 349, 350, 354, 358, 408, 412, 418, 423–429, 439, 457
  abstract, 100
  delusional, 153–161
  and the internal forward model, 254–258
  and interoception, 439
  probabilistic, 33, 69–75
  as propositions, 191
  self-representation, 227–237, 349
  of social reality, 350, 354
  and type-1 and type-1 processing of information, 73
  view-dependent, 100
Resonance, 100, 104, 105, 114, 117, 118, 230, 236, 242, 332
Reward, 11, 31, 44, 60, 65, 72, 74, 76, 87, 118, 120, 130, 243–245, 310, 392, 439
Ritual, 77, 78, 86, 127, 211, 223, 224, 259, 264, 265, 268, 270, 293, 302–305, 307, 308, 311, 312, 332, 334–336, 385

S

Salutogenetic, 91
Schema, 43, 63, 64, 72, 140–146, 148–150, 254, 294, 297, 299, 302, 349, 437, 457
Schizophrenia, 170, 171, 174–176, 312
Schizotypy, 173–175
Script, 10, 52–55, 57, 58, 60–66, 458
Secular, 4, 6, 9, 18, 21, 25, 77, 78, 91, 134, 140, 187, 200, 201, 210, 248, 249, 265, 300, 347
Selection, 45, 57, 75, 106, 115, 214, 250, 252, 280, 293, 294, 297, 300, 306, 308, 312, 313, 315, 326, 349, 351, 352, 380, 381, 383, 385, 457
Self, 11, 24, 29, 63, 73, 86, 105, 119, 127, 139–142, 146, 156, 172, 188, 227–245, 247, 263, 278–279, 282–285, 334, 344, 419, 421, 439, 447, 458
  brain and self, 227
  neuroanatomy
    contextual event representations, 114, 131
    motor representations, 98
    representation of beliefs, 258
  neurophilosophy
    experimental specificity, 242–243
    neuronal specificity, 241–242
    psychology specificity, 242–243
    self-specificity, 243–244
  self-awareness, 229, 439, 441
  self-identity, 12, 247–260, 458
  self-narrative, 256, 259
  self-reference effect (SRE)
    neurophysiological substrates, 228
    self-representation, 230–232
  self-transcendence, 141, 142, 145, 146, 148
  sense of self

empirical self, 228, 232–233
first-person perspective, 235
mental self, 228, 231
mind-body interaction, 231–232, 328–329
minimal self, 229, 233–234
second-person perspective, 235–236
self-representation, 232–234
third-person perspective, 235
Semantics, 64, 120, 230, 406, 407, 409, 412–414, 454
Sense, 19, 41, 63, 70, 84, 105, 146, 172, 211, 222, 227, 242, 253, 264, 281, 349, 365, 399, 439, 454, 455
Sensory processes, 333
Serotonin, 446, 448
Shannon formula, 420
Short-chain fatty acids, 447
Simulation theory, 11, 105, 107
Social anxiety disorders, 446
Social cognition, 84, 86, 87, 104, 105, 107, 116, 120, 161, 239, 282, 283, 293, 303, 307, 308
Social neuroscience, 84, 86, 90, 308
Social psychology, 39, 305, 306, 308, 313
Space of action, 24, 29, 31, 364, 366
Spirit, 11, 18, 77, 84, 130, 146, 168, 202, 212, 266, 302, 322, 332, 448, 454
Spirituality, 18, 25, 42, 44, 46, 89, 91, 130, 168, 169, 172, 173, 175, 176, 302, 303, 305, 311, 454
Spiritual Well-Being Scale, 172
existential well-being, 172
religious well-being, 172
Stabilizer function, 32, 106, 140, 145, 146, 150, 248, 249, 258, 349, 364
Stressor, 86
Structures, 418
dissipative structures (DS), 420, 427
equilibrium structures (ES), 420, 427
Subliminal, 25, 27, 28, 30, 74, 105, 106, 248, 258, 439
Suicide, 169
Supernatural, 119, 121, 173, 210, 211, 215, 293, 297, 303, 307–309, 311–313, 315
Supplementarity, 430–431
Supplementary motor area (SMA), 75, 77, 98
Survival, 41, 45, 48, 54, 58, 61, 84, 140, 141, 143, 144, 146, 147, 149, 151, 297, 308, 309, 314, 348
Symbolic language, 407, 412, 414
Symbolic systems
application, 59
dissociation of elements, 59–60, 64–65
elements of, 58
Symbols, 14, 43, 55–65, 75, 224–225, 265, 271, 291, 293–295, 298, 300, 303, 305, 314, 335, 354, 355, 357, 407, 412, 414, 415, 427, 431, 436

T

Temporo-parietal junction (TPJ), 103, 112, 115, 239, 249
Terminology, 24, 26, 217, 355, 547
Theology, 10, 12–13, 17, 19, 33, 190, 225, 266, 300, 329, 364, 369, 370, 373, 413, 460
Theory of mind (ToM), 32, 47, 59, 102, 103, 105, 106, 119, 156, 241, 296, 298, 304, 309, 310, 314, 423, 454
Theory of relativity, 196
Theory-theory, 11
Third-party punishment, 114, 115
Time, 4, 22, 42, 55, 70, 85, 98, 120, 127, 143, 155, 176, 187, 212, 222, 253, 266, 280, 290, 320, 332, 367, 378, 388, 410, 419, 438, 443
Tradition, 4, 5, 17, 76, 168, 183–185, 187–189, 204, 248, 260, 263, 264, 266, 268–270, 272, 294, 300, 303, 312, 313, 321, 322, 335, 345, 348, 355, 376, 385, 391, 392, 412, 415, 448, 454, 455, 458, 460
Transcendence, 24, 77, 85, 139–141, 145, 146, 148, 168, 302, 321
Transmitter, 86, 116, 132, 445, 448
Trust, 10, 18, 74, 83–90, 118, 126, 137, 158, 172, 185, 197, 264, 343–354, 364, 375–380, 388, 409, 454
Two-factor theory of emotion, 26, 222

U

Ulcerative colitis, 447

V

Vagus nerve, 438, 448
Valuation, 9, 10, 21, 29, 31, 33, 72–74, 214, 225, 244–245, 250, 378
Value, 26, 29, 31, 33, 44, 47, 65, 72, 73, 75, 78, 89, 106, 116, 139–140, 143–148, 150, 168, 186, 200, 205, 219, 224, 244, 249, 250, 258, 278, 286, 297, 302, 304, 312, 349, 353, 354, 356, 364, 371, 372, 378, 390, 408, 420, 440

Vasopressin (VP), 10, 86–88, 90
function, 86–87
production, 86
Ventral striatum (VS), 118, 243, 244
Ventromedial prefrontal cortex (vmPFC), 116–118, 236, 237, 243, 244
Vigilance, 87
Virome, 444
Voxel-based lesion symptom mapping (VLSM), 119

W
Whiteheadian metaphysics
actual occasions, 218
descriptive metaphysics, 218
higher phases of experience, 219
prehensions, 218–219
proposition, 219–220
revisionary, metaphysics, 218
reality, 217
religious intuition, 223–224
Worship, 89, 211, 335

MIX
Papier aus verantwortungsvollen Quellen
Paper from responsible sources
FSC® C105338

If you have any concerns about our products,
you can contact us on
ProductSafety@springernature.com

In case Publisher is established outside the EU,
the EU authorized representative is:
Springer Nature Customer Service Center GmbH
Europaplatz 3, 69115 Heidelberg, Germany

Printed by Libri Plureos GmbH
in Hamburg, Germany